ASTHMA IN THE WORKPLACE

ASTHMA IN THE WORKPLACE

FIFTH EDITION

Edited by

Susan M. Tarlo
Professor of Medicine
University Health Network and St Michael's Hospital, Toronto
Department of Medicine, University of Toronto
Ontario, Canada

Olivier Vandenplas
Professor of Medicine, Head Department of Chest Medicine
Centre hospitalier Universitaire UCL Namur
Université Catholique de Louvain
Yvoir, Belgium

David I. Bernstein
Professor Emeritus of Medicine
Division of Immunology, Allergy and Rheumatology
University of Cincinnati College of Medicine
Cincinnati, Ohio, USA

Jean-Luc Malo
Professor of Medicine (retired)
Hôpital du Sacré-Cœur de Montréal and Université de Montréal
Montréal, Canada

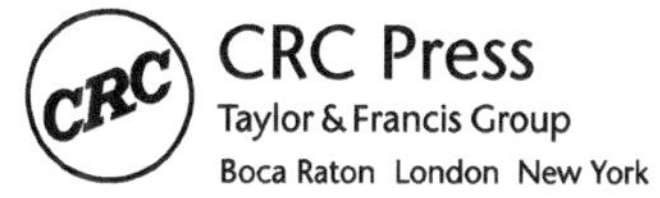

CRC Press
Taylor & Francis Group
Boca Raton London New York

CRC Press is an imprint of the
Taylor & Francis Group, an **informa** business

CRC Press
Boca Raton and London
Fifth edition published 2022
by CRC Press
6000 Broken Sound Parkway NW, Suite 300, Boca Raton, FL 33487-2742
and by CRC Press

2 Park Square, Milton Park, Abingdon, Oxon, OX14 4RN
© 2022 Taylor & Francis Group, LLC

Fourth Edition published by Informa Healthcare 2013

CRC Press is an imprint of Taylor & Francis Group, LLC

Library of Congress Cataloging-in-Publication Data

Names: Tarlo, Susan, editor. | Vandenplas, Olivier, editor. | Bernstein, David I., editor. |
Malo, Jean-Luc, editor.
Title: Asthma in the workplace / edited by Susan M. Tarlo, Olivier Vandenplas, David I. Bernstein,
Jean-Luc Malo.
Description: 5th edition. | Boca Raton, FL : CRC Press, 2021. | Includes bibliographical references
and index. | Summary: "This new edition focuses on recent developments that are reflected by an
impressive addition to the scientific literature. This fifth edition retains key elements that have made
the success of previous editions: world-wide contributors, variety of topics covered, presentation of
key aspects using workplace scenarios and case histories"–Provided by publisher.
Identifiers: LCCN 2021007704 (print) | LCCN 2021007705 (ebook) | ISBN 9780367430092
(hardback) | ISBN 9781032043425 (paperback) | ISBN 9781003000624 (ebook)
Subjects: MESH: Asthma–chemically induced | Asthma, Occupational–chemically induced |
Occupational Diseases–chemically induced
Classification: LCC RC591 (print) | LCC RC591 (ebook) | NLM WF 553 | DDC 616.2/38–dc23
LC record available at https://lccn.loc.gov/2021007704
LC ebook record available at https://lccn.loc.gov/2021007705

ISBN: 9780367430092 (hbk)
ISBN: 9781032043425 (pbk)
ISBN: 9781003000624 (ebk)

Typeset in Warnock Pro
by KnowledgeWorks Global Ltd.

The editors dedicate this book to our current and former students and fellows who trained in the field of asthma in the workplace, and also to our families for all their love and support.

CONTENTS

PART I: INTRODUCTION

PART II: ASSESSMENT

PART III: MANAGEMENT

PART IV: SPECIFIC AGENTS CAUSING IMMUNOLOGICAL OCCUPATIONAL ASTHMA

PREFACE

Preparation of the preface in this fifth edition of *Asthma in the Workplace* provided editors an opportunity to reflect on previous editions, from the first edition in 1993 to the fourth edition published in 2013. New editions have been published at 6- to 7-year intervals, an adequate time frame to update recent contributions to the literature. Looking back on the previous editions, the editors would like to emphasize key issues and themes that remain just as relevant to this new edition:

1. Over the years, the focus on occupational pneumoconiosis has changed to asthma in the workplace:
   The interest in occupational lung diseases used to be focused principally on infiltrative diseases caused by inhalation of mineral dusts (pneumoconiosis). As stated in the fourth edition, "Although occupational asthma was recognized as early as the eighteenth century by Ramazzini, its importance as a significant hazard in the workplace was not widely appreciated until the spurt in industrial technology after World War II. The literature concerning workplace asthma has steadily increased since the great impetus given by Professor Jack Pepys, who can be considered the father of occupational asthma and to whom the first three editions of this book were dedicated."
2. The frequency of asthma in the workplace and occupational asthma has increased since the second part of the twentieth century. Although there has been a diminution in the number of workers affected by the disease according to figures obtained from medicolegal agencies, meta-analyses suggest that approximately 15% of asthma is attributable to conditions in the workplace.
3. Asthma in the workplace can be manifested as asthma caused by a condition at work (i.e. occupational asthma) or aggravation of preexisting asthma:
   The term *asthma in the workplace* is not entirely synonymous with new-onset occupational asthma induced de novo by an occupational exposure as defined in the first two editions of this book. Since the third edition, the term has broadened to also include asthmatic workers with preexisting or concomitant nonoccupational asthma whose asthmatic symptoms worsen at work (i.e. work-exacerbated asthma).
4. Asthma in the workplace is a condition that has attracted the interests of a wide variety of disciplines: allergists, immunologists, pulmonologists, immunotoxicologists, public health and occupational health specialists, aerosol scientists, hygienists, epidemiologists, social workers, lawyers, and economists. Outbreaks of occupational asthma in specific work settings provide mini-epidemiological paradigms of asthma and excellent opportunities for investigating the sources, the characteristics of the emission–dispersion cycles, and the health impact of inciting agents. The ready access to such integrated data in a defined setting provides an ideal milieu for research and an investigational model for further advancement of knowledge about the pathophysiological pathways and natural history of asthma by specialists from various disciplines. At an individual level in addition, the economic and social hardships imposed on a worker with refractory symptoms associated with occupational asthma may require consultation with a psychologist and a legal counsel.
5. Asthma in the workplace and occupational asthma represent a satisfactory model of the development of asthma in humans: environmental and host susceptibility factors intervene in a complex way to incite the immunological process that will lead to the development of symptoms and disease. Moreover, subjects can be assessed after they leave exposure to the causal agent, a possibility that is not offered in asthma caused by numerous ubiquitous allergens. Finally, it is principally at the workplace that it has been shown that exposure to irritants at high (irritant-induced) or chronic low doses (viz. cleaning) have been demonstrated to cause asthma and airway obstruction.
6. The enthusiastic response to publication of the previous editions of this book and the number of literature citations attributed to it have more than justified preparation of a fifth edition.
7. Discovery and research in workplace-related asthma have continued at a rapid pace and have served as the impetus for this updated and revised edition.
8. This new edition retains its international nature in the coalition of editors and individual contributors. The common goal of this cooperative effort was to prepare an authoritative, educational resource for primary care physicians, occupational health specialists, allergists, and pulmonologists.
9. To make this reference book particularly germane for primary care providers to develop skills in the early recognition of the disease, we keep in this new edition a feature proposed in the previous edition: a clinical case history or a workplace scenario relevant to the main part of the chapter.
10. As the diagnosis of occupational asthma is often difficult because of multiple causalities in many occupational environments, the variability of symptoms, and patterns of late-phase asthmatic reactions, the requirements for special diagnostic procedures, and the unpredictability of onset and persistence of symptoms, special emphasis has been given to an algorithm of clinical diagnosis, immunological evaluation, and physiological methods of evaluation (Chapters 6–9) as a practical guide for primary care physicians.

As in the previous edition, the book is organized into five main parts:

Part I, "Introduction," contains chapters on definitions, historical background, epidemiology, genetics, pathophysiology, and animal models.

Part II, "Assessment," includes chapters that delineate guidelines for assessing the worker and the workplace.

Part III, "Management," includes chapters that propose guidelines for the management of workers and the workplace, including compensation aspects.

Part IV, "Specific Agents Causing Immunological Occupational Asthma," provides detailed information about specific agents (including a variety of high-molecular-weight and low-molecular-weight agents).

Part V, "Specific Disease Entities and Variants," covers other types of work-related asthma conditions, for example, irritant-induced asthma, asthma exacerbated at work, eosinophilic bronchitis as well as acute and chronic asthma-like syndromes. Occupational rhinitis, chronic obstructive pulmonary disease (COPD), as well as urticaria and allergic contact dermatitis are also covered in this section.

All chapters have been revised and the information as well as references have been updated. Some of the chapters have new or additional contributors. The editors were the same from the first to the third edition (I. Leonard Bernstein, Moira Chan-Yeung, Jean-Luc Malo, and David I. Bernstein) and their work praised and appreciated. The preparation of the fourth edition was sadly marked by the loss of one of our editors, Dr. I. Leonard Bernstein, a most renowned thought leader and authority in allergy and immunology and an attentive, stimulating, and cheerful colleague. Sadly, during the process of preparation of this new edition, the editors were informed of the unexpected passing of Professor Jean-Charles Dalphin,

from Besançon, France, who had enthusiastically and generously accepted to coauthor the chapter on hypersensitivity pneumonitis. The editors want to pay tribute to him for his outstanding career, becoming a world authority in hypersensitivity pneumonitis.

The remaining editors, Jean-Luc Malo and David I. Bernstein, are happy to welcome new editors for this fifth edition, Susan M. Tarlo and Olivier Vandenplas, who have generously agreed to join the team, bringing a refreshing wind of ideas in the preparation of the current edition.

Finally, we all want to pay tribute to and sincerely thank all authors of the previous editions (see the list below). We acknowledge their contributions that, on occasion, have been transmitted from one edition to the next as a "traditional" link that joins all editions of this book.

Susan M. Tarlo
Olivier Vandenplas
David I. Bernstein
Jean-Luc Malo

Asthma in the Workplace, First Edition, Marcel Dekker, Inc. New York, 1993. Editors: I. Leonard Bernstein, Moira Chan-Yeung, Jean-Luc Malo, David I. Bernstein

Contributors:

Margaret R. Becklake	David I. Bernstein	I. Leonard Bernstein
J. Bousquet	S. M. Brooks	P. Sherwood Burge
B.T. Butcher	A. Cartier	M. Chan-Yeung
A. Ciaccia	H. Dhivert	D. Enarson
L.M. Fabbri	P. Godard	S. Gordon
L.C. Grammer	S. Kennedy	J. Lesage
J.T.C. Li	J.-L. Malo	P. Maestrelli
C.E. Mapp	J.A. Merchant	F.B. Michel
A.J. Newman-Taylor	R. Patterson	J. Pepys
G. Perrault	B. Perrin	C.E. Reed
M. Saetta	P.J. Seligman	J.A. Seta
M.C. Swanson	R.O. Young	C.R. Zeiss

Asthma in the Workplace, Second Edition, Marcel Dekker, Inc. New York, 1999. Editors: I. Leonard Bernstein, Moira Chan-Yeung, Jean-Luc Malo, David I. Bernstein

Contributors:

M.R. Becklake	David I. Bernstein	I. Leonard Bernstein
J. A. Bernstein	P. Blanc	P. Boschetto
J. Bousquet	S. Brooks	S. Burge
B.T. Butcher	G. Caramori	A. Cartier
M. Chan-Yeung	B.L. Charous	D.C. Christiani
Y. Cormier	H. Dhivert-Donnadieu	L.M. Fabbri
W.G. Gaines	D. Gautrin	P. Godard
S. Gordon	L.C. Grammer	D. Heederik
A. Johnson	M. Karol	S.M. Kennedy
H. Keskinen	J. Lesage	J.T. Li
G.M. Liss	B.D. Lushniak	J.-L. Malo
C.E. Mapp	C.G. Toby Mathias	D. Menzies
J. A. Merchant	F.B. Michel	G. Moscato
B. Nemery	A.J. Newman-Taylor	R. Patterson
D.H. Pedersen	J. Pepys	G. Perrault
B. Perrin	A. Pickering	C.E. Reed
H.B. Richerson	C.S. Rose	K. Sarlo
D.A. Schwartz	J.A. Seta	M.C. Swanson
Susan M. Tarlo	O. Vandenplas	K.M. Venables
R.O. Young	C.R. Zeiss	

Asthma in the Workplace, Third Edition, Taylor & Francis, Inc. New York, 2006. Editors: I. Leonard Bernstein, Moira Chan-Yeung, Jean-Luc Malo, David I. Bernstein

Contributors:

X. Baur	M.R. Becklake	D. Beezhold
David I. Bernstein	I. Leonard Bernstein	J.A. Bernstein
R.E. Biagini	P.D. Blanc	S. Brooks
P.S. Burge	R.K. Bush	P. Campo
A. Cartier	M. Chan-Yeung	D.C. Christiani
Y. Cormier	L.M. Fabbri	D. Gautrin
S. Gordon	D. Heederik	P.K. Henneberger
E. Hnizdo	A. Johnson	V.J. Jonhson
S.M. Kennedy	H. Keskinen	K. Kreiss
C. Lemière	J. Lesage	G.M. Liss
B.D. Lushniak	M.I. Luster	P. Maestrelli
J.-L. Malo	C.E. Mapp	C.G. Toby Mathias
D. Menzies	R. Merget	G. Moscato
A.J. Newman-Taylor	M. Nieuwenhuijsen	H. Nordman
H.S. Park	J. Pepys	G. Perrault
S. Quirce	C.A. Redlich	K. Sarlo
M. Schuyler	D.A. Schwartz	J. Singh
A. Siracusa	M.C. Swanson	S.M. Tarlo
K. Toren	O. Vandenplas	S. Von Essen
G.R. Wagner	A.V. Wisnewski	B. Yucesoy
C.R. Zeiss		

Asthma in the Workplace, Fourth Edition, CRC Press, Taylor & Francis Group, Inc. New York, 2013. Editors: Jean-Luc Malo, Moira Chan-Yeung, David I. Bernstein

Contributors:

V.H. Arrandale	X. Baur	D.I. Bernstein
I. Leonard Bernstein	J.A. Bernstein	P.D. Blanc
N. Bourdeau	S.M. Brooks	L. Budnik
P.S. Burge	A. Cartier	R. Castano
M. Chan-Yeung	Y. Cormier	P. Cullinan
V. De Vooght	M. Desrosiers	M.S. Dykewicz
D. Gautrin	N. Goyer	L.C. Grammer
P. Harber	D. Heederik	P.K. Henneberger
E. Hnizdo	D.L. Holness	R. Houba
M.S. Jaakkola	M.F. Jeebhay	V.J. Johnson
M. Jones	K. Kreiss	M. Labrecque
Y. Lacasse	K.L. Lavoie	C. Lemière
G.M. Liss	A.L. Lopata	P. Maestrelli
Jean-Luc Malo	C.E. Mapp	C.G. Toby Mathias
R. Merget	J.D. Miller	M. Millerick-May
G. Moscato	D. Norbäck	K.A. Pacheco
H.S. Park	J. Pepys	P. Phénix
J.A. Poole	S. Quirce	C.A. Redlich
M. Ribeiro	B. Roberge	C. Rodriguez
K.D. Rosenman	K. Sarlo	J. Sastre
T. Sigsgaard	S.M. Tarlo	K. Toren
O. Vandenplas	J.A.J. Venoirbeek	S. Von Essen
G.R. Wagner	A.V. Wisnewski	B. Yucesoy

EDITORS

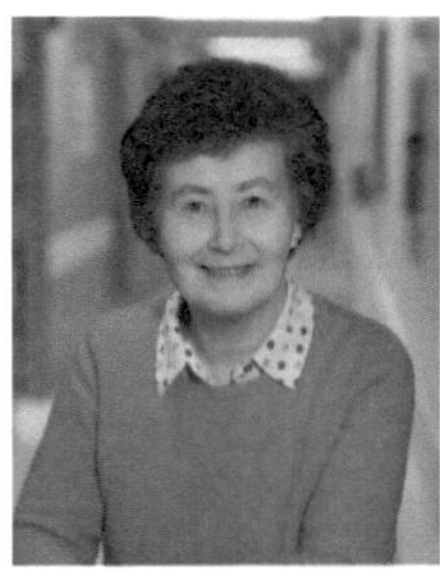

Susan M. Tarlo is a respiratory physician who went to medical school in London, UK at Westminster Medical School, completing her MBBS in 1969. She completed further training in England including at the Royal Brompton Hospital and Westminster Hospital before coming to Canada in 1974. She trained further at Queens University (allergy/immunology) then McMaster University (respirology) before her appointment at the University of Toronto in 1977. She is a Professor in the Department of Medicine at the University of Toronto with an academic cross-appointment in the University of Toronto, Dalla Lana Department of Public Health. Her main clinical staff appointment is at the University Health Network at Toronto Western Hospital where she is head of the Occupational Lung Disease Clinic and also has a focus on asthma and allergic respiratory disease. She has research appointments at the Gage Occupational and Environmental Health Unit, Li Ka Shing Research Institute, Toronto General Hospital Research Institute and University of Toronto Institute of Medical Science, and the Centre for Research Excellence in Occupational Disease at St. Michael's Hospital where she also has a WSIB occupational lung specialty clinic. Her research interests and publications are mainly in work related to asthma and occupational allergy.

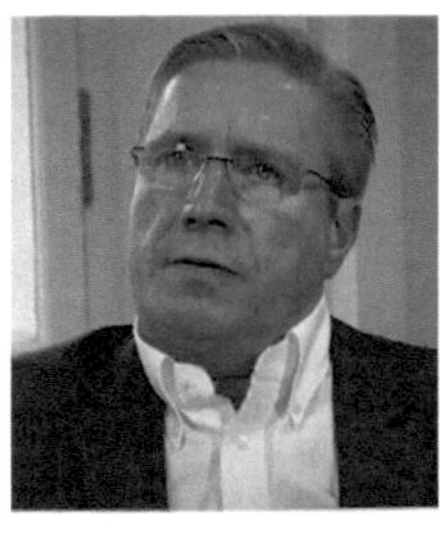

Olivier Vandenplas is Professor of Medicine, Faculty of Medicine, Université Catholique de Louvain and Head of the Chest Medicine Department at the University Hospital of Mont-Godinne, Belgium. After a fellowship with Professor Jean-Luc Malo at Hôpital du Sacré-Cœur de Montréal, Québec, Canada, he dedicated his clinical and research activities to the diagnosis and management of asthma and work related to asthma over the last three decades. He is the author or coauthor of over 120 research articles and book chapters, and a member of the European Academy of Allergy and Clinical Immunology, the Belgian Society of Allergy and Clinical Immunology, and the Belgian Respiratory Society. Dr. Vandenplas received his MD (1984) and PhD (1996) degrees from the Université Catholique de Louvain, Belgium and the MSc degree in Biomedical Sciences from Université de Montréal, Québec, Canada. Additionally, he serves as Expert Consultant at the Belgian Workers' Compensation Board (Agence fédérale des risques professionnels-Fedris).

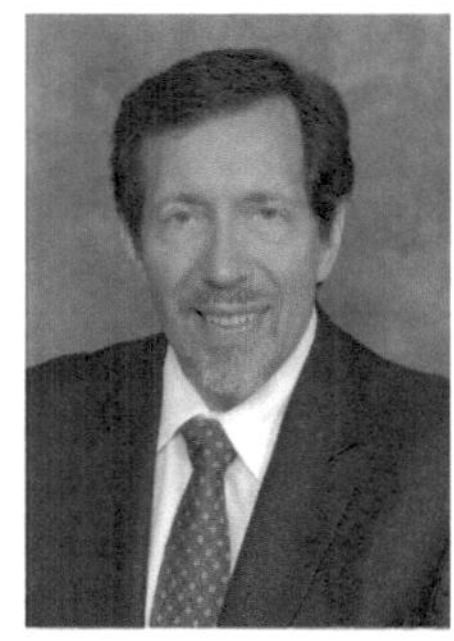

David I. Bernstein is Professor Emeritus of Medicine in the Division of Immunology and Allergy at the University of Cincinnati College of Medicine where he is also the Co-Director of the Allergy Fellowship training program. Dr. Bernstein has authored or coauthored over 260 original publications. His major clinical research interests include genetic and allergic mechanisms of occupational asthma, environmental determinants of allergic disorders in childhood, allergen immunotherapy, and new therapies for asthma and allergic diseases. He is former Chair of the American Board of Allergy and Immunology and the Occupational Disease Committee of the American Academy of Allergy Asthma and Immunology.

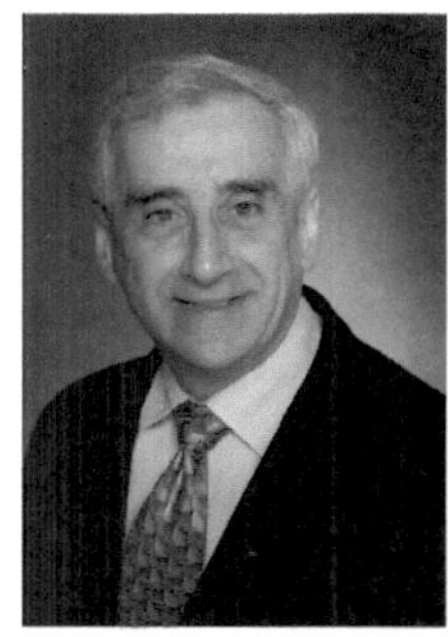

Jean-Luc Malo did his fellowship studies at the Brompton Hospital and Cardiothoracic Institute, London, UK, under late professor Jack Pepys, referred to as "the father of occupational asthma" from 1974 to 1976. Dr. Malo was the Professor of Medicine at the Faculté de Médecine of Université de Montréal, serving for a term as Vice-Dean, Research and Postgraduate Studies, and Clinical researcher at Service de Pneumologie of Hôpital du Sacré-Coeur de Montréal, Montreal, Canada, from 1976 to 2016. He is Specialist Consultant in Asthma in the Workplace for the Québec Commission des normes, de l'équité, de la santé et de la sécurité du travail (CNESST). He has published more than 350 original works as well as chapters and reviews, mainly in the field of occupational asthma, and was also the co-editor of the previous editions of *Asthma in the Workplace*. His clinical and research interest cover several aspects of asthma in the workplace focusing on means of investigation and diagnosis, natural history, as well as clinical and psychosocial outcomes.

CONTRIBUTORS

Victoria H. Arrandale
PhD, Assistant Professor
Dalla Lana School of Public Health
University of Toronto
Toronto, Ontario, Canada

Xaver Baur
MD, Professor Emeritus
University of Hamburg
Hamburg, Germany

Anne-Pauline Bellanger
PhD, Associate Professor
Parasitology-Mycology Department
University Hospital Besancon
Besançon, France

David I. Bernstein
MD, Professor Emeritus of Medicine
Division of Immunology, Allergy, and Rheumatology
University of Cincinnati College of Medicine
Cincinnati, Ohio, USA

Jonathan A. Bernstein
MD, Professor of Medicine
Division of Immunology, Allergy and Rheumatology
University of Cincinnati College of Medicine
Cincinnati, Ohio, USA

Paul D. Blanc
MD, Professor of Medicine
School of Medicine, University of California
San Francisco, California, USA

Nathalie Bourdeau
BSc, Clinical Nurse
Occupational Health, Direction de santé publique,
    CISSS de Lanaudière
Joliette, Québec, Canada

P. Sherwood Burge
MD, Consultant Physician
University Hospitals Birmingham
and
Honorary Professor
Birmingham University
Birmingham, United Kingdom

Christopher Carlsten
MD, MPH, Professor of Medicine
Head of Respiratory Medicine
Department of Medicine, Faculty of Medicine
University of British Columbia
Vancouver, British Columbia, Canada

André Cartier
MD, Clinical Professor of Medicine
Department of Medicine, Faculty of Medicine
University of Montréal
Montréal, Québec, Canada

Moira Chan-Yeung
MB, FRCP, FRCPC, Emeritus Professor
Department of Medicine, Faculty of Medicine
University of British Columbia
Vancouver, British Columbia, Canada

Maria Jesús Cruz Carmona
PhD, Professor, Head of the Pulmonology Research Laboratory
Department of Pulmonology
Vall d'Hebron Research Institute (VHIR) and University
    of Barcelona
Barcelona, Spain

Paul Cullinan
MD FRCP FFOM, Professor
Department of Occupational and Environmental Lung Disease
Imperial College (NHLI) and Royal Brompton Hospital
London, United Kingdom

Frédéric de Blay
MD, Professor of Pulmonology
Department of Pulmonology
Les Hôpitaux universitaires de Strasbourg, University
    of Strasbourg
Strasbourg, France

Katelynn E. Dodd
MPH, Associate Service Fellow
Respiratory Health Division
National Institute for Occupational Safety and Health (NIOSH)
Centers for Disease Control and Prevention
Morgantown, West Virginia, USA

Gert Doekes
PhD, Guest Researcher and Assistant Professor
Institute for Risk Assessment Sciences
Utrecht University
Utrecht, The Netherlands

Orianne Dumas
PhD
Université Paris-Saclay
UVSQ, Univ. Paris-Sud
Villejuif, France

Carole Ederlé
MD, Assistant Professor of Pulmonology
Department of Pulmonology, Les Hôpitaux universitaires de
    Strasbourg
University of Strasbourg
Strasbourg, France

David Fishwick
MD, FRCP, FFOM, FFOMI, Consultant Respiratory Physician
    and Honorary Professor
University of Sheffield and Centre for Workplace Health, Health
    and Safety Executive (HSE) Science and Research Centre
Buxton, United Kingdom

Ilenia Folletti
MD, Researcher
Department of Medicine and Surgery
Section Occupational Medicine, Respiratory Diseases,
    Occupational and Environmental Toxicology
University of Perugia
Terni Hospital
Terni, Italy

Sheiphali Gandhi
MD, MPH, Occcupational and Environmental Medicine
    Resident, Clinical Medicine Fellow
School of Medicine, University of California
San Francisco, California, USA

Denyse Gautrin
PhD, Retired Professor
Department of Medicine
Faculté de Médecine
Université de Montréal
Montréal, Québec, Canada

Brett James Green
PhD, Research Biologist
National Institute for Occupational Safety and Health (NIOSH)
Centers for Disease Control and Prevention
Morgantown, West Virginia, USA

Philip Harber
MD, MPH, Professor of Public Health
Mel and Enid Zuckerman College of Public Health
University of Arizona
Tucson, Arizona, USA

Dick Heederik
PhD, Professor of Health Risk Analysis
Institute for Risk Assessment Sciences
Utrecht University
Utrecht, The Netherlands

Paul K. Henneberger
MPH, ScD, ATSF, Senior Science Advisor
Respiratory Health Division
National Institute for Occupational Safety and Health
    (NIOSH)
Centers for Disease Control and Prevention
Morgantown, West Virginia, USA

D. Linn Holness
MD, MHSc, FRCPC, FFOM (Hon), Professor Emerita
Dalla Lana School of Public Health and Department of Medicine
University of Toronto
St. Michael's Hospital
Toronto, Ontario, Canada

Ryan Hoy
MBBS, FRACP, MOccEnvHlth, Respiratory and Sleep Disorders
    Physician, Senior Research Fellow
Monash Centre for Occupational and Environmental Health
School of Public Health & Preventive Medicine
Faculty of Medicine, Nursing and Health Sciences
Monash University
Melbourne, Australia

Mohamed F. Jeebhay
PhD, MBChB, Professor, Head of Occupational Medicine
    Division
Occupational Medicine Division and Centre for Family
    Environmental & Occupational Health Research (CEOHR)
School of Public Health and Family Medicine
University of Cape Town
Cape Town, South Africa

Amber N. Johnson
MD, Pulmonary-Critical Care Fellow, Pulmonary and Critical
    Care Medicine
University of Nebraska Medical Center
Omaha, Nebraska, USA

Athena Jolly
MD, MPH, Medical Consultant
Huntsman International LLC
West Chester, Pennsylvania, USA

Ambrose Lau
MD, MEd, Assistant Professor
University Health Network
Toronto Western Hospital
Toronto, Ontario, Canada

Kim L. Lavoie
PhD, Professor, Canada Research Chair in Behavioural
    Medicine
Department of Psychology
University of Quebec at Montréal (UQAM)
Montréal, Québec, Canada

Nicole Le Moual
PhD, Epidemiologist
Equipe d'épidémiologie respiratoire intégrative, INSERM
Univ. Paris-Saclay, Univ. Paris-Sud, UVSQ
CESP 94807
Villejuif, France

Catherine Lemière
MD, MSc, Hôpital du Sacré-Coeur de Montréal
CIUSSS du Nord de l'île de Montréal
Professeur titulaire
Université de Montréal
Montréal, Québec, Canada

Andreas L. Lopata
PhD (Medical Science), MSc (Biochemistry)
Professor, James Cook University, Australian Institute of
    Tropical Health and Medicine
Queensland, Australia

Piero Maestrelli
MD, Professor
University of Padova
Padova, Italy

Jean-Luc Malo
MD, Professor of Medicine (retired)
Department of Medicine
Hôpital du Sacré-Cœur de Montréal and Université
    de Montréal
Montréal, Québec, Canada

Jacek M. Mazurek
MD, MS, PhD, Branch Chief
Surveillance Branch, Respiratory Health Division
National Institute for Occupational Safety
    and Health (NIOSH)
Centers for Disease Control and Prevention
Morgantown, West Virginia, USA

Julie McKibben
MD, MS, Senior Director
Global Medical Operations Leader
Procter & Gamble Company
Cincinnati, Ohio, USA

Rolf Merget
MD, Prof. Dr.
Institute for Prevention and Occupational Medicine of the
    German Social Accident Insurance (IPA)
Institute of the Ruhr University
Bochum, Germany

Laurence Millon
PhD, Professor, Head of the Parasitology-Mycology
    Department
University Hospital of Besançon
Besançon, France

Vicky C. Moore
PhD, Clinical Scientist
Department of Respiratory Medicine, University Hospitals
    Birmingham NHS Foundation Trust
Birmingham, United Kingdom

Gianna Moscato
MD, Professor, Dr.
Specialization School in Occupational Medicine
University of Pavia
Pavia, Italy

Xaver Munoz
MD, PhD, Head of the Asthma Unit
Servei Pneumologia Hospital Vall d'Hebron
and
Professor of Cell Biology, Physiology and Immunology
    Department
Universidad Autonoma de Barcelona
Barcelona, Spain

Nicola Murgia
MD, PhD, Associate Professor
Section of Occupational Medicine, Respiratory Diseases and
    Toxicology
University of Perugia, Perugia, Italy

Karin Pacheco
MD, MSPH, Associate Professor
Division of Environmental & Occupational Health Sciences
Department of Medicine
National Jewish Health
and Division of Environmental & Occupational Health
University of Colorado School of Public Health
Colorado, USA

Hae-Sim Park
MD, PhD, Professor
Ajou Research Institute for Innovative Medicine
Suwon, South Korea

Pierre Phénix
MD, Physician Advisor (retired)
Direction Régionale de Santé Publique de Montréal
CIUSSS du Centre-Sud de l'Ile-de-Montréal
Montréal, Québec, Canada

Jill A. Poole
MD, Professor of Medicine, Chief
Division of Allergy and Immunology
University of Nebraska Medical Center
Omaha, Nebraska, USA

Santiago Quirce
MD, PhD, Head of the Department of Allergy
La Paz University Hospital
Associate Professor of Medicine
Universidad Autonoma de Madrid
Madrid, Spain

Monika Raulf
PhD, Prof. Dr. rer. nat., Head of the Department of German
    Allergology/Immunology of the Institute of Prevention and
    Occupational Medicine of the Social Accident Insurance
Institute of the Ruhr-University Bochum (IPA)
Bochum, Germany

Gabriel Reboux
PhD, Director
Research Team: UMR/CNRS Chrono-Environnement
Université Bourgogne Franche Comté
Parasitologie-Mycologie Department
University Hospital of Besançon
Besançon, France

Carrie A. Redlich
MD, MPH, Professor of Medicine
Director, Pulmonary Section & Occupational and
    Environmental Medicine Program
Yale Occupational and Environmental Medicine Program
Yale School of Medicine
New Haven, Connecticut, USA

                                     Contributors

Marcos Ribeiro
MD, PhD, Associate Professor
Section of Pulmonology
Department of Medicine
Health Science Centre
State University of Londrina
Parana, Brazil

Kenneth Rosenman
MD, Professor of Medicine and Chief
Division of Occupational and Environmental Medicine, College
    of Human Medicine
Michigan State University
East Lansing, Michigan, USA

Joaquin Sastre
MD, PhD, Head of the Allergology Department
Fundacion Jimenez Diaz
Facultad de Medicina
Universidad Autonoma de Madrid
Madrid, Spain

Vivi Schlünssen
MD, PhD, Professor
Department of Public Health, Environment, Occupation and
    Health
Danish Ramazzini Centre
Aarhus Universitet
Aarhus C, Denmark

Pierre Séguin
MD, Occupational Physician Specialist
Occupational Health, Direction régionale de Santé publique,
    CIUSSS du Centre-Sud de l'Ile-de-Montréal
Montréal, Québec, Canada

Dennis Shusterman
MD MPH, Professor of Clinical Medicine, Emeritus
Division of Occupational and Environmental Medicine
Faculty of Medicine, University of California
San Francisco, California, USA

Torben Sigsgaard
MD, Professor, FERS
Department of Public Health
Section for Environment, Work & Health
Aarhus University
Aarhus C, Denmark

Andrea Siracusa
MD, Formerly Professor of Occupational Medicine
University of Perugia
Perugia, Italy

Eva Suarthana
MD, MSc, PhD,
(Formerly) Département de Médecine Sociale et Préventive
École de Santé Publique
Université de Montréal
(Currently) Department of Obstetrics and Gynecology
McGill University
Montréal, Québec, Canada

Hille Suojalehto
MD, PhD, Chief Physician and Adjunct Professor
Finnish Institute of Occupational Health
University of Helsinki
Helsinki, Finland

Katri Suuronen
PhD, Senior Specialist and Adjunct Professor
Finnish Institute of Occupational Health
Helsinki, Finland

Susan M. Tarlo
MB, BS, Professor of Medicine
University Health Network and St Michael's Hospital, Toronto,
    Canada
Department of Medicine
University of Toronto, Ontario, Canada

Kjell Torén
MD, PhD, Senior Professor
School of Public Health and Community Medicine, Sahlgrenska
    Academy
University of Gothenburg
Gothenburg, Sweden

Hung- Chang Tsui
MD, PhD Student
Department of Public Health and Primary Care, Center for
    Environment and Health
KU Leuven, Leuven, Belgium

Vera van Kampen
Dr. rer. nat.
Institute for Prevention and Occupational Medicine of the
    German Social Accident Insurance (IPA)
Institute of the Ruhr University
Bochum, Germany

Olivier Vandenplas
MD, MSc, PhD, Professor of Medicine, Head of the Department
    of Chest Medicine
Centre hospitalier Universitaire UCL Namur
Université Catholique de Louvain
Yvoir, Belgium

Jeroen Vanoirbeek
PhD, Professor
Department of Public Health and Primary Care, Center for
    Environment and Health
Occupational, Environmental & Insurance Medicine
KU Leuven, Belgium

Gregory R. Wagner
MD, Adjunct Professor, Department of Environmental Health
Harvard T.H. Chan School of Public Health
Boston, Massachusetts, USA

Gareth I. Walters
MD, MMEd, FRCP(UK)
NHS Regional Occupational Lung Disease Service,
    Birmingham Chest Clinic
University Hospitals
Birmingham, United Kingdom

Jolanta Walusiak-Skorupa
MD, PhD, Professor of Medicine, Department of Occupational
    Diseases and Environmental Health, Department of
    Occupational Diseases and Environmental Health
Nofer Institute of Occupational Medicine
Lodz, Poland

David Weissman
MD, Director, Respiratory Health Division
CDC-NIOSH
Morgantown, West Virginia, USA

Adam Wisnewski
PhD, Senior Research Scientist in Medicine (Occupational
    Medicine)
Yale University School of Medicine
New Haven, Connecticut, USA

Marta Wiszniewska
MD, PhD, Professor
Department of Occupational Diseases and Environmental Health
Nofer Institute of Occupational Medicine
Lodz, Poland

Part I
Introduction

1

DEFINITION AND CLASSIFICATION OF ASTHMA IN THE WORKPLACE

Susan M. Tarlo,[1] Olivier Vandenplas,[2] David I. Bernstein,[3] and Jean-Luc Malo[4]
[1]Professor of Medicine, Department of Medicine, University Health Network and
St Michael's Hospital, University of Toronto, Toronto, Ontario, Canada
[2]Professor of Medicine, Head, Department of Chest Medicine, Centre Hospitalier Universitaire
UCL Namur, Université Catholique de Louvain, Yvoir, Belgium
[3]Professor Emeritus of Medicine, Division of Immunology, Allergy and Rheumatology,
University of Cincinnati College of Medicine, Cincinnati, Ohio, USA
[4]Professor of Medicine (retired), Hôpital du Sacré-Cœur de Montréal and Université de Montréal, Montréal, Québec, Canada

Contents

Introduction

Definitions vary with time according to the current status of evidence and changing diagnostic methods. Definitions also vary according to the purposes for which they are used, such as epidemiology, surveillance programs, public health (1), clinical diagnosis, and medicolegal jurisdiction. In the same way as the consensus definition of asthma has improved its recognition and management, precise and workable definitions of occupational asthma (OA) are required to improve its investigation and management.

Classification of asthma in the workplace

The workplace can trigger or induce asthma (Figure 1.1). In the broad spectrum of asthma conditions related to the workplace, some nosological entities can be identified based on the strength of the causal relationship, clinical and objective features, and/or pathophysiological mechanisms (Table 1.1) (2).

Definitions

Occupational asthma

To avoid ambiguity in defining OA in this book, an editorial consensus was sought by analyzing the essential content of prior definitions of OA of presumed allergic or immunological causation (3) (Table 1.1).

Any agent specific to the workplace

The word *specific* used in these definitions can easily be understood if it is contrasted to *nonspecific* stimuli to which all asthmatic subjects react (e.g. irritants, fumes, exercise, and cold air). Therefore, *specific* used in this context refers to any agent or exposure that is present in the workplace that directly causes OA.

Sensitizing agents specific to the workplace

Narrower definitions can be used to describe OA caused by "sensitizing agents specific to the workplace." These definitions specifically apply to agents that are present in the workplace and exert their effects through demonstrable (e.g. specific IgE) or presumed "sensitization" of the airways. In these definitions, the nature of the "sensitizing" mechanism is not always obvious, although it can be assumed in many cases as originating from a classical allergic process.

The workplace as the etiology of the condition

The key element common to all of the aforementioned definitions is the presence of a causal relationship between workplace exposure and the development of work-related asthma. It therefore seems logical to limit the definition of OA to those conditions in which the asthma is induced or caused by the occupation, as originally proposed by professor Jack Pepys: "Having made a diagnosis of asthma ("widespread airways obstruction reversible over short periods of time, either spontaneously or as a result of treatment"), it is then necessary in occupational asthma to establish a relationship to the work as recommended by Ramazzini in 1713" (4).

Agents causing sensitizer-induced OA can be referred to as inducers. Inducers cause airway obstruction, hyperresponsiveness, and inflammation but inciters (i.e. nonspecific asthma triggers) do not (5). All asthmatic subjects react to inciters (i.e. triggers) but only a minority to inducers.

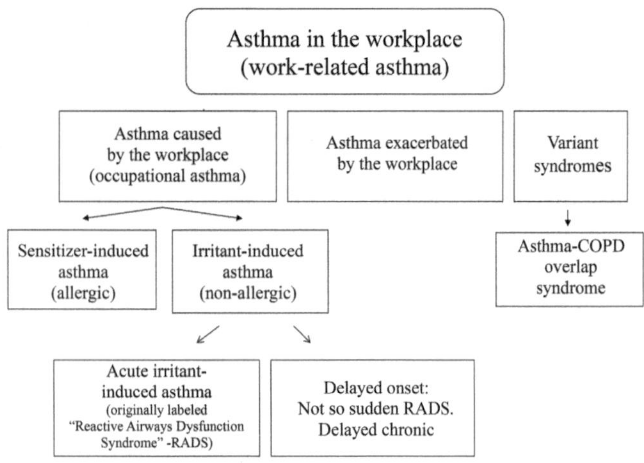

FIGURE 1.1 Phenotypic entities of asthma in the workplace.

Irritant-induced asthma or non-allergic OA is a condition that was described in the mid-twentieth century and initially labeled *reactive airways dysfunction syndrome* (RADS) (6). With time, it became more evident that RADS was induced by nonspecific irritants at work and therefore satisfied the definition of OA. Subsequently, the term *irritant-induced asthma* has been used to include both RADS and those (conditions) with incomplete criteria for RADS, but in whom it was nevertheless considered likely that irritant exposure(s) had caused asthma (7). In the first

edition of *Asthma in the Workplace*, therefore, the editors' consensus definition proposed that this condition be accepted as a type of OA.

Editorial consensus definition of OA

Several features of the definitions of sensitizer- and irritant-induced OA that have been proposed in the scientific literature warrant consideration in proposing an editorial consensus definition.

As mentioned in Table 1.1, *the exposure that causes OA should be related or "specific" to the workplace.* Whereas all asthmatic subjects react to nonspecific stimuli such as cold air, exercise, etc., only asthmatic subjects with OA will experience an asthmatic reaction on exposure to specific stimuli or sensitizers such as diisocyanates, flour, etc. In various proposed definitions, "specific" can be interpreted to mean that the agent that causes OA exists only at work and is not ubiquitous, which is the case in almost all instances of OA with a few exceptions open to debate. For example, should a chambermaid who develops sensitization to mites or a landscaper who is sensitized to summer molds with asthmatic symptoms worsening at work be compensated? In the case of irritant-induced asthma, the causal exposure should be documented as having occurred in the workplace and not in the general environment. Inhalational accidents also occur in domestic environments. Finally, the word *specific* might also refer to the evidence that the asthmatic reaction occurs only if the worker is at the workplace and is less severe in the general or domestic environment.

TABLE 1.1 Definitions of Sensitizer-Induced Occupational Asthma Proposed in the Literature

Any agent specific to the workplace

"Occupational asthma is a disorder in which there is generalized obstruction of the airways, usually reversible, caused by inhalation of a substance or a material that a worker manufactures or uses directly or is incidentally present at the worksite" (8).

"Although the term *occupational asthma* usually refers to new onset asthma caused by workplace exposure, exacerbations of preexisting asthma are an equally important cause of workplace morbidity … extreme sensitivity of airways to chemical, physical, and pharmacological stimuli is a characteristic feature of asthma. Thus many agents encountered in the workplace that have little or no effect on nonasthmatic workers can cause pronounced symptomatic bronchoconstriction in workers with asthma" (9).

"Occupational asthma, therefore, is caused by some specific agent or agents in the form of dust, fumes, or vapors in a industrial environment" (10).

"Occupational asthma is variable airways narrowing causally related to exposure in the working environment to airborne dust, gases, vapors, or fumes" (11).

"Occupational asthma will be defined as asthma caused by specific agents in the workplace. This will exclude bronchoconstriction induced by irritants at work, exercise, and cold air" (12).

Sensitizing agents specific to the workplace

"Occupational asthma is caused by exposure at a place of work to a sensitizing bronchoconstrictor agent" (13).

"Occupational asthma is asthma which is due in whole or in part to agents met at work. Once occupational sensitization has occurred … " (14).

"Occupational asthma refers to de novo asthma or the recurrence of previously quiescent asthma (i.e. asthma as a child or in the distant past that has been in remission) induced by either sensitization to a specific substance (e.g. an inhaled protein [high-molecular-weight (HMW) protein of >10 kd] or a chemical [low-molecular-weight (LMW) agent]), at work, which is termed *sensitizer-induced OA*, or by exposure to an inhaled irritant at work, which is termed *irritant-induced OA*" (15).

"It (OA) affects only a proportion (usually a minority) of those exposed to the agents (…) and develops only after an initial symptom-free period of exposure, which may vary between individuals from weeks to years (…). Such findings fulfill the classical clinical criteria of hypersensitivity (…) " (11).

The workplace as the etiology of the condition

"OA is a disease characterized by airway inflammation, variable airflow limitation, and airway hyperresponsiveness caused by conditions attributable to a particular occupational environment and not to stimuli encountered outside the workplace, (…) would be more appropriately labeled occupation-induced asthma to emphasize the determining causal relationship between asthma and the workplace" (2).

"occupational asthma, defined as asthma due to conditions attributable to work exposures and not to causes outside the workplace" (16).

Occupational asthma as a type of work-related asthma (that also encompasses work-exacerbated asthma)

"Occupational asthma (OA) is a form of work-related asthma characterized by variable airflow obstruction, airway hyperresponsiveness, and airway inflammation attributable to a particular exposure in the workplace and not due to stimuli encountered outside the workplace" (17).

Also, the *causal relationship should be established or suspected as a sensitizing process causing allergic inflammation* (often eosinophilic). For high-molecular-weight agents causing OA, this is through an IgE-mediated mechanism that can be documented by allergen skin testing or assessment of serum-specific IgE. Such proof has not been demonstrated for most low-molecular-weight agents. The causal agent therefore acts as an inducer and not as a trigger or inciter of asthma (5). Even in the case of RADS, airway inflammation (eosinophilic and neutrophilic) and remodeling share similarities with allergic inflammation. Airway inflammation and remodeling are not caused by exposure to most agents acting as triggers. Epidemiological studies have shown that chronic occupational exposure to irritant occupational agents leads to higher incidence of bronchial obstruction and nonspecific bronchial hyperresponsiveness (NSBH) that can be interpreted or misclassified as irritant-induced asthma (see Chapter 3).

OA is a phenotype of asthma, which is a condition characterized by variable airway obstruction, hyperresponsiveness, and inflammation. The clinical investigation of OA starts with establishing that the worker is affected with asthma before examining the role of possible causal agents present at work, and then proving that the asthma is caused by the workplace.

Finally, the *expression "OA with a latency period"* was used in previous editions in reference to sensitizer-induced OA in the context of an exposure period to aeroallergens during which IgE-dependent sensitization theoretically occurs prior to onset of clinical allergy (allergic rhinitis, asthma). Irritant-induced asthma with low-dose exposures also has a latency period (18). However, the presence of this characteristic does add some certainty to the diagnosis of sensitizer-induced OA, and the absence of latency greatly reduces its likelihood. Moreover, irritant-induced asthma with low-dose exposures is an entity that has been proposed in epidemiological studies and is not generally recognized as a clinical diagnosis by specialists and Workers' Compensation Board (WCB) authorities.

After considering the opinions mentioned in Table 1.1 and scientific evidence, the editors propose the following definition that allows sufficient latitude to include both allergic and non-allergic forms of OA:

Items in the Definition	Justification
• OA is a type of work-related asthma	Asthma in the workplace or work-related asthma includes OA and work-exacerbated asthma.
	OA is a phenotype of asthma, a condition characterized by reversible airway obstruction, hyperresponsiveness, and inflammation.
• that is caused by immunological (identified or presumed)	The mechanism of OA is immunological or allergic, shown as IgE-mediated for high-molecular-weight agents and presumed to be immunological or allergic for most low-molecular-weight agents. It is associated with a symptom-free latency period between the beginning of exposure and the onset of asthma.
• and non-immunological stimuli	This is the case for irritant-induced OA.
• present in the workplace.	The causal agent or exposure has to be at the workplace.

Occupational asthma is a type of work-related asthma that is caused by immunological (identified or presumed) and non-immunological stimuli present in the workplace.

Two types of OA are distinguished, based on the underlying mechanism:

1. OA caused by workplace sensitizers: allergic or immunological OA

This category encompasses (i) OA caused by most high- and certain low-molecular-weight agents for which an allergic (immunoglobulin E, IgE-mediated) mechanism has been proven, and (ii) OA induced by specific occupational agents (e.g. diisocyanates, Western red cedar) in which the responsible allergic and immunologic mechanisms have not yet been identified or fully characterized, though such mechanisms are probable.

2. OA caused by irritants: non-allergic or non-immunological OA, irritant-induced asthma

This category includes acute irritant-induced asthma, initially labeled RADS, which may occur rapidly after a single exposure to nonspecific irritants at high concentrations as originally described by Brooks (6) and not-so-sudden RADS in which onset of symptoms is delayed (19). This type of OA also includes what has been referred to as "possible irritant-induced asthma," a syndrome mainly identified in epidemiological studies that may follow chronic exposure to moderate or low levels of irritants at work (18). Activation of preexistent asthma or airway hyperresponsiveness by nontoxic irritants or physical and antigenic (antigens also present in the general environment) stimuli in the workplace ordinarily is excluded by this definition. (See definition in section "Work-Exacerbated Asthma.")

Besides OA, other conditions can be distinguished, as illustrated in Figure 1.1.

Work-exacerbated asthma

The term *work-exacerbated asthma* is used to describe the worsening of preexisting or coincident (adult new-onset) asthma because of workplace environmental exposure (15). Aggravation of asthma in the workplace can manifest as an increase in frequency or severity of asthma symptoms and/or increase in medication required to control symptoms on working days. These clinical features are similar to those encountered in OA; however, several studies have shown that subjects who experience exacerbation of asthma symptoms at work often fail to demonstrate significant objective evidence of the asthma worsening when they are exposed to the non-irritating levels of the suspected agent and monitored either in their workplace or in the laboratory (20, 21). Work-exacerbated asthma and OA are not mutually exclusive, and, rarely, both could coexist in certain workers (22). The prevalence of work-exacerbated asthma is not known, although it is likely to be a common condition, especially transient episodes that have been reported by up to 50% of working asthmatic subjects (22). It has been estimated that approximately 10% to 15% of all adult-onset asthma cases can be attributable to the workplace (23). This population-based data most likely includes both OA and work-exacerbated asthma cases. As the economic burden of work-exacerbated asthma to individuals and to society is similar to OA, a great deal of research on its physiopathology, optimal management, and long-term consequences is needed.

Asthma-like variant syndromes

Asthma-like disorders typically present with asthma-like symptoms associated with one or more objective asthmatic features, i.e., a significant cross-shift change in forced expiratory volume (FEV), "medium-range" or partial degree of reversibility in airway obstruction, bronchial hyperresponsiveness, and airway inflammation (eosinophilic and/or neutrophilic). Symptoms and functional evidence of partially reversible obstructive airflow limitation occur in workers who are exposed to grain dusts or in workers of aluminum potrooms. There is also evidence that exposure to inorganic dusts such as silica and silicon carbide may cause airway obstruction with some reversibility and bronchial hyperresponsiveness. More commonly, the workplace in "dusty trades" is responsible for a significant proportion of chronic obstructive pulmonary disease (COPD) (24, 25). An asthma-COPD overlap syndrome has been described in population studies (26) and in subjects with OA (27). Another condition, eosinophilic bronchitis, shows evidence of eosinophilic airway inflammation without evidence of reversible airway obstruction or bronchial hyperresponsiveness, which may represent a pre-asthmatic state in some subjects.

Nosological working definitions for diagnostic and epidemiological purposes

The strength and the nature of the causal relationship between exposure and onset of symptoms or disease vary according to the purpose (Table 1.2). The practicing physician must determine whether a subject referred as having "asthma in the workplace" has OA as discussed (28). For diagnosing OA, the physician therefore needs a more stringent association and will use more time-consuming, expensive, and invasive diagnostic procedures. The epidemiologist who conducts field studies is interested in identifying cases of "asthma in the workplace"; the epidemiologist's intention is not to diagnose OA but to identify disease susceptibility factors. For the occupational physician who runs a medical surveillance program, when early detection of disease is desirable, the requirements will again be different.

It is therefore convenient to have precise definitions for asthma in the workplace, similar to definitions for other conditions such as cardiovascular diseases (29). Such schemes for ascertaining asthma in the workplace have been proposed for clinical purposes previously (see the consensus panel of experts from the American College of Chest Physicians, Table 1.3) (30) and for epidemiological or surveillance surveys (see proposal by the National Institute for Occupational Safety and Health in Table 1.4) (31). These definitions incorporate different levels of evidence that result in

TABLE 1.2 Nosological Classification of Asthma in the Workplace

	Occupational Asthma (OA)		Work-Exacerbated Asthma
	Sensitizer-Induced OA	**Irritant-Induced OA**	
Causes	All high- and some low-molecular-weight agents	Single or multiple exposure to agents present at high concentrations or chronic exposure to "acceptable/moderate" levels of irritants	Agents with irritant properties
Mechanisms	IgE mediated for all high- and some low-molecular-weight agents (e.g. acid anhydrides, platinum salts, obeche wood)	Irritant injury to bronchi	Related to airway hyperresponsiveness caused by conditions that are not related to work
Essential features	Latency period of exposure and sensitization prior to onset of symptoms	Onset after sudden, single, or repetitive exposures to irritants; insidious development of asthma/COPD in workers exposed to irritants; variable levels of probability	Work-related asthma symptoms
Evidence of causal relationship	Demonstration of specific IgE by skin testing or in vitro assays	Temporal relationship between single or repeated exposure to agents present in high concentrations and the rapid onset of upper and/or lower respiratory symptoms	Exclusion of occupational asthma
		Epidemiological evidence of asthma in workers exposed to irritants	
Objective diagnosis	Assessment of airway caliber (PEFR), nonspecific airway responsiveness, and inflammation at work and away from work	Assessment of airway caliber and responsiveness after the inhalational accident(s)	Assessment of medication uses, airway caliber, airway responsiveness, and inflammation at work and away from work
	Specific inhalation challenges	Epidemiological probability	
Outcome	Improvement on removal from exposure; often with persistent airway hyperresponsiveness	Improvement on removal from exposure (sometimes); with persistent airway obstruction and/or hyperresponsiveness	Some improvement after avoidance

Abbreviations: COPD: chronic obstructive pulmonary disease; IgE: immunoglobin E; PEFR: peak expiratory flow rate.

TABLE 1.3 Criteria for Defining Occupational Asthma Proposed by the American College of Chest Physicians

A. Diagnosis of asthma
B. Onset of symptoms after entering the workplace
C. Association between symptoms of asthma and work
D. One or more of the following criteria:
  1. Workplace exposure to an agent or process known to give rise to occupational asthma
  2. Significant work-related changes in FEV_1 or PEFR
  3. Significant work-related changes in nonspecific airway responsiveness
  4. Positive response to specific inhalation challenge tests with an agent to which the patient is exposed at work
  5. Onset of asthma with a clear association with a symptomatic exposure to an irritant agent in the workplace RADS
Requirements
  Occupational asthma:
    Surveillance case definition: A + B + C + D1 or D2 or D3 or D4 or D5
    Medical case definition: A + B + C + D2 or D3 or D4 or D5
    Likely occupational asthma: A + B + C + D1
    Work-aggravated asthma: A + C (i.e. the subject was symptomatic or required medication before and had an increase in symptoms or medication requirement after entering a new occupational exposure setting)

Source: Information from reference (30).
Abbreviations: FEV_1, forced expiratory volume in 1 second; PEFR: peak expiratory flow rate; RADS, reactive airways dysfunction syndrome.

various positive and negative predictive values for recognizing the link between exposure and the defined condition.

TABLE 1.4 Surveillance Case Definition of Occupational Asthma Proposed by the Sentinel Event Notification System for Occupational Asthma (SENSOR)

A. Healthcare professional's diagnosis of asthma
B. An association between symptoms of asthma and work
C. One or more of the following criteria:
  1. Increased asthma symptoms or increased use of asthma medication (upon entering an occupational exposure setting) experienced by a person with preexisting asthma who was symptomatic or treated with asthma medication within the 2 years prior to entering that new occupational setting (work-aggravated asthma)
  2. New asthma symptoms that develop within 24 hours after a one-time high-level inhalation exposure (at work) to an irritant gas, fume, smoke, or vapor and that persist for at least 3 months (RADS)
  3. Workplace exposure to an agent or process previously associated with occupational asthma
  4. Work-related changes in serially measured FEV_1 or PEFR
  5. Work-related changes in bronchial responsiveness as measured by serial nonspecific inhalation challenge testing
  6. Positive response to specific inhalation challenge testing with an agent to which the patient has been exposed at work

Source: From reference (31). Public domain.
Abbreviations: FEV_1, forced expiratory volume in 1 second; PEFR: peak expiratory flow rate; RADS, reactive airways dysfunction syndrome.

Conclusion

This book aims to present the whole spectrum of asthma phenotypes related to the workplace. OA represents a condition in which the disease is asthma and the causal relationship of the disease with exposure is a key element. Therefore, this condition constitutes the principal part of the presentation. Because OA is often associated with involvement of other target organs (nose, eyes, and skin), these conditions are also addressed. Work-exacerbated asthma is relatively more common compared to OA and is associated with substantial socioeconomic impact. It represents a situation in which the causal relationship between the disease and the occupational environment is uncertain, borderline, not well characterized, or open to debate. Therefore, further research is needed. Finally, asthma-like conditions and conditions of confirmed (hypersensitivity pneumonitis), possible immunological (organic dust exposure), or apparently non-immunological (indoor or building-related conditions) etiologies that affect the airways and the lungs (including COPD) which partially share one or more features of asthma are presented in separate chapters and less extensively than OA.

References

1. Jaakkola MS, Jaakkola JJK. Assessment of public health impact of work-related asthma. BMC Med Res Methodol. 2012;12:22.
2. Malo JL, Vandenplas O. Definitions and classification of work-related asthma. Immunol Allergy Clin North Am. 2011;31:645–52.
3. Johansson SGO, Hourihane JOB, Bousquet J, et al. A revised nomenclature for allergy: An EAACI position statement from the EAACI nomenclature task force. Allergy. 2001;56:813–24.
4. Pepys J. Occupational asthma: Review of present clinical and immunologic status. J Allergy Clin Immunol. 1980;66:179–85.
5. Dolovich J, Hargreave FE. The asthma syndrome: Inciters, inducers, and host characteristics. Thorax. 1981;36:641–4.
6. Brooks SM, Weiss MA, Bernstein IL. Reactive airways dysfunction syndrome (RADS). Persistent asthma syndrome after high level irritant exposures. Chest. 1985;88:376–84.
7. Tarlo SM. Irritant-induced asthma in the workplace. Curr Allergy Asthma Rep. 2014 Jan;14(1):406.
8. Brooks SM. Occupational asthma. In: EB Weiss, MS Segal, M Stein, eds. Bronchial asthma. Boston, MA: Little, Brown, 1985: 461–9.
9. Sheppard D. Occupational asthma and byssinosis. In: JF Murray, JA Nadel, eds. Textbook of respiratory medicine. Philadelphia, PA: WB Saunders, 1988: 1593–605.
10. Parkes WR. Occupational asthma (including byssinosis). In: Occupational lung disorders. London: Butterworths, 1982: 415–53.
11. Newman-Taylor AJ. Occupational asthma. Thorax. 1980;35:241–5.
12. Chan-Yeung M, Malo JL. Occupational asthma. Chest. 1987;91:130S–6S.
13. Cotes JE, Steel J. Occupational asthma. In: Work-related lung disorders. Oxford: Blackwell Sc Publications, 1987: 345–72.
14. Burge PS. Occupational asthma. In: P Barnes, IW Rodger, NC Thomson, eds. Asthma: Basic mechanisms and clinical management. London: Academic Press, 1988: 465–82.
15. Tarlo SM, Balmes J, Balkisssoon R, et al. ACCP consensus statement: Diagnosis and management of work-related asthma. Chest. 2008;134:1S–41S.
16. Tarlo SM, Lemiere C. Occupational asthma. N Engl J Med. 2014;370:640–9.
17. Cartier A, Bernstein DI. Occupational asthma: definitions, epidemiology, causes, and risk factors. UptoDate. 2016.
18. Vandenplas O, Wiszniewska M, Raulf M, et al. EAACI position paper: Irritant-induced asthma. Allergy. 2014;69:1141–53.
19. Brooks SM, Hammad Y, Richards I, Giovinco-Barbas J, Jenkins K. The spectrum of irritant-induced asthma. Chest. 1998;113:42–9.
20. Malo JL, Ghezzo H, L'Archevêque J, et al. Is the clinical history a satisfactory means of diagnosing occupational asthma? Am Rev Respir Dis. 1991;143:528–32.
21. Tarlo SM, Leung K, Broder I, et al. Asthmatic subjects symptomatically worse at work: prevalence and characterization among a general asthma clinic population. Chest. 2000;118:1309–14.

22. Henneberger PK, Redlich CA, Callahan DB, et al. An official American Thoracic Society statement: Work-exacerbated asthma. Am J Respir Crit Care Med. 2011;184:368–78.

23. Toren K, Blanc P. Asthma caused by occupational exposures is common—A systematic analysis of estimates of the population-attributable fraction. BMC Pulm Med. 2009;9:7.

24. Trupin L, Earnest G, SanPedro M, et al. The occupational burden of chronic obstructive pulmonary disease. Eur Respir J. 2003;22:462–9.

25. Omland O, Würtz ET, Aasen TB, et al. Occupational chronic obstructive pulmonary disease: A systematic literature review. Scand J Work Environ Health. 2014;40:19–35.

26. de Marco R, Marcon A, Rossi A, et al. Asthma, COPD and overlap syndrome: A longitudinal study in young European adults. Eur Respir J. 2015;46:671–9.

27. Ojanguren I, Moulec G, Hobeika J, et al. Clinical and inflammatory characteristics of asthma-COPD overlap in workers with occupational asthma. PLOS ONE. 2018 Mar 2;13(3):e0193144.

28. Malo JL, Gautrin D. From asthma in the workplace to occupational asthma. Lancet. 2007;370:295–7.

29. Hurst JW, Morris DC, Alexander RW. The use of the New York Heart Association's classification of cardiovascular disease as part of the patient's complete Problem List. Clin Cardiol. 1999;22:385–90.

30. Chan-Yeung M. Assessment of asthma in the workplace. ACCP consensus statement. American College of Chest Physicians. Chest. 1995;108:1084–117.

31. Matte TD, Hoffman RE, Ronsenman KD, Stanbury M. Surveillance of work-related asthma in selected United States using surveillance guidelines for state health departments, California, Massachusetts, Michigan, and New Jersey, 1993-1995. Mor Mortal Wkly Rep CDC Surveill Summ. 1999;48:1–20.

2

HISTORICAL ASPECTS OF OCCUPATIONAL ASTHMA

Jack Pepys,[*] I. Leonard Bernstein[*] Jean-Luc Malo,[1] and Susan M. Tarlo[2]

[1]Hôpital du Sacré-Cœur de Montréal and Université de Montréal, Montréal, Québec, Canada
[2]Department of Medicine, University Health Network and St Michael's Hospital, University of Toronto, Toronto, Ontario, Canada

Contents

Introduction

The history of asthma in the workplace includes aspects related to asthma, allergy, and occupational medicine. The concept of occupational asthma (OA) has broadened to include not only a type of asthma induced at work by a sensitizing mechanism but also irritant-induced asthma and asthma in the workplace.

Historical aspects of asthma, allergy, and occupational respiratory diseases

History of asthma and allergy

Asthma translated literally means "panting," or a "shallow breathing" as proposed by Homer in the XVth song of the Iliad (850 BC), which describes the "terrible suffocation" of Hector lying in the plain (1). Early literature on asthma has distinguished intrinsic from extrinsic causal factors. Hippocrates (460–370 BC) cited its presence in metal workers, fullers, tailors, horsemen, farmhands, and fishermen. The Arabic physician Rhazes (864–930) was the first to identify allergic asthma followed by Maimonides (1138–1204), Saladin's physician, who, in a treatise on asthma comments on the influence of heredity, the wintery exacerbations of asthma, foods, hygiene, and emotion. The paroxysmal nature of the disorder was described by the Belgian physiologist and physician van Helmont (1) who, in his treatise *Ortus medicinae* published in 1648, proposed that allergy and heredity were involved. The role of extrinsic factors was also reported in Sir John Floyer's *A Treatise of the Asthma* (1698) in which the author who suffered from asthma reports improvement due to breathing the fresh air in Oxford. Floyer describes the case of a worker with asthma due to handling of wheat. Laennec (1781–1826) contributed to the understanding of asthma through the auscultation of wheezing in his famous *Traité de l'auscultation médiate*. Later, the role of secretions and bronchial inflammation was suspected. Curschmann (1846–1910) and Ernst von Leyden (1832–1910), respectively, discovered spirals and crystals in sputum of asthmatic subjects. Characterization of airway caliber by the French physiologist Tiffeneau in the 1950s, the so-called Tiffeneau index (FEV1/vital capacity), and its enhanced variability in asthma as assessed by serial peak expiratory flows (PEF) (2) represent major landmarks. Development of methodologies to assess nonspecific bronchial responsiveness with standardization contributed to a more precise clinical diagnosis of asthma and identification in epidemiological studies. Assessment of induced sputum and exhaled nitric oxide (NO) (3) provided a unique means to assess bronchial inflammation.

The development of immunology and allergy in the beginning of the twentieth century allowed identification of causative allergic factors leading to the proposed classification of intrinsic and extrinsic asthma by Rackeman in 1947 (4). Charles Harrison Blackley (1820–1900) (5) was the first physician to demonstrate that pollen allergy was the cause of seasonal hay fever. The beginning of the twentieth century marked the discovery of anaphylaxis by the French scientists Charles Richet and Paul Portier. Von Pirquet and Bela Schick first coined the word *allergy* to describe severe reactions to horse serum, from Greek words (*allos* or "other" combined with *ergon* or "reaction"). Years 1909–1910 represented an important historic milestone for asthma. Meltzer incriminated anaphylaxis in the pathogenesis of asthma (6). Leonard Noon prepared the first allergenic extracts used for desensitization in 1911. Blocking antibodies, later identified as IgG immunoglobulins, were described by Cooke in 1935 who also

9

began the first allergen injection immunotherapy clinic in North America. Histamine and the development of antihistaminic preparations also took place in the beginning of the twentieth century. The ability of serum from allergic subjects to be passively transferred to the skin of a naive subject and elicit an immediate skin test reaction to an allergen (the Prausnitz–Küstner test) was proposed to be caused by reaginic antibodies (5) later identified as IgE immunoglobulins by Ishizka in 1966–1967 (7). Johansson developed the radioallergosorbent test (RAST) (8). The leukotrienes cascade (formerly called slow-reactive substance of anaphylaxis) was elucidated in the 1970s (5) and followed by major breakthroughs in understanding the role of specific subsets of lymphocytes in driving (Th2 cells) and regulating allergic inflammation (T regulatory cells).

Occupational respiratory diseases and occupational asthma

The life-threatening effect of inhaled contaminants has been recognized very early, especially in miners, potters, and glass workers as well as flax, silk, and cotton handlers though it is principally at the time of the Industrial Revolution from 1750 onward that diseases caused by inhalants became apparent. Early examples of occupational respiratory problems can be seen in a citation from an ancient Egyptian papyrus (Papyrus Sallier) describing "the weaver engaged in home work (who) is worse off in the house than the women, doubled up with his knees drawn up to his stomach, he cannot breathe." Roman Pliny stated that "persons employed in the manufactories in preparing minimum (native cinnabar, red lead) protect the face with masks of loose bladder skin, to avoid inhaling the dust."

With the development of trade and the need for precious and other metals in the fifteenth century, occupational diseases became of medical interest and were mainly concerned with mining (9).

The Scandinavian monk Olaus Magnus described in 1555 the difficult breathing that could occur in grain handlers and might either represent farmer's lung or asthma (Figure 2.1). Occupational disease in general came of age when Bernardino Ramazzini published in 1713 his classic landmark in occupational diseases, *De morbis artificum diatriba* (10), reporting occupational respiratory diseases affecting bakers, handlers of old clothes, and workers with flax, hemp, and silk. Ramazzini made another contribution. He wrote: "The Divine Hippocrates informs us, that when a Physician visits a Patient, he ought to inquire into many things, To which I would presume to add one Interrogation more: namely, what Trade is he of?"

The next step in occupational diseases arose with the Industrial Revolution in the United Kingdom in the 1800s. Charles Turner Thackrah published in 1832 a book on the effects of arts, trades, and professional and civic status and habits of living on health and longevity (11). Thackrah used the term *asthma* only twice, with reference to maltsters and coffee roasters and to hatters and hairdressers. Thackrah described the usefulness of the "pulmometer" in diseases of the lungs, an instrument developed in 1836 to assess the "quantity of air expired."

Proteinaceous agents were the first to be described in the twentieth century as causes of OA. Castor bean dust was the first of these agents (12), followed by gums and insects. Although low-molecular-weight (LMW) agents such as metal salts, chromium and platinum, and anhydrides were also described as causes of OA in reports made early in the twentieth century, the first description of OA due to a chemical product, diisocyanates, a common cause of OA, was made in 1951 by Fuchs and Valade (13).

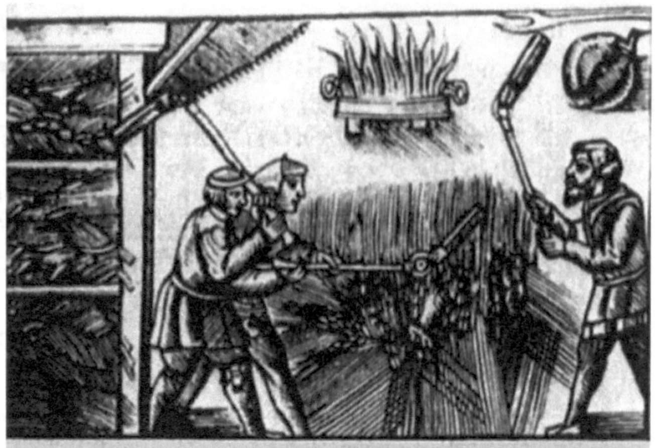

FIGURE 2.1 "When sifting the chaff from the wheat, one must carefully consider the time when a suitable wind is available that sweeps away the harmful dust. The fine-grained material readily makes its way into the mouth, congests in the throat, and threatens the life organs of the threshing men. If one does not seek instant remedy by drinking one's beer, one may never more, or only for a short time, be able to enjoy what one has threshed" Olaus Magnus, 1555. (From Pepys J, Bernstein IL, Malo JL. Historical aspects. In: Malo JL, Chan-Yeung M, Bernstein DI, eds. *Asthma in the Workplace.* 4th ed. Boca Raton, FL: CRC Press, 2013:8. By courtesy of late Professor Jack Pepys.)

Originally, the diagnosis of OA was mainly based on the clinical history. Skin testing to document possible IgE-mediated sensitization and spirometry were subsequently used, followed by evaluation of nonspecific bronchial responsiveness.

The use of bronchial provocation tests with common protein allergens was proposed in the mid-twentieth century. Late asthmatic reactions, that will later be incriminated in the physiopathology of asthma as the culprit cause of inflammation, were described by Herxheimer in 1952 (14). A new era in which such tests are made with LMW chemical compounds was opened by Gelfand (15). He elicited immediate skin and bronchial reactions to various amines. Gandevia reported on asthma caused by diisocyanates (16) and Western red cedar (17) by using specific inhalation challenges as well as Popa with amines (18). The development by Pepys, considered by many to be the father of OA, of an experimental type of simulated exposure to agents suspected to cause OA from 1970 onward, as summarized in a key article (19), enabled the identification of several agents causing OA, the description of the temporal patterns of asthmatic reactions and the inhibitory effect of drugs such as sodium cromoglycate and inhaled steroids on these reactions (Figure 2.2).

At-work and off-work monitoring of PEF rates was subsequently suggested (20). Other noninvasive means to document

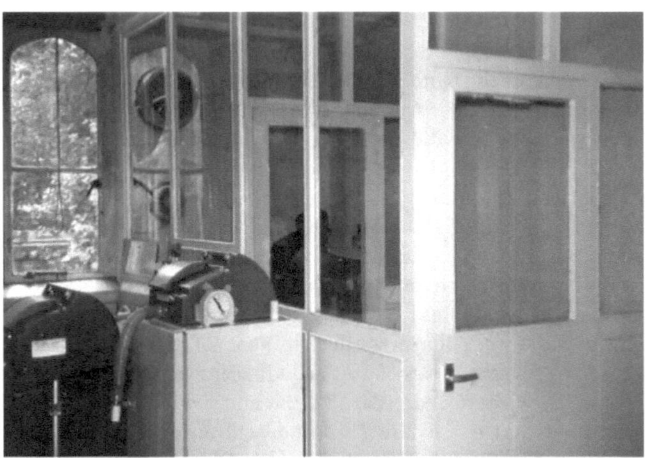

FIGURE 2.2 Cubicle used for specific inhalation challenges with occupational agents, Brompton Hospital 1975. (From Pepys J, Bernstein IL, Malo JL. Historical aspects. In: Malo JL, Chan-Yeung M, Bernstein DI, eds. *Asthma in the Workplace*. 4th ed. Boca Raton: CRC Press; 2013:9.)

airway inflammation, a key element included in definitions of asthma, have been added to the diagnostic arsenal while attempts to improve the methodology of laboratory challenges have been carried out.

From occupational asthma to asthma in the workplace

Under the general heading of "asthma in the workplace," several conditions can be distinguished. First, the workplace can cause asthma through a known, in the case of all high-molecular-weight (HMW) and some LMW agents, or apparently plausible, for most LMW agents, sensitizing process that needs to operate;

until recently this was the main focus of interest as reviewed above. Although it had been known since the early twentieth century that exposure to products with irritant properties could cause pulmonary edema and bronchial damages, the entity *irritant-induced asthma* or *reactive airway dysfunction syndrome* (RADS) was described by Brooks and coworkers in 1985 (21). This syndrome now represents the second type of OA. Study of exacerbations of asthma at the workplace became relevant as it encompasses socioeconomic consequences that are equivalent to OA. Finally, occupational eosinophilic bronchitis was identified (22).

Distinction between asthma in the workplace and OA has important impacts on the assessment of frequency. Estimates of frequency initially targeted OA and were based on cross-sectional workplace surveys with OA suspected or confirmed by objective findings and not only questionnaires: skin testing or specific IgE assessment with suspected HMW occupational agent; and/or lung function abnormalities: pre- and post-shift FEV1, serial PEFs, assessment of nonspecific bronchial responsiveness, and specific inhalation challenges with the suspected agent in some "screened" workers. Population-based epidemiological studies (23) and studies using population-based registries (24) provide an estimate of asthma in the workplace, not of OA because, even if asthma is suspected or confirmed, OA is not confirmed, as discussed and illustrated (Figure 2.3) (25).

Practice guidelines on asthma in the workplace have been issued in the United States (26, 27), Canada (28), and the United Kingdom (29).

Key advances from the first edition in 1993 to now

This fifth edition of *Asthma in the Workplace* appears more than 20 years after the first edition. Unfortunately, Dr. Jack Pepys can no longer personally witness the rapid evolution of the discipline he helped to pioneer, but some of his predictions about the future of OA either have already transpired or are beginning to emerge

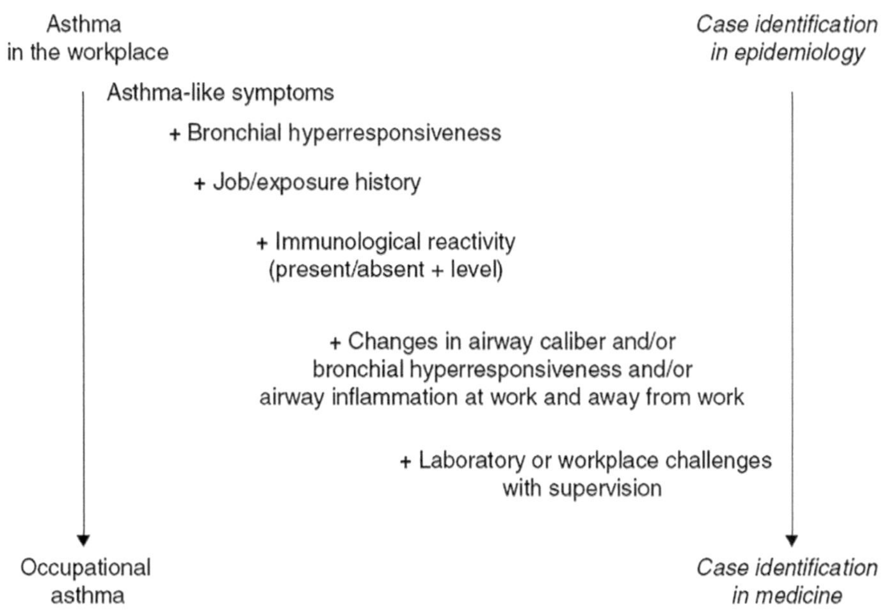

FIGURE 2.3 Steps in assessment of workplace asthma. (From Pepys J, Bernstein IL, Malo JL. Historical aspects. In: Malo JL, Bernstein DI, Chan-Yeung M, eds. *Asthma in the Workplace*. 4th ed. Boca Raton: CRC Press; 2013:10. Different graphical reinterpretation in reference [25].)

in the relatively short period of time since the original publication of this book.

As rates of asthma have risen and reached an apparent plateau, the perception that occupational allergens, nonspecific triggers, and irritants are important contributory factors has been noted in several evidence-based guideline documents on the diagnosis and management of asthma. Technological progress in the identification of HMW and LMW agents in the workplace environment has expanded, and the role of nonspecific irritants in the induction of nonimmunological OA has been explored more extensively since the first edition of this book was published. Better understanding of risk factors has evolved over the years with confirmation of the key role of exposure and its modulation by personal predisposition. Determination of "safe" exposure thresholds has been undertaken for some allergens causing OA.

In his historical review, Dr. Jack Pepys emphasized the interest of eliciting the mechanism of the development of allergenicity to various chemicals (19). Since then, there has been renewed interest in predictive structure–activity relationships. Genetic susceptibility has been explored further and may predispose individuals to sensitization. Both susceptibility and protective specific class II genes have been reported as well as an increase in specific nucleotide polymorphisms, certain gene/gene interactions, and haploid prevalences. The risk for upregulation of IgE sensitization to occupational allergens can be enhanced by exposure to various environmental contaminants such as ozone, nitrogen oxides, and diesel fumes.

In recent years, some information has also been provided on the psycho-socioeconomic aspects of asthma in the workplace, particularly in follow-up studies of workers removed from exposure. All these aspects are related to the compensation that is offered by medicolegal agencies. Emphasis should be put on readaptation programs that are essential for young workers.

Occupational asthma as a model for environmental asthma: what occupational asthma has taught us about environmental asthma

Asthma caused by allergy to agents inhaled at work has several advantages for investigation over asthma caused by allergy to environmental allergens, for which it has been considered a model (Figure 2.4).

These include: 1. a well-defined population at risk that can be followed prospectively with a pre-exposure assessment, an assessment at the time of sensitization, symptoms and disease, and, finally, serial assessments after cessation of exposure. This therefore provides an entirely experimental situation for which it is possible to assess individuals pre- and post-end of exposure; 2. immunological sensitization in the case of HMW allergens; 3. high risk of developing disease within a relatively short period from onset of exposure and the opportunity for well-characterized exposure.

A number of studies have exploited these advantages to investigate in workforce cohorts the determinants of allergy and asthma caused by several causes of OA, including enzymes used in detergents (31), Western red cedar (32), rat and mouse urine proteins (33), flour and α-amylase (34), and acid anhydrides (35). The strength of some of these studies has been the follow-up of a proportion of new employees not previously exposed to the relevant allergen to overcome the problems of survivor bias inherent in cross-sectional surveys and the ability to relate disease incidence to level of exposure (36). The use of an entirely prospective model has been particularly fruitful in examining apprentices before they enter a training program (37, 38) because this represents an experimental situation in which subjects can be examined before, during, and after stopping exposure.

Nature and intensity of allergenic exposure: exposure is a more important determinant than personal and genetic factors

Most ubiquitous inhaled allergens are proteinaceous material. The history of OA as reviewed in Section "Historical aspects of asthma, allergy, and occupational respiratory diseases" shows that chemicals can also induce sensitization, although the mechanism of such sensitization still remains unknown in most instances. An analysis of chemical structure in relation to the risk of causing sensitization has been developed (39). Several studies have consistently demonstrated the importance of the level of exposure to airborne allergen (enzyme, flour, α-amylase, detergent enzyme, acid anhydride, Western red cedar) as the major determinant of risk of developing specific IgE allergy and/or asthma. Factors such as atopy and cigarette smoking previously identified as risk factors for some agents (e.g. platinum salts) were found to be of lesser importance than intensity of exposure. The importance of exposure intensity as a determinant of OA and of its effect in reducing disease incidence is well demonstrated by examining the history

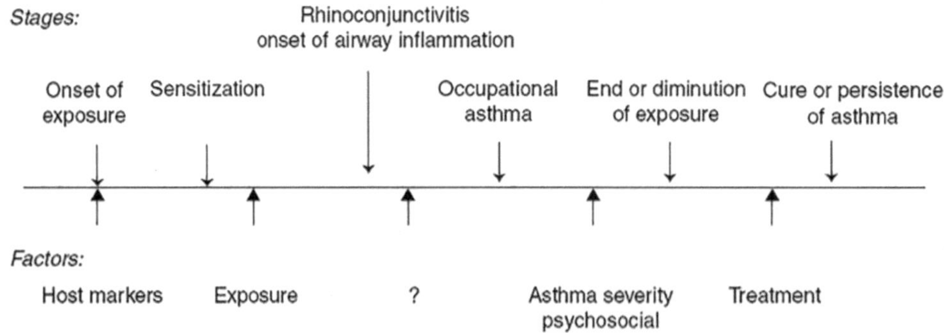

FIGURE 2.4 Stages in the natural history of occupational asthma with factors that may influence the progression. (From Pepys J, Bernstein IL, Malo JL. Historical aspects. In: Malo JL, Bernstein DI, Chan-Yeung M, eds. *Asthma in the Workplace.* 4th ed. Boca Raton: CRC Press; 2013:11. Derived from data in reference [30].)

of asthma caused by occupational exposures to enzymes in the detergent industry.

Irritant exposures can cause asthma: The example of RADS

It was generally thought that asthma invariably results from a sensitizing process. The description of irritant-induced asthma shows that asthma can result from a purely apparently traumatic event. Long-term follow-up of workers who experienced a RADS event shows the persistence of airway obstruction and pathologic features comparable to asthma, including the presence of eosinophils in the bronchial walls (40). It is therefore not excluded that a significant number of so-called intrinsic asthma cases might result from inhalation accidents, either single or multiple lower dose events (21, 41).

Asthmatic reactions on exposure

Late asthmatic reactions that have originally been described by Herxheimer in 1952 are common after exposure to agents that cause OA. Isolated late reactions have only been documented after exposure to occupational agents. The effect of anti-asthmatic preparations on late reactions has been examined through specific inhalation challenges (42).

The example of specific inhalation challenges carried out for the diagnosis of OA has also been useful in showing that both the level of nonspecific bronchial responsiveness, the degree of immunological reactivity, and the level of eosinophilic inflammation in the airways play a role in the likelihood of inducing immediate asthmatic reactions (43, 44).

Outcome after cessation of exposure

Examining the outcome of OA after cessation of exposure provides a unique opportunity to know whether asthma is a curable disease. Many thought naively that OA would be invariably cured after cessation of exposure. Moira Chan-Yeung was the first to show in the 1970s and 1980s (45) that this is not generally the case. Many follow-up studies have since demonstrated that clinical symptomatic asthma disappears in about 25% of subjects removed from exposure with normalization of bronchial responsiveness. Most studies have shown that the duration of symptomatic exposure is the key factor that predisposes to the persistence of asthma. The maximum improvement takes place in the first 2 years after stopping exposure with slower rate of improvement thereafter (46). Long-term studies have shown the presence of airway neutrophilic and eosinophilic inflammation 10 years or more after stopping exposure even in apparently cured subjects (47). Also, even after stopping exposure, the immunological memory still operates as re-exposure to the causal agent, even in workers apparently cured, generally still induces an asthmatic reaction (48). Finally, studies show that some subjects who acquired IgE-mediated sensitization to an occupational allergen lose sensitization if they are removed from exposure (30).

How to assess impairment/disability

Whereas means and scales for assessing pneumoconiosis have been developed, these tools could not be usually applied in the case of asthma, a disease characterized by variable airway obstruction. Different criteria had to be defined in the case of asthma, of which OA offered a model. Criteria based on need for medication to control asthma as well as levels of airway obstruction and hyperresponsiveness were therefore proposed by the American Thoracic Society in 1993 and later endorsed by the American Medical Association. Quality of life and general psychological questionnaires can be used to assess disability.

Can we prevent the disease and modify its outcome?

Studies evaluating the effectiveness of interventions to reduce exposure levels on disease incidence have now been reported for a number of the important causes of OA including enzymes in the detergent industry (49), flour (50), latex in healthcare workers (51), laboratory animal proteins in a pharmaceutical company (52), platinum (53), and isocyanates (54). In these studies, the environmental intervention has been accompanied by occupational health measures designed to identify cases at an early stage.

Conclusions and perspectives on research and societal needs

Asthma in the workplace is a condition that has been identified for centuries, although more in the twentieth century. Several issues now need to be considered as suggested by Malo and Newman Taylor (55):

- OA represents only a small proportion of asthma in the workplace, the rest being mostly asthma exacerbated by the workplace. Better characterization and assessment of this condition is necessary to reduce its important psycho-socioeconomic impact.
- The immunological mechanisms of asthma caused by the majority of chemicals still remain unknown.
- Means to assess frequency should allow for international comparisons, so as to assess overall prevalence trends of the disease and of causal agents.
- Reduction in the level of aeroallergen concentration that plays a key role in reducing the incidence of sensitization and asthma should be more generally advocated.
- OA should be more widely recognized as a valuable model of adult-onset asthma in particular in eliciting the role of irritants and the gene-environment interaction.
- Considering the existence of various efficient diagnostic means, clear decision trees have to be proposed for developing countries, health professionals responsible for running prevention programs in targeted workplaces, and family doctors.
- A satisfactory medicolegal management of cases should include readaptation programs with retraining and psychosocial interventions that should be included in addition to a lump-sum disability award. Scales to assess impairment have been proposed but tools to evaluate disability have to be further validated and used.
- Frequently associated with OA, occupational rhinitis is more common but has not been studied to the same extent. A "united airways" approach should be proposed.

References

1. Peumery JJ. Histoire illustrée de l'asthme. Paris: Les éditions Roger Dacosta, 1984.
2. Turner-Warwick M. Another look at asthma. Br J Dis Chest. 1977;71:73.
3. Quirce S, Lemière C, deBlay F, et al. Noninvasive methods for assessment of airway inflammation in occupational settings. Allergy. 2010;65:445–58.
4. Rackeman FM. A working classification of asthma. Am J Med. 1947;3:601–6.
5. Becker EL. Elements of the history of our present concepts of anaphylaxis, hay fever and asthma. Clin Exp Allergy. 1999;29:875–95.

6. Meltzer SJ. Bronchial asthma as a phenomenon of anaphylaxis. JAMA. 1910;55:1021–4.

7. Ishizaka K, Ishizaka T, Hornbrook MM. Physiochemical properties of reaginic antibody. IV. Presence of a unique immunoglobulin as a carrier of reaginic activity. J Immunol. 1966;97:75–85.

8. Johansson SGO, ed. Raised levels of a new immunoglobulin class (IgND) in asthma. Lancet; 1967.

9. Baxter PJ. Hunter's Diseases of Occupations. London: Hodder Arnold, 2010; Xth edition.

10. Ramazzini B. De morbis artificium diatribas. WC Wright, trans 1940. Chicago, IL: University of Chicago Press, 1940.

11. Thackrah CT. The effects of the principal arts, trades and professions, and of civic states and habits of living on health and longevity, with suggestions for the removal of many of the agents which produce disease and shorten the duration of life. Edinburgh: Livingstone, 1957 (Reprint) 1832.

12. Figley KD, Elrod RH. Endemic asthma due to castor bean dust. JAMA. 1928;90:79–82.

13. Fuchs S, Valade P. Étude clinique et expérimentale sur quelques cas d'intoxication par le Desmodur T (diisocyanate de toluylene 1-2-4 et 1-2-6). Arch Mal Profess. 1951;12:191–6.

14. Herxheimer H. The late bronchial reaction in induced asthma. Int Arch Allergy Appl Immunol. 1952;3:323–8.

15. Gelfand HH. Respiratory allergy due to chemical compounds encountered in the rubber, lacquer, shellac, and beauty culture industries. J Allergy. 1963;34:374–81.

16. Gandevia B. Respiratory symptoms and ventilatory capacity in men exposed to isocyanate vapour. Aust Ann Med. 1964;13:157–66.

17. Milne J, Gandevia B. Occupational asthma and rhinitis due to western (Canadian) red cedar. Med J Aust. 1969;2:741–4.

18. Popa V, Teculescu D, Stanescu D, et al. Bronchial asthma and asthmatic bronchitis determined by simple chemicals. Dis Chest. 1969;56:395–404.

19. Pepys J, Hutchcroft BJ. Bronchial provocation tests in etiologic diagnosis and analysis of asthma. Am Rev Respir Dis. 1975;112:829–59.

20. Burge PS, O'Brien IM, Harries MG. Peak flow rate records in the diagnosis of occupational asthma due to isocyanates. Thorax. 1979;34:317–23.

21. Vandenplas O, Wiszniewska M, Raulf M, et al. EAACI position paper: irritant-induced asthma. Allergy. 2014;69:1141–53.

22. Quirce S. Eosinophilic bronchitis in the workplace. Curr Opin Allergy Clin Immunol. 2004;4:87–91.

23. Kogevinas M, Zock JP, Jarvis D, et al. Exposure to substances in the workplace and new-onset asthma: an international prospective population-based study (ECRHS-II). Lancet. 2007;370:336–41.

24. Karjalainen A, Kurppa K, Martikainen R, et al. Exploration of asthma risk by occupation-extended analysis of an incidence study of the Finnish population. Scand J Work Environ Health. 2002;28:49–57.

25. Malo JL, Gautrin D. From asthma in the workplace to occupational asthma. The Lancet. 2007;370:295–7.

26. Bernstein DI, Cohn JR. Guidelines for the diagnosis and evaluation of occupational immunologic lung disease: preface. J Allergy Clin Immunol. 1989;84:791–3.

27. American Thoracic Society. Guidelines for assessing and managing asthma risk at work, school, and recreation. Am J Respir Crit Care Med. 2004;169:873–81.

28. Tarlo SM, Liss GM. Evidence based guidelines for the prevention, identification and, management of occupational asthma. Occup Environ Med. 2005;62:288–9.

29. Newman Taylor AJ, Cullinan P, et al. BOHRF guidelines for occupational asthma. Thorax. 2005;60:364–6.

30. Gautrin D, Ghezzo H, Infante-Rivard C, et al. Long-term outcomes in a prospective cohort of apprentices exposed to high-molecular-weight agents. Am J Respir Crit Care Med. 2008;177:871–9.

31. Greenberg M, Milne JF, Watt A. A survey or workers exposed to dusts containing derivatives of Bacillus subtilis. Br Med J. 1970;2:629–33.

32. Chan-Yeung M, Vedal S, Kus J, et al. Symptoms, pulmonary function, and bronchial hyperreactivity in Western Red Cedar workers compared with those in office workers. Am Rev Respir Dis. 1984;130:1038–41.

33. Hollander A, Van Run P, Spithoven J, et al. Exposure to laboratory animal workers to airborne rat and mouse urinary allergens. Clin Exp Allergy. 1997;27:617–26.

34. Houba R, Heederik DJJ, Doekes G, et al. Exposure-sensitization relationship for a-amylase allergens in the baking industry. Am J Respir Crit Care Med. 1996;154:130–6.

35. Barker RD, van Tongeren MJA, Harris JM, et al. Risk factors for sensitisation and respiratory symptoms among workers exposed to acid anhydrides: a cohort study. Occup Environ Med. 1998;55:684–91.

36. Cullinan P, Cook A, Nieuwenhuijsen MJ, et al. Allergen and dust exposure as determinants of work-related symptoms and sensitization in a cohort of flour-exposed workers; a case-control analysis. Ann Occup Hyg. 2001;45:97–103.

37. Gautrin D, Ghezzo H, Infante-Rivard C, et al. Incidence and determinants of IgE-mediated sensitization in apprentices: a prospective study. Am J Respir Crit Care Med. 2000;162:1222–8.

38. Walusiak J, Hanke W, Gorski P, et al. Respiratory allergy in apprentice bakers: do occupational allergies follow the allergic march? Allergy. 2004;59:442–50.

39. Seed MJ, Agius RM. Progress with Structure-Activity Relationship modelling of occupational chemical respiratory sensitizers. Curr Opin Allergy Clin Immunol. 2017;17:64–71.

40. Takeda N, Maghni K, Daigle S, et al. Long-term pathologic consequences of acute irritant-induced asthma. J Allergy & Clin Immunol. 2009;124:975–81.

41. Dumas O, Laurent E, Bousquet J, et al. Occupational irritants and asthma: an Estonian cross-sectional study of 34,000 adults. Eur Respir J. 2014;44:647–56.

42. Pepys J. Clinical and therapeutic significance of patterns of allergic reactions of the lungs to extrinsic agents. Am Rev Respir Dis. 1977;116:573–88.

43. Malo JL, Cardinal S, Ghezzo H, et al. Association of bronchial reactivity to occupational agents with methacholine reactivity, sputum cells and immunoglobulin E-mediated reactivity. Clin Exp Allergy. 2011;41:497–504.

44. Vandenplas O, Godet J, Hurdubaea L, et al. Are high- and low-molecular-weight sensitizing agents associated with different clinical phenotypes of occupational asthma? Allergy. 2019;74:261–72.

45. Chan-Yeung M, Lam S, Koerner S. Clinical features and natural history of occupational asthma due to western red cedar (thuja plicata). Am J Med. 1982;72:411–5.

46. Malo JL, Cartier A, Ghezzo H, et al. Patterns of improvement of spirometry, bronchial hyperresponsiveness, and specific IgE antibody levels after cessation of exposure in occupational asthma caused by snow-crab processing. Am Rev Respir Dis. 1988;138:807–12.

47. Sumi Y, Foley S, Daigle S, et al. Structural changes and airway remodelling in occupational asthma at a mean interval of 14 years after cessation of exposure. Clin Exp Allergy. 2007;37:1781–7.

48. Lemière C, Cartier A, Malo JL, et al. Persistent specific bronchial reactivity to occupational agents in workers with normal nonspecific bronchial reactivity. Am J Respir Crit Care Med. 2000;162:976–80.

49. Juniper CP, How MJ, Goodwin BFJ. Bacillus subtilis enzymes: a 7-year clinical, epidemiological and immunological study of an industrial allergen. J Soc Occup Med. 1977;27:3–12.

50. Smith TA. Preventing baker's asthma: an alternative strategy. Occup Med. 2004;54:21–7.

51. Tarlo SM, Easty A, Eubanks K, et al. Outcomes of a natural rubber latex control program in an Ontario teaching hospital. J Allergy Clin Immunol. 2001;108:628–33.

52. Fisher R, Saunders WB, Murray SJ, Stave GM. Prevention of laboratory animal allergy. J Occup Env Med. 1998;40:609–13.

53. Merget R, Caspari C, Kulzer SA et al. Effectiveness of a medical surveillance program for the prevention of occupational asthma caused by platinum salts: a nested case-control study. J Allergy Clin Immunol. 2001;107:707–12.

54. Tarlo SM, Liss GM, Yeung KS. Changes in rates and severity of compensation claims for asthma due to diisocyanates: a possible effect of medical surveillance measures. Occup Environ Med. 2002;59:58–62.

55. Malo JL, Newman-Taylor A. The history of research on asthma in the workplace-Development, victories and perspectives. In: Occupational Asthma. T Sigsgaard and D Heederik, eds. Progress in inflammation Research. MJ Parnham, Series editor. Basel, Switzerland: Birkhauser, 2010:1–15.

3

DISEASE OCCURRENCE AND RISK FACTORS

Mohamed F. Jeebhay,[1] Paul K. Henneberger,[2] Nicole Le Moual,[3] Jean-Luc Malo,[4] and Susan M. Tarlo[5]

[1]*Occupational Medicine Division and Centre for Environmental & Occupational Health Research (CEOHR), School of Public Health and Family Medicine, Faculty of Health Sciences, University of Cape Town, Cape Town, South Africa*
[2]*Respiratory Health Division, National Institute for Occupational Safety and Health, CDC, Morgantown, West Virginia, USA*
[3]*Université Paris-Saclay, UVSQ, Univ. Paris-Sud, Inserm, Équipe d'Épidémiologie respiratoire intégrative, Villejuif, France*
[4]*Hôpital du Sacré-Cœur de Montréal and Université de Montréal, Montréal, Québec, Canada*
[5]*University Health Network and St Michael's Hospital, Toronto, Department of Medicine, University of Toronto, Toronto, Ontario, Canada*

Contents

Introduction

The determinants of disease are usually considered under two broad headings—environmental and host factors. In the context of work-related asthma (WRA), all exposures encountered in the workplace, whether gaseous or airborne particulates of chemical (generally low-molecular-weight [LMW]) or biological (generally high-molecular-weight [HMW] vegetable/animal proteins) origin, physical stressors (manual work and/or cold temperatures), or factors related to workplace organization are of interest as they are considered to be either the main cause of occupational asthma (OA) or contribute to work-related aggravation/exacerbation of asthma (WEA). A determinant has been defined as "any physical, chemical, biological, social, cultural, or behavioral factor that influences the study outcome (in the present context, WRA)" (1). It may be causal or not, and can increase or decrease risk; risk factors may be primary (i.e. they increase incidence) or secondary (i.e. they increase the severity and/or trigger symptoms) (2). Host factors are generally modifiers, that is, they may modify the relationship between workplace exposure and the disease.

The increase in the frequency of OA among work-related lung diseases recognized by workers' compensation boards and surveillance systems in Europe and North America occurred over a period (1970–1990) when the prevalence, and probably the incidence, of asthma in the general population, particularly in children, had also been increasing, with a plateau being observed afterwards in some countries (Figure 3.1) (3). While environmental factors, particularly those associated with a "Westernized" lifestyle, have been implicated (4), support continues to grow for the view that societies are also becoming more susceptible (5). If so, this may also have contributed to the increasing rates of OA among work-related lung diseases in these societies. The relative contribution of host versus environmental factors in the development of the more ubiquitous adult-onset asthma compared to OA has increasingly been observed (6).

The classic approach to the study of occupational lung disease focuses on the environmental determinants with careful documentation of exposure levels by objective measurement. Objectives include characterizing the exposures and the adverse respiratory outcomes for the purposes of (i) establishing a causal relationship between an exposure and the respiratory effect under study, and/or (ii) providing the scientific basis for establishing workplace threshold exposure limits. The epidemiologic approach for the study of OA is hampered by the nature of the condition itself for several reasons. First, asthma is often a nonpermanent fluctuating condition, and its markers may be absent during the epidemiologic survey. Second, once sensitized to an asthmagenic agent or agents in the workplace, the individual reacts to a lower level of exposure, often because of the development and persistence of nonspecific bronchial hyperresponsiveness and underlying airway inflammation.

As a result, certain prevalence studies, and even incidence studies, may fail to identify levels responsible for provoking the onset of the condition (even if the affected individual has not quit the workplace location). Furthermore, this level is likely to differ according to the mechanism causing the asthma (allergic, or irritant induced).

Exposures responsible for WEA are usually identified by self-report and, similar to the exposures leading to OA, are usually difficult to quantify. More detail on WEA is provided in Chapter 20.

Methodological issues

Introduction

From the epidemiological and public health perspective, it would be important that studies of occupational and work-exacerbated asthma apply methods that are less influenced by country-specific factors, such as diagnostic practices, healthcare system, workers' compensation system, and reporting systems (7). This will provide an objective and comprehensive picture of the extent of occupational and work-aggravated asthma phenotypes, their causes, and their impact on the workforce and society.

There are two approaches for assessing occurrence of OA in a given population (8):

- Assessment of OA occurrence per se
- Assessment of adult-onset asthma and the attributable fractions (AFs) and population-attributable fractions (PAFs) due to specific occupational exposures

The former involves identifying individuals with diagnosed OA in a specified working population, while the latter provides an estimate of the occurrence of OA at the population level, without identifying specific individuals with OA.

Assessment of the occurrence of occupational asthma

For assessing the occurrence of OA, an estimate of the *numerator* representing cases of OA and the *denominator* representing the population at risk that produces the cases, expressed in person-time, is required. Two measures of occurrence are prevalence and incidence (cumulative incidence, incidence rate) (7, 8).

The numerator should be obtained from verified cases of OA. Incident (new) cases are more suitable than prevalent (being present at a particular point in time) cases for assessing the effect of occupational exposures on the development of asthma and for predicting future trends of public health burden resultant from OA. Prevalent cases may be more relevant when assessing the total disease burden from current cases. This can be evaluated by assessing the disease burden associated with increased symptoms, healthcare utilization, disability, healthcare costs, and other consequences of OA. A similar approach can be applied to groups of individuals and probabilities of developing asthma among exposed and unexposed populations.

The choice of the correct denominator is also dependent on the purpose of the assessment or study question to be addressed. For calculating the incidence of OA, the denominator should be person-time at risk of developing OA in the population for which the occurrence is assessed. This is easily calculated for a specific study population followed up over a period of time. When using existing population registries, the appropriate population at risk

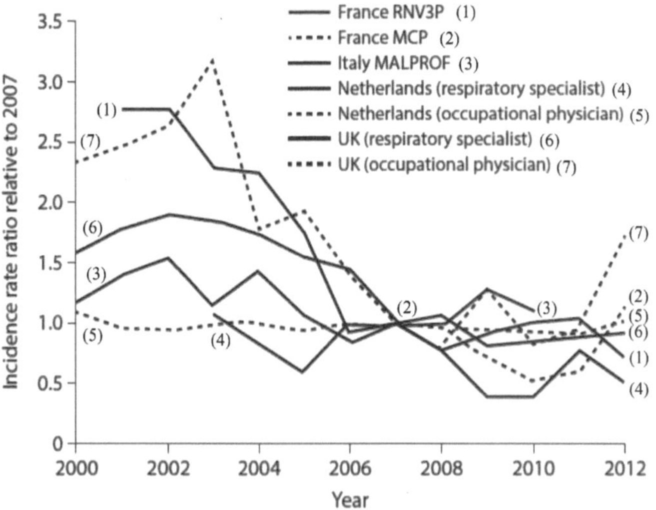

FIGURE 3.1 Estimated annual changes in incidence of occupational asthma in Europe based on national reporting surveillance data. RNV3P: Le Réseau national de vigilance et de prévention des pathologies professionnelles; MCP: Programme de surveillance des maladies à caractère professionnel (French surveillance system); MALPROF: Malattie Professionali (Italian surveillance system). (From Reference (3) in which the figure is presented as a modified version of Figure 2 in Stocks SJ, McNamee R, van der Molen HF, et al. *Occup Env Med* 2015;72:294-303, with permission.) Since the original version of the figure was published in colour, each line denoting the seven studies has been numbered at both upper and lower ends. For improved readability please refer to the original publication.

for calculating incidence of OA is the adult population that has ever been at work. OA may be detected even after a person has quit their job, although in such a case, the relevant time period at risk may be limited to a few years. Since new causes of OA are constantly being identified even among workforces that have traditionally not been considered as high-risk occupations, it is not recommended to limit the denominator to certain known "high-risk" occupational groups. When assessing OA incidence for certain specific exposures, individuals ever exposed to those specific exposures form the relevant denominator.

The issues related to the accuracy and comparability of this type of assessment of occurrence of OA include: (i) How should OA be verified? (ii) What is the coverage of the identification system for OA? (iii) What is the access to (occupational) health services? (iv) What are the workers' compensation practices and their influence on diagnostic practices? (v) How does the whole social security system influence all of these?

The identification and diagnostic procedures for OA vary between countries with well-developed occupational healthcare systems tending to have broader coverage, leading to higher estimates of occurrence. A well-functioning workers' compensation system may enhance detection of OA, but on the other hand, it may influence the diagnostic procedures and decisions such that OA cases that are not compensable may not be diagnosed at all. In irritant-induced asthma, diagnostic procedures are less standardized than for sensitizer-induced OA and may therefore not be reported should the compensation system require very specific diagnostic tests, such as specific bronchial inhalation challenges.

On the other hand, if there are poor compensation and social security systems for OA, workers may not report their symptoms or seek medical assistance, resulting in continued exposure while working until such time that their asthma becomes severe and debilitating.

National or regional voluntary registries that receive data from routine healthcare practices provide useful information for assessing the trends in OA over time at the national or regional level, but they may not provide very useful data for international comparisons or for etiologic research due to reporting biases.

Assessment based on the occurrence of adult-onset asthma and attributable fractions (AF) and population-attributable fractions (PAF) due to specific occupational exposures

For assessing the occurrence of OA based on AFs and PAFs due to specific occupational exposures, the following estimates are needed (7, 8):

1. an effect estimate for a specific or all occupational exposures, in the form of incidence rate ratio (IRR), which is obtained by computing the incidence rate (IR) in the exposed divided by IR in the unexposed;
2. an estimate of AF calculated based on this; and
3. an estimate of PAF calculated based on AF and the prevalence of occupational exposure(s) of interest in the population for which the assessment is made (P_e).

IRR gives an estimate of the risk of developing asthma in relation to the exposure of interest. The AF is used to estimate the proportion of exposed cases for which the disease could be attributable to the exposure. This approach applies to a population rather than to an individual case. The methodological issues related to the accuracy and comparability of assessment based on AF include: (i) Is the estimate of exposure used for assessing the effect valid? And (ii) is the effect estimate valid? The estimate of exposure should be accurate in terms of giving a valid effect estimate, but it does not need to be representative of the entire population. To ensure a valid effect estimate, this should be based on a high-quality study or on a meta-analysis if available. A high-quality study should be based on incident cases and be free of any major biases and confounding. Assessment of AF is comparable between populations that have similar exposure, making it less dependent on country-specific healthcare and insurance systems.

PAF is defined as the reduction in incidence that would be achieved if the population were entirely unexposed (7). It is usually interpreted as the proportion of cases in the population that could be prevented if exposure would be reduced to zero. The additional question to be asked is: Is the estimate of exposure representative of the population? The estimate of exposure should be valid in relation to the effect estimate used and it should also be representative of the exposure of the population for which the assessment is made.

The final step in assessing the occurrence of OA based on PAF due to specific occupational exposure(s) is calculating excess burden of disease (EBD). The additional question to be asked is: Is the estimate of incidence of asthma valid for the population of interest? A valid estimate of the incidence of asthma for the population(s) may be attained from a high-quality study or in some countries from existing registries.

The method based on assessment of PAF and EBD provides good and comparable estimates of excess incidence due to specific

TABLE 3.1 Summary of the Methods to Assess Occurrence of Occupational Asthma: The Method, Its Advantages and Limitations, and Recommended Applications

Method	Advantages	Limitations	Recommended Applications
Assessment of occurrence of diagnosed occupational asthma per se, for example, registries	Data collection takes place as part of the routine healthcare practices	Influenced heavily by country-specific differences in diagnostic practices, healthcare system, workers' compensation system, and reporting system	Can be used in countries with well-functioning occupational health services Suitable for assessing national or regional trends over time Not very useful for international comparisons
Assessment of occurrence (i.e. excess cases) based on population-attributable fraction due to occupational exposures	Gives good and internationally comparable estimates of excess incidence attributable to occupational exposures Not affected much by country-specific practices or healthcare or compensation systems	Needs valid, high-quality estimates of exposure prevalence, health effect of exposure, and incidence of adult-onset asthma	Works well at population level Suitable for assessing occurrence of occupational asthma for etiologic studies and for planning healthcare and health policies Suitable for international comparisons

Source: Adapted from Reference (7).

occupational exposures or specific occupational groups. This approach is not affected as much by country-specific practices as is the assessment based on identifying cases of diagnosed OA.

The advantages and disadvantages of the two methods for assessing the occurrence of OA are summarized in Table 3.1 (7).

Study approaches and designs

The purpose of epidemiological research on WRA is to explain patterns of the disease occurrence, its causation (i.e. etiology), or life course of an existing disease (i.e. prognosis). The approach for conducting a study on asthma in the workplace is selected primarily based on the study question, but the choice is also influenced by resources and other factors related to feasibility. Different study designs are accompanied by different strengths and limitations. When planning the study, it is important to be aware of these and their potential influence on the interpretation of the results. Table 3.2 lists these in increasing order of the strength of the study design in making causal inferences (7).

Target populations

Introduction

The term *target population* usually refers to the population a study seeks to describe and/or to which the results can be generalized. It is also used to describe the group of individuals about whom the study will make inferences. For a population at risk of OA with high employment turnover, and/or job change or redeployment, particularly in the short term, the survivor effect is likely to be strong. It is important to consider what the appropriate denominator (or target population) for prevalence and/or incidence studies should be (ever exposed, currently exposed, or average workforce over a given period of time) and the appropriate time frame for data collection (months, years, or decades).

Apprentices

Apprentices in trades or professions with increased risks for developing OA due to exposure to HMW or LMW agents represent a population of choice for inception cohort studies of WRA since the individuals are mostly naïve in terms of prior contact with work-specific allergens (9). Although the time frame for the follow-up is usually short (training period) to detect the incidence

of disease, 2 or 3 years are sufficient to identify early markers of OA, such as immunologic sensitization in the case of HMW agents (10). The survivor effect is low in these populations since individuals who quit their apprenticeship tend to do so for non-health-related reasons, such as economic or personal (11). The results may be generalizable to other populations of apprentices and newly hired workers with similar exposure. However, the intensity of exposure is likely to be lower for apprentice populations, and may act as a modifying factor. Cohort members can be assessed periodically for several years. Similar to birth cohort studies, information on risk factors and possible modifiers for OA can be collected prospectively from baseline onward.

Workforce-based and community-based studies

There is a rich literature of workforce-based surveys, some initiated by the identification of clusters of cases, through physician referral or sentinel programs, and others seeking a priori to examine risk factors. These studies are epidemiological in concept, that is, population (workforce) based.

Studies of individuals of a specific workforce also offer a number of advantages. There is usually common exposure to known agent(s) albeit with varying intensity according to job title and work task (12); and the probability is also high for detecting occurrence of OA. Possible approaches using workforce-based OA studies include: cross-sectional prevalence studies, incidence studies among individuals that are initially free of disease, evaluative studies to assess the effects of intervention programs to reduce the exposure (13, 14), and case-control studies in workplaces where health and exposure information is collected routinely (15). However, use of apprentice populations of workforces at risk presents some challenges such as a high turnover rate and attrition, introducing a healthy survivor effect in prevalence studies, and some lost-to-follow-up over time in longitudinal incidence and evaluative intervention studies.

Environmental factors examined are generally exposure level and duration and/or occupation (as an estimate of exposure). Host factors have examined age, gender, smoking status, and atopy (family history, immunological reactivity generally assessed by skin prick testing) as illustrated in the study of supermarket bakeries (16).

TABLE 3.2 Study Designs for the Study of Work-Related Asthma

Type of Study Design	Purpose/Description	Advantages/Strengths	Limitations/Pitfalls
Case series	First observations to identify potential new causes of occupational asthma (OA) Identification of clusters of cases Important for clinical practice	Carefully conducted and individually described exposure and outcome	No assessment of occurrence or estimate of risk Do not assess numerator or denominator
Registry-based studies	Extensions of case series where OA cases are reported systematically to a registry or a surveillance scheme	Give a good picture of the trend in magnitude of the problem and of the spectrum of causes of OA Good to assess regional or national trends	Influenced by country-specific factors (diagnostic practices, health care, compensation and reporting systems) Not useful for international comparisons or etiologic studies
Cross-sectional studies	Address the relationship between exposure and outcome in a defined population at a particular point in time	Can be conducted in a relatively short period of time Can be applied to large population sample, improving generalizability All information on exposure and outcome obtainable for all participants	Impossible to infer temporal sequence between exposure and outcome "Healthy worker survivor effect" with underestimation of the risk. Those with disease represent a selected proportion of cases with possible misclassification of cases and exposure.
Case-control studies	Compare exposure and risk factor distribution between those with a specified outcome, such as OA (cases) and those who are free of the outcome (controls)	The controls (referents) provide information on the exposure distribution in the source population. Efficient study design as it is possible to gather more detailed information on exposure and disease status, especially for rare outcomes Suitable for etiologic research Not as time-consuming as cohort studies	Recall bias with possible overestimation of risk Exposure and disease not necessarily confirmed in a similar way in cases and controls "Healthy worker survivor effect"
Case-crossover studies	Compare the exposure distribution during a hazard period Cases serve as their own controls.	Good for assessing work-exacerbated asthma Eliminate potential confounding by subject characteristics Eliminate the concern about potential differences in selection of cases and controls	Not suitable for the study of factors causing OA
Clinical or preventive trials	To assess the beneficial effect of preventive or treatment measures Intervention study with randomization of subjects	The strongest study design to prove a causal relationship or treatment effect	Unethical to randomize subjects to harmful exposures Potential noncompliance with the preventive measures Possible unequal distribution of confounders High cost

Source: Reproduced and adapted from Reference (7).

Community-based studies have proved surprisingly powerful in bringing to attention associations between occupational exposures and wheezing complaints despite the fact that, in such studies, the potential for misclassification, both of exposure and outcomes (which are of necessity self-reported), is considerable. The strength of community-based studies derives from the fact that they reach all individuals ever exposed in workplaces at risk, as distinct from only those currently exposed or only those exposed long enough to be registered in any workforce-based survey (17).

Practical issues associated with occupational surveys

The implementation of occupational surveys is strongly influenced by laws and practices that vary by country and potentially by jurisdictions within the same country. Ideally, investigators can obtain cooperation from all relevant stakeholders, including representatives from management, labor, occupational health and safety committees at the involved companies, local or regional health departments, and patient groups. The survey organizers should conduct meetings before the survey to address the concerns of stakeholders and answer questions.

Ideally, monitoring of the workplace environment should be carried out at the time of the survey to provide appropriate estimates when studying the association of relevant health outcomes with current exposure. Questionnaire surveys and medical tests in the field should be conducted under optimal conditions. Calibration of lung function equipment should be done daily before testing or twice daily if a large number of workers are to be tested. It is preferable to have the survey conducted at the worksite, which assumes that the employer will allow workers to participate either during the workday or directly before or after. However, some employers find this type of arrangement unacceptable, and it is necessary to conduct the survey offsite, for example in a union hall or community building. Performing tests in an organized and efficient manner minimizes time lost from work if the survey takes place during normal working hours and respects the sacrifice made by participants if the survey occurs away from work. At the end of the study, it is a good practice to send individual results directly to the worker and offer to give further explanation if necessary. It is also advisable to present the group results to management, workers, and other stakeholders for further input before preparing a final report.

WRA identified among patients in specialized clinics or hospitals, and by Sentinel case surveillance

A major concern of studying WRA among asthma patients treated in specialized outpatient settings (e.g. an asthma clinic or pulmonary medicine practice) or in hospitals is that the cases tend to be more severe than those treated by primary care physicians. One approach to address this issue is to evaluate the association of asthma with occupational exposures among patients from a variety of treatment settings. For example, a study conducted in Italy surveyed asthma patients identified in records of the national health system (18). Asthma cases were classified as WRA if they provided a positive response to at least one of seven questions that inquired about work-related patterns in symptoms and medication use, and whether they had been told their asthma was induced by work. The frequencies were 40.8% for WEA and 7.2% for OA. A potential weakness of conducting studies in either specialized or general care settings is that WRA status may not have been systematically confirmed with the same criteria in all cases and those criteria may not have been based on objective tests.

The Sentinel Event Notification System for Occupational Risks (SENSOR), introduced in several states in the United States in the 1980s (19), was based on mandatory and/or voluntary reporting of suspected work-related disease by physicians, as well as identification of cases from existing sources such as workers' compensation and healthcare records. State-based public health officials responded to the reports by investigating workplaces thought to be at risk. While this program is no longer called SENSOR, it continues with state-based surveillance of occupational diseases, with coordination and guidance provided by the National Institute for Occupational Safety and Health. In the United Kingdom, a sentinel-type system called Surveillance of Work-related and Occupational Respiratory Disease (SWORD), modeled on the informal reports of communicable diseases submitted by its Public Health Laboratory Service, was introduced in 1989 (20) and based on voluntary reporting by selected physicians across the country. Systems based on this model were at least attempted elsewhere, for instance in Canada, in the provinces of Quebec (21) and British Columbia (22), in France (23), South Africa (24), and Australia (25). As with infectious disease notification, underreporting is a persistent problem. However, as cases are not necessarily confirmed by objective findings, overreporting might also occur and distort estimates of frequency (21). Therefore, the magnitude of the balance between under- and overreporting is unknown and likely varies considerably from one country or jurisdiction to the next.

General and specific registries (agencies)

Registries focusing on occupational diseases in general or specific occupational diagnoses like WRA have been used for investigating trends over time in occurrence and distribution of causal workplace agents within a country, a region within a country, or a specified subcategory of a population. The reporting system may include mandated or voluntary reporting, and medicolegal statistics can also be applied. The benefits of registries include the fact that they yield developing data produced by everyday inpatient and outpatient healthcare practice and related systems such as for health insurance and workers' compensation. Such data can provide an estimate of public health impact and be used to inform health policy and healthcare planning. If the diagnostic procedures for occupational diseases can be standardized well with national guidelines, the data within the system can be reasonably comparable over time. However, changes in the diagnostic procedures, structures of health care, sources of reports, reporting system itself, or compensation systems will lead to changes in occurrence that do not necessarily reflect any true changes in the magnitude of disease prevalence or occurrence or relative importance of exposures. Because these country- and region-specific factors have a strong influence on the occurrence of WRA, registry-based data are often not very useful for international or inter-regional comparisons (8). In addition, such routine registries more accurately reflect diseases caused by well-known occupational agents, while underreporting is more likely with novel causes and causes for which the diagnosis is more difficult to establish, for example, irritant-induced OA (26).

A good example of a national registry on occupational diseases, including OA, is the Finnish Registry of Occupational Diseases that was established in 1964 and gets its data through reporting required by law (27). The registry changed into the Finnish Registry of Work-Related Diseases in the early 2000s and started to register separately confirmed occupational diseases and suspicions of occupational disease. The reporting system also changed to facilitate electronic submission and the data comes now through the Federation of Accident Insurance Institutions and Farmers' Social Insurance Institution, which receive reports from individual insurance companies or physicians. In Finland, all employees are covered by insurance and compensation for a confirmed occupational disease by law, but for self-employed people this insurance is voluntary, which means that even this rather comprehensive register does not represent all Finnish adults encountering potentially harmful exposures at work.

Looking at trends over time in the occurrence of OA in the Finnish Registry of Work-Related Diseases demonstrates well how changes in medicolegal practices and other societal factors have influenced the estimates of incidence. In Finland, the diagnosis of OA has been strongly influenced by the rather good compensation system covering the costs of treatment, retraining, and pension for confirmed OA. The disadvantage has been that cases not likely to be compensated by the medicolegal system may have remained underdiagnosed. Inclusions of farmers into the same compensation scheme in 1982 led to a significant increase in OA, especially because of cow dander and flour exposures (28). Since the mid-1990s, indoor mold problems emerged as a major occupational hazard in Finnish workplaces after the economic recession in the early 1990s was accompanied by a reduction in building maintenance activities and an increase in mold-induced OA (8, 29, 30). Since 2005, more emphasis was dedicated to producing statistics that separate confirmed OA from the suspicions, and in 2009, a dramatic change in the diagnostic protocol for indoor mold-induced OA was introduced as it seemed that specific inhalation challenges did not work well for this type of OA. Since 2005, a considerable decline in confirmed OA was observed with about 100–150 new cases reported annually since then, while the numbers of suspicions increased during the same period to 600–700 each year (31). There has been discussion about potential causes of this change. Does it reflect changes in the healthcare structures and consequent underdiagnosis of OA or does it reflect a real decline in OA due to improvements in exposure control measures in the workplaces? These trends were confirmed in a more recent publication based on the frequency of occupational diseases in Finland during 1975–2013 (32). Asthma was included with allergic rhinitis, allergic alveolitis, and chronic laryngitis in the category of allergic respiratory diseases (ARDs). From 2005 to 2013, the average annual change in incidence for ARDs was negative (–7.8%) for recognized disease and positive (+2.8%) for suspected disease.

Other studies using specific registries include the Ontario Workers' Compensation Board database that has been utilized since 2010 for assessing how a cleaners' strike impacted compensation claims for asthma submitted by teachers (33) and changes in the frequency of diisocyanate and non-diisocyanate sensitizer-induced OA during 2003–2007 (34). In the United Kingdom, there are statistics on OA available from the Industrial Injuries Scheme and the Health and Safety Executive that receives reporting under the Reporting of Injuries, Diseases and Dangerous Occurrences Regulations (RIDDOR), but these have been found to be subject to serious underreporting (28).

General registries can also provide information useful for studies in WRA. In the section describing assessment of occurrence of OA based on PAF, it was mentioned that combining PAF with high-quality registries on (adult) asthma will give an estimate of excess number of cases (i.e. EBD) attributable to the occupational exposure(s) of interest (8). Studies from Finland have also utilized the Medication Reimbursement Register of the National Social Insurance Institution to identify cases of diagnosed asthma and combine that data with information on occupation from census data to estimate the risk of adult-onset asthma related to specific occupations (35). Such an approach is vulnerable to potential sources of error related to registry data in general (e.g. some degree of misclassification of outcome and exposure status and lack of individual level information on confounders), but it does provide an opportunity to utilize large datasets to address important study questions related to asthma in the workplace.

Tools to measure health outcomes
Questionnaire
Community-based studies allow evaluation of the burden of the disease and are opportunities for a better understanding of the occupational determinants of the clinical activity of the disease (36). In community-based surveys, it is difficult to identify participants with OA in contrast to clinical identification of asthma cases (7). Recording complete asthma activity histories with precise definitions of outcomes is crucial (37, 38), and it is important to favor specificity over sensitivity for asthma definitions. Disease activity and status have been mostly recorded by standardized questionnaires, which are easy to administer, especially in large community-based epidemiological surveys (7).

Standardized dichotomous definition of ever asthma has been mostly evaluated in epidemiological surveys by a positive response to the question: "Have you ever had asthma attacks?", with or without complementary questions ("Have you ever had attacks of breathlessness at rest with wheezing?" "Was asthma confirmed by a doctor?") (37, 38). Current asthma was commonly defined among participants with ever asthma, and with the presence over the past 12 months of asthma attacks, an asthma treatment or at least one asthma attack or respiratory symptoms (wheezing, nocturnal chest tightness, attack of breathlessness following activity, at rest or at night time) (38).

However, these dichotomous definitions of asthma may not be optimal when studying risk factors of asthma. A continuous asthma symptom score has been proposed (39). This score ranges from 0 to 5 and represents the numbers of positive answers to the five following items, recorded in the last 12 months: (i) breathless while wheezing, (ii) woken up with a feeling of chest tightness, (iii) attack of shortness of breath at rest, (iv) attack of shortness of breath after exercise, and (v) woken by attack of shortness of breath. Interestingly, this asthma symptom score was constructed independently of the asthma status. In addition, this score allows increasing power, compared to a dichotomous definition of asthma, when studying asthma risk factors (39).

In clinical studies, asthma control is often defined through Global Initiative for Asthma (GINA) guidelines (https://gina-asthma.org/gina-reports/), but it is difficult in epidemiological surveys to strictly use this definition (40). Therefore, standardized questionnaires designed to measure the multidimensional nature of asthma control have been proposed, such as the Asthma Control Test (ACT) (41), which has been validated both in clinical and epidemiological surveys (42). Asthma control defined by ACT is based on the sum of response (0/1) to five questions in the past 4 weeks: (i) activity limitation, (ii) symptom frequency, (iii) sleep interference, (iv) use of rescue treatment, and (v) a self-reported rate of control level, resulting in a score ranging from 5 to 25 (fully controlled). A dichotomous definition based on a 19-threshold is often used to identify participants with uncontrolled asthma (≤19) (43).

WRA, which includes both OA and WEA, may be evaluated through standardized questionnaires (7, 44–46). A strategy has been proposed to classify participants as "suspected occupational asthma," "suspected work-exacerbated asthma," or "non-work-related asthma" (45).

Immunological assessment
Immunological assessment is important in identifying symptomatic individuals with OA due to HMW agents (proteins) and some LMW chemicals. In such individuals, tests such as skin-prick tests (SPT) or in vitro allergen-specific immunoglobulin E (IgE) assays can be used to identify sensitization to specific occupational allergens when these tests are technically reliable and available (47). Standardization and validation of SPT solutions is highly recommended since studies show a wide variability in SPT solutions from a similar allergen source. The sensitivity of several SPT solutions, especially those for LMW agents, is low compared to HMW protein antigens. For several food allergens, fresh natural raw extracts are often used. The positive and negative predictive value of immunological tests for OA varies depending on the allergen. Overall, a negative SPT does not exclude the diagnosis of OA, whereas a positive test supports the diagnosis but is not definitive for the diagnosis. In general, SPTs can test many allergens at once, provide immediate results, and are cheaper, but they are more labor intensive to perform and have some contraindications. Specific IgE tests are logistically easier to perform and relatively without adverse reactions but are more expensive per allergen extract.

Functional assessment
Measurement of lung function

Lung function tests can be conducted at a worksite or nonmedical off-site location, and can present special problems not usually encountered in hospitals or clinic laboratories (48). It is important to have trained technicians to calibrate the equipment and deal with problems. The technicians should also be trained to recognize poor subject performance. Poor performance, in particular, poor reproducibility, may also be a marker of airway dysfunction (49).

Several factors need to be considered in choosing the lung function tests: the cost of equipment, the testing time, the simplicity of the test, and analysis of results, reproducibility, acceptability, and the degree of standardization of the instrument and test procedures. Instrument requirements, calibration techniques, test procedures, measurement of test results, and data interpretation should conform to the 2019 update of the American Thoracic Society (ATS)/European Respiratory Society (ERS) guidelines for standardization of spirometry (50). For most epidemiologic studies of WRA, measurements of peak expiratory flow (PEF), FEV_1, FVC, and FEV_1/FVC are sufficient.

Pre- and post-shift spirometric measurement

Assessment of pre- and post-shift (cross-shift) FEV_1 has been used to confirm the work-relatedness of asthma. Initial reports suggested that it is neither specific nor sensitive for case identification, due to factors such as diurnal variation (levels lowest in early hours of morning, highest in early hours of afternoon), measurement or technical errors, and intermittent exposures to the sensitizing agent (51). However, it has proved useful in detecting acute nonallergic airway responses associated with exposure to agents such as cotton dust and grain dust. The cross-shift change in lung function with these agents is directly proportional to the level of exposure (52).

Serial measurements of peak expiratory flows

Although serial measurements of PEF have proven to be a valuable tool in assessment of patients with OA in a clinical setting (53) and show a reasonable correlation with the results of specific challenge testing, their role in the assessment of OA in prevalence surveys is challenging. Serial PEF monitoring has been used successfully in several epidemiological surveys (54–57). Subjects' compliance is a problem because the subjects are usually asked to monitor their PEF at least four times a day at work and at home for a period of 3 to 4 weeks, a commitment that many find hard to keep. More time is needed in field studies in comparison with the usual clinical setting, to explain to and instruct the subjects how to measure their own PEF properly. Former concerns about the falsification of patient-recorded readings have been addressed by using testing devices that automatically record and date and time stamp results. The between-observer reproducibility of the interpretation of peak flow rate recordings obtained from surveys is good (58) and comparable to the interpretation carried out in a clinical setting (59). Moreover, there is an online program for analyzing serial PEF data that is relatively easy to use and yields a decision about work-relatedness (60).

Exhaled nitric oxide

Exhaled nitric oxide (FeNO) is a simple noninvasive tool that can be used as a surrogate marker of predominantly eosinophilic airway inflammation in asthma. It can easily be measured in the workplace using a small portable device using American Thoracic Society/European Respiratory Society recommendations (61). It

has been assessed as a screening tool in several populations of workers exposed to HMW and LMW agents (62). There are many confounding factors to consider in interpreting FeNO, the most common being smoking and atopy. Some studies of workers exposed to HMW agents have shown that an increase in FeNO over time has been associated with the development of bronchial hyperresponsiveness (BHR). Workers with high allergen-specific IgE have higher FeNO levels. In a clinical setting increases in FeNO show high positive predictive values for a positive specific inhalation challenge (SIC) to HMW agents. For LMW agents, changes in FeNO have less frequently been observed, except for isocyanate-induced OA. In terms of serial changes in FeNO, a delayed (post 24 hours) work-related increase has been observed in an epidemiological study of spice mill workers (63). It has also been used to assess the effect of an intervention in supermarket bakeries, in which a significant decline in FeNO ($\geq$10%) was observed following intervention in bakers with baseline work-related ocular–nasal symptoms (14).

Nonspecific challenge tests

Measurement of nonspecific bronchial responsiveness has been used by a number of investigators in epidemiologic surveys of general populations (64, 65) and workplace populations (66–69). These studies have shown that methacholine, histamine, and hyperventilation of dry or cold air challenge tests can be carried out in epidemiologic settings safely without the presence of physicians, the occurrence of severe bronchoconstriction being rare and reversible (70). As discussed in another chapter, measurement of nonspecific bronchial responsiveness is not specific enough to be used alone in identifying subjects with asthma. The epidemiological definition of asthma includes specific answers to a respiratory questionnaire and bronchial hyperresponsiveness to a pharmacological agent (71). When combined with questionnaire information and immunologic tests (when feasible), this test is very useful for identifying subjects with possible OA and WEA in the workplace (69).

Specific bronchial challenge tests

Specific bronchial challenge tests with the suspected offending agent have been used successfully in the clinical setting to confirm the diagnosis of OA. It is not practical to include specific challenge testing in field studies carried out at the workplace in the same way as this can be done in clinical settings for the confirmation of OA (72). These tests can be used to confirm the diagnosis in subjects suspected of OA identified through surveillance. However, in some countries like the United States, specific challenge is used infrequently due, in part, to concerns about liability if the patient experiences an extreme reaction to the test.

Algorithm for case identification (decision tree) in epidemiologic studies

An example of a stepwise approach (Figure 3.2) proposed elsewhere has been used successfully in several studies that assessed the frequency of OA at the workplace. Subjects who require further investigation for the confirmation of the diagnosis of OA include those who have questionnaire responses compatible with WRA, evidence of immunologic sensitization, and/or nonspecific bronchial responsiveness. Serial monitoring of PEF and nonspecific challenge tests should also be conducted on these subjects. It is highly unlikely that subjects without evidence of nonspecific bronchial responsiveness and immunologic sensitization will react on specific challenge testing to the offending agent.

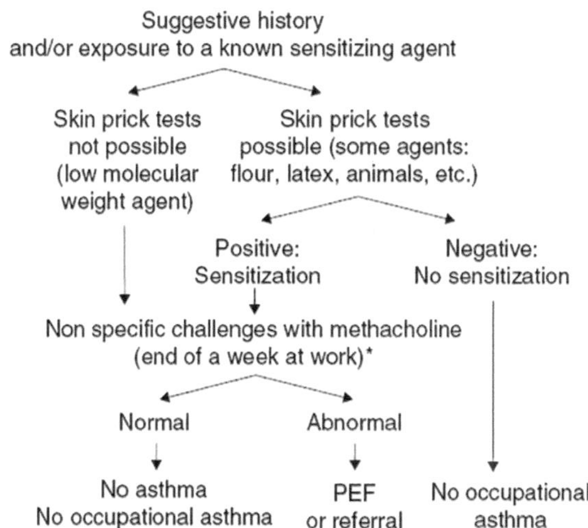

FIGURE 3.2 Scheme of investigation of WRA in workforces. (From Reference [7].)

Biases and pitfalls

Introduction

The aim of epidemiological surveys is to produce valid and precise results (7). In occupational epidemiology, associations between exposure and asthma may be influenced by random error, which affects the precision of the estimate but may be reduced by increasing the size of the population (7, 73). Another source of inaccurate results is bias, which is a systematic error that should always be minimized. Biases are often difficult to take fully into account and may compromise the estimates of the associations between exposure and disease. In case of biases, associations between exposure and disease may not reflect the causal impact of exposure in the source population (74). Potential sources of bias should be taken into account in the interpretation of the results. Three types of biases are classically described in occupational epidemiology: selection bias, information bias, and confounding, in addition to modifiers. Selection bias can be avoided in the design phase of a study whereas confounding can be reduced during data analysis.

Selection bias

The study design, self-selection of people who accepted to participate, and incomplete follow-up may induce selection bias in work-related epidemiological surveys. Such bias may distort the estimate of the association between exposure and disease (7). Selection bias and confounding are not always clearly distinguished (73). An important selection bias named the "healthy worker effect" (HWE) (75), which may occur commonly in WRA surveys, may be also considered as a confounder (and may be taken into account by appropriate statistical models). The HWE is a reverse causation phenomenon that may mask or underestimate the associations with WRA in epidemiological surveys (75). The HWE can be induced by the fact that sicker workers may choose a job/task with low exposures or may not be hired, especially in exposed jobs (healthy worker hire effect). In addition, once hired, these workers may decide to move to less exposed jobs or leave their job (healthy worker survival effect). The impact of this phenomenon in population-based studies on WRA has been evaluated recently in some studies using appropriate statistic methods (76).

Information bias

Information biases include recall (memory) and misclassification biases and may concern both exposure and disease (73). We will focus this part on exposure misclassification (the phenomenon is similar for disease misclassification). Two types of exposure misclassification are classically described: nondifferential and differential. A nondifferential bias appears when the likelihood of exposure misclassification is the same whatever the disease status. In case of nondifferential bias, the relative risk ratio is mostly biased toward the null for dichotomous exposure (73, 77). Such bias may induce an underestimate of the burden of OA in case of an underreport of exposures by workers, which may be partly explained by lack of knowledge especially for specific products or ingredients (78). Otherwise, when exposure is evaluated through a multilevel scale, exposure-response trends may be disrupted (77). A differential bias is a major challenge in epidemiology as the association between exposure and disease is biased in an unknown way (73). Some methods used to assess exposure and especially self-report may induce differential misclassification biases (78). Recall bias may be important, especially in case-control surveys, when asthmatics could remember their exposures in a different way than controls (7). The use of more objective tools, as the one suggested recently based on bar codes of the products and an associated ingredients database (79), should reduce differential misclassification. Missing data may also bias the results and this potential bias should be taken into account (7).

Confounding

Confounding is defined by Schwartz et al. (74) as a bias caused by noncomparability arising from "nature" (e.g. exposed and non-exposed groups are not comparable also in the source population due to social structures or health behavior). A confounder is a factor related to both the exposure and the outcome (Figure 3.3) (77). When strong associations between the potential confounder and exposure or disease are recognized, the confounders have much more of an impact on the association between exposure and disease. By contrast to selection bias, confounders could be taken into account either through stratification or appropriate adjusted analyses. Misclassification in the evaluation of confounders may result in an underestimation of the impact of the confounding (77). The most profound effects of misclassification of confounders seem to occur when the exposure is a weak risk factor compared with the confounder. Potential residual confounding may also occur and should be discussed to improve the interpretation of the results, especially in the case of substantial differences between crude and adjusted estimates (77). To evaluate the

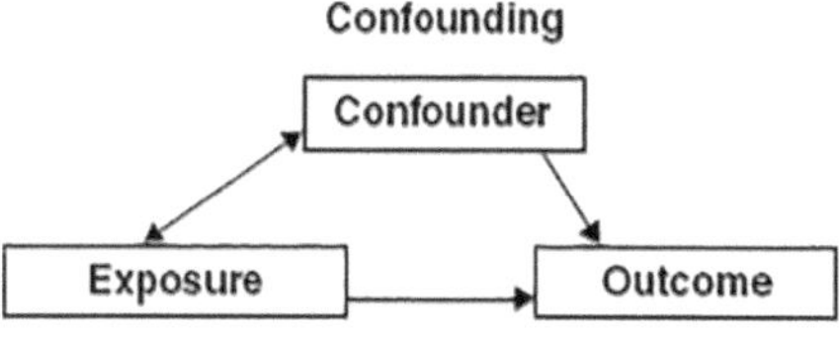

FIGURE 3.3 Illustration of a confounding variable associated both with the exposure of interest and the outcome. (From Reference [7].)

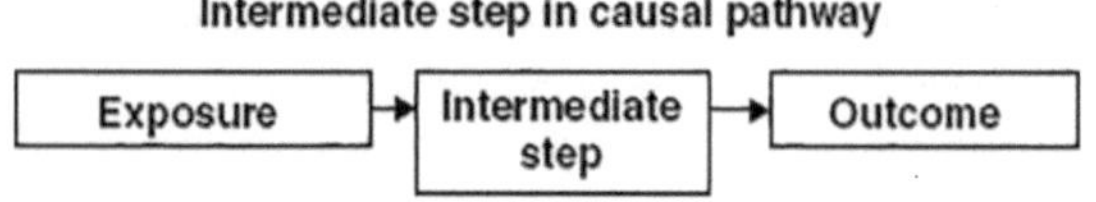

FIGURE 3.4 Illustration of an intermediate step (not a confounder) between exposure and outcome (disease). (From Reference [7].)

potential impact of unmeasured confounding, a sensitivity analysis, based on calculation of the E-value, has been proposed (80). This method is easy to perform and may strengthen the interpretation of the results by evaluating evidence of causation in the face of unmeasured confounders. It has been suggested that the interpretation of the results from epidemiological surveys may suffer more misclassification biases than confounding ones (77).

It is important to note that a risk factor (that is affected by the exposure) that may be an intermediate factor (Figure 3.4) in the causal pathway between exposure and disease should not be treated as a confounder (7, 73).

Effect modification

A modifier is associated with both exposure and disease (like a confounder) but the association between exposure and disease is modified according to this modifier factor status/level (Figure 3.5). In the presence of an effect modification, risk ratio estimates for the association between exposure and disease vary according to the modifier status/level. Therefore, a modifier should not be treated as a confounder (7). Association should be stratified according to the modifier status/level and the presence of an interaction between this factor and exposure should be statistically tested. Estimates of risk ratios should be calculated for each level of the modifier. Atopy, smoking, and asthma treatment (especially anti-inflammatory inhaled corticosteroid treatment) should be considered as potential modifiers in the relation between occupation exposure and asthma (7, 40).

Occurrence (incidence and prevalence) of asthma in the workplace and occupational asthma

Workforce- and apprentice-based studies

The first workforce-based studies were mostly cross-sectional and designed to estimate the *prevalence* of WRA and related endpoints such as work-related lower respiratory symptoms suggestive of asthma, nasal and ocular symptoms, and, where appropriate, specific allergic sensitization to work-related asthmagens. In the 1990s, longitudinal studies were initiated in specific

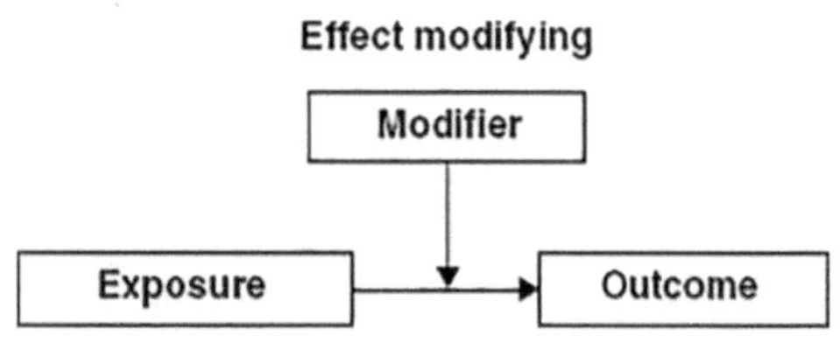

FIGURE 3.5 Illustration of the effect of a modifier (not a confounder) between exposure and outcome (disease). (From Reference [7].)

populations of workers and apprentices to estimate the *incidence* of WRA and associated outcomes. The study of inception cohorts in populations of apprentices enabled detailed description of the *time course* of WRA and related outcomes.

There is a rich literature of workforce-based surveys, some initiated by the identification of workplace case clusters, through physician referral or sentinel programs, and others seeking a priori to examine risk factors associated with particular asthmagenic exposures. Table 3.3 summarizes the findings from selected cross-sectional studies of workplaces between 1971 and 2018, known for their exposure to high- and low-molecular-weight asthmagens. The studies listed estimated the *prevalence* by identifying the number of cases and related them to the number of subjects at risk. The table, while not comprehensive, is illustrative of the type of information available to guide both clinical and public health practice. The studies are listed in decreasing order of prevalence using questionnaire markers of OA. In several studies, the algorithm for clinical case identification (Figure 3.2) was followed and the differences in the rates between the two definitions, the first essentially for epidemiological (public health) purposes and the second for clinical use, are illustrated (55, 81–83).

In Table 3.3, which describes workforces exposed to HMW asthmagens, it is evident that the estimates of prevalence vary considerably, from rates as high as 50% for workers of an Australian plant manufacturing enzyme detergents, when the process was first introduced (84) to as low as 2% in hospital workers exposed to latex (83). While these between-workforce differences are no doubt due in part to methodological issues, such as differences in the questions used in studies to define OA, the intensity of the exposures of the different workforces, and the asthmagenic potential of the agents involved may have also played a role.

Furthermore, Table 3.3 also describes workforces exposed to LMW asthmagens, with estimates of prevalence also varying over a wide range. It is of interest that in all the studies listed in Table 3.3 and for cross-sectional studies, in general, the questionnaire markers of asthma were related to exposure.

Incidence studies

Table 3.4 shows the distribution of the incidence of OA and related outcomes in selected longitudinal (cohort) studies in apprentices and workers with exposure to HMW and LMW agents carried out between 1988 and 2020. The central and long-term outcomes considered in the published cohorts of apprentices were OA, probable OA, and its variants such as work-aggravated respiratory symptoms (97). After a relatively short follow-up of 3 years, cases of OA were confirmed objectively in a Polish cohort study (98). The nearest outcome to OA was a combination of (i) a significant increase in bronchial responsiveness defined as a 3.2-fold (or 2-fold) decrease in PC_{20} in a methacholine challenge test, and (ii) sensitization to training-specific allergens when the causal agent is a HMW allergen (99) or incident WRA-like symptoms in the case of LMW agents when an immunologic mechanism has not been confirmed (99, 100). The term *probable OA* has been used to denote these groupings of outcomes. Work-exacerbated respiratory symptoms were defined as asthma-like symptoms or rhinitis that became worse in the occupational environment in the Danish apprentice bakers study (97), and asthma-like symptoms aggravated by dust or fumes among apprentices in the Canadian province of British Columbia were tested 2 years after baseline (101). The investigators consulted medical records for the apprentices who took part in the 2-year study and determined

TABLE 3.3 Results from Selected Cross-Sectional (Prevalence) Studies of Workers Exposed to Occupational Asthmagens

Exposure/Industry/ Occupation	Number Studied	Exposure Before the Diagnosis (months)	Prevalence of Work-Related Asthma (%): Symptoms[a]/ BCT[b]	References
High-molecular-weight agents				
Enzymes/detergent	98	Intermittent	50	(84)
Guar gum/carpet industry	162	Up to 108	23 (2)[b]	(81)
Snow-crab/food processing	303	Several months	21 (16)	(55)
Laboratory animal workers	238	26	7	(85)
Flour/bakery workers	264	12	6	(82)
Latex/hospital workers	289	120	2 (3)	(83)
Latex/dental health workers	454	120	7	(86)
Fish processing workers	594	84	16	(87)
Spice mill workers	150	36	17	(88)
Poultry farm workers	230	60	23	(89)
Table grape farm workers	207	108	26	(90)
Low-molecular-weight agents				
Platinum refinery	91	12–24	54	(91)
Colophony/electronic plants	924	24	22	(92)
Isocyanates/secondary industry	51	54	20 (11.8)	(93)
Spiramycin/pharmaceutical	51	n/a	9 (8)	(56)
Plicatic acid/forestry workers	652	n/a	4	(94)
Cleaning chemicals/professional medical center cleaners	142	72	59	(95)
Cleaning chemicals/health professionals	3650	n/a	3	(96)

Source: Reproduced and updated from Reference (7).

[a] Based on work-related symptoms.

[b] Occupational asthma confirmed by bronchial challenge testing.

Abbreviations: BC, British Columbia; n/a, not available.

a new annual asthma incidence rate of 3.6 per 1000 in this group of machining, electrician, insulator and construction painting apprentices. Other endpoints related to OA have also been evaluated and include occupational rhinitis, confirmed through nasal specific inhalation tests as performed in symptomatic persons in the Polish cohort (98) and probable occupational rhinitis defined as the incidence of both specific sensitization to an occupational allergen and work-related symptoms of rhinitis (102). Occupational rhinitis was confirmed in 12.5% of Polish apprentice bakers, a slightly higher proportion than for OA in the same population (98); the incidence of probable occupational rhinitis among Canadian pastry-making apprentices was low (1.3 per 100 per year (PY)) compared to the incidence of work-related symptoms of rhinoconjunctivitis without specific sensitization to flour (13.1 per 100 PY) (103).

It is interesting to note in Table 3.4 that after a rather short follow-up of apprentices of 4 years or less, the incidence of endpoints suggestive of WRA reached 6.1 per 100 PY. The time course of symptoms suggestive of WRA and other associated relevant outcomes has been described through repeated assessments in apprentice studies (98, 99). The rate of incident work-related rhinoconjunctivitis symptoms and sensitization to training-specific allergens assessed among apprentice animal-health technicians was over 10% after 1 year of training and remained high after 2 and 3 years; however, the rate of new work-related chest symptoms was highest only after 2 and 3 years (99). Similarly, the incidence of respiratory symptoms to bakers' allergens was higher in the second year of training; the incidence of skin reactivity to these allergens also increased from 4.6% to 8.2% between the first and second year in training (98). Almost one-third (31.5%)

of apprentices in British Columbia without symptoms at baseline reported asthma-like symptoms aggravated by dust or fumes when tested 2 years later (101). Differences in the time course of occurrence of these outcomes are difficult to interpret. Nevertheless, the implications for setting the timing of surveillance programs are the same and would be to screen for sensitization and symptoms in the first 2–3 years of apprenticeship.

The long-term follow-up of the Canadian inception cohort of apprentices exposed to HMW agents, 8 years after ending their training, was the first long-term study of such population of apprentices after entering a workforce (104). It has revealed that the incidence values of work-related skin sensitization, rhinoconjunctivitis symptoms, chest symptoms, and bronchial hyperresponsiveness (BHR) were 1.3, 1.7, 0.7, and 2.0 per 100 PY, respectively, in individuals who at any time during the follow-up held a job related to their training (78%). These incidence figures were lower compared to those found during the apprenticeship for the same endpoints, that is, 7.3, 12.9, 1.7, and 5.8 per 100 PY, respectively. It can be hypothesized that the most vulnerable individuals acquired these features early after starting exposure to specific sensitizers. Of interest, high proportions of apprentices who developed these outcomes during training were in remission at the follow-up assessment even if they were still working in the same field; and more so in participants with a work history not related to their apprenticeship. In this cohort, 30 incident cases of probable OA (2.7 per 100 PY) had been identified during apprenticeship. Among these, 23 of 277 (8.3%) were identified at the 8-year follow-up and six incident cases among the 201 (3%) were identified at the follow-up assessment of individuals still working in the same type of work (104).

TABLE 3.4 Results from Selected Longitudinal (Incidence) Studies of Workers Exposed to Occupational Asthmagens

Exposure/Occupation/Apprenticeship	Number	Duration of Follow-Up (years)	Endpoint for WRA	Incidence of WRA Endpoint (% or rate)	References
Occupational asthma					
Flour/apprentice bakers	287	2	Confirmed OA by inhalation tests	8.7%	(98)
Apprentice animal health technicians	417	Up to 4	SPT+ to specific training-related allergen and BHR	2.7/100 PY	(69)
Apprentice dental hygienists	122	Up to 2.5	SPT+ to latex and BHR	1.8/100 PY	(110)
Metalworking fluids/apprentice machinists	95	2	WRA-like symptoms and BHR	7%	(111)
Diisocyanates/apprentice car painters	385	1.5	WRA-like symptoms and BHR	6.1/100 PY	(112)
Apprentice welders	286	1.25	WRA-like symptoms and BHR	3%	(100)
Nurses; self-reported use of disinfectants to clean surfaces or medical instruments; JTEM for specific disinfecting/cleaning agents	61,539 (277,744 PY)	Up to 6	Self-reported incident physician-diagnosed asthma	0.13/100 PY; asthma not associated with self-reported or JTEM exposures	(109)
Work-aggravated symptoms					
Baking allergens/apprentice bakers	187	2	Asthma-like symptoms aggravated at work	10%	(97)
Machining, electrician, insulator, and construction painting apprentices	197[a]	2	Onset of asthma-like symptoms aggravated by dust or fumes during 2 years after baseline	31.5%	(101)
Asthma-like symptoms					
Flour/bakers and millers	300	Up to 7	Symptoms suggestive of asthma/physician's diagnosis of asthma/ hospitalized for asthma	12%	(107)
Sensitizing materials with irritant exposure/apprentice hairdressers	297	Up to 3	Wheezing, change in FEV_1 (predicted)	10%	(113)
Flour/apprentice bakers	125	2.5	Work-related respiratory symptoms	9% (cumulative incidence)	(114)
Bakery and flour mill workers	300	3	Work-related respiratory symptoms	4.1/100 PY	(108)

Source: Reproduced and updated from Reference (7).

Abbreviations: BHR, bronchial hyperresponsiveness; FEV_1, forced expiratory volume in 1 second; JTEM, job-task-exposure matrix; PY, person-years; SPT, skin-prick test; WRA, work-related asthma.

[a] The 197 apprentices had no symptoms at baseline.

Cohort studies of the incidence of laboratory animal allergy (LAA) have been carried out in groups of workers (105). In the Netherlands, a retrospective cohort study of laboratory animal workers used pre-employment screening data to assess the incidence of LAA symptoms in "naïve" individuals at the time they were accepted for a job in a research institute; it showed that the risk of developing LAA was still present after 3 years or more of exposure (106).

Adjusted estimates of incidence of work-related respiratory symptoms among other cohorts of workers ranged from 12% in a 2004 UK study of 300 bakers and millers (107) to 4.1 per 100 PY in a 2001 UK study of 300 new employees in three large, modern bakeries, two flour mills, and a flour packing station (108).

A large longitudinal cohort study of late career nurses in the United States provided the opportunity to examine the association of incident physician-diagnosed asthma with self-reported cleaning and disinfecting activities and exposures to specific products related to these activities as assigned by a job-task-exposure matrix (109) (Table 3.4). Incident asthma (370 cases) during 6 years of follow-up was not significantly associated with any of the occupational exposure metrics.

Community-based studies

Workplace exposures are still important contributors to the burden of asthma and are an important cause of disability around the world (115, 116). The number of recognized asthmagens (>500 currently) (117) has increased fourfold in the past three decades (118, 119). However, most recognized occupational asthma cases were induced by exposure to a small number of agents, both

HMW (flour, animals) and LMW agents (diisocyanates, alde-hydes). Whereas OA induced by "older" well-known asthmagens (such as latex) has decreased, an increasing impact of cleaning products/disinfectants on WRA has been observed (46, 119). Around 1 out of 6 adult-onset asthma cases are attributable to occupational exposures (46). Several studies have shown an increase in both the prevalence and incidence of OA over the past few decades (120). The reported annual incidence of OA ranged from 13 to 178 new cases per million workers and strongly varied according to industries (121). In addition, occupational exposure to asthmagens has been associated with more severe or uncon-trolled asthma (40, 117, 122). Two physiopathology mechanisms have been proposed for OA: immunological asthma (with a latency period) and nonimmunological asthma (without latency period), classically induced by a single exposure to a high level of irritants (but the mechanism is unknown) (121, 123). Recent epi-demiological surveys suggest that exposures to irritants (which are also LMW agents) at a low-to-moderate level may also induce asthma, with unknown underlying mechanisms (124).

Occupational exposure to cleaning products has been recently recognized as an important asthma risk factor that may induce or exacerbate asthma (46, 125, 126). However, out of nearly 30 pub-lished epidemiological studies on the impact of cleaning products/tasks in WRA, few of them have studied new-onset asthma (109, 127). An increased risk of incident asthma was observed in one sur-vey for some categories of workers (in healthcare, cleaners) and for workers occupationally exposed to cleaning products (127). Specific involved products are not well known, partly due to the lack of accu-rate evaluation of exposure in epidemiological surveys (46).

General and specific registries

Table 3.5 provides a summary of some reported occurrence rates for OA based on surveillance schemes and national or workers' compensation board (WCB) registries. Surveillance schemes have benefited from high participation of medical physicians but many no longer exist, except in the United Kingdom (SWORD) (128). Figures of frequency from WCB represent the tip of the iceberg, being affected by biases such as workers not following claims because compensation is insufficient or they fear losing jobs, and diagnostic criteria more or less stringent to accept claims. Contrary to results in community-based studies, there is a general consensus on a declining frequency of OA worldwide (129).

Risk factors and markers or modifiers

Occupational exposure

Exposure assessment methods

In community-based epidemiological surveys, to assure unbi-ased results, it is crucial to record complete occupational his-tories including exposure windows linked to asthma onset (46, 75). Most common methods used to assess exposures are self-reports, expert assessments, or job-exposure matrices. The lack of accurate methods to evaluate exposure to specific agents, such as cleaning/disinfecting products, is an important limitation in epidemiological surveys. In most studies, assessment of expo-sure to specific cleaning products or disinfectants at workplaces is mostly based on standardized questionnaires, which may be prone to bias. Occupational exposure assessed through a job-exposure matrix (JEM) is less prone to differential misclassifica-tion bias than self-report. Few studies on WRA have evaluated occupational exposures to specific agents through case-by-case expertise or job-task-exposure matrices (130).

Recent findings from epidemiological surveys

For a better understanding of the underlying mechanisms in OA and to identify specific chemicals involved, a key challenge would be to improve assessment methods, especially to evaluate specific chemical compounds. JEMs are tools easy to apply and frequently used especially in large epidemiological cohorts. A new occupational asthma-specific JEM (OAsJEM, http://oasjem. vjf.inserm.fr/) (131), an update of the previous asthma-specific JEM (132), was recently developed to evaluate exposure to 30 spe-cific known or suspected asthmagens (seven large groups, includ-ing sensitizers and irritants). However, a JEM does not take into account the variability of exposure between workers within the same occupation, whereas exposure may be heterogeneous for a given occupation depending on the tasks performed. To reduce exposure misclassification biases, the tasks may be taken into account through a job-task-exposure matrix (JTEM). Recently, a JTEM has been proposed to evaluate occupational exposures to disinfectants and cleaning products among US nurses (130).

Compounds of products such as cleaning/disinfecting agents may evolve rapidly. These agents are complex mixture of vari-ous ingredients, partly available on various detergent companies' websites, but often unknown by participants. More accurate exposure assessment methods such as smartphone applications with sensors (e.g. bar code reader) are increasingly used in epi-demiology. A new tool, based on a smartphone application that allows scanning barcodes and a corresponding products' data-base, has been developed to evaluate occupational exposure to cleaning/disinfecting agents among hospital workers (79). The development of such easy-to-use and unbiased tools may improve occupational assessment. In addition, Carder et al. recently pro-posed a "quantitative structure activity relationship" (QSAR) to predict respiratory sensitizing potentials for LMW compounds of cleaning agents (126). They classified compounds of disinfec-tants and cleaning products in 12 categories based on taxonomy of cause.

Host-associated factors

In this section, we will describe host susceptibility factors such as genetic factors, atopy, immunological sensitization to specific ubiquitous allergens, rhinitis, bronchial responsiveness, and psy-chological and socioeconomic factors that may increase the risk of WRA in individuals exposed at work to etiologic agents (6).

Genetic

Important advances have been made to understand the role of genetics as part of the multifactorial pathogenesis of OA. One main focus of research is to determine how environmental and/or occupational factors interact with genes and how this influences disease susceptibility (133, 134). Studies on genetic factors in OA have disclosed significant associations between specific agents and genetic markers (135). This is the case for Western red cedar asthma; asthma due to acid anhydrides, platinum salts and latex; and laboratory animal proteins and their association with HLA class II molecules. Associations between confirmed diisocyanate asthma, and some HLA class II alleles as well as single nucleo-tide polymorphisms (SNPs) of antioxidant enzymes have been shown (136, 137) as well as genetic variants in TNF alpha, TGFB1, PTGS1, and PTGS2 (138) and genetic variants of gene regulatory effects (139). Other studies in populations of workers exposed to hexamethylene diisocyanate (HDI) with either a confirmed diagnosis of HDI asthma or without have shown an association

TABLE 3.5 Incidence of Occupational or Work-Aggravated Asthma in Different Countries According to Surveillance Schemes and Registries

Source	Country	Time Period	No. of Cases	Trend over Time	Annual Incidence Rate per 1,000,000 Employed	Top Causal Exposure	Reference or Source
Surveillance scheme							
Surveillance of	UK	2015–2017	1215 total	—	—	Flour	*1. Zhou, 2019*
work-related and occupational respiratory disease (SWORD)[a]	UK	1999–2017	2630 total	Increasing 2014–2017	—	Diisocyanates	*2. Seed, 2019*
West Midlands Midland Thoracic Society voluntary surveillance scheme (SHIELD)	UK	1991–2011	135 to 34 annually	Declining	58 to 14	Diisocyanates	*3. Walter, 2015*
Physician reporting and compensation programs							
Réseau national de vigilance et de prevention des pathologies Professionnelles (RNV3P)	France	2001–2009	502–242	Declining	—	Flour Diisocyanates Hairdressing	*4. Paris, 2012*
Belgium WCB	Belgium	1993–2002	971 accepted claims	Declining	—	Flour Diisocyanates	*5. Vandenplas, 2011*
Ontario WSIB	Ontario, Canada	2003–2007	971 accepted claims	Declining overall, but increasing for WAA	—	Flour Diisocyanates	*6. Ribeiro, 2014*
Québec CNESST (WCB)	Québec, Canada	1987–2015	97–43	Declining	—	Diisocyanates Flour Seafood	Québec CNESST WCB
Finnish Institute of Occupational Health (FIOH)	Finland	2005–2015	—	—	0.52–0.31	Indoor mold Flour and grain Bovine	Dr. Hille Suojalehto, FIOH
Tunisia National Medical Care Fund (CNAM)	Tunisia	2000–2008	361 cases	—	24.4, average	Textile industry	*7. Maoua, 2016*
Worldwide trends	Claims	2001–2010	—	Declining 1.7% to 7.7% annually[b]	—	—	*8. Stocks, 2016*

Source: Reproduced from Reference (7) and updated with legend references:
1. Zhou AY, et al. *Occup Med (Lond). 2019;70(1):52-59.* **2.** Seed M, et al. *Occup Env Med. 2019;76:396-7.* **3.** Walters G, et al. *Occup Environ Med. 2015;72:304-10.* **4.** Paris C, et al. *Occup Environ Med. 2012;69:391-7.* **5.** Vandenplas O, et al. *Respir Med. 2011;105:1364-72.* **6.** Ribeiro M, et al. *J Occup Environ Med. 2014;56(9):1001-7* **7.** Maoua M, et al. *Occup Diseases and Env Med. 2016;4:27-36.* **8.** Stocks SJ, et al. *Curr Opin Allergy Clin Immunol. 2016;16:113-9.*

Abbreviations: WCB, workers' compensation board; WSIB, Workplace Safety and Insurance Board.

[a] Derived from UK Health and Occupation Research (THOR) network.

[b] Rate of decline varies by country.

between genotype combinations associated with TH2 and innate immunity, and HDI-induced asthma (140). Most studies on genetics of OA have not been replicated. It has been suggested that this difficulty may be due to the lack of consideration of the interaction between environmental and occupational exposures on one hand, and genetic markers on the other (Chapter 4).

Gender

Some studies have suggested that the incidence of OA is higher in men; for example, in the United Kingdom, for the period between 1992 and 2001 (141). In contrast a longitudinal population-based study of all employed Finns without preexisting asthma, aged between 25 and 59 years, followed between 1986 and 1998 showed that the number of incident cases of confirmed OA was almost identical for men and women (142). Studies of some specific workforces, for example Canadian snow crab processors, found that the risk of probable OA was significantly greater in women; of note, in that industry, women were overrepresented in job categories associated with high levels of measured snow crab aeroallergens that may explain this difference (12, 143). A 2020 European Academy of Allergy Asthma and Clinical Immunology Taskforce report concluded that "differing rates of work-related asthma as well as the risk of respiratory work disability and job change are more likely related to specific occupational exposures than to gender-specific reaction patterns" (144).

Obesity and diet

There is little information as to the role of diet and obesity in WRA separate from the role of these in general asthma (6). A nested case-control study (145) was performed among bakers, pastry-makers, and hairdressers. Among bakers and pastry makers, only atopy was a significant independent predictive factor for development of OA, but among hairdressers, body mass index (BMI) was a significant predictive factor for OA, and intake of vitamin A and vitamin D were significantly higher in hairdressing cases after adjustment for BMI and obesity. In contrast, a cross-sectional study of patients with OA (146) found a reduced vitamin D intake especially in the milder asthmatics and a relationship between BMI and irritant OA.

Atopy and sensitization to specific allergens

In epidemiological studies, atopy is defined as at least one (or two) positive skin-test reaction or specific IgE to common allergens, or a history of atopic diathesis (e.g. personal asthma, allergic rhinitis, or eczema). Atopy is common in the general population: as defined as one or more positive skin tests it has been reported in 32% of young Danish adults (males 43%, females 23% p<0.001) (147). Atopy has been consistently shown to be associated with sensitization to HMW agents. However, the positive predictive value of atopy for OA is low and variable according to the etiologic agent. In laboratory animal workers it was 33%, which was very similar to the general population at the time (148). Atopy was only marginally associated with the development of probable OA in laboratory animals in a prospective study (85) but among bakers/pastry makers atopy was a strong risk factor. In the case of LMW agents, the relation between atopy, specific sensitization, and OA is still controversial, for example, in workers exposed to acid anhydrides or platinum salts (149). Among young bakers and pastry makers, atopy was a strong risk factor for incidence of OA but among bakers/pastry makers and also hairdressers, atopy did not affect the timing of onset of OA (150). On the whole, these findings do not justify routine screening for atopy among workers in high-risk workplaces. Atopic individuals should be advised of this potential risk in advance and regular follow-up examinations for early detection of sensitization and development of NSBH (i.e., surveillance for case identification) should be carried out.

Sensitization to specific ubiquitous allergens

Interestingly, pre-exposure sensitization to specific common allergens increases the risk of developing probable OA when there is cross-reactivity with specific occupational allergens. This was shown for sensitization to pets and the risk of probable OA in apprentices exposed to laboratory rats (69). Other examples come from the pastry making and bakery trades (103). In an experimental study, Merget et al. (151) showed that subjects with a pronounced sensitization to grass or tree pollen but without prior occupational exposure to flour could demonstrate specific sensitization and a positive asthmatic reaction after flour inhalation. More studies are needed, with a prospective design, to assess the predictive value of sensitization to specific common allergens likely to demonstrate cross-reactivity with workplace allergens.

Rhinitis

Subjects seen in the clinic for suspected OA frequently also report symptoms of rhinitis. The occurrence of these symptoms is greater for OA due to HMW versus LMW agents (72% versus 52 p<0.001, in a French study) and was more likely to precede OA due to HMW agents (152, 153). In a series of 43 workers with work-related respiratory symptoms assessed concomitantly by bronchial- and nasal-specific inhalation challenge, a significant association was demonstrated between nasal and bronchial responses (RR = 1.7, 95% CI 1.0–2.4) (154). Interestingly, the prevalence of symptoms of rhinitis at work in individuals with a diagnosis of work-exacerbated asthma (83%) was roughly the same as in those with OA (90%) (155).

Prospective epidemiological studies performed in cohorts of apprentices exposed to HMW agents have revealed that symptoms of rhinitis often occurred earlier than respiratory symptoms suggestive of WRA (99) and were associated with long-term development of bronchial hyperresponsiveness (104). However, this time course of symptoms occurrence known as the "allergic march" was not observed in a Polish prospective study where nasal symptoms more often developed at the same time as lower respiratory symptoms among apprentice bakers who developed OA, which was confirmed by specific inhalation challenge (98).

A large Finnish study using data from the Finnish Registry for Occupational Diseases and the Medication Reimbursement Register–Social Insurance Institution of Finland, has demonstrated a high risk for asthma (RR = 4.8; 95% CI, 4.35.4) in workers with a diagnosis of occupational rhinitis. Among the 420 cases of asthma identified, 156 were confirmed cases of OA, and the incidence of asthma was markedly increased in the year after occupational rhinitis was reported (156). While several studies indicate that symptoms of rhinitis or occupational rhinitis increase the risk of OA, it should be noted that the impact is modest; indeed, in the Finnish study only 4.3% of workers with occupational rhinitis developed OA within a follow-up period of 7.7 years on average (156); in the Canadian study of apprentices in animal health technology, the predictive value of work-related nasal symptoms for probable OA was only 11.4% (99).

A systematic review concluded that limited data do support the development of occupational rhinitis preceding OA especially related to HMW agents (157). As outlined in a position paper by the International Task Force on Occupational Rhinitis, occupational rhinitis diagnosed according to the recommended guidelines should be considered as an early marker for OA (158).

Bronchial hyperresponsiveness

Prospective cohort studies of apprentices at risk of OA showed that nonspecific bronchial hyperresponsiveness evaluated when starting exposure to HMW allergens was strongly associated with the incidence of work-related respiratory symptoms in the short term and with a significant increase in bronchial hyperresponsiveness 8 years later (104).

Socioeconomic factors, environment, and lifestyle

Socioeconomic status (SES), environmental, and lifestyle conditions may play an important role in asthma (6). Interrelationships between these various factors and activity of asthma disease are complex. SES is associated with various well-known asthma risk factors such as occupation and some lifestyle factors (smoking, BMI, diet) (159). In addition, poor adherence to asthma treatment seems associated with lower income and lower educational level (160). Galobardes et al. suggested that understanding the socioeconomic patterns of asthma phenotypes may help distinguish which exposures are preventable (161). In most studies, SES is often evaluated only in terms of educational level or job category estimates (162). Such evaluation of SES is difficult to take into account when studying associations between occupational exposures and asthma.

Some studies suggested that low SES plays a role in adult-onset asthma, but this topic is still a matter of debate (163). Regarding asthma control, lower SES was associated with more symptomatic/severe asthma or poorly controlled asthma (164). A recent survey suggested a deleterious impact of both low education level and low deprivation indices on asthma control (164). Various deprivation indices are now available and might be proposed in WRA epidemiological research to take into account SES (159, 165).

Others: Smoking and exposure to pollutants

Not only smoking, but also the occupational environment, contributes a substantial burden to chronic obstructive lung diseases (166, 167). The total pollutant burden of dusts, dusts previously considered as nuisance dusts, fumes, gases, and vapors even at quite low levels (168), diesel and ozone (169), weather and temperature conditions in the general and occupational environments as well as damp and moldy workplaces (170) have also been examined with regard to their role in determining the outcome of airway function and adult-onset asthma in the general population.

The effect of smoking on OA appears to be dependent on the type of occupational agent. When the agent induces asthma by producing specific IgE antibodies, cigarette smoking may enhance sensitization. Venables et al. (171) found an interaction between smoking and atopy in workers exposed to laboratory animals and platinum salts (91); atopic smokers had the highest and the nonatopic nonsmokers the lowest prevalence of sensitization. Among platinum refinery workers, smoking, not atopy, is the most important determinant for sensitization (172). Smoking was found to be a significant determinant of OA and probable OA among snow crab processors (12, 55). Cigarette smoking, however, was not associated with increased work-related asthmatic symptoms in workers exposed to detergent enzymes (84). It appeared that when the agent induces asthma independent of IgE antibodies, nonsmokers may be more frequently affected than smokers as in diisocyanate-induced asthma (173), colophony (92), and red cedar asthma (174). In an exhaustive review of the relationship between smoking and OA, occupational rhinitis, or occupational sensitization covering a wide range of occupational agents and occupations, Siracusa et al. (175) highlighted the controversies and uncertainties still existing on the role of smoking on the development of OA, while they showed there was some evidence that smokers are at increased risk of occupational sensitization in occupations with exposures to both HMW and LMW agents.

Microbial exposures in the farm environment in children and adults are protective against atopy, allergic rhinitis, and atopic asthma (176). In adults, paradoxically, this effect has been found in conjunction with an increase in nonatopic asthma (177). In a large study of farmers and agricultural industry workers, in which objective health and endotoxin measurements were made, it was shown that high endotoxin exposure was a risk factor for BHR and wheeze characterized mostly by a nonatopic phenotype, and also that endotoxin exposure was associated with a reduced risk for atopy and specific IgE to grass pollen (178).

Occupational asthma as a model to study the natural history of asthma

As presented in Chapter 2, OA offers a unique opportunity to get information on the natural history of asthma, the principal reason being the existence of a well-defined population at risk that can be followed prospectively with a preexposure assessment, an assessment at the time of sensitization, symptoms, and disease, and, finally, serial assessments after cessation of exposure, as illustrated in Figure 2.4 of Chapter 2.

This therefore provides an entirely experimental situation, which is not possible in the case of environmental asthma for which it is impossible to assess individuals' pre- and post-end of exposure. Because there is no difference between occupational HMW allergens and common inhalant allergens in inducing host response, studies of the natural history of OA due to HMW allergens will likely reflect the origin and progression of non-occupational allergic asthma.

The use of an entirely prospective model has been particularly fruitful in examining apprentices before they enter a training program (98, 179). This provides a useful insight on the timing of events that play a role in the "allergic march" from the onset of sensitization to rhinoconjunctivitis symptoms, the onset of lower airway inflammation, and asthma (98).

Studies of the natural history of OA due to LMW compounds and/or irritant-induced asthma will be useful in our understanding of adult-onset or intrinsic asthma. The example of irritant-induced asthma is particularly relevant as it demonstrates that an acute or multiple recurrent insults to the bronchi can lead to asthma that has been labeled intrinsic due to the lack of knowledge on the initiating event. It is therefore possible that many cases of so-called intrinsic asthma are due to initial exposure to irritants.

Conclusion

Information about the epidemiology (distribution and determinants) of asthma associated with occupational exposures is used for several purposes (180, 181). These include:

1. Establishing prevalence and/or incidence data for public health purposes and as a guide to the need for preventive services and/or surveillance of industries at risk.
2. Addressing etiologic questions relating to exposures and host risk factors.
3. Establishing exposure-response relationships to provide the scientific basis for setting threshold exposure limits.
4. Evaluating preventive services or control measures.

Although none of this information can be furnished by clinical case studies, they all inform the various steps in the clinical evaluation of a case of OA, namely establishing the diagnosis, understanding prognosis, planning and evaluating management approaches, and taking appropriate steps in notification of OA cases.

In the application of epidemiology to the study of OA, the importance of selecting the design most appropriate for answering the particular study question cannot be overemphasized. Equally important is to identify the appropriate definition of the study outcome (usually asthma or some surrogate of asthma), and of careful selection of the study population to minimize underestimation of the exposure-response effect due to selection bias due to the "healthy worker" effect, whether due to "healthy hire" or "survivor" effects. These studies provide information on the host and environmental determinants of OA, including specific exposure factors and, in some studies, exposure-response relationships. This represents an important step toward appreciation of the potential of environmental measurements for evaluating workplace exposures and practices as well as the effectiveness of environmental control measures (181).

Research needs

The important questions to be addressed by research should include the following:

- What is the best estimate of the PAF of WRA as a whole and its two entities, WEA and OA?
- What is the prevalence and incidence of irritant-induced asthma?
- What is the value of FeNO in the surveillance of workers at risk of developing OA and is it the same for HMW versus LMW agents?
- What are the host markers and genetic susceptibility factors for WRA, OA, and occupational rhinitis (OR), related to different types of exposure and in populations of diverse origins?
- What are the permissible exposure limits for common agents responsible for occupational sensitization, OA, and OR?
- What are the interactions between host susceptibility factors and environmental exposure?
- What are the most effective interventions for OA due to common agents?

Acknowledgments

This chapter was developed from an earlier edition of this book, written by Maritta S. Jaakkola, Denyse Gautrin, and Jean-Luc Malo—to whom we are indebted.

References

1. Last JM. A Dictionary of Epidemiology, 3rd edn. New York: Oxford University Press, 1995: 1–180.
2. Becklake MR, Ernst P. Environmental factors. Lancet 1997; 350: 10–13.
3. De Matteis S, Heederik D, Burdorf A, et al. Current and new challenges in occupational lung diseases. Eur Respir Rev 2017; 26(146): 170080.
4. Platts-Mills TAE, Carter MC. Asthma and indoor exposure to allergens. N Engl J Med 1997; 336: 1382–4.
5. Seaton A, Godden DJ, Brown K. Increase in asthma: a more toxic environment or a more susceptible population? Thorax 1994; 49: 171–4.
6. Jeebhay MF, Ngajilo D, Le Moual N. Risk factors for non-work-related adult-onset asthma and occupational asthma – A comparative review. Curr Opin Allergy Clin Immunol 2014; 14(2): 84–94.
7. Jaakkola MS, Gautrin D, Malo JL. Disease occurrence and risk factors. In: Malo JL, C-YM, Bernstein DI, eds. Asthma in the workplace, 4th edn. Boca Raton, FL: CRC Press, 2013: 18–39.
8. Jaakkola MS, Jaakkola JJK. Assessment of public health impact of work-related asthma. BMC Med Res Methodol 2012; 12: 22.
9. Gautrin D, Malo JL. Asthma in apprentice workers. The birth cohort parallel: using apprentices as a powerful cohort design for studying occupational asthma. In: Sigsgaard T, Heederik D, eds. Occupational Asthma, 1st edn. Basel: Birkhäuser Basel/Springer Basel AG, 2010: 229–48.
10. Moscato G, Pala G, Boillat MA, et al. EAACI Position Paper: prevention of work-related respiratory allergies among pre-apprentices or apprentices and young workers. Allergy 2011; 66: 1164–73.
11. Monso E, Malo JL, Infante-Rivard C, et al. Individual characteristics and quitting in apprentices exposed to high-molecular-weight agents. Am J Respir Crit Care Med 2000; 161: 1508–12.
12. Gautrin D, Cartier A, Howse D, et al. Occupational asthma and allergy in snow crab processing in Newfoundland and Labrador. Occup Environ Med 2010; 67: 17–23.
13. Tarlo SM, Easty A, Eubanks K, et al. Outcomes of a natural rubber latex control program in an Ontario teaching hospital. J Allergy Clin Immunol 2001; 108: 628–33.
14. Al Badri F, Baatjies R, Jeebhay MF. Assessing the health impact of interventions for baker's allergy and asthma in supermarket bakeries: a group randomised trial. Int Arch Occup Environ Health 2020; 93: 589–99.
15. Brant A, Upchurch S, van Tongeren M, et al. Detergent protease exposure and respiratory disease: case-referent analysis of a retrospective cohort. Occup Environ Med 2009; 66: 754–8.
16. Baatjies R, Lopata AL, Sander I, et al. Determinants of asthma phenotypes among supermarket bakery workers. Eur Respir J 2009; 34(4): 825–33.
17. Demir A, Joseph L, Becklake MR. Work-related asthma in Montreal, Quebec: population attributable risk in a community-based study. Can Respir J 2008; 15(8): 406–12.
18. Talini D, Ciberti A, Bartoli D, et al. Work-related asthma in a sample of subjects with established asthma. Respir Med 2017; 130: 85–91.
19. Matte TD, Hoffman RE, Rosenman KD, Stanbury M. Surveillance of occupational asthma under the SENSOR model. Chest 1990; 98: 173S–8S.
20. Meredith SK, Taylor VM, McDonald JC. Occupational respiratory disease in the United Kingdom 1989: a report to the British Thoracic Society and the Society of Occupational Medicine by the SWORD project group. Br J Ind Med 1991; 48: 292–8.
21. Provencher S, Labrèche FP, De Guire L. Physician based surveillance system for occupational respiratory diseases: the experience of PROPULSE, Québec, Canada. Occup Environ Med 1997; 54: 272–6.
22. Contreras GR, Rousseau R, Chan-Yeung M. Occupational respiratory diseases in British Columbia, Canada in 1991. Occup Environ Med 1994; 51: 710–12.
23. Ameille J, Pauli G, Calastreng-Crinquand A, et al. Reported incidence of occupational asthma in France, 1996–99: the ONAP programme. Occup Environ Med 2003; 60: 136–42.
24. Hnizdo E, Esterhuizen TM, Rees D, Lalloo UG. Occupational asthma as identified by the Surveillance of Work-related and Occupational Respiratory Diseases programme in South Africa. Clin Exp Allergy 2001; 31: 32–9.
25. Elder D, Abranson M, Fish D, et al. Surveillance of Australian workplace based respiratory events (SABRE): notifications for the first 3.5 years and validation of occupational asthma cases. Occup Med 2004; 54: 395–9.
26. Karjalainen A, Kurppa K, Virtanen S, et al. Incidence of occupational asthma by occupation and industry in Finland. Am J Ind Med 2000; 37: 451–8.
27. Keskinen H, Alanko K, Saarinen L. Occupational asthma in Finland. Clin Allergy 1978; 8: 569–79.
28. Meredith S, Nordman H. Occupational asthma: measures of frequency from four countries. Thorax 1996; 51: 435–40.
29. Jaakkola MS, Nordman H, Piipari R, et al. Indoor dampness and molds and development of adult-onset asthma: a population-based incident case-control study. Env Health Perspect 2002; 110: 543–7.
30. Piipari R, Keskinen H. Agents causing occupational asthma in Finland in 1986–2002: cow epithelium bypassed by moulds from moisture-damaged buildings. Clin Exp Allergy 2005; 35: 1632–7.
31. Oksa P. Occupational asthma in Finland according to the Finnish register of work-related diseases (ammattiastmat suomessa rekisteritietojen valossa. in Finnish). Duodecim 2011; 127: 2225–30.
32. Oksa P, Sauni R, Talola N, et al. Trends in occupational diseases in Finland, 1975–2013: a register study. BMJ Open 2019; 9: e024040. doi:10.1136/bmjopen-2018-024040.
33. Ribeiro M, Buyantseva LV, Liss GM, et al. Impact of a cleaners' strike on compensation claims for asthma among teachers in Ontario. Can Respir J 2013; 20(3): 171–74.

34. Ribeiro M, Tarlo SM, Czyrka A, et al. Diisocyanate and non-diisocyanate sensitizer-induced occupational asthma frequency during 2003 to 2007 in Ontario. Canada. JOEM 2014; 56(9): 1001–1007.

35. Karjalainen A, Kurppa K, Martikainen R, et al. Work is related to a substantial portion of adult-onset asthma incidence in the Finnish population. Am J Respir Crit Care Med 2001; 164: 565–8.

36. Henneberger PK, Redlich CA, Callahan DB, et al. An official American Thoracic Society Statement: work-exacerbated asthma. Am J Respir Crit Care Med 2011; 184(3): 368–78.

37. Pekkanen J, Sunyer J, Anto JM, Burney P, et al. Operational definitions of asthma in studies on its aetiology. European Community Respiratory Health Study. Eur Respir J 2005 Jul; 26(1): 28–35.

38. Siroux V, Boudier A, Bousquet J, et al. Asthma control assessed in the EGEA epidemiological survey and health-related quality of life. Respir Med 2012; 106(6): 820–8.

39. Sunyer J, Pekkanen J, Garcia-Esteban R, et al. Asthma score: predictive ability and risk factors. Allergy 2007; 62(2): 142–8.

40. Le Moual N, Carsin AE, Siroux V, et al. Occupational exposures and uncontrolled adult-onset asthma in the ECRHS II. Eur Respir J 2014; 43(2): 374–86.

41. Nathan RA, Sorkness CA, Kosinski M, et al. Development of the asthma control test: a survey for assessing asthma control. J Allergy Clin Immunol 2004; 113(1): 59–65.

42. Schatz M, Sorkness CA, Li JT, et al. Asthma Control Test: reliability, validity, and responsiveness in patients not previously followed by asthma specialists. J Allergy Clin Immunol 2006; 117(3): 549–56.

43. Thomas M, Kay S, Pike J, et al. The Asthma Control Test (ACT) as a predictor of GINA guideline-defined asthma control: analysis of a multinational cross-sectional survey. Prim Care Respir J 2009; 18(1): 41–9.

44. Pralong JA, Moullec G, Suarthana E, et al. Screening for occupational asthma by using a self-administered questionnaire in a clinical setting. J Occup Environ Med. 2013; 55(5): 527–31.

45. Mevel H, Demange V, Penven E, et al. Assessment of work-related asthma prevalence, control and severity: protocol of a field study. BMC Public Health 2016; 16(1): 1164.

46. Dao A, Bernstein DI. Occupational exposure and asthma. Ann Allergy Asthma Immunol 2018; 120(5): 468–75.

47. van Kampen V, de Blay F, Folletti I, et al. EAACI position paper: skin prick testing in the diagnosis of occupational type I allergies. Allergy 2013; 68(5): 580–4.

48. Redlich C, Tarlo SM, Hankinson JL, et al. An Official American Thoracic Society Document: spirometry in the occupational setting. Am J Respir Crit Care Med 2014; 189: 984–94.

49. Becklake MR. Epidemiology of spirometric test failure. Br J Ind Med 1990; 47: 73–4.

50. Graham BL, Steenbruggen I, Miller MR, et al. Standardization of spirometry 2019 update. An Official American Thoracic Society and European Respiratory Society Technical Statement. Am J Respir Crit Care Med 2019; 200(8): e70–e88. doi:10.1164/rccm.201908-1590ST.

51. Burge PS. Single and serial measurements of lung function in the diagnosis of occupational asthma. Eur J Respir Dis 1982; 63: 47–59.

52. Corey P, Hutcheon M, Broder I, Mintz S. Grain elevator workers show work-related pulmonary function changes and dose-effect relationships with dust exposure. Br J Ind Med 1982; 39: 330–7.

53. Moscato G, Godnic-Cvar J, Maestrelli P, et al. Statement on self-monitoring of peak expiratory flows in the investigation of occupational asthma. J Allergy Clin Immunol 1995; 96: 295–301.

54. Blair Smith A, Bernstein DI, London MA, et al. Evaluation of occupational asthma from airborne egg protein exposure in multiple settings. Chest 1990; 98: 398–404.

55. Cartier A, Malo JL, Forest F, et al. Occupational asthma in snow crab-processing workers. J Allergy Clin Immunol 1984; 74: 261–9.

56. Malo JL, Cartier A. Occupational asthma in workers of a pharmaceutical company processing spiramycin. Thorax 1988; 43: 371–7.

57. Bardy JD, Malo JL, Séguin P, et al. Occupational asthma and IgE sensitization in a pharmaceutical company processing psyllium. Am Rev Respir Dis 1987; 135: 1033–8.

58. Venables KM, Burge PS, Davison AG, Newman Taylor AJ. Peak flow rate records in surveys: reproducibility of observers' reports. Thorax 1984; 39: 828–32.

59. Malo JL, Cartier A, Ghezzo H, Chan-Yeung M. Compliance with peak expiratory flow readings affects the within- and between-reader reproducibility of interpretation of graphs in subjects investigated for occupational asthma. J Allergy Clin Immunol 1996; 98: 1132–4.

60. Moore VC, Jaakkola MS, Burge CBSG, et al. A new diagnostic score for occupational asthma: the area between the curves (ABC score) of peak expiratory flow on days at and away from work. Chest 2009; 135: 307–14.

61. American Thoracic Society/European Respiratory Society. ATS/ERS recommendations for standardized procedures for the online and offline measurement of exhaled lower respiratory nitric oxide and nasal nitric oxide. Am J Respir Crit Care Med 2005; 171(8): 912–30.

62. Coman I, Lemiere C. Fractional exhaled nitric oxide (FeNO) in the screening and diagnosis work-up of occupational asthma. Curr Treat Options Allergy 2017; 4: 145–59.

63. van der Walt A, Singh T, Baatjies R, Jeebhay M. Environmental factors associated with baseline and serial changes in fractional exhaled nitric oxide (FeNO) in spice mill workers. Occup Environ Med 2016; 73: 614–20. doi:10.1136/oemed-2015-103005.

64. Burney PGJ, Britton JR, Chinn S, et al. Descriptive epidemiology of bronchial reactivity in an adult population: results from a community study. Thorax 1987; 42: 38–44.

65. Woolcock AJ, Peat JK, Salome CM, et al. Prevalence of bronchial hyper-responsiveness and asthma in a rural adult population. Thorax 1987; 42: 361–8.

66. Hendrick DJ. Epidemiological measurement of bronchial responsiveness in polyurethane workers. Bull Eur Physiopathol Respir 1988; 23: 555–9.

67. Pham QT, Mur JM, Chau N, et al. Prognostic value of acetylcholine challenge test: a prospective study. Br J Ind Med 1984; 41: 267–71.

68. Vedal S, Enarson DA, Chan H, et al. A longitudinal study of the occurrence of bronchial hyperresponsiveness in western red cedar workers. Am Rev Respir Dis 1988; 137: 651–5.

69. Gautrin D, Infante-Rivard C, Ghezzo H, Malo JL. Incidence and host determinants of probable occupational asthma in apprentices exposed to laboratory animals. Am J Respir Crit Care Med 2001; 163: 899–904.

70. Troyanov S, Malo JL, Cartier A, Gautrin D. Frequency and determinants of exaggerated bronchoconstriction during shortened methacholine challenge tests in epidemiological and clinical set-ups. Eur Respir J 2000; 16: 9–14.

71. Toelle BG, Peat JK, Salome CM, Mellis CM, Woolcock AJ. Toward a definition of asthma for epidemiology. Am Rev Respir Dis 1992; 146: 633–7.

72. Rioux JP, Malo JL, L'Archevêque J, et al. Workplace specific challenges as a contribution to the diagnosis of occupational asthma. Eur Respir J 2008; 32: 997–1003.

73. Pearce N, Checkoway H, Kriebel D. Bias in occupational epidemiology studies. Occup Environ Med 2007; 64(8): 562–8.

74. Schwartz S, Campbell UB, Gatto NM, Gordon K. Toward a clarification of the taxonomy of "bias" in epidemiology textbooks. Epidemiology 2015; 26(2): 216–22.

75. Le Moual N, Kauffmann F, Eisen EA, Kennedy SM. The healthy worker effect in asthma: work may cause asthma, but asthma may also influence work. Am J Respir Crit Care Med 2008; 177(1): 4–10.

76. Dumas O, Le Moual N, Siroux V, et al. Work related asthma. A causal analysis controlling the healthy worker effect. Occup Environ Med 2013; 70: 603–10.

77. Blair A, Stewart P, Lubin JH, Forastiere F. Methodological issues regarding confounding and exposure misclassification in epidemiological studies of occupational exposures. Am J Ind Med 2007; 50(3): 199–207.

78. Dumas O, Donnay C, Heederik DJ, et al. Occupational exposure to cleaning products and asthma in hospital workers. Occup Environ Med 2012; 69(12): 883–9.

79. Quinot C, Amsellem-Dubourget S, Temam S, et al. Development of a bar code-based exposure assessment method to evaluate occupational exposure to disinfectants and cleaning products: a pilot study. Occup Environ Med 2018; 75(9): 668–74.

80. VanderWeele TJ, Ding P. Sensitivity analysis in observational research: introducing the e-value. Ann Intern Med 2017; 167(4): 268–74.

81. Malo JL, Cartier A, L'Archevêque J, et al. Prevalence of occupational asthma and immunological sensitization to guar gum among employees at a carpet-manufacturing plant. J Allergy Clin Immunol 1990; 86: 562–9.

82. Cullinan P, Lowson D, Nieuwenhuijsen MJ, et al. Work related symptoms, sensitisation, and estimated exposure in workers not previously exposed to flour. Occup Environ Med 1994; 51: 579–83.

83. Vandenplas O, Delwich JP, Evrard G, et al. Prevalence of occupational asthma due to latex among hospital personnel. Am J Respir Crit Care Med 1995; 151: 54–60.

84. Mitchell CA, Gandevia B. Respiratory symptoms and skin reactivity in workers exposed to proteolytic enzymes in the detergent industry. Am Rev Respir Dis 1971; 104: 1–12.

85. Cullinan P, Lowson D, Nieuwenhuijsen MJ, et al. Work related symptoms, sensitisation, and estimated exposure in workers not previously exposed to laboratory rats. Occup Environ Med 1994; 51: 589–92.

86. Singh T, Bello B, Jeebhay MF. Risk factors associated with asthma phenotypes in dental healthcare workers. Am J Ind Med 2013; 56(1): 90–3.

87. Jeebhay MF, Robins TG, Miller ME, et al. Occupational allergy and asthma among salt water fish processing workers. Am J Ind Med 2008; 51(12): 899–910.

88. van der Walt A, Singh T, Baatjies R, et al. Work-related allergic respiratory disease and asthma in spice mill workers is associated with inhalant chili pepper and garlic exposures. Occup Environ Med 2013; 70(7): 446–52.

89. Ngajilo D, Singh TS, Ratshikopa E, et al. Risk factors associated with allergic sensitisation and asthma phenotypes in poultry farm workers. Am J Ind Med 2018; 61(6): 515–23.

90. Jeebhay MF, Baatjies R, Chang YS, et al. Risk factors for allergy due to the two-spotted spider mite (Tetranychus urticae) among table grape farm workers. Int Arch Allergy Immunol 2007; 144: 143–9.

91. Venables KM, Dally MB, Nunn AJ, et al. Smoking and occupational allergy in workers in a platinum refinery. BMJ 1989; 299: 939–42.

92. Burge PS, Perks WH, O'Brien IM, et al. Occupational asthma in an electronics factory: a case control study to evaluate aetiological factors. Thorax 1979; 34: 300–7.

93. Séguin P, Allard A, Cartier A, Malo JL. Prevalence of occupational asthma in spray painters exposed to several types of isocyanates, including polymethylene polyphenylisocyanates. JOM 1987; 29: 340–4.

94. Chan-Yeung M, Vedal S, Kus J, et al. Symptoms, pulmonary function, and bronchial hyperreactivity in Western red cedar workers compared with those in office workers. Am Rev Respir Dis 1984; 130: 1038–41.

95. Lipińska-Ojrzanowska A, Wiszniewska M, Świerczyńska-Machura D, et al. Work-related respiratory symptoms among health centres cleaners: a cross-sectional study. Int J Occup Med Environ Health 2014; 27(3): 460–6.

96. Arif AA, Delclos Gl. Association between cleaning-related chemicals and work-related asthma and asthma symptoms among healthcare professionals. Occup Environ Med 2012; 69(1): 35–40.

97. Skjold T, Dahl R, Juhl B, Sigsgaard T. The incidence of respiratory symptoms and sensitisation in baker apprentices. Eur Respir J 2008; 32: 452–9.

98. Walusiak J, Hanke W, Gorski P, Palczynski C. Respiratory allergy in apprentice bakers: do occupational allergies follow the allergic march? Allergy 2004; 59: 442–50.

99. Gautrin D, Ghezzo H, Infante-Rivard C, Malo JL. Natural history of sensitization, symptoms and diseases in apprentices exposed to laboratory animals. Eur Respir J 2001; 17: 904–8.

100. El-Zein M, Malo JL, Infante-Rivard C, Gautrin D. Incidence of probable occupational asthma and of changes in airway calibre and responsiveness in apprentice welders. Eur Respir J 2003; 22: 513–8.

101. Peters CE, Demers PA, Sehmer J, Karlen B, Kennedy SM. Early changes in respiratory health in trades' apprentices and physician visits for respiratory illnesses later in life. Occup Environ Med 2010; 67: 237–43.

102. Rodier F, Gautrin D, Ghezzo H, Malo JL. Incidence of occupational rhinoconjunctivitis and risk factors in animal-health apprentices. J Allergy Clin Immunol 2003; 112: 1105–11.

103. Gautrin D, Ghezzo H, Infante-Rivard C, Malo JL. Incidence and host determinants of work-related rhinoconjunctivitis in apprentice pastry-makers. Allergy 2002; 57: 913–8.

104. Gautrin D, Ghezzo H, Infante-Rivard C, et al. Long-term outcomes in a prospective cohort of apprentices exposed to high-molecular-weight agents. Am J Respir Crit Care Med 2008; 177: 871–9.

105. Cullinan P, Cook A, Gordon S, et al. Allergen exposure, atopy and smoking as determinants of allergy to rats in a cohort of laboratory employees. Eur Respir J 1999; 13: 1139–43.

106. Kruize H, Post W, Heederik D, et al. Respiratory allergy to laboratory animal workers: a retrospective cohort study using pre-employment screening data. Occup Environ Med 1997; 54: 830–5.

107. Brisman J, Nieuwenhuijsen MJ, Venables KM. Exposure-response relations for work related respiratory symptoms and sensitisation in a cohort exposed to alpha-amylase. Occup Environ Med 2004; 61: 551–3.

108. Cullinan P, Cook A, Nieuwenhuijsen MJ, et al. Allergen and dust exposure as determinants of work-related symptoms and sensitization in a cohort of flour-exposed workers; a case-control analysis. Ann Occup Hyg 2001; 45: 97–103.

109. Dumas O, Boggs KM, Quinot C, et al. Occupational exposure to disinfectants and asthma incidence in U.S. nurses: a prospective cohort study. Am J Ind. Med 2020; 63(1): 44–50.

110. Archambault S, Malo JL, Infante-Rivard C, et al. Incidence of sensitization, symptoms and probable occupational rhinoconjunctivitis and asthma in apprentices starting exposure to latex. J Allergy Clin Immunol 2001; 107: 921–3.

111. Kennedy SM, Chan-Yeung M, Teschke K, Karlen B. Change in airway responsiveness among apprentices exposed to metalworking fluids. Am J Respir Crit Care Med 1999; 159: 87–93.

112. Dragos M, Jones M, Malo JL, et al. Specific antibodies to diisocyanate and work-related respiratory symptoms in apprentice car-painters. Occup Environ Med 2009; 66: 227–34.

113. Iwatsubo Y, Matrat M, Brochard P, et al. Healthy worker effect and changes in respiratory symptoms and lung function in hairdressing apprentices. Occup Environ Med 2003; 60: 831–40.

114. De Zotti R, Bovenzi M. Prospective study of work related respiratory symptoms in trainee bakers. Occup Environ Med 2000; 57: 58–61.

115. Collaborators GBDOCRRF. Global and regional burden of chronic respiratory disease in 2016 arising from non-infectious airborne occupational exposures: a systematic analysis for the Global Burden of Disease Study 2016. Occup Environ Med 2020; 77(3): 142–50.

116. Blanc PD, Annesi-Maesano I, Balmes JR, et al. The Occupational Burden of Nonmalignant Respiratory Diseases. An Official American Thoracic Society and European Respiratory Society Statement. Am J Respir Crit Care Med 2019; 199(11): 1312–34.

117. Meca O, Cruz MJ, Sanchez-Ortiz M, et al. Do low molecular weight agents cause more severe asthma than high molecular weight agents? PLOS ONE 2016; 11(6): e0156141.

118. Chan-Yeung M, Malo JL. Table of major inducers of occupational asthma. In: Bernstein IL, Chan-Yeung M, Malo JL, Bernstein DI, eds. Asthma in the workplace. New-York: Marcel Dekker, Inc. 1993: 595–623.

119. Dumas O, Le Moual N. Do chronic workplace irritant exposures cause asthma? Curr Opin Allergy Clin Immunol 2016; 16: 75–85.

120. Vandenplas O, Dressel H, Nowak D, Jamart J. What is the optimal management option for occupational asthma? Eur Respir Rev 2012; 21(124): 97–104.

121. Cormier M, Lemiere C. Occupational asthma. Int J Tuberc Lung Dis 2020; 24(1): 8–21.

122. Dumas O, Wiley AS, Quinot C, et al. Occupational exposure to disinfectants and asthma control in US nurses. Eur Respir J 2017; 50(4).

123. Tarlo SM, Lemiere C. Occupational asthma. N Engl J Med 2014; 370(7): 640–9.

124. Vandenplas O, Wiszniewska M, Raulf M, et al. EAACI position paper: irritant-induced asthma. Allergy 2014; 69(9): 1141–53.

125. Folletti I, Siracusa A, Paolocci G. Update on asthma and cleaning agents. Curr Opin Allergy Clin Immunol 2017; 17(2): 90–5.

126. Carder M, Seed MJ, Money A, et al. Occupational and work-related respiratory disease attributed to cleaning products. Occup Environ Med 2019; 76(8): 530–6.

127. Lillienberg L, Andersson E, Janson C, et al. Occupational exposure and new-onset asthma in a population-based study in Northern Europe (RHINE). Ann Occup Hyg 2013; 57(4): 482–92.

128. Zhou AY, Seed M, Carder M, et al. Sentinel approach to detect emerging causes of work-related respiratory diseases. Occup Med (Lond) 2020; 70(1): 52–9.

129. Stocks SJ, Bensefa-Colasb L, Berkd SF. Worldwide trends in incidence in occupational allergy and asthma. Curr Opin Allergy Clin Immunol 2016; 16: 113–9.

130. Quinot C, Dumas O, Henneberger PK, et al. Development of a job-task-exposure matrix to assess occupational exposure to disinfectants among US nurses. Occup Environ Med 2017; 74(2): 130–7.

131. Le Moual N, Zock JP, Dumas O, et al. Update of an occupational asthma-specific job exposure matrix to assess exposure to 30 specific agents. Occup Environ Med 2018; 75(7): 507–14; available from: http://oasjem.vjf.inserm.fr/. Date last accessed April, 2020.

132. Kennedy SM, Le Moual N, Choudat D, Kauffmann F. Development of an asthma specific job exposure matrix and its application in the epidemiological study of genetics and environment in asthma (EGEA). Occup Environ Med 2000; 57: 635-41; available from: http://asthmajem.vjf.inserm.fr/. Date last accessed: April 8, 2020.

133. Bernstein DI. Genetics of occupational asthma. Curr Opin Allergy Clin Immunol 2011; 11(2): 86–9.

134. Rava M, Ahmed I, Kogevinas M, et al. Genes interacting with occupational exposures to low molecular weight agents and irritants on adult-onset asthma in three European studies. Environ Health Perspect 2017; 125(2): 207–14.

135. Vandenplas O. Occupational asthma: etiologies and risk factors. Allergy Asthma Immunol Res 2011; 3: 157–67.

136. Maestrelli P, Boschetto P, Fabbri LM, Mapp CE. Mechanisms of occupational asthma. J Allergy Clin Immunol 2009; 123: 531–42.

137. Yucesoy B, Johnson VJ, Lummus ZL, et al. Genetic variants in antioxidant genes are associated with diisocyanate-induced asthma. Toxicol Sci 2012; 129(1): 166–73.

138. Yucesoy B, Kashon ML, Johnson VJ, et al. Genetic variants in TNFalpha, TGFB1, PTGS1 and PTGS2 genes are associated with diisocyanate-induced asthma. J Immunotoxicol 2016; 13(1): 119–26.

139. Bernstein DI, Lummus ZL, Kesavalu B, et al. Genetic variants with gene regulatory effects are associated with diisocyanate asthma. J Allergy Clin Immunol 2018; 142: 959–69.

140. Bernstein DI, Kissling GE, Khurana Hershey G, et al. Hexamethylene diisocyanate asthma is associated with genetic polymorphisms of CD14, IL-13, and IL-4 receptor alpha. J Allergy Clin Immunol 2011; 128: 418–20.

141. McDonald JC, Chen Y, Zekveld C, Cherry NM. Incidence by occupation and industry of acute work related respiratory diseases in the UK, 1992–2001. Occup Environ Med 2005; 62: 836–42.

142. Karjalainen A, Kurppa K, Martikainen R, et al. Exploration of asthma risk by occupation-extended analysis of an incidence study of the Finnish population. Scand J Work Environ Health 2002; 28: 49–57.

143. Howse D, Gautrin D, Neis B, et al. Gender and snow crab occupational asthma in Newfoundland and Labrador, Canada. Environ Res 2006; 101: 163–74.

144. Moscato G, Apfelbacher C, Brockow K, et al. Gender and Occupational Allergy, EAACI Task Force Report. Allergy April 12, 2020. doi:10.1111/all.14317.

145. Remen T, Acouetey DS, Paris C, Zmirou-Navier D. Diet, occupational exposure and early asthma incidence among bakers, pastry makers and hairdressers. BMC Public Health 2012; 12: 387.

146. Otelea MR, Rascu A. Vitamin D intake and obesity in occupational asthma patients and the need for supplementation. Endocr Metab Immune Disord Drug Targets 2018; 18(6): 565–72.

147. Von Linstow ML, Porsbjerg CS, Ulrik S, et al. Prevalence and predictors of atopy among young Danish adults. Clin Exp Allergy 2002; 32(4): 520–5.

148. Slovak AJ, Hill RN. Laboratory animal allergy: a clinical survey of an exposed population. Br J Ind Med 1981; 3: 123.

149. Merget R, Kulzer R, Dierkes-Globisch A, et al. Exposure-effect relationship of platinum salt allergy in a catalyst production plant: conclusions from a 5-year prospective cohort study. J Allergy Clin Immunol 2000; 105: 364–70.

150. Remen TDS, Acouetey C, Paris B, et al. Early incidence of occupational asthma is not accelerated by atopy in the bakery/pastry and hairdressing sectors. Int J Tuberc Lung Dis 2013; 17(7): 973–81.

151. Merget R, Sander I, van Kampen V, et al. Allergic asthma after flour inhalation in subjects without occupational exposure to flours: an experimental pilot study. Int Arch Occup Environ Health 2011; 84: 753–60.

152. Ameille JK, Hamelin P, Andujar L, et al. Occupational asthma and occupational rhinitis: the united airways disease model revisited. Occup Environ Med 2013; 70(7): 471–5.

153. Malo JL, Lemière C, Desjardins A, Cartier A. Prevalence and intensity of rhinoconjunctivitis in subjects with occupational asthma. Eur Respir J 1997; 10: 1513–5.

154. Castano R, Gautrin D, Thériault C, et al. Occupational rhinitis in workers investigated for occupational asthma. Thorax 2009; 64: 50–4.

155. Vandenplas O, Van Brussel P, D'Alpaos V, et al. Rhinitis in subjects with work-exacerbated asthma. Respir Med 2010; 104: 497–503.

156. Karjalainen A, Martikainen R, Klaukka T, et al. Risk of asthma among Finnish patients with occupational rhinitis. Chest 2003; 123: 283–8.

157. Balogun RA, Siracusa A, Shusterman D. Occupational rhinitis and occupational asthma: association or progression? Am J Ind Med 2018; 61(4): 293–307.

158. Moscato G, Vandenplas O, Van Mijk GR, et al. Occupational rhinitis. Allergy 2008; 63: 969–80.

159. Temam S, Varraso R, Pornet C, et al. Ability of ecological deprivation indices to measure social inequalities in a French cohort. BMC Public Health 2017; 17(1): 956.

160. Davidsen JR, Sondergaard J, Hallas J, et al. Impact of socioeconomic status on the use of inhaled corticosteroids in young adult asthmatics. Respir Med 2011; 105(5): 683–90.

161. Galobardes B, Granell R, Sterne J, et al. Childhood wheezing, asthma, allergy, atopy, and lung function: different socioeconomic patterns for different phenotypes. Am J Epidemiol 2015; 182(9): 763–74.

162. Li X, Sundquist J, Sundquist K. Socioeconomic and occupational groups and risk of asthma in Sweden. Occup Med (Lond) 2008; 58(3): 161–8.

163. Beasley R, Semprini A, Mitchell EA. Risk factors for asthma: is prevention possible? Lancet 2015; 386(9998): 1075–85.

164. Temam S, Chanoine S, Bedard A, et al. Low socioeconomic position and neighborhood deprivation are associated with uncontrolled asthma in elderly. Respir Med 2019; 158: 70–7.

165. Galobardes B, Shaw M, Lawlor DA, Lynch JW, Davey Smith G. Indicators of socioeconomic position (part 1). Epidemiol Community Health 2006; 60; 7–12.

166. Trupin L, Earnest G, SanPedro M, et al. The occupational burden of chronic obstructive pulmonary disease. Eur Respir J 2003; 22: 462–9.

167. Balmes J, Becklake M, Blanc P. Environmental and Occupational Health Assembly, American Thoracic Society. American Thoracic Society Statement: occupational contribution to the burden of airway disease. Am J Respir Crit Care Med 2003; 167: 787–97.

168. Chan-Yeung M, Malo JL. Occupational asthma. N Engl J Med 1995; 333: 107–12.

169. D'Amato G, Liccardi G, D'Amato M, Holgate S. Environmental risk factors and allergic bronchial asthma. Clin Exp Allergy 2005; 35: 1113–24.

170. Karvala K, Toskala E, Luukkonen R, et al. Prolonged exposure to damp and moldy workplaces and new-onset asthma. Int Arch Occup Environ Health 2011; 84: 713–21.

171. Venables KM, Upton JL, Hawkins ER, et al. Smoking, atopy and laboratory animal allergy. Br J Ind Med 1988; 45: 667–71.

172. Calverley AE, Rees D, Dowdeswell RJ, et al. Platinum salt sensitivity in refinery workers: incidence and effects of smoking and exposure. Occup Environ Med 1995; 52: 661–6.

173. Paggiaro PL, Loi AM, Rossi O, et al. Follow-up study of patients with respiratory disease due to toluene diisocyanate (TDI). Clin Allergy 1984; 14: 463–9.

174. Chan-Yeung M, Lam S, Koerner S. Clinical features and natural history of occupational asthma due to Western red cedar (thuja plicata). Am J Med 1982; 72: 411–5.

175. Siracusa A, Marabini A, Folletti I, Moscato G. Smoking and occupational asthma. Clin Exper Allergy 2006; 36: 577–84.

176. Heederik D, Sigsgaard T. Respiratory allergy in agricultural workers: recent developments. Curr Opin Allergy Clin Immunol 2005; 5: 129–34.

177. Eduard W, Douwes J, Omenaas E, Heederik D. Do farming exposures cause or prevent asthma? Results from a study of adult Norwegian farmers. Thorax 2004; 59: 381–6.

178. Smit LA, Heederik D, Doekes G, et al. Occupational endotoxin exposure reduces the risk of atopic sensitization but increases the risk of bronchial hyperresponsiveness. Int Arch Allergy Immunol 2010; 152: 151–8.

179. Gautrin D, Ghezzo H, Infante-Rivard C, et al. Incidence and determinants of IgE-mediated sensitization in apprentices: a prospective study. Am J Respir Crit Care Med 2000; 162: 1222–8.

180. Becklake MR. Population studies in risk assessment: strengths and weaknesses. In: Mohr U, ed. Inhalational Toxicology the Design and Interpretation of Inhalational Studies and their use in Risk Assessment. New York: Springer-Verlag. 1988: 263–72.

181. Smith AB, Castellan RM, Lewis D, Matte T. Guidelines for the epidemiologic assessment of occupational asthma. Report of the subcommittee on the epidemiologic assessment of occupational asthma, occupational lung disease committee. J Allergy Clin Immunol 1989; 84: 794–805.

4

MECHANISMS, GENETICS, AND PATHOPHYSIOLOGY

Piero Maestrelli,[1] Adam V. Wisnewski,[2] Christopher Carlsten,[3] Xavier Munoz,[4]
Hung-Chang Tsui,[5] Jeroen Vanoirbeek,[6] Jean-Luc Malo,[7] and David I. Bernstein[8]
[1]University of Padova, Padova, Italy
[2]Yale University School of Medicine, New Haven, CT, USA
[3]Respiratory Medicine, University of British Columbia, Vancouver, British Columbia, Canada
[4]Pneumology Department, Hospital Vall d'Hebron, and Cell Biology, Physiology and
Immunology Department, Universidad Autonoma de, Barcelona, Spain
[5]Department of Public Health and Primary Care, Center for Environment and Health, KU Leuven, Leuven, Belgium
[6]Department of Public Health and Primary Care, Center for Environment and Health,
Occupational, Environmental & Insurance Medicine, KU Leuven, Leuven, Belgium
[7]Hôpital du Sacré-Cœur de Montréal and Université de Montréal, Montréal, Québec, Canada
[8]Division of Immunology, Allergy and Rheumatology, University of Cincinnati College of Medicine, Cincinnati, Ohio, USA

Contents

Introduction

Occupational asthma (OA), like non-OA, is a multifactorial disease with complex genetic, environmental, and behavioral interactions. Clinical, functional, and pathological alterations in OA show several similarities to those found in non-OA; however, mechanisms of "induction" or sensitization do not necessarily overlap in OA and non-OA. There are several hundred causes of sensitizer-induced OA, which can be classified as high-molecular-weight (HMW) or low-molecular-weight (LMW) compounds. In most cases, sensitizer-induced OA is the result of a specific immunoglobulin E (IgE) dependent hypersensitivity to a workplace-sensitizing agent, although there may also be important accessory mechanisms in the case of LMW-induced OA. This type of OA is distinguished from *irritant-induced asthma,* which is the term used to describe OA caused by exposure at work to substances that cause asthma through an irritant mechanism rather than by immunologic sensitization. Also, there is evidence of interaction between the immune-based inflammatory reaction and disease (OA) on the one hand and occupation-based environmental factors on the other hand, as examined in epigenetic studies.

Most HMW allergens, such as flours, enzymes, and animal proteins, can induce IgE-mediated responses that cause work-related symptoms in exposed workers. However, the characteristics of immune responses induced by LMW agents and the nature of the effector mechanisms in chemical respiratory allergy are more controversial. This chapter also examines the current understanding of the role of genetic factors and their interaction with environmental factors in the development of OA as well as recent advances in OA pathophysiology.

Specific immunologic mechanisms of occupational asthma

Most HMW agents elicit IgE-dependent allergic reactions for which allergy skin-prick tests (SPTs) and measurements of serum specific antibodies can be useful for diagnosis (1). Specific IgE antibodies have been detected in OA induced by some LMW agents, such as acid anhydrides, diisocyanates, platinum salts, and reactive dyes (1, 2). Several studies have demonstrated significant associations between major histocompatibility complex (MHC) alleles and LMW-induced OA (see section "Role of Genetics in Occupational Asthma"), suggesting that immunologic mechanisms are involved in this type of OA.

IgE-mediated response

Most HMW allergens can induce IgE-mediated sensitization and elicit work-related symptoms in exposed workers (Table 4.1). Thus, for HMW allergens, allergy SPTs and/or measurements of allergen-specific IgE antibodies are useful for predicting OA phenotype and identifying asymptomatic, sensitized workers among exposed workers.

Some LMW allergens also induce IgE-mediated responses (Table 4.1). An IgE-mediated mechanism is one possible pathogenic mechanism in a minority of workers with OA induced by diisocyanates and acid anhydride chemicals. Detection of the diisocyanate-specific IgE antibody may be improved through optimization of methods used in preparation of chemical-protein conjugate antigens for in vitro serology (3).

Several kinds of reactive dyes can induce IgE-mediated OA in exposed workers (Table 4.1).

IgG-mediated and autoimmune mechanisms

Consistent with other antigenic exposures (e.g. infectious agents), exposure to occupational allergens can induce specific immunoglobulin G (IgG) responses. However, antigen-specific IgG may represent an immunological response to current or previous exposure that is not directly related to the pathogenic mechanism of OA (Table 4.1). Autoimmune mechanisms have also been suggested in the pathogenesis of LMW-induced OA (see Table 4.1).

Nonspecific mechanisms

Multiple mechanisms involving inflammation, airway epithelial injury-repair, structural remodeling, oxidative stress, and neurogenic factors may also contribute to asthma pathogenesis. Some have theorized that the unifying characteristic of asthma is a functionally impaired *barrier* function of the airway epithelium, resulting in greater penetration of allergens, microorganisms, and toxicants, which in turn triggers allergic-type inflammation (4). A similar process at skin epithelial cell surfaces underlies certain allergic skin diseases and has been linked to environmental asthma (5).

Innate mechanisms

While the adaptive immune system clearly plays an important role in OA, nonadaptive (innate) immune responses also play a role. For example, the intrinsic effects of diisocyanates might include the production of proinflammatory cytokines. In a previous study, a diisocyanate-HSA conjugate challenge of peripheral mononuclear cells from patients with isocyanate-induced OA revealed enhanced production of histamine-releasing factors and monocyte chemoattractant protein 1 (MCP-1) (6) which could initiate an immune response. Using human peripheral blood mononuclear cells stimulated in vitro with a hexamethylene diisocyanate (HDI)-albumin conjugate or control albumin antigens, Wisnewski et al. (7) demonstrated isocyanate moiety-specific changes in gene/protein expression. Significant changes were noted in lysosomal genes, and the expression of certain chemokines, including migration inhibitory factor and MCP-1, which attract mononuclear cells, chitinases (pattern recognition receptors), and oxidized low-density lipoprotein (CD68), was increased. Furthermore, studies of the gene expression profile of macrophages derived from the THP-1 human cell line and cultured with solubilized HDI have identified altered expression of genes involved in detoxification, oxidative stress, cytokine signaling, and apoptosis (8). Thus, there is evidence to suggest that isocyanates stimulate nonadaptive immune responses that contribute to respiratory sensitization, airway inflammation, and the clinical expression of OA. Other in vitro studies have demonstrated that

TABLE 4.1 Specific Immunological Mechanisms of OA

Mechanism		References
IgE mediated		
Antigen-presenting cells, such as dendritic cells, process inhaled allergens with subsequent presentation to CD4 T-helper cells, initiating an immune response		*1. Lummus, 2011*
Skin as a sensitizing route		*2. Redlich, 2010*
		3. Kim, 2010
HMW agents		*4. Wisnewski, 2011*
Most HMW occupational allergens induce an IgE-mediated response, examples:		
Wheat flour	In 392 bakery workers, IgE-mediated sensitization rate of 6.5%. Sensitization was closely associated with lower respiratory symptoms	*5. Hur, 2008*
Digestive enzymes	Levels of allergen-specific IgE and skin-prick positivity was significantly higher in exposed workers with work-related respiratory symptoms	*6. Bahn, 2006*
Herbal agents		*7. Lee, 2006*
Spider mites		*8. Kim, 1999*
Atopy as an important risk factor for the development of IgE-mediated sensitization and OA to HMW agents.		*9. Palihke, 2011*
		10. Sastre, 2003
LMW agents		
Diisocyanates		
Leading hypothesis: Diisocyanate act as a hapten that undergoes nucleophilic addition reactions with airway proteins to form conjugates in vivo.		*9. Palihke, 2011*
An IgE-mediated mechanism may play a pivotal role.		*11. Kimber, 2014*
Levels of allergen-specific IgG antibodies to a HSA conjugate of TDI significantly higher in asymptomatic exposed subjects and in subjects with allergic asthma than in unexposed, healthy control subjects.		*12. Park, 1999*
		13. Ye, 2006
Prevalence of allergen-specific IgE antibody highly variable, related to conjugate preparation and diisocyanate ligand-protein ratios.		*12. Park, 1999*
		13. Ye, 2006
		14. Baur, 1984
		15. Tee, 1998
		16. Maestrelli, 2009
Controversial: IgE-mediated sensitization to LMW agents enhanced by smoking or atopy.		*17. Maestrelli, 2009*
		9. Palihke, 2011
Increased specific IgE antibodies not always present in workers with TDI-induced OA but when this is the case, is significatnly associated with a greater likelihood of OA.		*15. Tee, 1998*
		18. Budnik, 2013
Workers with the AA genotype of the 46 A>G polymorphism have significantly higher serum levels of TDI-albumin-specific IgE than those with the GG genotype, suggesting that ADRB2 polymorphisms may affect IgE-specific sensitization.		*19. Ye, 2010*
In confirmed MDI-OA workers, levels of MDI-(albumin-specific IgE antibodies higher than in control groups, although test of sensitivity was low.		*20. Hur, 2008*
IgE may not play a role: Absence of bronchial RNA message for Cε and IL-4, the cytokine that promotes the B lymphocyte switch to IgE synthesis, after positive SIC in patients sensitized to diisocyanates.		*21. Jones, 2006*
Reactive dyes		
A study of 309 exposed workers in the reactive dye industry revealed that 17% had high levels of specific IgE antibodies against Black GR- and Orange 3R-HSA conjugate, and that the presence of these antibodies was significantly associated with work-related respiratory symptoms and the OA phenotype.		*22. Park, 1991*
Pharmaceutical compounds: *Antibiotics*		
A study of 161 healthcare workers exposed to three major cephalosporins (cefotiam, ceftriaxone, and ceftizoxime reported an IgE sensitization rate for cephalosporin-HSA conjugates of 17.4%.		*23. Kim, 2012*
		(Continued)

TABLE 4.1 Specific Immunological Mechanisms of OA (*Continued*)

Mechanism	References
IgG-mediated	
HMW agents	
Studies of HMW agents, such as spider mites or wheat flour, have demonstrated significantly higher levels of allergen-specific IgG_1 and IgG_4 antibodies in workers with greater exposure intensity.	*5. Hur, 2008* *24. Park, 2000*
LMW agents	
Diisocyanates	
IgG specific for TDI- or MDI-albumin HSA conjugates are readily detectable in serum of exposed workers.	*12. Park, 1999* *20. Hur, 2008*
Association of personal levels of exposure to HDI and specific HDI-specific IgG.	*25. Pronk, 2007*
Reactive dyes	
IgG and IgG_4 specific for a reactive dye-HSA conjugate were detected in 23% and 14%, respectively, of workers exposed to reactive dyes.	*26. Park, 1991*
Autoimmune mechanisms	
Some TDI-OA patients have been found to have two serum IgG autoantibodies, which recognize cytokeratin 19 (CK19 and transglutaminase (tTG.	*27. Choi, 2004* *28. Pham, 2014*
The prevalence of anti-CK19 and tTG IgG was significantly higher in workers with TDI-OA than in asymptomatic exposed subjects or unexposed control subjects.	*28. Pham, 2014*
Workers with high serum levels of anti-CK19 or tTG IgG were significantly more sensitive to inhaled methacholine challenge, suggesting an association with airway inflammation.	*29. Hur, 2009*

References: 1. Lummus ZL, et al. Immunol Allergy Clin North Am. 2011;31:699–716. 2. Redlich CA. Proc Am Thorac Soc. 2010;2:134–7. 3. Kim JE, et al. Allergy. 2010;65:791–2. 4. Wisnewski AV, et al. J Occup Med Toxicol. 2011;6:6. 5. Hur GY, et al. Respir Med. 2008;102:548–55.6. Bahn JW, et al. Clin Exp Allergy. 2006;36:352–8. 7. Lee LY, et al. Allergy. 2006;61:392–3. 8. Kim YK, et al. Ann Allergy Asthma Immunol. 1999;82:223–8. 9. Palikhe NS, et al. Allergy Asthma Immunol Res. 2011;3:21–6. 10. Sastre J, et al. Eur Respir J. 2003;22:364–73. 11. Kimber I, et al. J Appl Toxicol. 2014;34:1073–7. 12. Park HS, et al. J Allergy Clin Immunol. 1999;104:847–51. 13. Ye YM, et al. J Allergy Clin Immunol. 2006;118:885–91. 14. Baur X, et al. J Allergy Clin Immunol. 1984;73:610–8. 15. Tee RD, et al. J Allergy Clin Immunol. 1998;101:709–15. 16. Cartier A, et al. J Allergy Clin Immunol. 1989;84:507–14. 17. Maestrelli P, et al. J Allergy Clin Immunol. 2009;123:531–42. 18. Budnik LT, et al. Int Arch Occup Environ Health. 2013;86:417–30. 19. Ye YM, et al. Allergy Asthma Immunol Res. 2010;2(4:260–6. 20. Hur GY, et al. Clin Exp Allergy. 2008;38:586–93. 21. Jones MG, et al. J Allergy Clin Immunol. 2006;117:663–9. 22. Park HS, et al. J Allergy Clin Immunol. 1991;87:639–49. 23. Kim JE, et al. Allergy Asthma Immunol Res. 2012;4:85–91 24. Park HS, et al. J Korean Med Sci. 2000;15:407–12. 25. Pronk A, et al. Am J Respir Crit Care Med. 2007;176:1090–7. 26. Park HS, Hong CS. Clin Exp Allergy. 1991;21:357–62. 27. JH Choi, et al. Ann Allergy Asthma Immunol. 2004;93:293–8. 28. Pham le D, et al. Ann Allergy Asthma Immunol. 2014;113:48–54. 29. Hur GY, et al. J Clin Immunol. 2009;29:786–94.

toluene diisocyanate (TDI) exposure induces the production of interleukin-8 (IL-8) and other chemokines by bronchial epithelial cells with activation of proinflammatory cytokines. In vivo, increased levels of myeloperoxidase (MPO), IL-8, matrix metalloproteinase-9 (MMP-9), and vascular endothelial growth factor (VEGF) have been found in the airway secretions or serum of TDI-OA patients, indicating that these cytokines might be involved in airway inflammation, as well as airway remodeling, in these workers (9, 10).

Epithelial injury

The airway epithelium constitutes the interface between the internal milieu of the lung and the external environment. As the first point of contact for respirable particles, vapors, and aerosols, it is highly susceptible to their damaging effects. It was previously thought that only high-level exposures, such as those associated with reactive airways dysfunction syndrome (RADS), were able to sufficiently damage the epithelium to the point of clinical significance, but less dramatic and yet repeated irritant exposures are better appreciated as damaging (11, 12) (Chapter 19). Some compounds that cause OA are intrinsically cytotoxic (diisocyanates, anhydrides), while other sources, such as detergents/baking flour, contain enzymes capable of directly disrupting cell-cell or cell-matrix interactions. Damage to the airway epithelium is known to stimulate cell turnover through pathways that involve a number of autocrine growth factors as well as paracrine mediators from the adjacent mesenchyme (13). Epidermal growth factor (EGF), fibroblast growth factor (FGF), transforming growth factor-β, platelet-derived growth factor (PDGF), and VEGF, and their corresponding receptors are recognized as critical mediators in this process (14, 15). Extracellular traps, released from neutrophils (and/or other granulocytes) in the context of occupational exposures, can stimulate the epithelium toward increased inflammation (16, 17). Continuing cycles of epithelial damage and repair, as might be caused by occupational exposures, have been hypothesized to disrupt epithelial barriers, increasing the risks for the development of allergic sensitization. The smallest particles, including engineered nanoparticles that are cause increasingly for occupational exposure concerns, may interact with the epithelium and stimulate NK-kB to cause inflammation but also may pass relatively easily through the epithelium to cause systemic effects (18).

Airway wall remodeling

When epithelial injury and repair become a chronic cycle, the anatomical structure of the airway wall may become remodeled, including changes that further increase the opportunity for tissue penetration by allergens/toxins/viruses (19). Structural changes observed in OA include hyalinization/thickening of the laminar reticularis, epithelial denudation/desquamation, increased numbers of myofibroblasts, and hypertrophy/metaplasia of smooth muscle. Goblet cell hyperplasia and increased mucin have been observed (20). As mentioned above, the characteristic "thickening of the basement membrane" is due to the deposition of interstitial cross-linked collagens (types I, III, and IV) produced by myofibroblasts, noted for example in swimmers, more so than deposition of more appropriate collagen IV (20). A significant correlation has been reported between the thickness of the basement membrane's reticular layer and the severity of asthma (21). Cessation of workplace exposure may reduce subepithelial fibrosis and disease severity; however, structural remodeling and nonspecific airway hyperresponsiveness (AHR) may persist in some workers (22).

In some asthma pathology studies, increased intercellular spaces between basal epithelial cells have been observed, consistent with an abnormality of intercellular adhesion, and increased the chances for epithelial desquamation (21). Glycoprotein adhesion molecules, known to modulate the migration of inflammatory cells through endothelial intercellular spaces, may also be aberrantly expressed in OA, increasing the potential for tissue infiltration by leukocytes. Epithelial cells, damaged by occupational exposures, may produce increased amounts of proinflammatory signals, and decrease the amounts of epithelial-derived relaxant factors, which modulate the bronchoconstricting effects of exogenous and/or endogenous substances (23). Furthermore, desquamation of the airway epithelium may expose afferent nerve endings, and potentiate neuronal release of compounds that incite neuroinflammation (see section "Neurogenic Inflammation").

In animal models, profibrotic cytokines, especially IL-13, can mediate many of the structural changes associated with asthma. Metalloproteinases and their inhibitors, whose expression is downstream of IL-13 signaling, have been described as important enzymes in this process. The appearance of airway remodeling during the natural history of OA in humans remains unclear. However, in patients with environmental asthma, such architectural changes occur early in the course of disease and may precede inflammatory changes (24).

Oxidative stress

Evidence of increased oxidative stress during asthma, both locally within the airways, as well as systemically, has been derived from a number of different studies (25). Bronchoalveolar lavage (BAL) and exhaled breath condensate from affected individuals show increased levels of 8-isoprostane and other well-established, markers of oxidative stress. Peripherally, additional biomarkers of oxidative stress (lipid peroxidation, superoxide anion generation, nitrates/nitrites, and protein carbonyls/sulfhydrils) may be increased, concomitant with decreased levels of specific antioxidants (glutathione, glutathione peroxidase activity, superoxide dismutase, catalase activity, etc.) (26). Increased levels of oxidative stress are thought to aggravate asthmatic airway inflammation via multiple mechanisms, including inflammation and effects on smooth muscle and mucus (27).

Molecular mechanisms by which oxidative stress induces such responses are beginning to be deciphered. Oxidative stress prompts the transcription factor Nrf2 to translocate to the nucleus where it triggers expression of an array of antioxidant response element driven genes that regulate the balance of outcomes of oxidant exposure (28). When the oxidative stress exceeds the protective capacity of Nrf2-induced genes, additional intracellular signaling cascades (e.g. NF-κB) may be triggered, eventually resulting in expression of proinflammatory cytokines, chemokines, and adhesion molecules (29). Studies in animal models suggest that mitochondria may be important intracellular sources of reactive oxygen species that drive redox-sensitive cellular responses to respiratory exposures (30).

Certain occupational exposures (e.g. diesel exhaust) are well recognized for their ability to induce oxidative stress, and have been shown to act as adjuvants for the development of allergic-type respiratory responses in animal and human models (31, 32). Other important occupational exposures (isocyanates, phthalates, metallic nanoparticles, disinfectants, and exposure to sewage) may also induce oxidative stress (33, 34). Both ferritin and transferrin appear involved in oxidant-mediated airway inflammation due to diphenylmethane diisocyanate (MDI) exposure, which may worsen in the context of depleted antioxidant resources (35). Isocyanates may operate through leukocyte NADPH oxidase to generate inflammation. Isocyanate-induced oxidative stress may cause further harm by enhancing auto-antibody generation (36).

Thiols, especially glutathione (GSH), play a major role in protecting the airway against oxidant damage. Airway fluid GSH is normally maintained at high levels (>100 μM), ˜100-fold above systemic blood levels, and is intimately connected to redox-sensitive (proinflammatory) intracellular signaling cascades (37). In vitro, GSH reversibly reacts with some LMW occupational allergens (e.g. isocyanates), among other inhaled vapors, to carbamoylate other proteins (38). In animal studies, systemic GSH levels modulate TH-1 versus TH-2 priming by dendritic cells, and subsequent asthmatic response in animal models (39). In vivo studies of animal models and in vitro studies of human cells have demonstrated that isocyanates have marked effects on airway thiols (40) such as GSH, which play a major role in protecting the airway against oxidative damage. In humans, genetic associations of GSH-dependent enzyme polymorphisms (GST-P1, GST-M) with occupational and environmental asthma further support a potentially important role for airway GSH in asthma pathogenesis (41).

Neurogenic inflammation

Innervation of the human airways is complex and involves cholinergic, adrenergic, nonadrenergic, and noncholinergic (NANC) nerves. Some nerve cells penetrate the basement membrane, reaching into the epithelial cell layer, where they sense external signals via specific receptors, and secrete factors capable of eliciting inflammation and modulating bronchoconstriction (Chapter 19). Critical soluble mediators released by nerve cells include the neuropeptides, substance P (SP), neurokinins (NK), calcitonin gene-related, and vasoactive intestinal peptides (GCRP and VIP), which trigger responses from immune, vascular, and smooth muscle cells via specific receptors. Further cross-talk between neuronal and immune cells may be modulated through the epithelial-derived enzyme, NEP, which breaks down proinflammatory neuropeptides and can be modulated by occupational and/or environmental exposures (Chapter 19). Thus, neuronal cells produce potent mediators that may interact with other cell types to influence exposure-induced asthmatic responses.

A striking increase of SP-like, and decrease in VIP-like immunoreactive nerves has been reported in the airways of asthmatics in some studies but not confirmed in others. Several workplace stimuli (i.e. sulfur dioxide, dust, and cold air) may trigger reflex bronchoconstriction by directly stimulating sensory receptors in the airways of both normal and asthmatic subjects (42). Diisocyanates (e.g. TDI) have been further shown to stimulate release of SP and GCRP and inhibit neutral endopeptidase in experimental animals and in vitro preparations. A study demonstrated that genetic polymorphism of the NK2R gene among TDI-exposed workers affects serum VEGF levels (43).

A single neuronal receptor, transient receptor potential cation channel subfamily A member 1 (TRPA1), which recognizes a wide variety of "noxious" stimuli, including occupational allergens (diisocyanates), environmental irritants (cigarette smoke, chlorine), and endogenous compounds (reactive oxygen/nitrogen species, arachidonic acid derivatives) has now been molecularly cloned (44). In animal studies, TRPA1 expression colocalizes with SP, NK, and GCRP in nerve fibers in the airways, and TRPA1 knockout mice exhibit reduced inflammation in an ovalbumin asthma model (45). TRPV1 and TRPV4 may also be implicated in workplace settings (46). Support for the role of TRP channels in OA has been further augmented by the finding that TRPM8 stimulation by TDI causes inflammation and that cough is increased in workers with susceptibility variants in TRPV1 (47, 48).

While neurogenic inflammation and release of neuropeptides are well-established amplifying mechanisms in rodent models of airway inflammation and asthma, evidence that the same mechanisms are operative in human asthma is much less convincing. Tachykinins and their antagonists have shown limited pharmacologic benefits in human asthma and marked species differences in general innervation of the human (versus laboratory animal) lung are well noted, limiting translation of animal models (49).

Animal models

Introduction
Despite the disparity in the anatomy and the physiology between animals and humans, animal models remain essential tools to study different aspects of asthma, including relevant routes, dosages and duration of exposure, including respiratory and/or skin, exposure dosage, exposure duration as well as relevant epitopes of causative agents. With the transgenic techniques and antibody neutralization strategies that target specific molecular pathway, animal models can be used to investigate the underlying innate and adaptive immune responses and the disease mechanism, thereby providing translational value to clinical treatment modalities (50).

Animal species and strains
Numerous animal species have been proposed for asthma studies, from small animals like mice, rats, guinea pigs, and hamsters, to larger animals like cats, dogs, and primates (51). Though each species possesses certain advantages and disadvantages, mice have become the most widely used animal for asthma experiments because of the low cost, short gestation time, and low difficulty for transgenic manipulation.

The most frequently used strains of mouse are BALB/c, NC/Nga, and C57BL/6. By comparing various mouse strains, the immune profiles upon exposure to the offending agent showed that BALB/c strain induced: (1) the strongest Th2 reaction to toluene-2,4-diisocyanate (TDI) (52); (2) the strongest effect in IgE

increase, inflammatory cell influx in BAL, and cytokine production from hilar lymph nodes (LNs) in a glutaraldehyde-induced model of OA (53); (3) more pronounced AHR and higher mast cell number and histamine in BAL, but lower serum IgE and Th2-related cytokines in BAL in a trimellitic anhydride (TMA) model of OA (54); and (4) higher interleukin-9 (IL-9) and IL-17 gene expression in lung, which are known to interact with Th2 cell, innate lymphoid cells group 2 (ILC2) and group 3 (ILC3) in a model of OA due to chemicals (55).

Methodology of sensitization and elicitation
The typical design for an asthma study with animals involves two phases: sensitization and elicitation. Animals first receive the exposure to allergens via skin or airway in the sensitization phase, followed by the exposure via airways in the elicitation phase (56). The majority of murine studies involving LMW chemicals use skin exposure as the sensitization route, by means of intradermal injection, epicutaneous application, or occlusion on the trunk (57). Intranasal instillation and inhalation have also been applied.

Although inhalation is the most natural way of exposure, it is cost- and time-consuming, and requires large amounts of the studied agent. Intranasal application is easy to perform in repetition, but the distribution between upper and lower airway is largely influenced by the instilled volume, the anesthesia, and the vehicle dissolving allergens (58). Intratracheal instillation has the advantage of administering the exact amount of the agent into the lung, but the technique may injure the trachea. Pharyngeal aspiration has been introduced in recent years and is capable to simulate the characteristics of asthma without the limitation of the techniques described above (59).

The thresholds of respiratory sensitization (concentration × exposure time) to TDI, methylene diphenyl diisocyanate (MDI), and HDI have been examined in Brown Norway rats (60). The dose-response of respiratory sensitization to TDI has also been reviewed (61).

For both sensitization and elicitation, researchers have observed nonlinear dose-responses: sensitizing agents may induce a paradoxical weaker effect after the dosage exceeds a certain point. Dermal exposure with lower concentration (0.3%) of TDI induced a stronger sensitization than higher concentration (3%) in mice (62). Mice sensitized to 1% MDI via skin showed a stronger respiratory inflammation than mice exposed to 10% MDI (63). At the elicitation stage, consecutive longer exposure blunted airway hyperresponsiveness, despite higher serum IgE levels and lung inflammation (eosinophils and neutrophils) (64).

Assessment of asthma-like characteristics in animals exposed to low-molecular-weight agents
Physiological markers
The physiological endpoints generally consist of airway resistance, airflow, or breathing patterns that are assessed via invasive or noninvasive approaches, with or without the stimulation with bronchoconstricting agents (e.g. methacholine). Although this is mostly performed as an end stage analysis, efforts have been made to do repeated invasive lung function measurements (65). Noninvasive approaches, such as whole-body plethysmographs, enable longitudinal measurements of enhanced pause (Penh) in live animals (66).

Fractional FeNO has been suggested as a reliable marker reflecting the airway inflammation in Brown Norway rats exposed to TDI (67). Micro-computed tomography (μ-CT) has been introduced in asthma animal models, reflecting enlarged lung volume after the mice received naphthalene, an epithelial damaging agent (68). With the ex vivo method of precision-cut lung slices (PCLS), several samples can be taken from one animal to measure the airway contraction, thus reducing the need for larger animal samples (69).

Inflammatory and immunological markers

Typical endpoints of airway inflammation include cell influx (e.g. eosinophils and neutrophils) in the airway, which is evaluated at the microscopic level or via flow cytometry. Pathological changes of the airways usually include epithelium thickening/damage, goblet cell metaplasia, airway smooth muscle hypertrophy, and fibrosis.

Several cytokines, noncytokine markers, and specific immunoglobulins have been measured in animal models of asthma, either regarding the protein or the mRNA levels as summarized in Table 4.2.

Proteomic and genomic markers

Proteomic (Table 4.2) and genomic techniques have been applied to identify key routes of asthma. Whole genome analysis is typically conducted via mRNA microarrays that have identified a series of genes regulating lung inflammation in rats exposed to TMA, as regards both the sensitization and the elicitation processes (70). Whole genome analysis from mice exposed to MDI has identified substantial increase of calcium-activated chloride

channel regulator 1 (CLCA1), suggesting that Cl⁻ channels are involved in diisocyanate-induced asthma (71).

In addition to proteomic and mRNA genomic analysis, circulating microRNAs have become a study target. Up- or down-regulation of specific circulating microRNAs has been identified from blood of mice exposed to MDI (72) with several mediators, including cytokines, acting on their expression as shown in mice exposed to TDI (Table 4.2). These microRNAs are involved in the transcription of inducible nitric oxide synthases (iNOs), which have several roles in asthma.

Skin-lung relationship

Numerous studies have verified that dermal and respiratory sensitizers do not represent exclusive categories. For example, skin exposure to 2,4-dinitrochlorobenzene (DNCB), known as a dermal sensitizer, was able to change the airway susceptibility (evidenced by neutrophilic inflammation) to the following intranasal DNCB challenge in mice exposed to TMA (73). From the genomic analysis, oxazolone (known as a dermal sensitizer) showed comparable pattern as TMA (74).

Skin exposure to chemicals has become the predominant route for inducing sensitization in asthma animal models. Several chemicals have been tested based on the design that animals first received skin exposure and then respiratory elicitation as systematically reviewed, the majority of agents demonstrating airway hyperresponsiveness via skin exposure (57).

The conjugation of LMW hapten with other proteins after skin exposure has been studied in mice sensitized to MDI. Respiratory

TABLE 4.2 Inflammatory and Immunological Markers in Animal Models of Chemical-Induced Asthma, Including Diisocyanates

Types	Comments	References
Cytokines		
Interferon gamma	Representative of Th1 response	*1. Tarkowski, 2008*
IL-4, IL-5, IL13	Representative of Th2 response	*2. Kuper, 2008*
		3. Ban, 2006
		4. Sun, 2007
IL-13	Crucial mediator in TDI-induced model	*5. Devos, 2017*
IL-17	Directly linked to Th17 response and neutrophil recruitment	
IL-17F	Crucial for the airway hyperresponsiveness and respiratory neutrophilic inflammation	*6. Chen, 2019* *7. Pollaris, 2020*
IL-33	Activation of ILC2 and expression of micro-RNA-155	*8. Blomme, 2020*
KC (CXCL1) MIP-2 (CXCL2)	Linked to neutrophil recruitment	
MCP1 (CCL2)	Involved in mast cell degranulation	
Noncytokine markers		
GATA binding protein 3 (GATA3)	Increased in a model exposed to 2,4-d-butyl or TMA	*9. Fukuyama, 2010*
Signal transduction and activator of transcription 6 (STAT6)	Increased in a model exposed to 2,4-d-butyl or TMA	*9. Fukuyama, 2010*
C-C chemokine receptor type 4 (CCR4)	Increased in a model exposed to 2,4-d-butyl or TMA	*9. Fukuyama, 2010*
Serine-like protease inhibitor 6	Protein involved in tissue repair and downregulation of inflammation	*10. Kuper, 2008*
Various	Various proteins related to inflammation	*11. Haenen, 2010*
Specific antibodies	Hapten conjugation with mouse serum proteins	*12. Wisnewski, 2011* *13. Ruwona, 2010*

References: 1. Tarkowski M, Kur B, Polakowska E, et al. Int J Occup Med Environ Health. 2008;21(3):253–62. 2. Kuper CF, Stierum RH, Boorsma A, et al. Toxicology. 2008;246(2–3):213–21. 3. Ban M, Morel G, Langonne I, et al. Toxicology. 2006;218:39–47. 4. Sun LZ, Elsayed S, Bronstad AM, et al. Scand J Immunol. 2007;65(2):118–25. 5. Devos FC, Pollaris L, Cremer J, et al. PLOS ONE. 2017;12(7):e0180690. 6. Chen R, Zhang Q, Chen S, et al. Eur Respir J. 2019;53(4). 7. Pollaris L, Decaesteker T, Van Den Broucke S, et al. Allergy Asthma Immunol Res [Internet]. Accepted for publication. 2020. 8. Blomme EE, Provoost S, Bazzan E, et al. Eur Respir J. 2020 Jun 4. 9. Fukuyama T, Tajima Y, Ueda H, et al. Toxicol Lett. 2010;195(1):35–43. 10. Kuper CF, Heijne WH, Dansen M, et al. Toxicol Pathol.;36(7):985–98. 11. Haenen S, Vanoirbeek JA, De Vooght V, et al. J Proteome Res. 2010;9(11):5868–76. 12. Wisnewski AV, Xu L, Robinson E, et al. J Occup Med Toxicol. 2011;6:6. 13. Ruwona TB, Johnson VJ, Schmechel D, et al. Hybridoma (Larchmt).;29(3):221–9.

challenge with MDI conjugated with GSH, the major antioxidant of airway fluid, induced a greater respiratory eosinophilic inflammation than MDI respiratory challenge alone (63). This GSH-MDI conjugate can be identified in urine for up to 6 days (75).

Modulating factors

In mouse models with dermal sensitization and intranasal elicitation with TDI or persulfate salts, the effect of sensitization persisted up to 2 months as regards airway hyperresponsiveness and inflammation, and up to 3 months for the increase of serum immunoglobulins (IgE, IgG1, IgG2a) (76). In a rat model using TMA dermal sensitization, the effect of sensitization on airway susceptibility to elicitation persisted for 18–24 months (77).

The effects of causative agents in animal asthma experiments are also determined by the dissolving vehicles. This is possibly due to the irritating or lipophilic characteristics that help causative agents to penetrate the epithelium of exposed area. In an irritant-induced asthma study, mice receiving prior airway damaging agent, naphthalene, were more susceptible to the intranasal hypochlorite exposure (68). Nevertheless, co-exposure to irritants does not always aggravate the effects of causative agents. In a rat model of TMA-induced asthma, prior exposure to amorphous silica or sulfur dioxide (SO_2) did not enhance the airway hyperresponsiveness or inflammation, but even diminished those effects (78).

It remains uncertain whether chemicals with similar functional groups have cross-reactivity in asthma development. For mice receiving respiratory challenge of TDI, prior dermal exposure with toluene diamine (TDA) or MDI had no significant effects in changing airway susceptibility (79). However, in regards to mice receiving respiratory challenge with ammonium tetrachloroplatinate (ATCP), prior exposure to either ATCP or ammonium hexachloroplatinate (AHCP) enhanced airway hyperresponsiveness and eosinophilic infiltration, suggesting cross-reactivity (80).

Mechanistic findings from animal models

The typical design of mechanistic studies examining pathogenesis is to switch off/on a certain target mechanism by using animals with specific genetic background or by applying depletion agents (e.g. neutralizing antibodies), and observe whether the downstream physiologic or inflammatory responses are up- or downregulated.

Immunological determinants

Lymphocytes play crucial roles in asthma development. Mice with severe combined immunodeficiency disease (SCID), thus lacking functional lymphocytes, showed less severe airway hyperresponsiveness upon TDI exposure (81). When mice received lymph node cells from other mice having already been exposed to TDI, they showed greater airway hyperresponsiveness (82). B lymphocytes isolated from TDI treated mice showed higher antigen presenting capacity as evidenced by upregulation of costimulatory molecules. Reduced airway hyperresponsiveness upon TDI exposure was found in CD4 or CD8 knockout mice (83), or in mice receiving blocking antibodies against CD4 (84), indicating the importance of CD4[+] and CD8[+] T cell.

In addition to lymphocytes, several types of immune cells have been investigated in animal models. Depletion of neutrophils diminished airway hyperresponsiveness in mice exposed to TDI (85). Alveolar macrophages did not influence the early asthmatic response in rats exposed to TMA, but rather protected the non-specific inflammation (86).

The roles of innate immunity in asthma have been emphasized as different subtypes of dendritic cells (DCs) and innate lymphoid cells (ILCs) were identified. Group 2 ILC (ILC2) can be activated by cytokine like IL-33 and thymic stromal lymphopoietin (TSLP), and induce allergic eosinophilic inflammation (87). Elevation of IL-33 in BAL and ILC2 level in lung tissue has been observed in mice exposed to TDI (Table 4.2). Neutralization of TSLP was shown to alleviate airway inflammation induced by TDI (88). Group 3 ILC (ILC3) can induce neutrophilic inflammation. In terms of DCs, conventional type 2 DC (cDC2, typically identified by CD8a⁻CD11c^hi or CD11b⁺) and monocyte-derived DCs (moDC, typically identified by additional CD64⁺) are most relevant for Th2 cell development and attraction (89). Elevated level of moDC has been observed in mice with TDI-induced asthma (90).

Signaling pathways to inflammation

Airway inflammation is correlated with the oxidative/antioxidative process. Mice deficient in the expression of leukocyte nicotinamide adenine dinucleotide phosphate-reduced (NADPH) oxidase, an enzyme producing reactive oxygen species (ROS), failed to show airway hyperresponsiveness or inflammation to TDI exposure (84). AMP-activated protein kinase (AMPK) has been known to suppress NADPH oxidase. Upon TDI exposure, activation of AMPK alleviated the airway hyperresponsiveness and reduced the generation of ROS and Th2 related cytokines (91).

The maintenance of cell structure has become a focus in asthma animal studies, since LMW agents may alter airway epithelium. Airway epithelium of mice exposed to TDI showed abnormal distribution of E-cadherin, a transmembrane protein maintaining the cell adhesion (92). Examining the airway epithelial cells of mice exposed to TDI, researchers also found abnormal cytoplasmic retention of β-catenin, a protein maintaining the cell adhesion along with E-cadherin (93). The blockade of β-catenin activity was shown to downregulate the expression of β-catenin-targeted genes and alleviate the airway hyperresponsiveness (94). The cytoplasmic retention of β-catenin relies on signalization from the receptor for advanced glycation end products (RAGE), which is a multiligand receptor of the immunoglobulin superfamily. Inhibition of RAGE reversed the abnormal distribution of β-catenin and modified airway hyperresponsiveness induced by TDI (95).

The dysregulation of β-catenin is also dependent on the induction of phosphatidylinositol 3-kinase (PI3K), a multifunctional enzyme involving several aspects of asthma pathogenesis. PI3K inhibition restored β-catenin distribution and affected airway hyperresponsiveness to TDI (93). Besides β-catenin, PI3K also regulated NOD-like receptor protein 3 (NLRP3)/caspase-1 pathway that involved IL-1β cleavage (96). Blockade of NLRP3/caspase-1 pathway modifies airway hyperresponsiveness and inflammation due to TDI exposure (97).

Stimulation of cholinergic and sensory nerves

The vagus nerve, which regulates bronchial smooth muscle, is tightly associated with the airway hyperresponsiveness seen in asthma. The neural activation triggers irritation, neurogenic inflammation, mucus secretion, and reflex responses, with the signaling via transient receptor potential (TRP) ion channels. Different types of TRP ion channels involving cough via the vagus nerve have been identified. The two major families of TRP channels are ankyrin subtype (TRPA) and vanilloid subtype (TRPV).

TABLE 4.3 Transient Receptor Potential Ion Channels in Animal Models of Occupational Asthma

Agent	Effect	References
Trimellitic anhydride (TMA)	Exacerbates gene and protein expression of TRPA1, TRPV1, TRPV2	*1. Li, 2019*
Toluene diisocyanate (TDI)	Induces bronchial inflammation by activating TRP melastatin 8	*2. Kim, 2017*
	Suppression of airway hyperresponsiveness in TRPA1 and TRPV1 deficient mice	*3. Devos, 2016*
	Inhibition of TRPA1 and TRPV4 restores the aberrant distribution of E-cadherin and beta-catenin on cell membrane (cell contact dysfunction)	*4. Yao, 2019*
Hypochlorite and hydrogen peroxide	TRPA1 initiates Ca^{2+} influx and membrane currents in chemosensory neurons	*5. Bessac, 2008*
Formaldehyde	TRPA1 and TRPV1 inhibits airway inflammation and hyperresponsiveness as well as restores the upregulation of proinflammatory neuropeptides	*6. Wu, 2013*

References: 1. Li M, Fan X, Ji L, et al. Int Immunopharmacol. 2019;69:159–68. 2. Kim JH, Jang YS, Jang SH, et al. Exp Mol Med. 2017;49(3):e299. 3. Devos FC, Boonen B., Alpizar YA, et al. Eur Respir J. 2016;48(2):380–92. 4. Yao L, Chen S, Tang H, et al. Toxicol Sci. 2019;168(1):160–70. 5. Bessac BF, Sivula M, von Hehn CA, et al. J Clin Invest. 2008;118(5):1899–910. 6. Wu Y, You H, Ma P, et al.PLOS ONE. 2013;8(5):e62827.

Animal models have been used to study the role of different TRP ion channels upon the exposure to allergic or irritant chemicals. Some results of these studies are summarized in Table 4.3.

Asthma model using high-molecular-weight allergens

We have so far addressed some results of studies performed in animals exposed to LMW agents, mainly diisocyanates. OA due to HMW agents shares similar mechanisms with nonoccupational allergic (IgE-mediated) asthma, therefore explaining why animal studies with HMW agents have been less numerous.

Latex

Latex was a common cause of OA, although it has now become a rare condition due to much improved environmental control. Intraperitoneal sensitization of either recombinant Hevb5, a defined major latex allergen, or latex glove protein extract, followed by airway challenge, elicited antigen-specific IgE, eosinophilic pulmonary infiltration, elevated IL-5 and IL-13 in BAL, and mucus hypersecretion in airway (98). Compared with intradermal or intraperitoneal routes, the intranasal route showed relative weak sensitization effects (99).

Mouse models of latex-induced asthma were also used to search novel pharmacological treatments. Cytosine-phosphate-guanosine (CpG DNA) treatment was shown to reduce eosinophilic inflammation and Th2 cytokine level; nevertheless, it also induced higher levels of IFN-γ and hyperresponsiveness (100), suggesting that different mechanisms may exist separately in Th2/eosinophilic inflammation and airway hyperresponsiveness.

Flour dust

Baker's asthma induced by flour dust is still one of the most frequently reported respiratory diseases (see Chapter 12). Mice exposed to flour dust or extracts of flour dust showed higher neutrophilic airway inflammation, independent of the presence of toll-like receptor 4 (TLR4), indicating that the inflammation from flour dust may not be induced via endotoxin (101). Gliadins are the protein fraction containing major wheat allergens. With the B-cell epitope mapping in a mouse model, wheat gliadins were identified as targets of IgE antibodies in patients with baker's asthma and sensitized mice (102). Wheat gliadins that were modified by deamidation possessed higher water solubility and induced stronger Th2 allergic responses than native gliadins after intraperitoneal sensitization and challenge (103).

The research interests of wheat gliadins also focused on the gut-lung crosstalk. In a dust mite induced allergy model, mice receiving prior oral deaminated gliadins showed higher histamine, wheat-specific IgE, and HDM-specific IgE in serum (104). When spleen $CD4^+$ T cell from mice receiving prior oral intake of deaminated gliadins were transferred to other mice, the mice receiving transfer showed increase pulmonary resistance and a higher Th17/Treg cytokine ratio in BAL. This phenomenon was depleted in mice deficient in C-C chemokine receptor type 9 (CCR9), a receptor important for T cell gut-homing.

Detergent enzymes

Bacterial origin proteolytic enzymes, also termed as subtilisins, are important causes of detergent-induced asthma. Different endpoints, including serum antibodies, pulmonary inflammation, and airway hyperresponsiveness, have been assessed in BDF1 mice strain via intranasal exposure (105). A study using subcutaneous sensitization of mice and intranasal challenge of subtilisin indicated that the allergic responses were dependent on protease-activated receptor-2 (PAR2), a G-protein-coupled receptor, and on IL-33/ST2 coupled with MyD88 signaling pathways. In addition, mice deficient in PAR2 failed to show increased group 2 innate lymphoid cells (ILC2) in lung after subtilisin exposure (106).

Papain

Papain is a proteolytic enzyme extracted from papaya and used in the food industry. With gene knockout strategy, papain-promoted asthma via respiratory sensitization was identified as an innate inflammation dependent on IL-33, but not on T or B lymphocytes (107). The IL33/ILC2 pathway and the role of mast cells may differ depending on the mode of administration (respiratory vs. epicutaneous) (108).

ILC2-mediated inflammation from papain was shown to be stimulated by thymic stromal lymphopoietin (TSLP) via TSLP receptor (108). In a mouse model using a single intranasal exposure to papain, the signaling pathway of ILC2 via T1/ST2 (also known as interleukin 1 receptor 1, IL-1R1) was dependent on downstream MYD88 protein (109). Lung inflammation to papain is coordinated by microRNA (miRNA) in ILC2, especially miR-17-92 cluster (110).

Asthma model with nanoparticles

With the rapid advance of nanotechnology, the respiratory toxicology of nanoparticles attracts research focuses. Important nanoparticles include TiO_2, SiO_2, carbon nanotubes, as well as metals (zinc, copper, and cerium). Recently, the allergenicity of different nanoparticles has been assessed based on ovalbumin animal models, and most of these findings have been reviewed (111, 112). Nanoparticles not only aggravate preexisting asthma but also directly initiate airway allergy.

Advances have been made in studying the involvement of neuromediators, neurogenic receptors, and inflammasomes in the process of nanoparticle-induced airway hyperresponsiveness. Four neurogenic receptors lung tissue, including transient receptor potential vanilloid 1 (TRPV1), TRPV4, P2X purinoceptor 4 (P2X4), and P2X7, were augmented by inhalation of TiO_2 (113). Silica dioxide nanoparticles (SiONPs) exposure aggravated airway inflammation and mucus secretion, with the increase of NOD-like receptor pyrin domain-containing 3 (NLRP3), an inflammasome protein, and the increase of thioredoxin-interacting protein (TXNIP), an inflammatory mediator, in the lung tissue (114).

Summary and future directions of animal experimentation

Multiple advances to identify the allergenicity of causative agents through the physiological and immunological changes in animals have been realized. The occupational allergens have been tested for the induction of respiratory sensitization via different routes other than airways. It is thus worthwhile to investigate the role of carriers and antigen presenting cells binding the allergens after they enter the body. The roles of hapten-specific antibodies remained unclear for most LMW agents, thereby requiring further research.

The use of noninvasive techniques and markers is necessary to monitor the development and recovery of airway hyperresponsiveness. Apart from Th2 responses, several occupational asthmagens can induce Th17/neutrophilic inflammation or reaction via mast cells. Besides lymphocytes and granulocytes, the roles of innate lymphoid cells and dendritic cells, as well as the cell signaling and neural transmitters in the OA development, will be the focus at the next research stage.

Genetic background has been known to influence the effects of sensitization and elicitation. The advance of genomic and proteomic analyses may help to identify important mediators in the inflammatory process. These mediators may exert their influence on different steps in the process of asthma development: from the innate/adaptive immune response and the inflammatory cell recruitment to the intracellular signaling and gene regulation. The roles of these mediators upon exposure of different types of allergic or irritant asthmagens need further validation.

Role of genetics in occupational asthma

Genetic variations and their interaction with environmental factors may play a critical role in the pathogenesis of complex diseases such as asthma. Most of the variation in the genome is in the form of SNPs, which result from single base changes that substitute one nucleotide for another. SNPs that affect phenotype are referred to as "functional" variants. Most functional SNPs do not directly affect expression but rather interfere with transcriptional regulation and may influence disease susceptibility through complex interactions with other genes, host, and environmental factors.

Most genetic studies of asthma are hindered by vaguely defining phenotypes. OA is a unique asthma phenotype that can be more precisely defined by SIC testing (115). Gene-environment interactions can be evaluated as the causal agent can be identified (116). Identification of susceptibility variants could provide new opportunities for therapeutic and preventive strategies. Although many genetic association studies have been published on asthma and associated phenotypes, there is limited research on OA. The unavailability of large sample sizes needed to reach statistical significance has been a limitation of OA genetic studies. Most studies have examined associations with alleles or SNPs located on genes associated with: (1) immunoregulation (HLA class I and II genes); (2) Th1 and Th2 cytokines; (3) innate immune responses (e.g. Toll receptors, CD14); (4) antioxidant-enzymes including glutathione-S-transferases (GST), N-acetyl transferase (NAT); and (5) epithelial proteins. Characteristics of these studies are listed in Tables 4.4 and 4.5.

Associations with HLA Genes

HLA class II molecules play a role in presenting intracellularly processed peptides to CD4+ T-helper cells. These molecules are highly polymorphic and variation in their structure may determine the specific epitopes presented to T cells. Genetic studies to date have documented significant associations between OA and HLA class II as well as class I molecules.

In individual studies a greater prevalence of various HLA class I or class II genotypes were reported in workers with laboratory animal allergy versus controls, although these findings have not been replicated (117–119). The majority of published studies thus far have focused on OA induced by LMW agents (Table 4.4) (120). Bignon et al. (121) demonstrated that HLA DQB1'0503 and the allelic combination DQB1'0201/0301 were associated with susceptibility to diisocyanate asthma (DA), whereas the DQB1'0501 allele and the DQA1'0101-DQB1'0501-DR1 haplotype appeared to be protective. Mapp et al. (122) confirmed the association with HLA-DQB1'0503 and reported that the DQA1'0104 allele was increased in DA. The DA "protective" allele, HLA-DQB1'0501, was confirmed in this cohort. In another study, confirmed DA was significantly associated with aspartic acid residue at position 57 of HLA-DQB1'0503 (123). It is noteworthy that HLA allele-DA reported in European workers were not replicated in Asian workers. DRB1'15-DPB1'05 and HLA DRB1'1501-DQB1'0602-DPB1'0501 were reportedly associated with TDI-asthma in Koreans (124).

Horne et al. (125) investigated the association between HLA class II alleles and susceptibility to Western red cedar induced asthma. Workers with red cedar asthma had a higher frequency of HLA DQB1'0603 and DQB1'0302 alleles compared to asymptomatic exposed subjects. In workers exposed to acid anhydrides, the DQB1'0501 allele was more prevalent in workers with elevated serum specific IgE to anhydride antigens versus nonsensitized exposed referents (126). Protective effect of DQB1'0501 for other LMW sensitizers (isocyanates and plicatic acid) suggests differential affinities of these chemicals for specific class II molecules. Newman Taylor et al. (127) also found an excess of HLA-DR3 and a deficit of HLA-DR6 in cases with a positive SPT to ammonium hexachloroplatinate compared to controls.

Genes associated with innate immunity, Th-2 immunity, oxidative stress, and epithelial cells

In a study investigating association between toll-like receptor 4 (TLR-4) variants (TLR4/8551 and TLR4/8851) and sensitization to laboratory animal asthma, the TLR4/8551 G variant was significantly associated with atopy and laboratory animal sensitization (128). Other TLR4 variants, -2027A>G and -1608T>C, have been studied as potential risk factors for work-related respiratory

TABLE 4.4 HLA Genes Involved in Susceptibility to OA

Exposure	Sample Size (case/control)	Gene/Variant	Effect Size (OR, RR, or p)	References
Acid anhydrides	30/30	HLA-DR3	OR 6.0	*1. Young, 1995*
	52/73	HLA-DQ5	OR 4.3 (1.7–11.0)	*2. Jones, 2004*
		HLA-DQB1/*0501	OR 3.0 (1.2–7.4)	
		HLA-DQ-DR1	OR 3.0 (1.2–11.0)	
Laboratory animals	109/397	HLA-DR1/*07	OR 1.8 (1.1.–2.9)	*3. Jeal, 2003*
		HLA-DR1/*03	OR 0.5 (0.3–1.0)	
	27/0	HLA-B15 and DR4		*4. Low, 1988*
Platinum salts	44/57	HLA-DR3	OR 2.3 (1.0–5.6)	*5. Newman Taylor, 1999*
		HLA-DR6	OR 0.4 (0.2–0.8	
Red cedar	56/63	HLA-DQB1/*0302	OR 4.9 (1.3–18.6)	*6. Horne, 2000*
		HLA-DQB1/*0603	OR 2.9 (1.0–8.2)	
		HLA-DQB1/*0501	OR 0.3 (0.1–0.8)	
		HLA-DRB1/*O401 DQB1*0302	OR 10.3	
		HLA-DRB1/*0101 DQB1/*0501	OR 0.3	
Diisocyanates (TDI)	28/16	HLA-DQB1/*0503	RR 9.8	*7. Bignon, 1994*
		HLA-DQB1/*0201/ 0301	RR 9.5	
		HLA-DQB1/*0501	RR 0.1	
		HLA-DQA1/*0101 *0102	RR 0.04	
Diisocyanates (TDI)	30/126	HLA-DQB1/*0503	RR 2.9	*8. Balboni, 1996*
		HLA-DQB1/*0501	RR 0.04	
		HLA-DQB1/*0503	p = 0.009	
		HLA-DQA1/*0501	p = 0.01	
		HLA-DQA1/*0101	p = 0.004	
		HLA-DQA1/*0104	p = 0.005	
Diisocyanates (TDI)	84/127	HLA-DRB1/*1501 DQB1/*0602-DPB1/	OR 4.4 (1.5–13.1)	*9. Choi, 2009*
Diisocyanates (MDI, TDI, HDI)	73/67	HLA-E rs1573294	OR 6.3 (2.4–17)	*10. Yecesoy, 2014*
		HLA-B rs1811197,	OR 7.7 (2.3–26)	
		HLA-DOA rs3128935	OR 20 (2.9–135)	
		HLA-DQA2 rs7773955	OR 8.4 (3–23)	
Trimellitic anhydride	11/14	HLA-DR3	OR 16.0	*1. Young, 1995*

Abbreviations: OR: odd ratio; RR: relative risk.

References: 1. Young RP, et al. Am J Respir Crit Care Medicine. 1995;151:219–21. 2. Jones MG, et al. Clin Exper Allergy. 2004;34:812–6. 3. Jeal H, et al. J Allergy Clin Immunol. 2003;111:795–9. 4. Low B, et al. Tissue antigens. 1988;32:224–6. 5. Newman Taylor AJ, et al. Am J Respir Crit Care Med. 1999;160:435–8. 6. Horne C, et al. Eur Respir J. 2000;15:911–4. 7. Bignon JS, et al. Am J Respir Crit Care Med. 1994;149:71–5. 8. Balboni A, et al. Eur Respir J. 1996;9:207–10. 9. Choi JH, et al. Int Arch Allergy Immunol. 2009;150:156–63. 10. Yucesoy B, et al. J Occup Environ Med. 2014; 56(4):382–7.

symptoms and sensitization to wheat flour. Homozygotes for the -2027G and -1608C alleles exhibited a lower prevalence of work-related lower respiratory symptoms than carriers of the other genotypes (129). In a study investigating CD14 polymorphisms (-159, -1619, and -550) in laboratory animal workers, an interactive variable of cumulative endotoxin exposure and the CD14/-1619 G allele was associated with lower FEVI and FEF 25-75 (130). Homozygosity for CD14/-159T or CD14/-1619G alleles was also associated with lower lung function and wheeze among agricultural workers (131). A study showed an interaction between CD14/-260 SNP and endotoxin exposure in farmers. The carriers of the CD14/-260 C allele were found to be more susceptible to the effects of endotoxin exposure than T allele homozygotes (132).

SNPs associated with immune response genes (IL-4Rα, IL-13, and CD14) were evaluated in workers with confirmed DA. Increased frequencies of IL-4RA I50V allele and combinatorial genotypes of IL4RA (I50V), IL-13 (R110Q), and CD14 (C159T) were associated with DA in those workers exposed to HDI, suggesting an exposure-specific interaction (133, 134).

Since isocyanates are known to cause oxidative injury to respiratory epithelial cells, antioxidant defense genes have been examined in workers with DI. GSH protects epithelial cells against toxicity from isocyanates (135, 136). Piirila et al. (41) examined the

TABLE 4.5 Non-HLA Genes Involved in Susceptibility to OA

Exposure	Sample Size (Case/Control)	Gene/Variant	Effect Size (OR, p-value)	References
Laboratory	335	TLR4/8551G	OR 2.5 (1.5–5.5)	1. Pacheco, 2008
Diisocyanates (HDI)	103/115	IL-4RA(150V)II +CD14 (C159T) CT	OR 3.08 (1.2–7.6)	2. Bernstein, 2011
		IL-4RA(150V)II +IL-13(R110Q) RR + CD14 (C159T) CT	OR 3.86 (1.26–12.0)	2. Bernstein, 2011
Diisocyanates (TDI, HDI, MDI)	109/73	GSTM1 null	OR 1.9 (1.0–3.5)	3. Piirila, 2011
Diisocyanates (TDI)	109/73	NAT1 slow acetylator	OR 2.5 (1.3–4.9)	4. Wikman, 2002
Diisocyanates	90/102	NAT2 rs4271002	OR 2.77 (1.45, 5.30)	5 Yucesoy, 2015
Diisocyanates (TDI)	92/39	GSTP1 Val/Val	OR 0.2 (0.1–1.1)	6. Mapp, 2002
Diisocyanates (TDI)	84/263 GWAS	CTNNA3/rs 10762058	OR 4.9 (2.3–10.5)	7. Kim, 2009
		CTNNA3/rs 7088181	OR 4.9 (2.3–10.6)	
		CTNNA3/rs 4378283	OR 4.4 (2.1–9.2)	
Diisocyanates	74/824 GWAS	HERC2 rs12913832	$p = 6.9 \times 10^{-14}$	8. Yucesoy, 2015
		ODZ3 rs908084	$p = 8.6 \times 10^{-9}$	
Diisocyanates (TDI)	103/60	ADR/Arg16Gly A>G Leu134Leu G>A + Arg175 Arg C>A	OR 15.4 (1.81–131.1)	9. Ye, 2010
Diisocyanates	132/147 exposed asymptomatic/132 exposed negative challenges	CTNNA3 alpha catenin rs7088181	OR 9.05 (1.69–48.54) vs. asymptomatic workers	10. Bernstein, 2012
		CTNNA3 alpha catenin rs10762058	OR 6.82 (1.65–28.24) vs. vs. asymptomatic workers	
Diisocyanates	95/116 exposed symptomatic negative challenges/142 exposed asymptomatic	SOD2		11. Yucesoy, 2012
		rs4880	p = 0.004	
		GSTM1 (null)	p = 0.047	
		GSTP1		
		rs762803	p = 0.021	
		EPHX1		
		rs2854450 + various genotype combinations	p < 0.001	
Diisocyanates	95/142 asymptomatic exposed	PTGS1 rs5788	OR = 0.38 (0.17–0.89)	12. Yucesoy, 2016
		TGFB1 rs1800469	OR = 0.38 (0.18–0.74)	
		TNF rs1800629	OR = 2.08 (1.03–4.17)	
		PTGS2 rs20417	OR = 6.40 (1.06–38.75)	
Low-molecular weight agents + irritants	2539 adults in 3 European cohorts	PLA2G4A rs932476	p < 0.005	13. Rava, 2017
		near PLA2R1 rs26667026	p < 0.005	
		near RELA rs931127	p < 0.005	
		PRKD1 rs1958980 + rs11847351 + rs1958987	p < 0.005	

		PRKCA rs6504453	p < 0.005	
Diisocyanates (TDI, HDI, MDI)	91 OA 238 unexposed controls	130 risk variants significantly associated with OA; 5 regulatory nucleotide polymorphisms, 3 with luciferase reporter activity	p ≤ 0.05	*14. Bernstein, 2018*
Wheat flour	381	TLR4/-2727/GG	OR 0.163 (0.04–0.73)	*15. Cho, 2011*
	379	ADRB2/GAA Haplotype of 46A>G 252 G>A + 523 C>A	p < 0.05	*16. Hur, 2011*

Abbreviations: GWAS: genome-wide association study; OR: odd ratio.

References: **1.** Pacheco K, et al. *J Allergy Clin Immunol.* 2008;122:896–902. **2.** Bernstein DI, et al. *J Allergy Clin Immunol.* 2011;128:418–20. **3.** Piirila P, et al. *Pharmacogenetics.* 2001;11:437–45. **4.** Wikman et al. 2002;12:227–33. **5.** Yucesoy B, et al. *J Occup Environ Med.* 2015;57(12):1331–6. **6.** Mapp CE, et al. *J Allergy Clin Immunol.* 2002;109:867–72. **7.** Kim SH, et al. *Clin Exp Allergy.* 2009;39:203–12. **8.** Yucesoy B, et al. *Toxicol Sci.* 2015 Jul;146(1):192–201. **9.** Ye YM, et al. *Allergy Asthma Immunol Res.* 2010;2(4):260–6. **10.** Bernstein DI, et al. *Toxicol Sci.* 2012;131:242–6. **11.** Yucesoy B, et al. *Toxicol Sci.* 2012;129:166–73. **12.** Yucesoy B, et al. *J Immunotoxicol.* 2016;13:119–26. **13.** Rava M, et al. *Environ Health Perspect.* 2017;125:207–14. **14.** Bernstein DI, et al. *J Allergy Clin Immunol.* 2018;142(3):959–69. **15.** Cho HJ, et al. *Ann Allergy Asthma Immunol.* 2011;107:57–64. **16.** Hur GY, et al. *Yonsei Med J.* 2011;52(3):488–94.

polymorphisms of the GSH S-transferase (GST) genes (GSTM1, GSTM3, GSTP1, and GSTT1) in workers with DA. GSTM1 null genotype was associated with an increased risk of DA. Mapp et al. (137) reported a lower frequency of the GSTP1 Ile105Val Val/Val genotype in subjects with TDI-asthma and AHR. In another study, the N-acetyltransferase (NAT1) slow acetylator genotype was found to be associated with an increased risk of DA (OR, 2.5; 95% CI, 1.32–4.91). The risk of DA was higher among workers exposed to TDI (OR, 7.8; 95% CI, 1.18–51.6), suggesting an exposure-specific association (138).

Genome-wide association studies (GWAS) offer a powerful approach to scan the entire genome for disease associated SNPs. In a GWAS conducted in Korean workers with DA, significant associations were reported between catenin alpha 3 (CTNNA3) polymorphisms (rs10762058, rs7088181, rs4378283, and rs1786929) and TDI-asthma (139). CTNNA3 proteins play an important role in cell-cell adhesion thereby having potential to impact the effects of TDI exposure on airway epithelial cells. A GWAS study performed in Caucasian workers with confirmed DA did not confirm the findings (i.e. CTNNA3 SNPs) in the Korean study but did identify 11 OA-associated SNPs exceeding genome-wide significance ($p < 5×10^{-8}$) (140). Next-generation sequencing (NGS) was performed in 91 DA cases of 14 loci containing DA-associated SNPs identified in the GWAS. NGS and bioinformatic analysis was used to detect and prioritize 21 DA-associated SNPs; four of these SNPs located on ATF, CDH17, TACR1, and FAM71A exhibited functional effects on gene regulation (141).

Pathophysiology

Clinical, functional, and pathological alterations in OA share many similarities with those found in non-OA (142) this being irrespective of whether OA is caused by HMW, LMW, or workplace irritants. Respiratory symptoms (i.e. recurrent episodes of cough, wheeze, shortness of breath, and chest tightness) are suggestive of OA when temporally related to workplace exposure (143). The episodes are usually associated with variable airflow limitation that is often reversible, either spontaneously or with treatment. Nonspecific bronchial hyperresponsiveness (NSBH), which is an excessive reaction to bronchoconstrictor stimuli, is the hallmark of both occupational and non-OA. The pathologic alterations of the airways in OA are characterized by infiltration of the airway mucosa by inflammatory cells, including eosinophils, mast cells, and activated lymphocytes. Subepithelial fibrosis, which is another specific histologic feature of asthma, is also observed in OA. The relationship between these pathologic alterations and the clinical and functional features of asthma is only partially understood.

Airflow limitation

Airway smooth muscle contraction and mucosal edema are probably the main causes of acute airflow obstruction during immediate asthmatic reactions, whereas late asthmatic reactions are also associated with the accumulation of inflammatory cells and exudate in the airway walls and lumen. The relative proportion of airflow obstruction due to each mechanism remains to be established.

Airflow limitation upon specific inhalation challenge

Various temporal patterns of asthmatic reactions can occur after controlled exposure to the offending agent, including typical (immediate, late, and dual) and atypical (progressive, square waved, and prolonged immediate) reactions. Late asthmatic responses occur more frequently with specific inhalation challenge (SIC) to LMW agents. This may be a consequence of the single-dose challenge protocol that is commonly used, or of the intensity and type of inflammatory response induced by these agents (144). The degree of NSBH is the best variable for predicting the fall of FEV1 during a SIC regardless of whether the patient is exposed to HMW or LMW agents, or whether the reaction occurs early or late during SIC (145).

Airflow limitation under workplace exposure

Airflow limitation in the workplace can be monitored by serial measurements of PEF. Temporal patterns that resemble those occurring after SIC can be identified. However, the pattern of airflow limitation may be complex and may not involve merely immediate and/or late reactions. PEF deterioration may occur each day of exposure and return to baseline values before the next work shift. Progressive daily deterioration with repeated exposures has also been observed. Continuous low PEF values may develop on repeated exposure, with a slow recovery that can take several days after cessation of exposure.

Accelerated FEV1 declines have been demonstrated in general population studies of subjects with asthma (146). It is well established that persistence of work exposure to causal agents is associated with increased loss of lung function in subjects with OA (147) and that this loss of FEV1 is more marked in patients exposed to HMW agents (115). Whether subjects with OA continue to exhibit an accelerated decline in FEV1 after cessation of exposure is more controversial. Some studies do not find a decline (148, 149), while others do (150, 151).

Airway hyperresponsiveness

NSBH can be tested with either a direct-acting stimulus, such as methacholine, or indirectly by physical or pharmacological stimuli (e.g. mannitol).

Nonspecific bronchial hyperresponsiveness upon SIC

NSBH increases after a positive SIC with a sensitizing agent, particularly in subjects who develop a late asthmatic reaction (152). Clinical investigations indicate that the increase in NSBH may begin as early as two hours after challenge with either HMW or LMW sensitizing agents (153, 154). The increase in NSBH induced by sensitizing agents may last for days or even longer (152). Although some authors attribute the increase in NSBH to an acute inflammatory reaction (155), other studies have reported a lack of correlation between NSBH and the inflammatory reaction, NSBH lasting for many years (156).

Nonspecific bronchial hyperresponsiveness upon workplace exposure

In subjects with OA, the degree of NSBH to methacholine or histamine is usually, but not invariably, increased. The proportion of subjects with OA who have normal NSBH in a large cohort ($n = 129$) of OA was 27% (157). However, a number of studies have shown that NSBH may improve rapidly and even return to normal, sometimes within a few days, after cessation of exposure to the offending agent and may recur on reexposure (158). Pralong et al. (159) demonstrated in a retrospective large cohort (n = 1012) that 98% of patients with OA show NSBH while at work. NSBH present during the asymptomatic stage of OA seems to be long lasting and only partly reversible or irreversible even after treatment (150, 160). The pathogenesis of this long-lasting, poorly reversible NSBH in OA remains unknown.

Airway inflammation

Airway inflammation in all variants of asthma is thought to sustain NSBH and other sequelae, which result in limitation in airway caliber. The pathology of workers who died as a direct consequence of OA was remarkably similar to postmortem changes of non-OA. In two fatal cases caused by diisocyanate and powdered shark cartilage, there was thickening of collagen beneath the true basement membrane, massive infiltration of inflammatory cells, particularly eosinophils. In addition, the lungs showed edematous airways plugged by mucoid material with numerous eosinophils (161).

Airway inflammation upon SIC

Bronchoalveolar lavage studies

Bronchoalveolar lavage (BAL) samples obtained during various time intervals after asthmatic reactions induced by HMW or LMW agents demonstrated a significant increase of neutrophils and/or eosinophils upon exposure to flour (162), TDI (163), and plicatic acid (164), respectively. Leukotrienes, histamine, and tryptase were also detected in BAL fluid after early asthmatic reactions induced by occupational agents (162, 164), while eosinophil cationic protein (ECP) was identified during late asthmatic reactions in bakers sensitized to flour (162).

Induced sputum studies

There is fairly good agreement between the eosinophil count in induced sputum and in bronchial biopsies (165). At 8 and 24 hours after inhalation challenge with diisocyanates, Maestrelli et al. (166) reported sputum eosinophilia in patients with early and late reactions (Figure 4.1). Several subsequent studies confirmed the eosinophilic airway response in OA induced by both HMW and LMW occupational agents (115). In addition, Lemiere et al. observed that eosinophils, eotaxin, and IL-5 were detectable in induced sputum after SIC when concentrations of the causal agents were unable to elicit changes in functional parameters (FEV1 and PC20) (167). These findings were more pronounced after exposure to LMW agents than to HMW agents.

Neutrophilic airway inflammation in OA is less common and is presumably explained by interfering factors unrelated to the pathophysiology of the disease: treatment with corticosteroids, endotoxin contamination, and relatively high levels of exposure

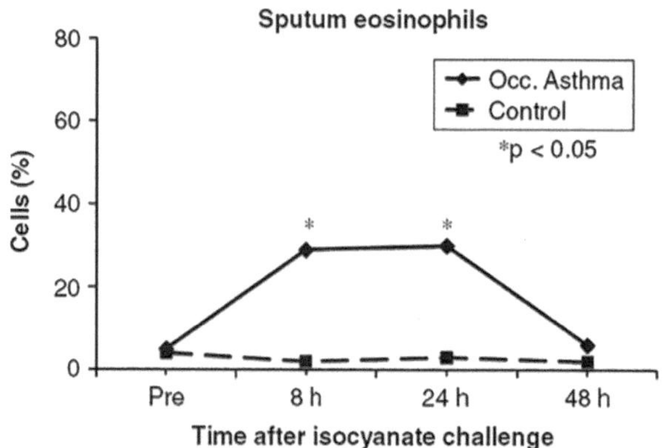

FIGURE 4.1 Time course of eosinophilic inflammation of the airways induced by exposure to isocyanates. Eosinophils were quantified in induced sputum before and 8, 24, and 48 hours after specific inhalation challenge in the laboratory in subjects with occupational asthma and control subjects not exposed previously to isocyanates. (From Maestrelli P, Yucesoy B, Park HS, Wisnewski AV. Mechanisms, genetics and pathophysiology. In: Malo JL, Chan-Yeung M, Bernstein DI. *Asthma in the Workplace.* 4th ed. Boca Raton: CRC Press; 2013. Data from Maestrelli P, et al. Sputum eosinophilia after asthmatic responses induced by isocyanates in sensitized subjects. *Clin Exp Allergy.* 1994;24:29–34.)

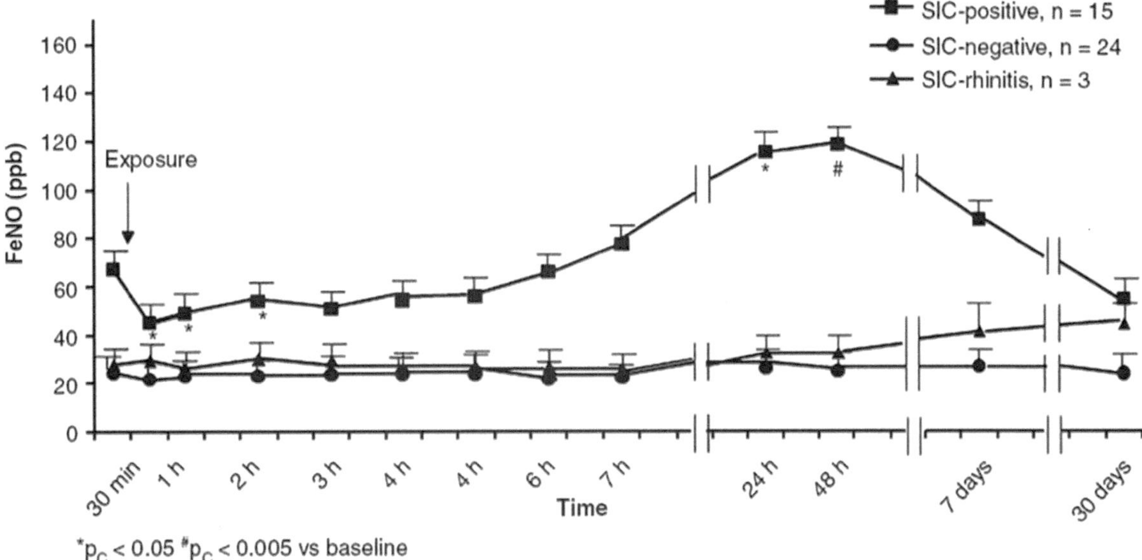

FIGURE 4.2 Time course of FeNO after SIC with isocyanates in sensitized subjects (SIC positive; $n = 15$), nonsensitized subjects (SIC negative; $n = 24$), and sensitized subjects with rhinitic responses only (SIC rhinitis; $n = 3$). Data are presented as the geometric mean $\pm$ SE; p_c = values corrected for multiple comparisons; *Abbreviations*: FeNO, fractional exhaled nitric oxide; ppb, parts per billion; SIC, specific inhalation challenge. (Data from Ferrazzoni S, et al. Exhaled nitric oxide and breath condensate pH in asthmatic reactions induced by isocyanates. *Chest.* 2009;136:155–62. With permission.)

to reactive chemicals able to produce irritant effects. However, in the case of diisocyanates, a preponderant neutrophil response has been elicited (168).

Exhaled nitric oxide (FeNO)

Nitric oxide (NO) is produced in the respiratory tract by activation of NO synthase in various cell types and is considered a biomarker of eosinophilic airway inflammation. Initial studies examining the usefulness of FeNO in the investigation of OA gave inconsistent results (169). A study showed that isocyanate-induced asthmatic reactions were associated with a consistent increase in FeNO, which was maximal at 48 hours post exposure, while FeNO did not vary with isocyanate exposure in workers with occupational rhinitis or in nonsensitized subjects (Figure 4.2) (170). More recent investigations established that subjects with OA caused by HMW agents showed a greater increase in post-SIC FeNO as compared to subjects with OA due to LMW agents (115). A large European, multicenter, retrospective cohort of subjects with OA showed that postchallenge FeNO increase was higher in acrylate- and isocyanate-induced OA, than in OA induced by other LMW agents (171). Several issues should be considered when interpreting studies of FeNO induction by SIC with occupational agents. One is the duration of patient monitoring as maximum increase in FeNO occurred 24–48 hours after SIC. Second, corticosteroids, which inhibit NO synthase, may blunt FeNO responses if administered at the time of investigation. Finally, an increase of NO production might have been underestimated, when FeNO is measured in the presence of bronchoconstriction (172).

Airway inflammation in sensitized subjects

Quantitative analysis of bronchial biopsies from patients with OA induced by TDI showed an increased number of inflammatory cells compared to biopsies of normal control subjects (Figure 4.3) (173). Eosinophils were increased in mucosal and

submucosal layers, while mast cells were increased only in the epithelium. Both eosinophils and lymphocytes showed evidence of activation. Biopsy specimens also revealed that the thickness of the subepithelial reticular layer was increased (Figure 4.3). This phenomenon is due to the deposition of interstitial cross-linked collagens (types I, III, and IV) produced by myofibroblasts and not of collagen IV, which is one of the specific components of the "true" basement membrane. This

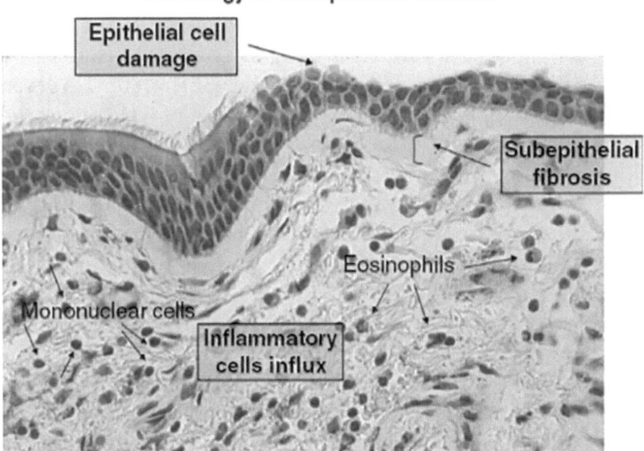

FIGURE 4.3 Light micrograph of bronchial biopsy from a patient with occupational asthma induced by toluene diisocyanate showing characteristic pathologic features. (From Maestrelli P, Yucesoy B, Park HS, Wisnewski AV. Mechanisms, genetics and pathophysiology. In: Malo JL, Chan-Yeung M, Bernstein DI. *Asthma in the Workplace.* 4th ed. Boca Raton: CRC Press; 2013.)

observation has been made both in non-OA and OA including OA caused by Western red cedar.

Somewhat different findings were obtained in biopsies from subjects who developed OA after acute exposure to irritants: the airway epithelium was extensively damaged, the submucosa was infiltrated predominantly by mononuclear cells, and, more importantly, the basement membrane thickness was more evident with values up to 20–30 μm (174) compared to 6–15 μm reported in isocyanate asthma and 3–8 μm in normal subjects (22, 175). However, bronchial biopsies taken 4–20 years after the acute exposure revealed the persistence of pathologic changes consistent with asthma, characterized by eosinophilic inflammation and subepithelial fibrosis (176). In potroom OA, associated with repeated irritant exposures to fume in the aluminium industry, nonsmoking asthmatics had higher density of regulatory T cells (Treg) and activated effector T cells in bronchial submucosa (177). These findings suggest an immune modulation by a functional balance between regulatory and effector T cell systems in this type of asthma.

Cessation of exposure was associated with some improvement at the histologic level, as suggested by a decrease of the number of inflammatory cells in the airway mucosa, and reversal of the subepithelial fibrosis present at the time of diagnosis (22). Interestingly, the decrease in thickness of the subepithelial reticular layer was also associated with a decrease in the number of fibroblasts in the submucosa. However, airway inflammation was still present in subjects with OA after cessation of exposure in a large follow-up study of 133 subjects with a mean period of follow-up of 8.7 years (178). The persistence of NSBH, found in 73% of subjects, was associated with more eosinophils and neutrophils in sputum.

Changes in sputum eosinophil counts (Chapter 7) are satisfactory predictors of a positive SIC to occupational agents. A >2% increase in sputum eosinophil counts at work, compared with away from work, led to a diagnostic sensitivity of 52% and specificity of 80%. The addition of work-related changes in eosinophil counts to serial PEF measurements increased the specificity of the latter by 27% when using an eosinophil threshold increase of >2%; the sensitivity, however, was not significantly changed (179).

The relationship between FeNO and workplace exposure (Chapter 7) has been variable in different studies. Baseline FeNO measurement has less sensitivity than NSBH (180). However, combining a FeNO ≥25 ppb to the presence of AHR increased the sensitivity from 87% to 91% in predicting a positive SIC (180). The diagnostic value of serial measurements of FeNO at and away from work in predicting OA has not been sufficiently investigated, although some reports suggest that they may give some complementary information (181, 182).

Future research directions

Although mechanisms underlying OA caused by large protein allergens is well understood, the pathogenesis of OA caused by LMW agents is uncertain. Apart from Th2 responses, understanding alternate immune pathways relevant to OA is an unmet need that can be addressed using experimental models. This could include defining the impact of causative chemicals (and protein allergens) on generation of innate immune responses in the respiratory epithelium. As with non-OA, it is important to understand if such exposures generate regulatory cytokines (e.g. TSLP, IL-25) from epithelial cells leading to enhancement of type 2 inflammation (i.e. mast cells, eosinophils) via adaptive Th2 and/or innate lymphoid cells (ILC2). Non-type 2 inflammatory pathways via generation of other regulatory cytokines (e.g. IL-33 or IL-6) could be investigated to better understand neutrophilic airway inflammation in OA (183).

Future research may also focus on roles of dendritic cells, cell signaling, and neural transmitters in the pathogenesis of OA.

Human genetic studies of OA are empowered by the ability to precisely define a specific phenotype via SIC testing, unlike many other asthma phenotypes. Such studies of workers with confirmed OA employing GWAS, NGS, and bioinformatic analysis of big datasets could assist in finding variant SNPs that bind transcription factors or have direct functional effects on gene expression. Such discoveries could better define underlying disease mechanisms and lead to identification of novel disease biomarkers or high-risk genotypes for poorly understood forms of OA (e.g. diisocyanate asthma). Many clinical, genetic, and mechanistic studies of workers with specific OA phenotypes are limited by the small numbers of workers with confirmed OA. Now and in the future, these can only be accomplished via multicenter, international collaborative efforts.

References

1. Maestrelli P, Boschetto P, Fabbri LM, et al. Mechanisms of occupational asthma. J Allergy Clin Immunol. 2009;123:531–42.
2. Palikhe NS, Kim JH, Park HS. Biomarkers predicting isocyanate-induced asthma. Allergy Asthma Immunol Res. 2011;3:21–6.
3. Kimber I, Dearman RJ, Basketter DA. Diisocyanates, occupational asthma and IgE antibody: implications for hazard characterization. J Appl Toxicol. 2014;34(10):1073–7.
4. Holgate ST, Roberts G, Arshad HS, et al. The role of the airway epithelium and its interaction with environmental factors in asthma pathogenesis. Proc Am Thorac Soc. 2009;6(8):655–9.
5. Kubo A, Nagao K, Amagai M. Epidermal barrier dysfunction and cutaneous sensitization in atopic diseases. J Clin Invest. 2012;122(2):440–7.
6. Lummus ZL, Alam R, Bernstein JA, et al. Diisocyanate antigen-enhanced production of monocyte chemoattractant protein-1, IL-8, and tumor necrosis factor by peripheral monocuclear cells of workers with occupational asthma. J Allergy Clin Immunol. 1998;102:265–74.
7. Wisnewski AV, Liu Q, Liu J, et al. Human innate immune responses to hexamethylene diisocyanate (HDI) and HDI-albumin conjugates. Clin Exp Allergy. 2008;38(6):957–67.
8. Verstraelen S, Wens B, Hooyberghs J, et al. Gene expression profiling of in vitro cultured macrophages after exposure to the respiratory sensitizer hexamethylene diisocyanate. Toxicol In Vitro. 2008;22(4):1107–14.
9. Choi JH, Suh YJ, Lee SK, et al. Acute and chronic changes of vascular endothelial growth factor (VEGF) in induced sputum of toluene diisocyanate (TDI)-induced asthma patients. J Korean Med Sci. 2004;19(3):359–63.
10. Kim JH, Kim JE, Choi GS, et al. Serum cytokines markers in toluene diisocyanate-induced asthma. Respir Med. 2011;105:1091–4.
11. Vandenplas O, Wiszniewska M, Raulf M, et al. EAACI position paper: irritant-induced asthma. Allergy. 2014;69:1141–53.
12. Dumas O, Le Moual N. Do chronic workplace irritant exposures cause asthma? Curr Opin Allergy Clin Immunol. 2016;16(2):75–85.
13. Zahm JM, Chevillard M, Puchelle E. Wound repair of human surface respiratory epithelium. Am J Respir Cell Mol Biol. 1991;5(3):242–8.
14. Hoshino M, Takahashi M, Aoike N. Expression of vascular endothelial growth factor, basic fibroblast growth factor, and angiogenin immunoreactivity in asthmatic airways and its relationship to angiogenesis. J Allergy Clin Immunol. 2001;107(2):295–301.
15. Vignola AM, Chanez P, Chiappara G, et al. Transforming growth factor-B expression in mucosal biopsies in asthma and chronic bronchitis. Am J Respir Crit Care Med. 1997;156:591–9.
16. Choi Y, Lee Y, Park HS. Neutrophil activation in occupational asthma. Curr Opin Allergy Clin Immunol. 2019;19:81–5.
17. Wooding DJ, Ryu MH, Li H, et al. Acute air pollution exposure alters neutrophils in never-smokers and at-risk humans. Eur Respir J. 2020;55(4).
18. Hussain S, Vanoirbeek JA, Hoet PH. Interactions of nanomaterials with the immune system. Wiley Interdiscip Rev Nanomed Nanobiotechnol. 2012;4(2):169–83.

19. Holgate ST. Epithelium dysfunction in asthma. J Allergy Clin Immunol. 2007;120(6):1233–44; quiz 45-6.

20. Bougault V, Loubaki L, Joubert P, et al. Airway remodeling and inflammation in competitive swimmers training in indoor chlorinated swimming pools. J Allergy Clin Immunol. 2012;129(2):351–8, 8.e1.

21. Montefort S, Roberts JA, Beasley R, et al. The site of disruption of the bronchial epithelium in asthmatic and non-asthmatic subjects. Thorax. 1992;47:499–503.

22. Saetta M, Maestrilli P, Turato G, et al. Airway wall remodeling after cessation of exposure to isocyanates in sensitized asthmatic subjects. Am J Respir Crit Care Med. 1995;151:489–94.

23. O'Byrne PM. Leukotrienes in the pathogenesis of asthma. Chest. 1997;111:27S–34S.

24. Barbato A, Turato G, Baraldo S, et al. Epithelial damage and angiogenesis in the airways of children with asthma. Am J Respir Crit Care Med. 2006;174(9):975–81.

25. Dozor AJ. The role of oxidative stress in the pathogenesis and treatment of asthma. Ann N Y Acad Sci. 2010;1203:133–7.

26. Garcia-Larsen V, Chinn S, Rodrigo R, et al. Relationship between oxidative stress-related biomarkers and antioxidant status with asthma and atopy in young adults: a population-based study. Clin Exp Allergy. 2009;39(3):379–86.

27. Mishra V, Banga J, Silveyra P. Oxidative stress and cellular pathways of asthma and inflammation: therapeutic strategies and pharmacological targets. Pharmacol Ther. 2018;181:169–82.

28. Ma Q. Role of nrf2 in oxidative stress and toxicity. Annu Rev Pharmacol Toxicol. 2013;53:401–26.

29. Liu T, Zhang L, Joo D, et al. NF-κB signaling in inflammation. Signal Transduct Target Ther. 2017;2:17023.

30. Aguilera-Aguirre L, Bacsi A, Saavedra-Molina A, et al. Mitochondrial dysfunction increases allergic airway inflammation. J Immunol. 2009;183(8):5379–87.

31. Hosseini A, Hirota JA, Tillie L, et al. Morphometric analysis of inflammation in bronchial biopsies following exposure to inhaled diesel exhaust and allergen challenge in atopic subjects. Part Fibre Toxicol. 2016;13(2).

32. Dumas O, Wiley AS, Quinot C, et al. Occupational exposure to disinfectants and asthma control in US nurses. Eur Respir J. 2017;50:1700237.

33. Eom HJ, Choi J. Oxidative stress of CeO2 nanoparticles via p38-Nrf-2 signaling pathway in human bronchial epithelial cell, Beas-2B. Toxicol Lett. 2009;187:77–83.

34. Shadab M, Agrawal DK, Aslam M, et al. Occupational health hazards among sewage workers: oxidative stress and deranged lung functions. J Clin Diagn Res. 2014;8(4):Bc11–2.

35. Hur GY, Choi GS, Sheen SS, et al. Serum ferritin and transferrin levels as serologic markers of methylene diphenyl diisocyanate-induced occupational asthma. J Allergy Clin Immunol. 2008;122(4):774–80.

36. Shin YS, Kim MA, Pham LD, et al. Cells and mediators in diisocyanate-induced occupational asthma. Curr Opin Allergy Clin Immunol. 2013;13(2):125–31.

37. Fitzpatrick AM, Teague WG, Holguin F, et al. Airway glutathione homeostasis is altered in children with severe asthma: evidence for oxidant stress. J Allergy Clin Immunol. 2009;123(1):146–52.e8.

38. Wisnewski AV, Hettick JM, Siegel PD. Toluene diisocyanate reactivity with glutathione across a vapor/liquid interface and subsequent transcarbamoylation of human albumin. Chem Res Toxicol. 2011;24:1686–93.

39. Koike Y, Hisada T, Utsugi M, et al. Glutathione redox regulates airway hyperresponsiveness and airway inflammation in mice. Am J Respir Cell Mol Biol. 2007;37(3):322–9.

40. Biswas SK, Rahman I. Environmental toxicity, redox signaling and lung inflammation: the role of glutathione. Mol Aspects Med. 2009;30:60–76.

41. Piirila P, Wikman H, Luukkonen R, et al. Glutathione S-transferase genotypes and allergic responses to diisocyanate exposure. Pharmacogenetics. 2001;11:437–45.

42. Nadel JA. Neutral endopeptidase modulates neurogenic inflammation. Eur Respir J. 1991;4:745–54.

43. Ye YM, Kang YM, Kim SH, et al. Relationship between neurokinin 2 receptor gene polymorphisms and serum vascular endothelial growth factor levels in patients with toluene diisocyanate-induced asthma. Clin Exp Allergy. 2006;36(9):1153–60.

44. Bessac BF, Jordt SE. Sensory detection and responses to toxic gases: mechanisms, health effects, and countermeasures. Proc Am Thor Soc. 2010;7:269–77.

45. Caceres AI, Brackmann M, Elia MD, et al. A sensory neuronal ion channel essential for airway inflammation and hyperreactivity in asthma. Proc Natl Acad Sci USA. 2009;106(22):9099–104.

46. Geppetti P, Patacchini R, Nassini R. Transient receptor potential channels and occupational exposure. Curr Opin Allergy Clin Immunol. 2014;14(2):77–83.

47. Kim JH, Jang YS, Jang SH, et al. Toluene diisocyanate exposure induces airway inflammation of bronchial epithelial cells via the activation of transient receptor potential melastatin 8. Exp Mol Med. 2017;49(3):e299.

48. Smit LA, Kogevinas M, Anto JM, et al. Transient receptor potential genes, smoking, occupational exposures and cough in adults. Respir Res. 2012;13:26.

49. Barnes PJ. Airway neuropeptides and their role in asthma. In: Holgate ST, Busse WW, eds. Inflammatory Mechanisms in Asthma. Marcel Dekker. 1998; Chapter 24.

50. Sagar S, Akbarshahi H, Uller L. Translational value of animal models of asthma: challenges and promises. Eur J Pharmacol. 2015;759:272–7.

51. Aun MV, Bonamichi-Santos R, Arantes-Costa FM, et al. Animal models of asthma: utility and limitations. J Asthma Allergy. 2017;10:293–301.

52. de Vooght V, Vanoirbeek JA, Luyts K, et al. Choice of mouse strain influences the outcome in a mouse model of chemical-induced asthma. PLOS ONE. 2010;5(9):e12581.

53. Nishino R, Fukuyama T, Watanabe Y, et al. Effect of mouse strain in a model of chemical-induced respiratory allergy. Exp Anim. 2014;63(4):435–45.

54. Nishino R, Fukuyama T, Watanabe Y, et al. Detection of respiratory allergies caused by environmental chemical allergen via measures of hyperactivation and degranulation of mast cells in lungs of NC/Nga mice. J Immunotoxicol. 2016;13(5):676–85.

55. Nishino R, Fukuyama T, Watanabe Y, et al. Significant upregulation of cytokine secretion from T helper type 9 and 17 cells in a NC/Nga mouse model of ambient chemical exposure-induced respiratory allergy. J Pharmacol Toxicol Methods. 2016;80:35–42.

56. Russjan E, Kaczyńska K. Murine models of hapten-induced asthma. Toxicology. 2018;410:41–8.

57. Tsui HC, Ronsmans S, De Sadeleer LJ, et al. Skin exposure contributes to chemical-induced asthma: what is the evidence? A systematic review of animal models. Allergy Asthma Immunol Res. 2020;12(4):579–98.

58. Southam DS, Dolovich M, O'Byrne PM, et al. Distribution of intranasal instillations in mice: effects of volume, time, body position, and anesthesia. Am J Physiol Lung Cell Mol Physiol. 2002;282:L833–9.

59. de Vooght V, Vanoirbeek JA, Haenen S, et al. Oropharyngeal aspiration: an alternative route for challenging in a mouse model of chemical-induced asthma. Toxicology. 2009;259(1-2):84–9.

60. Pauluhn J, Poole A. Brown Norway rat asthma model of diphenylmethane-4,4'-diisocyanate (MDI): determination of the elicitation threshold concentration of after inhalation sensitization. Toxicology. 2011;281:15–24.

61. Schupp T, Collins MA. Toluene diisocyanate (TDI) airway effects and dose-responses in different animal models. EXCLI J. 2012;11:416–35.

62. Vanoirbeek JA, Tarkowski M, Ceuppens JL, et al. Respiratory response to toluene diisocyanate depends on prior frequency and concentration of dermal sensitization in mice. Toxicol Sci. 2004;80:310–21.

63. Wisnewski AV, Xu L, Robinson E, et al. Immune sensitization to methylene diphenyl diisocyanate (MDI) resulting from skin exposure: albumin as a carrier protein connecting skin exposure to subsequent respiratory responses. J Occup Med Toxicol. 2011;6:6.

64. Vanoirbeek JA, de Vooght V, Nemery B, et al. Multiple challenges in a mouse model of chemical-induced asthma lead to tolerance: ventilatory and inflammatory responses are blunted, immunologic humoral responses are not. Toxicology. 2009;257:144–52.

65. Devos FC, Maaske A, Robichaud A, et al. Forced expiration measurements in mouse models of obstructive and restrictive lung diseases. Respir Res. 2017;18(1):123.

66. Frazer DG, Reynolds JS, Jackson MC. Determining when enhanced pause (Penh) is sensitive to changes in specific airway resistance. J Toxicol Environ Health A. 2011;74:287–95.

67. Liu F, Li W, Pauluhn J, et al. Rat models of acute lung injury: exhaled nitric oxide as a sensitive, noninvasive real-time biomarker of prognosis and efficacy of intervention. Toxicology. 2013;310:104–14.

68. Van Den Broucke S, Pollaris L, Vande Velde G, et al. Irritant-induced asthma to hypochlorite in mice due to impairment of the airway barrier. Arch Toxicol. 2018;92(4):1551–61.

69. Henjakovic M, Martin C, Hoymann HG, et al. Ex vivo lung function measurements in precision-cut lung slices (PCLS) from chemical allergen-sensitized mice represent a suitable alternative to in vivo studies. Toxicol Sci. 2008;106(2):444–53.

70. Kuper CF, Heijne WH, Dansen M, et al. Molecular characterization of trimellitic anhydride-induced respiratory allergy in Brown Norway rats. Toxicol Pathol. 2008;36(7):985–98.

71. Wisnewski AV, Liu J, Redlich CA. Analysis of lung gene expression reveals a role for Cl- channels in diisocyanate induced airway eosinophilia in a mouse model of asthma pathology. Am J Respir Cell Mol Biol. 2020 February 26.

72. Lin CC, Law BF, Hettick JM. Acute 4,4'-methylene diphenyl diisocyanate exposure-mediated downregulation of miR-206-3p and miR-381-3p activates inducible nitric oxide synthase transcription by targeting calcineurin/NFAT signaling in macrophages. Toxicol Sci. 2020;173(1):100–13.

73. Vanoirbeek JA, Tarkowski M, Vanhooren HM, et al. Validation of a mouse model of chemical-induced asthma using trimellitic anhydride, a respiratory sensitizer, and dinitrochlorobenzene, a dermal sensitizer. J Allergy Clin Immunol. 2006;117(5):1090–7.

74. Kuper CF, Radonjic M, van Triel J, et al. Oxazolone (OXA) is a respiratory allergen in Brown Norway rats. Toxicology. 2011;290(1):59–68.

75. Wisnewski AV, Nassar AF, Liu J, et al. Dilysine-methylene diphenyl diisocyanate (MDI), a urine biomarker of MDI exposure? Chem Res Toxicol. 2019;32(4):557–65.

76. Cruz MJ, Olle-Monge M, Vanoirbeek JA, et al. Persistence of respiratory and inflammatory responses after dermal sensitization to persulfate salts in a mouse model of non-atopic asthma. Allergy Asthma Clin Immunol. 2016;12:26.

77. Zhang XD, Hubbs AF, Siegel PD. Changes in asthma-like responses after extended removal from exposure to trimellitic anhydride in the Brown Norway rat model. Clin Exp Allergy. 2009;39:1746–53.

78. Arts JH, Jacobs EJ, Kuper CF. Pre-exposure to sulfur dioxide attenuates most allergic reactions upon trimellitic anhydride challenge in sensitized Brown Norway rats. Inhal Toxicol. 2010;22(3):179–91.

79. Pollaris L, Devos F, De Vooght V, et al. Toluene diisocyanate and methylene diphenyl diisocyanate: asthmatic response and cross-reactivity in a mouse model. Arch Toxicol. 2016;90(7):1709–17.

80. Lehmann DM, Williams WC. Cross-reactivity between halogenated platinum salts in an immediate-type respiratory hypersensitivity model. Inhal Toxicol. 2018;30(11-12):472–81.

81. Tarkowski M, Vanoirbeek JA, Vanhooren HM, et al. Immunological determinants of ventilatory changes induced in mice by dermal sensitization and respiratory challenge with toluene diisocyanate. Am J Physiol Lung Cell Mol Physiol. 2007;292(1):L207–14.

82. de Vooght V, Haenen S, Verbeken E, et al. Successful transfer of chemical-induced asthma by adoptive transfer of low amounts of lymphocytes in a mouse model. Toxicology. 2011;279:85–90.

83. Matheson JM, Johnson VJ, Luster MI. Immune mediators in a murine model for occupational asthma: studies with toluene diisocyanate. Toxicol Sci. 2005;84:99–109.

84. Liu SY, Wang WZ, Yen CL, et al. Leukocyte nicotinamide adenine dinucleotide phosphate-reduced oxidase is required for isocyanate-induced lung inflammation. J Allergy Clin Immunol. 2011;127(4):1014–23.

85. de Vooght V, Smulders S, Haenen S, et al. Neutrophil and eosinophil granulocytes as key players in a mouse model of chemical-induced asthma. Toxicol Sci. 2013;131:406–18.

86. Valstar DL, Schijf MA, Arts JH, et al. Alveolar macrophages suppress nonspecific inflammation caused by inhalation challenge with trimellitic anhydride conjugated to albumin. Arch Toxicol. 2006;80(9):561–71.

87. Jonckheere AC, Bullens DMA, Seys SF. Innate lymphoid cells in asthma: pathophysiological insights from murine models to human asthma phenotypes. Curr Opin Allergy Clin Immunol. 2019;19(1):53–60.

88. Yu G, Zhang Y, Wang X, et al. Thymic stromal lymphopoietin (TSLP) and Toluene-diisocyanate-induced airway inflammation: alleviation by TSLP neutralizing antibody. Toxicol Lett. 2019;317:59–67.

89. Voskamp AL, Kormelink TG, van Wijk RG, et al. Modulating local airway immune responses to treat allergic asthma: lessons from experimental models and human studies. Semin Immunopathol. 2020;42(1):95–110.

90. Pollaris L, Van Den Broucke S, Decaesteker T, et al. Dermal exposure determines the outcome of repeated airway exposure in a long-term chemical-induced asthma-like mouse model. Toxicology. 2019;421:84–92.

91. Park SJ, Lee KS, Kim SR, et al. AMPK activation reduces vascular permeability and airway inflammation by regulating HIF/VEGFA pathway in a murine model of toluene diisocyanate-induced asthma. Inflamm Res. 2012;61:1069–83.

92. Song J, Zhao H, Dong H, et al. Mechanism of E-cadherin redistribution in bronchial airway epithelial cells in a TDI-induced asthma model. Toxicol Lett. 2013;220(1):8–14.

93. Yao L, Zhao H, Tang H, et al. Phosphatidylinositol 3-kinase mediates β-catenin dysfunction of airway epithelium in a toluene diisocyanate-induced murine asthma model. Toxicol Sci. 2015;147(1):168–77.

94. Yao L, Zhao H, Tang H, et al. Blockade of β-catenin signaling attenuates toluene diisocyanate-induced experimental asthma. Allergy. 2017;72(4):579–89.

95. Yao L, Zhao H, Tang H, et al. The receptor for advanced glycation end products is required for β-catenin stabilization in a chemical-induced asthma model. Br J Pharmacol. 2016;173(17):2600–13.

96. Liang J, Zhao H, Yao L, et al. Phosphatidylinositol 3-kinases pathway mediates lung caspase-1 activation and high mobility group box 1 production in a toluene-diisocyanate induced murine asthma model. Toxicol Lett. 2015;236(1):25–33.

97. Chen S, Yao L, Huang P, et al. Blockade of the NLRP3/Caspase-1 axis ameliorates airway neutrophilic inflammation in a toluene diisocyanate-induced murine asthma model. Toxicol Sci. 2019;170(2):462–75.

98. Hardy CL, Kenins L, Drew AC, et al. Characterization of a mouse model of allergy to a major occupational latex glove allergen Hev b 5. Am J Respir Crit Care Med. 2003;167:1393–9.

99. Lehto M, Haapakoski R, Wolff H, et al. Cutaneous, but not airway, latex exposure induces allergic lung inflammation and airway hyperreactivity in mice. J Invest Dermatol. 2005;125(5):962–8.

100. Haapakoski R, Karisola P, Fyhrquist N, et al. Intradermal cytosine-phosphate-guanosine treatment reduces lung inflammation but induces IFN-gamma-mediated airway hyperreactivity in a murine model of natural rubber latex allergy. Am J Respir Cell Mol Biol. 2011;44(5):639–47.

101. Marraccini P, Brass DM, Hollingsworth JW, et al. Bakery flour dust exposure causes non-allergic inflammation and enhances allergic airway inflammation in mice. Clin Exp Allergy. 2008;38:1526–35.

102. Denery-Papini S, Bodinier M, Pineau F, et al. Immunoglobulin-E-binding epitopes of wheat allergens in patients with food allergy to wheat and in mice experimentally sensitized to wheat proteins. Clin Exp Allergy. 2011;41(10):1478–92.

103. Gourbeyre P, Denery-Papini S, Larre C, et al. Wheat gliadins modified by deamidation are more efficient than native gliadins in inducing a Th2 response in Balb/c mice experimentally sensitized to wheat allergens. Mol Nutr Food Res. 2012;56(2):336–44.

104. Bouchaud G, Gourbeyre P, Bihouée T, et al. Consecutive food and respiratory allergies amplify systemic and gut but not lung outcomes in mice. J Agric Food Chem. 2015;63(28):6475–83.

105. Krieger SM, Boverhof DR, Woolhiser MR, et al. Assessment of the respiratory sensitization potential of proteins using an enhanced mouse intranasal test (MINT). Food Chem Toxicol. 2013;59:165–76.

106. Florsheim E, Yu S, Bragatto I, et al. Integrated innate mechanisms involved in airway allergic inflammation to the serine protease subtilisin. J Immunol. 2015;194(10):4621–30.

107. Oboki K, Ohno T, Kajiwara N, et al. IL-33 is a crucial amplifier of innate rather than acquired immunity. Proc Natl Acad Sci U S A. 2010;107(43):18581–6.

108. Kamijo S, Suzuki M, Hara M, et al. Subcutaneous allergic sensitization to protease allergen is dependent on mast cells but not IL-33: distinct mechanisms between subcutaneous and intranasal routes. J Immunol. 2016;196(9):3559–69.

109. Agoro R, Piotet-Morin J, Palomo J, et al. IL-1R1-MyD88 axis elicits papain-induced lung inflammation. Eur J Immunol. 2016;46(11):2531–41.

110. Singh PB, Pua HH, Happ HC, et al. MicroRNA regulation of type 2 innate lymphoid cell homeostasis and function in allergic inflammation. J Exp Med. 2017;214(12):3627–43.

111. Di Giampaolo L, Di Gioacchino M, Mangifesta R, et al. Occupational allergy: is there a role for nanoparticles? J Biol Regul Homeost Agents. 2019;33(3):661–8.

112. Ihrie MD, Bonner JJ. The toxicology of engineered nanomaterials in asthma. Curr Environ Health Rep. 2018;5(1):100–9.

113. Kim BG, Park MK, Lee PH, et al. Effects of nanoparticles on neuro-inflammation in a mouse model of asthma. Respir Physiol Neurobiol. 2020;271:103292.

114. Ko JW, Shin NR, Je-Oh L, et al. Silica dioxide nanoparticles aggravate airway inflammation in an asthmatic mouse model via NLRP3 inflammasome activation. Regul Toxicol Pharmacol. 2020;112:104618.

115. Vandenplas O, Godet J, Hurdubaea L, et al. Are high- and low-molecular-weight sensitizing agents associated with different clinical phenotypes of occupational asthma? Allergy. 2019;74:261–72.

116. Frew AJ. What can we learn about asthma from studying occupational asthma? Ann Allergy Asthma Immunol. 2003;90(5 Suppl 2):7–10.

117. Low B, Sjostedt L, Willis S. Laboratory animal allergy-possible association with HLA B15 and DR4. Tissue Antigens. 1988;32:224–6.

118. Sjostedt L, Willers S, Orbaek P. Human leukocyte antigens in occupational allergy: a possible protective effect of HLA-B16 in laboratory animal allergy. Am J Ind Med. 1996;30:415–20.

119. Jeal H, Draper A, Jones M, et al. HLA associations with occupational sensitization to rat lipocalin allergens: a model for other animal allergies? J Allergy Clin Immunol. 2003;111:795–9.

120. Kelada SN, Eaton DL, Wang SS, et al. The role of genetic polymorphisms in environmental health. Environ Health Perspect. 2003;111(8):1055–64.

121. Bignon JS, Aron Y, Ju LY, et al. HLA class II alleles in isocyanate-induced asthma. Am J Respir Crit Care Med. 1994;149:71–5.

122. Mapp CE, Beghè B, Balboni A, et al. Association between HLA genes and susceptibility to toluene diisocyanate-induced asthma. Clin Exp Allergy. 2000;30:651–6.

123. Balboni A, Baricordi OR, Fabbri LM, et al. Association between toluene diisocyanate-induced asthma and DQB1 markers: a possible role for aspartic acid at position 57. Eur Respir J. 1996;9:207–10.

124. Kim SH, Oh HB, Lee KW, et al. HLA DRB1*15-DPB1*05 haplotype: a susceptible gene marker for isocyanate-induced occupational asthma? Allergy. 2006;61:891–4.

125. Horne C, Quintana PJE, Keown PA, et al. Distribution of HLA class II DQB1 alleles in patients with occupational asthma due to Western red cedar. Eur Respir J. 2000;15:911–4.

126. Jones MG, Nielsen J, Welch J, et al. Association of HLA-DQ5 and HLA-DR1 with sensitization to organic acid anhydrides. Clin Exp Allergy. 2004;34:812–6.

127. Newman Taylor AJ, Cullinan P, Lympany PA, et al. Interaction of HLA phenotype and exposure intensity in sensitization to complex platinum salts. Am J Respir Crit Care Med. 1999;160:435–8.

128. Pacheco K, Maier L, Siulveira L, et al. Association of TLR4 alleles with symptoms and sensitization to laboratory animals. J Allergy Clin Immunol. 2008;122:896–902.

129. Cho HJ, Kim SH, Kim JH, et al. Effect of toll-like receptor 4 gene polymorphisms on work-related respiratory symptoms and sensitization to wheat flour in bakery workers. Ann Allergy Asthma Immunol. 2011;107:57–64.

130. Pacheco KA, Rose CR, Silveira LJ, et al. Gene-environment interactions influence airways function in laboratory animal workers. J Allergy Clin Immunol. 2010;126:232–40.

131. LeVan TD, Von Essen S, Romberger DJ, et al. Polymorphisms in the CD14 gene associated with pulmonary function in farmers. Am J Respir Crit Care Med. 2005;171(7):773–9.

132. Smit LA, Heederik D, Doekes G, et al. Occupational endotoxin exposure reduces the risk of atopic sensitization but increases the risk of bronchial hyperresponsiveness. Int Arch Allergy Immunol. 2010;152:151–8.

133. Bernstein DI, Kissling GE, Khurana Hershey G, et al. Hexamethylene diisocyanate asthma is associated with genetic polymorphisms of CD14, IL-13, and IL-4 receptor alpha. J Allergy Clin Immunol. 2011;128:418–20.

134. Bernstein DI, Wang N, Campo P, et al. Diisocyanate asthma and gene-environment interactions with IL4RA, CD-14, and IL-13 genes. Ann Allergy Asthma Immunol. 2006;97:800–6.

135. Lantz RC, Lemus R, Lange RW, et al. Rapid reduction of intracellular glutathione in human bronchial epithelial cells exposed to occupational levels of toluene diisocyanate. Toxicol Sci. 2001;60(2):348–55.

136. Wisnewski AV, Liu Q, Liu J, et al. Glutathione protects human airway proteins and epithelial cells from isocyanates. Clin Exp Allergy. 2005;35:352–7.

137. Mapp CE, Fryer AA, DeMarzo N, et al. Glutathione S-transferase GSTP1 is a susceptibility gene for occupational asthma induced by isocyanates. J Allergy Clin Immunol. 2002;109:867–72.

138. Wikman H, Piirila P, Rosenberg C, et al. N-Acetyltransferase genotypes as modifiers of diisocyanate exposure-associated asthma risk. Pharmacogenetics. 2002;12:227–33.

139. Kim SH, Cho BY, Park CS, et al. Alpha-T-catenin (CTNNA3) gene was identified as a risk variant for toluene diisocyanate-induced asthma by genomewide association analysis. Clin Exp Allergy. 2009;39:203–12.

140. Yucesoy B, Kaufman KM, Lummus ZL, et al. Genome-wide association study identifies novel loci associated with diisocyanate-induced occupational asthma. Toxicol Sci. 2015;146(1):192–201.

141. Bernstein DI, Lummus ZL, Kesavalu B, et al. Genetic variants with gene regulatory effects are associated with diisocyanate-induced asthma. J Allergy Clin Immunol. 2018;142(3):959–69.

142. Ginasthma.org. Global strategy for asthma management and prevention. Updated 2020. https://ginasthmaorg/wp-content/uploads/2020/04/GINA-2020-full-report_-final-_wmspdf. 2020.

143. Tarlo SM, Lemiere C. Occupational asthma. N Engl J Med. 2014;370:640–9.

144. Dufour MH, Lemière C, Prince P, et al. Comparative airway response to high- versus low-molecular weight agents in occupational asthma. Eur Respir J. 2009;33:734–9.

145. Hu C, Cruz MJ, Ojanguren I, et al. Specific inhalation challenge: the relationship between response, clinical variables and lung function. Occup Environ Med. 2017;74:586–91.

146. Lange P, Parner J, Vestbo J, et al. A 15-year follow-up study of ventilatory function in adults with asthma. N Eng J Med. 1998;339:1194–200.

147. Maestrelli P, Schlünssen V, Mason P, et al. Contribution of host factors and workplace exposure to the outcome of occupational asthma. ERS Task Force on the Management of Work-related Asthma. Eur Respir Rev. 2012;21:88–96.

148. Anees W, Moore VC, Burge PS. FEV1 decline in occupational asthma. Thorax. 2006;61:751–5.

149. Padoan M, Pozzato V, Simon M, et al. Long-term follow-up of toluene diisocyanate-induced asthma. Eur Respir J. 2003;21:637–40.

150. Piirila PL, Nordman H, Keskinen HM, et al. Long-term follow-up of hexamethylene diisocyanate-, diphenylmethane diisocyanate-, and toluene diisocyanate-induced asthma. Am J Respir Crit Care Med. 2000;162:516–22.

151. Munoz X, Viladrich M, Manso L, et al. Evolution of occupational asthma: does cessation of exposure really improve prognosis? Respir Med. 2014;108(9):1363–70.

152. Cartier A, L'Archevêque J, Malo JL. Exposure to a sensitizing occupational agent can cause a long-lasting increase in bronchial responsiveness to histamine in the absence of significant changes in airway caliber. J Allergy Clin Immunol. 1986;78:1185–9.

153. Thorpe JE, Steinberg D, Bernstein IL, et al. Bronchial reactivity increases soon after the immediate response in dual-responding asthmatic subjects. Chest. 1987;91:21–5.

154. Durham SR, Graneek BJ, Hawkins R, et al. The temporal relationship between increases in airway responsiveness to histamine and late asthmatic responses induced by occupational agents. J Allergy Clin Immunol. 1987;79:398–406.

155. Chan-Yeung M, Leriche J, Maclean L, et al. Comparison of cellular and protein changes in bronchial lavage fluid of symptomatic and asymptomatic patients with red cedar asthma on follow-up examination. Clin Allergy. 1988;18:359–65.

156. Ollé-Monge M, Muñoz X, Vanoirbeek JA, et al. Persistence of asthmatic response after ammonium persulfate-induced occupational asthma in mice. PLOS ONE. 2014;9(10):e109000.

157. Malo JL, Cardinal S, Ghezzo H, et al. Association of bronchial reactivity to occupational agents with methacholine reactivity, sputum cells and immunoglobulin E-mediated reactivity. Clin Exp Allergy. 2011;41:497–504.

158. Vandenplas O, Suojalehto H, Cullinan P. Diagnosing occupational asthma. Clin Exp Allergy. 2017;47:6–18.

159. Pralong JA, Lemière C, Rochat T, et al. Predictive value of nonspecific bronchial responsiveness in occupational asthma. J Allergy Clin Immunol. 2016;137:412–6.

160. Rachiotis G, Savani R, Brant A, et al. Outcome of occupational asthma after cessation of exposure: a systematic review. Thorax. 2007;62:147–52.

161. Saetta M, Di Stefano A, Rosina C, et al. Quantitative structural analysis of peripheral airways and arteries in sudden fatal asthma. Am Rev Respir Dis. 1991;143:138–43.

162. Górski P, Krakowiak A, Ruta U. Nasal and bronchial responses to flour-inhalation in subjects with occupationally induced allergy affecting the airway. Int Arch Occup Environ Health. 2000;73(7):488–97.

163. Fabbri LM, Boschetto P, Zocca E, et al. Bronchoalveolar neutrophilia during late asthmatic reactions induced by toluene diisocyanate. Am Rev Respir Dis. 1987;136:36–42.

164. Chan-Yeung M, Chan H, Salari H, et al. Histamine, leukotrienes and prostaglandins release in bronchial fluid during plicatic acid-induced bronchoconstriction. J Allergy Clin Immunol. 1989;84:762–8.

165. Maestrelli P, Saetta M, Di Stefano A, et al. Comparison of leukocyte counts in sputum, bronchial biopsies, and bronchoalveolar lavage. Am J Respir Crit Care Med. 1995;152:1926–31.

166. Maestrelli P, Calcagni PG, Saetta M, et al. Sputum eosinophilia after asthmatic responses induced by isocyanates in sensitized subjects. Clin Exp Allergy. 1994;24:29–34.

167. Lemière C, Chaboilliez S, Trudeau C, et al. Characterization of airway inflammation after repeated exposures to occupational agents. J Allergy Clin Immunol. 2000;106:1163–70.

168. Lemière C, Romeo P, Chaboillez S, et al. Airway inflammation and functional changes after exposure to different concentrations of isocyanates. J Allergy Clin Immunol. 2002;110:641–6.

169. Quirce S, Lemière C, deBlay F, et al. Noninvasive methods for assessment of airway inflammation in occupational settings. Allergy. 2010;65:445–58.

170. Ferrazzoni S, Scarpa MC, Guarnieri G, et al. Exhaled nitric oxide and breath condensate pH in asthmatic reactions induced by isocyanates. Chest. 2009;136:155–62.

171. Suojalehto H, Suuronen K, Cullinan P, et al. Phenotyping occupational asthma caused by acrylates in a multicenter cohort study. J Allergy Clin Immunol Pract. 2020;8(3):971–9.e1.

172. Mason P, Scarpa MC, Guarnieri G, et al. Exhaled nitric oxide dynamics in asthmatic reactions induced by diisocyanates. Clin Exp Allergy. 2016;46(12):1531–9.

173. Saetta M, di Stefano A, Maestrelli P, et al. Airway mucosal inflammation in occupational asthma induced by toluene diisocyanate. Am Rev Respir Dis. 1992;145:160–8.

174. Gautrin D, Boulet LP, Boutet M, et al. Is reactive airways dysfunction syndrome a variant of occupational asthma? J Allergy Clin Immunol. 1994;93:12–22.

175. Redington AE, Howarth PH. Airway wall remodeling in asthma. Thorax. 1997;52:310–2.

176. Takeda N, Maghni K, Daigle S, et al. Long-term pathologic consequences of acute irritant-induced asthma. J Allergy Clin Immunol. 2009;124:975–81.

177. Sjåheim TB, Bjørtuft Ø, Drabløs PA, et al. Increased bronchial density of CD25+Foxp3+ regulatory T cells in occupational asthma: relationship to current smoking. Scand J Immunol. 2013;77(5):398–404.

178. Maghni K, Lemière C, Ghezzo H, et al. Airway inflammation after cessation of exposure to agents causing occupational asthma. Am J Respir Crit Care Med. 2004;169:367–72.

179. Girard F, Chaboillez S, Cartier A, et al. An effective strategy for diagnosing occupational asthma: use of induced sputum. Am J Respir Crit Care Med. 2004;170:845–50.

180. Florentin A, Acouetey DS, Remen T, et al. Exhaled nitric oxide and screening for occupational asthma in two at-risk sectors: bakery and hairdressing. Int J Tuberc Lung Dis. 2014;18:744–50.

181. van Kampen V, Brüning T, Merget R. Serial fractional exhaled nitric oxide measurements off and at work in the diagnosis of occupational asthma. Am J Ind Med. 2019;62:663–71.

182. Merget R, Sander I, van Kampen V, et al. Serial measurements of exhaled nitric oxide at work and at home: a new tool for the diagnosis of occupational asthma. Adv Exp Med Biol. 2015;834:49–52.

183. Israel E, Reddell HK. Severe and difficult-to-treat asthma in adults. N Engl J Med. 2017;377:965–76.

Part II
Assessment

5

ASSESSMENT OF THE WORKER

André Cartier,[1] Kenneth D. Rosenman,[2] Nathalie Bourdeau,[3] Pierre Phénix,[4]
Pierre Séguin,[5] David Fishwick,[6] and Jean-Luc Malo[7]
[1]University of Montréal, Montréal, Québec, Canada
[2]Division of Occupational and Environmental Medicine, College of Human Medicine, Michigan State University, Michigan, USA
[3]Occupational Health, Direction de santé publique, CISSS de Lanaudière, Joliette, Québec, Canada
[4]Occupational Health, Direction régionale de Santé publique, CIUSSS du Centre-Sud de l'Ile-de-Montréal, Montréal, Québec, Canada
*[5]Occupational Health, Direction régionale de Santé publique , CIUSSS du Centre-
Sud de l'Ile-de-Montréal, Montréal, Québec, Canada*
[6]University of Sheffield and Centre for Workplace Health, Health and Safety Executive (HSE) Science and Research Centre, Buxton, UK
[7]Hôpital du Sacré-Cœur de Montréal and Université de Montréal, Montréal, Québec, Canada

Contents

CASE HISTORY

A 25-year-old worker has been employed for 2 years in a small family bakery that employs three other bakers and two helpers.

1. During his apprenticeship course, the worker received information on possible allergies to cereals, enzymes, and other products in flour.
2. He started having sneezing at work 1 year before you see him, and his wife noticed some wheezy breathing at home in the evening in the past few months.
3. The local public health department had started a surveillance program in bakeries in the area. After some hesitation, the employer allowed an industrial hygienist from that department to visit the workplace and a nurse to meet with the workers.
4. An information session was offered and two short self-administered questionnaires (one for occupational asthma [OA], and one for occupational rhinitis [OR]) were completed by all attending workers.
5. Because the worker had positive responses on the self-administered questionnaires, he met with the occupational nurse, who inquired about the details of his symptoms with more detailed medical questionnaires, one for OA and one for OR. The results of these two questionnaires indicated that the worker had symptoms consistent with work-related rhinitis and asthma.
6. The worker was seen by the occupational physician of the local health department. The worker had been seen (without being referred) by an allergy specialist who had performed skin-prick tests (SPTs) to various cereals, which were positive. He was given inhaled salbutamol on demand.
7. The nurse and physician suggested that the worker make an appointment at a specialized center for further testing.
8. The worker, a recent immigrant with two children, feared losing his job because he had no other formal training but followed the advice and scheduled an appointment.
9. The worker mentioned that one coworker who was not at the meeting and had not completed the initial questionnaire had nasal symptoms and coughing. The industrial hygienist's evaluation showed that the flour dust levels in the bakery were quite high, but within the legal standards.

Introduction

Occupational asthma (OA) is an almost entirely preventable condition (1), and should be suspected in all adult patients with asthma. Developing such workplace and healthcare approaches, which primarily aim to prevent cases or identify possible cases early for further diagnostic assessment, is consequently of upmost importance.

How these approaches develop will depend on local and national expertise and will vary by resource available and medical practice in different countries. Some countries link claims for compensation, for example Finland (1), with investigations for OA, while others separate these requirements (2). Others have well-developed local protocols that consider in detail local allergen types (3) and diagnostic processes. It is likely that in other countries of lower economic development, systems may be less developed, although details are sparse (4).

Despite differences in approach by country, it is likely that globally the diagnosis of OA remains underreported, delayed when the diagnosis is made, and undercompensated (5, 6).

Health surveillance: The role of health surveillance for occupational asthma at work

The objective of health surveillance for OA in the workplace is to identify sensitized workers or those with the disease at an early and reversible stage, because clinical outcome is better when OA is diagnosed earlier (6, 7).

The optimal content of a surveillance program for OA is still a matter of debate despite the fact that such a program is mandated in many countries. In their review, Szram and Cullinan (8) state that almost all surveillance programs include a questionnaire that is generally self-completed. They concur that no questionnaires have been formally validated although it is likely that those which include standardized questions on asthma with an inquiry into any work relationship will have appropriately high sensitivity and specificity if they are completed accurately. They add that questionnaires should also include items relating to work-related rhinitis, which is not only a significant associated risk factor for asthma, but itself an indicator of failed exposure control.

The question of the accuracy with which questionnaires are completed has been raised, thus affecting the sensitivity of the test. Nicholson et al. (7) concluded that surveillance questionnaires may lead to an underestimation of the prevalence of asthmatic symptoms. Szram and Cullinan (8) state that there is good evidence that a high proportion of employees are unwilling to divulge their symptoms, because of uncertainties over confidentiality or the perceived consequences leading to job loss (9). They propose that several determinants are likely to influence the accuracy of responses: the employees' judgment on the relative importance of their health versus their employment, dependent on the severity of their symptoms and their individual attitudes; the circumstances and setting of their employment; and the attitudes of their employer. Fishwick and Forman (6) comment that despite the caveat of accuracy, questionnaires remain the key component of respiratory health surveillance schemes, as they are inexpensive and foster the culture of reporting new symptoms between surveillance visits.

Spirometry testing is a frequent tool in surveillance programs for OA, but it probably detects only few cases that would not otherwise be detected by a questionnaire (7). Szram and Cullinan (8) opine that it seems premature to reject all surveillance spirometry, but that it must be interpreted appropriately. Similarly, Fishwick and Forman (6) are in favor of including high-quality workplace spirometry, in workplaces with at least a moderate risk of OA.

Immunological testing is helpful in some settings, particularly for workers exposed to high-molecular-weight (HMW) occupational allergens. Combined with assessment of nonspecific bronchial hyperresponsiveness (NSBH), the yield of immunological testing in terms of positive predictive value for OA (as confirmed by specific inhalation challenge [SIC]), is high (10, 11) as also shown in earlier studies (12).

Induced sputum (13) and exhaled nitric oxide (FeNO) (14) have been used in epidemiological surveys but their relevance and benefit, alone or combined with other tests, within a health surveillance program are unknown.

Health surveillance: What is the role of the occupational nurse in health surveillance for occupational asthma in the workplace?

The occupational nurse has a preventive and clinical role. The occupational nurse should be involved in the identification and assessment of health risks at work, and their prevention through health education and the surveillance program. The occupational nurse's actions must be based on rigorous methods and follow professional ethics and confidentiality standards.

In the province of Québec (Canada), public health departments are mandated by law to provide preventive occupational health services in targeted workplaces of all sizes, mostly in resources, manufacturing, and construction sectors. In Montréal, a standardized program was initiated in 2013 for the surveillance of OA and occupational rhinitis (OR) where there is a risk of sensitization (15). The occupational nurse plays a pivotal role in this context, as she/he is responsible for initiating and carrying out the program activities (16) (Figure 5.1). For the sake of efficiency, the program adopts a collective

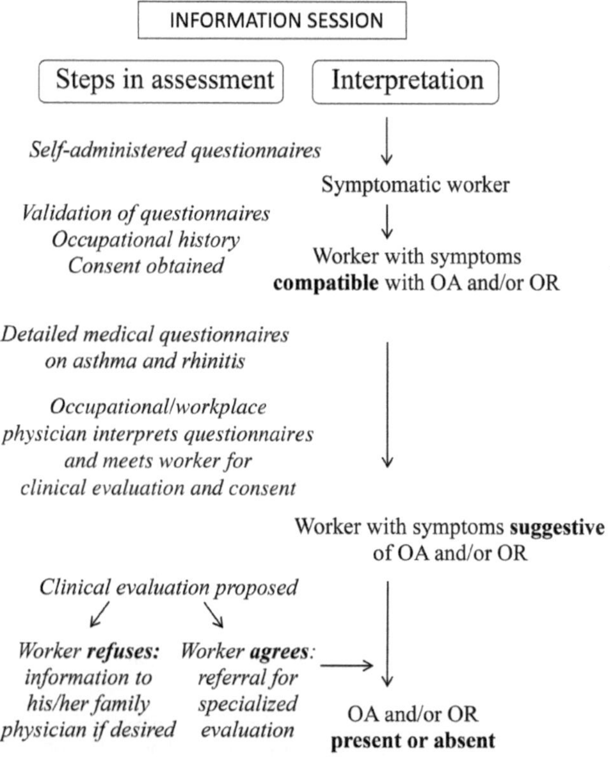

FIGURE 5.1 Severity of asthma symptoms by duration of exposure to allergenic substance.
Abbreviations: OA: occupational asthma; OR: occupational rhinitis.

approach (group information sessions for workers and employer's representatives), followed if needed by personal interactions with each worker. This strategy aims to ensure respect of each worker's autonomous decision in regards to issues that concern their health.

The occupational nurse's first task, in collaboration with industrial hygiene professionals, is to perform a risk assessment according to task and workstation, leading to stratification of workers into groups that receive a targeted information. The presentation starts with a clear explanation of the purpose of the surveillance program and items communicated are sensitizing agent(s), risky tasks/locations and exposure levels, and preventive measures (respiratory protection, ventilation, maintenance). Workers are informed about symptoms of OR and OA, their usual onset and progression, and the temporal relation with work exposure. Workers are also advised to be aware if any of these symptoms arise at work.

Self-administered questionnaires are given to workers and each question might be explained by the occupational nurse, if needed. (English questionnaires are available on pages 75 [OR] and 89 [OA] of the program document (15).) Workers are invited to meet or call the occupational nurse if they have difficulties reading and understanding the self-administered questionnaire.

It is of utmost importance to keep the content simple and at the appropriate educational level of the workers, because according to international surveys, a significant proportion of adults do not necessarily have the capacity to properly understand and use health information in written documents.

In the Montréal program, the occupational nurse meets only workers who make a request because of a self-administered questionnaire compatible with OA and/or OR. In other types of programs proposed by occupational health and safety administrations, it might be necessary to evaluate each worker individually, even after a group information session.

If the self-administered questionnaires are compatible with OR and/or OA, the occupational nurse meets the worker and gets an occupational history, with a focus on exposure to sensitizing agents. In order to obtain informed consent to proceed with further evaluation, the occupational nurse gives the worker relevant information about the advantages/disadvantages of the different options, using the standardized documentation of the program. The occupational nurse should validate that the worker understands the information, allow the worker to ask questions, and give them an appropriate period of time to decide whether or not they want further clinical investigation. In Québec, consent is legally required for any investigation required in the context of a surveillance program in occupational health. In other jurisdictions, such as the United States, the employer can require further evaluation if the worker wishes to maintain employment.

If the worker agrees to further evaluation, the occupational nurse completes more detailed medical questionnaires on OA and OR with them. The occupational nurse then forwards a request to the occupational health physician, who reviews with the worker the information already collected, interprets the two questionnaires (self-administered and detailed medical questionnaires), assesses the clinical condition, and revalidates the worker's consent to further evaluation, if needed. Workers with symptoms suggestive of OA or OR are referred for a specialized evaluation (Figure 5.1). If the diagnosis of OA/OR and causative agent are confirmed and a worker's compensation claim is accepted, the occupational nurse and the occupational health physician can assist in the relocation of the affected worker in their workplace, if that is the preferred option.

The situation at the workplace is revised every 1–2 years, with new workers invited to the full session, while the continuing workers complete the self-administered questionnaires.

The role of the occupational health physician

The role of the occupational health physician in relation to OA is to provide an expertise aimed at reducing the risk through prevention and implementation of health surveillance programs, with the help of a team of professionals that include nurses and industrial hygiene professionals. The specific tasks of the occupational health and safety department vary significantly depending on the organizational structure of the occupational health service at the workplace. In the internal model, which is increasingly rare, the surveillance is more readily integrated with the other elements of a primary preventive strategy (17). By comparison, the occupational health physician providing consultant work for many small-size industries might be asked to perform only the activities that comply with the regulatory requirements.

In 1979, a reform of the Québec occupational health and safety system put under the same umbrella the different facets of prevention (including standards setting and enforcement/inspection) and the workers' compensation system, which is a public administration (Commission des normes, de l'équité, de la santé et sécurité du travail—CNESST) financed by the employers. The specificity is that the occupational health physician, who devises and puts into action the occupational health program in a workplace, must be associated with the public health department of the region and accepted by the employer and workers' representatives sitting on the local occupational health and safety committee. Furthermore, the occupational nurse and industrial hygiene professionals who operate the program are employees of the public health department. In Québec, there are no specific standards for health surveillance of workers. To foster efficiency and coherence, occupational health physicians in Montréal generally ask the regional team to coordinate the development of practice guidelines for frequently encountered risks such as asbestos, silica, noise, etc. The guide for sensitizer-induced OA was issued in 2013 (15) addressing also OR because it is often associated with OA (Chapter 22) (17, 18). The self-administered questionnaire used for OA was initially prepared by Labrecque et al. for a prospective diisocyanate surveillance project (19). It has been described and shown to have satisfactory discriminative qualities elsewhere (20). A detailed self-administered questionnaire for OR (not published) was prepared with the same rationale as for OA. Three of the authors of the present chapter (Bourdeau, Phénix, Seguin) were the lead initiators of the surveillance program and the Section "Health surveillance: what is the role of the occupational nurse in health surveillance for, occupational asthma in the workplace?" describes the main elements of the program carried out by the occupational nurse.

This surveillance program proposes a pragmatic approach, with different recommendations from expert groups available in 2013, this including among others the European Respiratory Society (21), the British Occupational Health Research Foundation (7), and the European Academy of Allergy and Clinical Immunology (18) while being compatible with the public health principles of empowerment and benevolence. Lately, the elements of the program pertaining to OA became the basis of the provincial program prioritizing the risk associated with exposure to wood dust.

The main objective is to offer workers exposed to a known sensitizer the most relevant information and tools, so they can recognize the early symptoms of OA/OR (17) and ask for guidance if they choose to. From the start, workers make autonomous decisions as to what conduct is in their best interest, and the role of the occupational nurse and the occupational health physician is to foster their decision process by highlighting the advantages/disadvantages of the different options available. The worker has control of the sequential process and can refuse to proceed further if they foresee unfavorable socioeconomic consequences (21, 22) mainly on employment and insurance.

The program follows the suggestions of the World Health Organization, cited by Wilken et al. (23): it addresses a significant health problem (OA) that has a better prognosis if diagnosed early; OR has a significant impact on quality of life and productivity (24) and can be inferred as a proxy to early or coexisting OA (25); the process is acceptable to the worker, who is asked for their consent at all times; the different questionnaires have an interpretation grid that provide explicit criteria for proposing a presumptive diagnosis. Each question of the 11-item self-administered questionnaire as well as the whole questionnaire used in the Québec program show high sensitivity and negative predictive value (20), and therefore represents a satisfactory preliminary triage followed by the sequential use of a detailed questionnaire and occupational health physician's evaluation, all these means increasing the predictive value of the surveillance method (23); the cost/benefit ratio is favorable, because the occupational nurse already has the mandate to give information sessions on health risks and only symptomatic workers will require occupational nurse and occupational health physician attention/time. The utilization of more costly specialized resources is also limited to workers with a significant probability of being diagnosed with OA/OR.

Skin-prick tests (SPTs) have been integrated in epidemiological studies of asthma (26) and OA for many years (27) but they are not generally part of the surveillance program, for different reasons: availability of extracts with satisfactory allergenic quality, time required, quality control for SPT (Chapter 7), but, mostly, these tests need consent that addresses the possible consequences of a positive test on employment. They are reserved for workers whose symptoms are suggestive of OA/OR and want further evaluations. It is the same for spirometry, which, besides the logistical aspect, does not add any significant benefit over questionnaires (25).

In small workshops, employers are not always aware of the health risks in their workplace and of their obligations; the intervention of the public health department team increases their knowledge and hopefully helps change their attitudes, although this represents an ongoing challenge. If the employer has a satisfactory occupational health and safety organization, new employees are likely to receive appropriate health information. When the risk evaluation shows an unacceptable level of exposure, a link is made with the inspection agent who has the enforcement power for improving the situation.

In Québec, public health regulation specifies that OA is an occupational disease that should be notified, and each case is investigated by the public health department to ascertain whether other workers are also at risk and if exposure levels are acceptable. If appropriate, the program is applied to a specific workplace, even though it might not be in a prioritized sector of economic activity. OR is not an occupational disease that needs to be notified but this diagnosis is likely to increase the attention given to reducing exposure to possible causal agents present in the workplace (24).

A large proportion of Québec workers exposed to sensitizers do not have access to the surveillance program described here, because their workplace is not on the priority list. In these situations, it is the role of the family physician (primary healthcare provider, see below) to identify respiratory symptoms, see whether they might be work-related, and, if so, advise on proper referral. Suojalehto et al. make the point that an OA surveillance program increases awareness of OA symptoms and encourages workers to seek health care (25). In the Montréal program, a worker that refuses to go ahead with the evaluation is given a copy of their file, so she/he can bring it to a family physician.

Initial assessment of workers with possible occupational asthma by primary healthcare providers

Workers presenting to primary care physicians with recurrent respiratory symptoms need to be assessed for asthma and the possible relationship of their symptoms to work. A joint statement of the European and American Thoracic Societies concluded that the estimated population-attributable fraction (PAF) for the occupational contribution to incident asthma was 16% (95% CI = 10%–22%) (28) and another 21.5% of asthma in adults is aggravated by workplace exposures (29). Despite these estimates that work is an important contributor to the cause and exacerbation of asthma in adults, Mazurek and coworkers reported that only 9% of 50,000 working American adults with asthma were ever told by a physician that their asthma could be related to any job they ever had (30). An audit that included nearly 400 UK patients selected from a general practice population of 27,000 patients showed that occupation was recorded in only 14% of cases (31).

The American College of Chest Physicians (ACCP) consensus statement recommends the following four key questions for adult patients with new-onset asthma or with asthma that becomes more symptomatic (32):

1. Were there changes in work processes in the period preceding the onset of symptoms?
2. Was there an unusual work exposure within 24 hours before the onset of initial asthma symptoms?
3. Do asthma symptoms differ during times away from work such as weekends or holidays or other extended times away from work?
4. Are there symptoms of allergic rhinitis and/or conjunctivitis symptoms that are worse with work?

The medical history provided by the patient is not specific for the diagnosis of work-related asthma (WRA) but is sensitive, a quality also required for a tool to be kept in surveillance programs (33). If the symptoms involve loss of voice, then vocal cord dysfunction should be considered (34).

Recommended question 1 elicits whether there have been changes in the process such that a new chemical has been introduced or levels of exposure have changed. Question 2 asks about a previous acute exposure that immediately (within 24 hours) preceded the onset of symptoms to uncover the development of irritant-induced asthma and reactive airways dysfunction syndrome

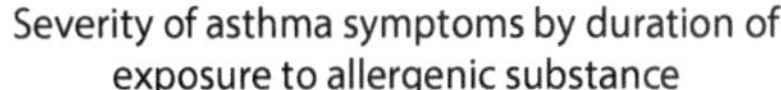

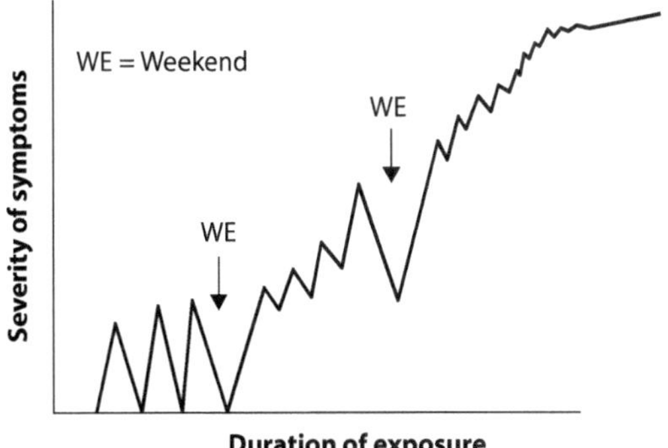

FIGURE 5.2 Typical temporal pattern of respiratory symptoms of OA with marked improvement away from work diminishing or even ceasing if the patient continues to be exposed to the substance causing the OA. (From Cartier A, Bourdeau N, Phénix P, Rosenman KD. Assessment of the worker. In: Malo JL, Chan-Yeung M, Bernstein DI, eds. *Asthma in the Workplace*. 4th ed. Boca Raton FL: CRC Press; 2013:77.)
Abbreviation: OA, occupational asthma.

(RADS) (see Chapter 19). The typical response obtained from a patient with OA to question 3 is improvement of symptoms on weekends or vacations or even complete resolution after a prolonged time away from work for 1–2 weeks. This is particularly true early in the course of OA. Figure 5.2 illustrates the typical temporal pattern of symptoms related to work with continued exposure over weeks, months, and years after the onset of symptoms. As duration of exposure and symptoms increases, the patient is less likely to have symptoms resolve when away from work, to the point where there may be no improvement away from work. It is important to ask about temporal relationship of symptoms with work exposure at the time symptoms first began since temporal relationships may become less obvious or disappear with time (Figure 5.2).

Question 3 is the key question that assesses improvement away from the workplace. If a patient's asthma symptoms improve away from work, it is important to assess what the patient does and the potential exposures at work. The patient should be asked to describe precisely the tasks accomplished and what activities or exposures are associated with respiratory symptoms that either develop immediately and/or occur later even at home after work. Asking the patient to draw a floor plan of the workspace can be helpful to better understand potential exposures. The use of personal protective equipment and the patient's perception of the ventilation should be assessed. The frequency of spills and leaks, what the patient was doing at the time, whether the patient was responsible for cleaning up the spilled material, and whether they wore special protective equipment should be evaluated. Industrial hygiene reports of previous air sampling studies when available can be useful to document particular substances in the workplace and exposures levels. However, since the allowable air level standards for most workplace substances causing asthma were not implemented to prevent sensitization, measured levels that are below allowable Occupational Safety and Health Administration (OSHA) standards are no assurance that the suspected agent is not potentially causative.

Safety Data Sheet

1. Product Identification

PRODUCT NAME..INSTANT-LOK (R)

2. HAZARDOUS INGREDIENTS

INGREDIENT NAME/CAS NUMBER/PERCENTAGE	EXPOSURE LIMITS
PARAFFIN WAX	OSHA......2 mg/m3
CAS NUMBER.......................8002-74-2	ACGIH....2 mg/m3
OSHA PERCENTAGE...............>1	STEL.......6 mg/m3
	CEILING..none

FIGURE 5.3 Example of an SDS of an adhesive, which provided only a partial listing of ingredients because the chemical company that wrote the SDS did not include colophony, a well-accepted cause of OA, as a hazardous ingredient. (From Cartier A, Bourdeau N, Phénix P, Rosenman KD. Assessment of the worker. In: Malo JL, Chan-Yeung M, Bernstein DI, eds. *Asthma in the Workplace*. 4th ed. Boca Raton, FL: CRC Press; 2013:78.)
Abbreviations: OA, occupational asthma; SDS, safety data sheet.

Patients should be asked to provide the names of the substances and the material safety data sheets (SDSs) of products they work with or are used by others around them. Exposures from nearby processes may be more important than the patient's own activity. SDSs are required to be made available to all workers but patients may not know how to access them or are afraid to request these from their employer. When patients can provide them, healthcare providers should be wary of their completeness (35). SDSs are prepared by the manufacturer or formulator of the product, who is not required to list all the ingredients in the product below 1%, Figure 5.3 shows the top half of the first page of an SDS of an adhesive used in a bottling plant to glue the labels. The SDS did not indicate that the adhesive contained 70% colophony, a well-known cause of OA. The developer of the SDS is required to provide a complete list of the ingredients even if they are trade secrets after the treating physician contacts address/phone number on the SDS. Chapters 12 to 19 discuss known asthma-causing agents. A comprehensive list of asthma-causing agents is regularly updated and can be consulted on the Association of Occupational and Environmental Clinics website (36) and elsewhere: https://reptox.cnesst.gouv.qc.ca/en/occupational-asthma/Pages/occupational-asthma.aspx

Since new substances causing asthma are described each year, the absence of exposure to a substance known to cause asthma in a patient with symptoms suggestive of WRA should not preclude further workup for OA. Guidelines for taking a complete occupational history have been prepared by the Centers for Disease Control and Prevention (CDC) Agency for Toxic Substances and Disease Registry (ATSDR) (https://www.atsdr.cdc.gov/csem/exphistory/docs/exposure_history.pdf).

The fourth recommended question asks about allergic rhinitis and conjunctivitis since these symptoms are common in subjects with OA (37).

The time between first exposure and development of symptoms may vary from weeks to years but is generally more common in the first 2 years after exposure (38). Symptoms that begin immediately or within days after initiation of work are not consistent with OA unless the patient has had similar exposures in a previous job. Symptoms that begin so soon after initiation of work are more likely secondary to preexisting asthma or to upper airway irritation in the absence of asthma. Sensitization has been reported after an acute spill or leak but this is more commonly the history in a patient with RADS (see Chapter 19).

Other relevant items in the history include nonoccupational factors such as cigarette smoking and exposure to secondhand smoke, hobbies of the patient or members of the household, presence of pets, and a personal or family history of allergies. The presence or absence of these factors does not preclude the diagnosis of WRA, but the acquisition of a pet or the initiation of a hobby coincidental with a new job or work exposure may confound the evaluation of WRA. Chronic cigarette smoking may cause chronic obstructive pulmonary disease (COPD) that may be difficult to distinguish from asthma, especially in the asthma-COPD overlap (ACO). Cigarette smoking is not generally reported as being associated with OA except for very few agents (39). Atopy has been associated with an increased risk of sensitization to many HMW compounds and a few low-molecular-weight (LMW) agents (see Chapter 3). However, the risks associated with atopy or cigarette smoking are not sufficient to guide decisions regarding placement for new employees starting in work environments with known sensitizers.

The physical examination is of secondary importance to the history and pulmonary function studies (see section "Confirming the Diagnosis of OA"). A chest radiograph is generally sufficient to exclude nonasthmagenic causes of respiratory symptoms. A high-resolution computed tomography (CT) scan may be indicated when considering conditions such as hypersensitivity pneumonitis or bronchiolitis obliterans (see Chapter 24).

In some countries where there is a mandatory duty to report confirmed or suspected occupational diseases such as OA, the role of the primary care physician includes the reporting of patients to the public health agency. Notification helps to achieve more precise surveillance of the incidence of WRA and to identify trends and new causal agents. The notification may initiate an inquiry in the workplace with primary and secondary prevention objectives. The inquiry may help to identify sentinel cases (40) and other workers affected by the disease as well as to promote prevention initiatives.

Confirming the diagnosis of OA

A suggestive history, even in the presence of a known sensitizer, is not enough to confirm the diagnosis neither of asthma (41) nor of OA (42). The diagnosis needs to be confirmed objectively. The

---

CASE HISTORY FOLLOW-UP

Following the administration of detailed medical questionnaires, the occupational nurse referred the worker to the occupational physician. The worker had been seen by an allergy specialist (without being referred) and SPTs to various cereals and enzymes had revealed immediate skin reactions to wheat and soy flour allergens. Following a second interview with the occupational physician and the positive results of the skin tests, the worker agreed to be referred to a specialized center for evaluation of OA.

(SEE CASE HISTORY, ITEM NO. 7)

The worker described in the case history was subsequently seen at the OA clinic of the local university hospital. He had spirometry performed in the clinic, which was within normal values, but his methacholine challenge showed mild increased bronchial responsiveness with a PC20 of 2 mg/mL. Monitoring of PEF at and off work showed significant changes in PEF while at work with 20% fall in PEF on several occasions improving during weekends, particularly on Sundays. On Sundays, he had minimal variation in his PEF values. Sputum induction showed moderate eosinophilia (5% eosinophils for a total cell count of 2.5×10^6 cells/g) at the end of a working week. After 2 weeks off work, his PC20 improved to 9 mg/mL and he had 1% eosinophils in sputum for a total cell count of 1.9 cells/g. These data confirmed the diagnosis of OA, and the patient was taken off work as there were no jobs available where he would not be exposed to flour. The necessary information was also provided to the appropriate authorities for evaluation of the worker's right to compensation and reassignment services.

---

various tests used to confirm or exclude the diagnosis are outlined in the following paragraphs. Although specific inhalation challenges are considered the diagnostic reference standard, all steps involved in the investigation have their own value and contribute to establishing the diagnosis. Combining the various elements strengthens the likelihood of a proper diagnosis (11).

Confirming the diagnosis of asthma

The diagnosis of asthma is based on history and objective evidence of reversible airflow obstruction or increased nonspecific bronchial responsiveness (NSBR) (43).

Simple spirometry is often not performed early in the medical evaluation of workers suspected of OA. Although documentation of reversible airflow limitation confirms the diagnosis of asthma, most workers investigated for OA have normal spirometry when seen in the clinic. Furthermore, pre- and postshift monitoring of forced expiratory volume in 1 second (FEV$_1$) has not proven sensitive or specific enough to be a useful tool in the evaluation of OA (7).

Even if increased NSBR is the hallmark of asthma, its presence does not alone establish a diagnosis of OA. The absence of increased NSBR assessed shortly (minutes, hours) after a work shift in a worker with symptoms virtually excludes OA (44). Even in workers with confirmed OA, NSBR may normalize after several days (a weekend may be enough [45] or weeks to months away from work). Subsequent return to work or even exposure via a specific inhalation test may be adequate to cause increased NSBR (46, 47).

Use of investigations to confirm or exclude occupational asthma

Workers with OA must fulfill the diagnostic requirements for asthma, and further assessment is needed to confirm an occupational cause.

Symptoms and lung function

Most patients with OA complain of typical WRA symptoms, but some may not. For example, there may be evidence of work-related changes in lung function (such as PEF, FEV_1, airway responsiveness, or an accelerated annual decline in FEV_1 [48]) in the absence of symptoms that might suggest further investigation is necessary. The intent is to identify symptoms, or other features as above, that suggest the need for further investigation. In the case of sensitizer-induced OA, symptoms should also have a latency, that is a period of sensitization between the beginning of exposure and the onset of symptoms. Rhinitis is a common accompanying feature. It should always be inquired of, as the likelihood of developing OA is higher in the first few years after starting exposure to HMW agents such as laboratory animals.

Questionnaires are highly sensitive (although not specific) tools to collect this information. Measuring lung function with spirometry should always be carried out. All measures should be quality controlled and conform to relevant guidelines (49). Whenever possible, further confirmatory tests are required to make a diagnosis of OA, guided by a multidisciplinary approach.

IgE-mediated immunity: Skin testing and specific IgE assessment

SPTs and specific IgE testing to occupational agents are useful diagnostic tools to confirm sensitization to an occupational allergen, particularly HMW agent. A meta-analysis of specific IgE assessment identified a 74% sensitivity and 71% specificity for HMW agents and of 28% and 89%, respectively, for LMW agents (10). The lack of availability and immunological validity for a wide range of allergens also limits their use (Chapter 7).

Tests to assess airway inflammation: Sputum eosinophils and FeNO

These tests are markers of airway inflammation and are useful in the investigation of OA (Chapter 7). Measured alone, a high (≥2%) sputum eosinophil count or an elevated FeNO (≥ 25 ppb) each has a low sensitivity for OA (50). However, when used in combination and together with the assessment of NSBR, their sensitivity is significantly improved (50). One study suggests that this may predict accelerated lung function decline in continually exposed workers (51).

Functional tests

Peak expiratory flow (PEF) measurement Serial measures of PEF are regarded as the next important investigation (Chapter 8). A meta-analysis has identified pooled sensitivity and specificity of serial PEF measurements of 75% and 79%, respectively, for a diagnosis of OA (52), with more complete data improving these indicators. Workers will need to be taught the importance of making these recordings and encouraged, ideally through the period of data collection.

NSBR testing Achieved by provoking the airway with a variety of inhaled agents that can cause transient airway narrowing (principally methacholine), is useful for confirming a diagnosis of asthma. The presence of NSBR well may support a diagnosis of asthma, and thus OA, but its absence does not exclude OA if the worker has been away from work or has become asymptomatic (53). Assessment of NSBR may further be improved by measures of FeNO and sputum eosinophilia.

Specific inhalation challenges (SIC) (Chapter 8) Are still considered the reference standard to confirm the diagnosis of OA (54–56), although not widely available given the expertise required. Originally done in the laboratory and aiming to mimic work exposure, these are also done in the workplace (57). They are indicated when there is discrepancy between results of PEF monitoring and PC20 or sputum induction or when history is highly suggestive of OA despite negative monitoring. Specific challenges in the workplace are particularly useful when the worker is exposed to several sensitizers or when the offending agent is unknown.

SICs are safe when performed under the close supervision of an expert physician and by trained personnel and are thus limited to specialized centers. A statement (55) and handbook (58) on methodology have been proposed. Further details on the method of specific challenges are given in Chapter 8. A positive test is generally defined by a fall of ≥ 15%–20% from baseline, although another means of interpretation has been suggested in the case of late reactions (59), and confirms the diagnosis of OA, whereas a negative test in the workplace, or in the laboratory, does not absolutely rule out the diagnosis of OA in a worker who has not been exposed to work for several months as they may have become "desensitized." This is particularly true if there is a change in methacholine PC20 following a negative response to SICs. Such a worker should return to work for serial monitoring of PEF and bronchial responsiveness for at least a few weeks before excluding the diagnosis. False-negative challenges in the laboratory may also be due to exposure to the wrong agent or inadvertent administration of a forbidden drug (e.g. inhaled β-2 agonist) before the test. Indeed, Rioux et al. showed that as high as 20% of challenges done in the laboratory may be false negative, particularly when workers are exposed to LMW agents (57). However, if the subject experiences their usual symptoms during the challenge procedure without any spirometric changes, these tests are conclusive in excluding the diagnosis of OA.

Workplace challenges collect serial physiology during normal work activities, comparing airway responses between periods of exposure and nonexposure (or not at work). They may be useful if SIC is not available, and in the context of mixed or complicated exposures that are difficult to re-create in the laboratory setting (57). Again, analysis can use the 95% CI of all measures taken on nonexposed days (59), with a significant fall in FEV_1 on an active day defined as one that falls below the lower bound of the confidence limit from control days.

Figure 5.4 illustrates the algorithm for the investigation of OA summarizing the various steps required to exclude or confirm the diagnosis depending on the level of certainty required.

What other diagnosis should be considered when investigating a worker for work-related asthma?

Workers presenting with symptoms suggestive of WRA may require consideration of alternate or coexisting diagnoses, given the relatively low diagnostic specificity of common respiratory symptoms:

i. *Occupational hypersensitivity pneumonitis* (HP) (Chapter 24) should always be considered in workers with work-related respiratory symptoms. It is plausible that HP could present in a similar manner to WRA, given that respiratory complaints are commonly seen in HP, often along with systemic features such as fever and weight loss. Previous workplace outbreaks of occupational lung disease have described both conditions occurring that were attributed to the same cause (60). More focused airway inflammation, such as seen in (ii) *eosinophilic bronchitis* (Chapter 21),

INVESTIGATION OF WORK-RELATED ASTHMA

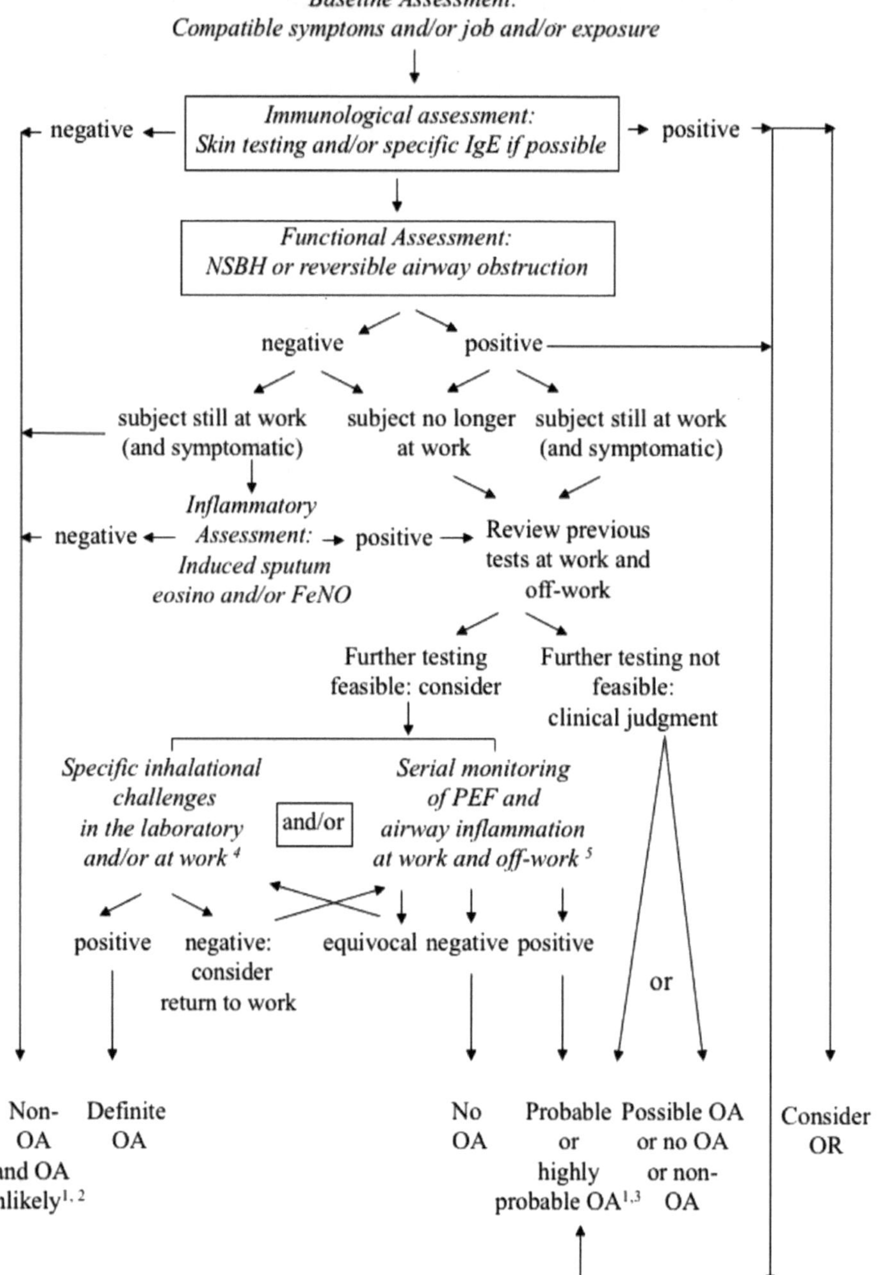

FIGURE 5.4 Proposed stepwise algorithm for diagnosing occupational asthma. (Adapted from Cullinan, P, Vandenplas O, Bernstein D. Assessment and management of occupational asthma. *J Allergy Clin Immunol Pract.* 2020;8(10):3264–3275. By permission.) *Abbreviations:* eosino: eosinophils; FeNO: exhaled nitric oxide level; NSBH: nonspecific bronchial hyperresponsiveness; OA: occupational asthma; OR: occupational rhinitis; PEF: peak expiratory flow.

1. High negative predictive value (NPV) and positive predictive value (PPV) are applicable only for selected populations of subjects with a high pretest probability of OA (i.e. investigated in tertiary centers).
2. NPV >95% for the combination of absence of immunological reactivity and NSBH.
3. In subjects with NSBH (when immunological tests have been validated by comparison with specific inhalation challenge) increasing the cutoff value for a positive sIgE test ≥ 2.22 kU$_A$/L for wheat flour, ≥ 9.64 kU$_A$/L for rye flour, and ≥ 4.41 kU$_A$/L for latex provides a PPV for a positive specific inhalation challenge result > 95%.
4. Especially useful when: SIC can be performed efficiently and safely; the subject is no longer exposed at work; the highest level of diagnostic confidence is required; there is need to identify a particular agent; PEF records are inconclusive.
5. Especially useful when: the subject is exposed to multiple asthmagens at work; no agent known as causing OA has been identified at work; facility for SIC is not easily available; the conditions of exposure at work cannot be reproduced in the laboratory.

considered as a potential precursor of asthma, may also need consideration; (iii) *Chronic obstructive pulmonary disease* should also be considered in a worker being investigated for OA, although it is relatively easily distinguished from asthma (Chapter 25). COPD itself may be related or unrelated to workplace exposures, but irrespective of causation can still cause work-related symptoms. Workers may display features of both asthma and COPD (asthma-COPD overlap). Other less common respiratory conditions that affect the airway (and/or the parenchyma) should always be considered in the differential diagnosis. These include (iv) *obliterative bronchiolitis* (Chapter 25) (61), seen most notably following diacetyl exposure, or rarely (v) *organizing pneumonia* with an occupational attribution (61). Episodes of shortness of breath associated with systemic features should also raise the possibility of (vi) a *fume fever*; such as caused by metal (Chapter 16) or polymer fume (62). Similarly, such episodes might, in the correct occupational context, suggest that bioaerosols, or specifically endotoxin exposure, might be responsible for an (vii) *inhalation fever* (Chapters 23 and 24) that may mimic OA. Long known to influence breathing and important to exclude, (viii) *disorders of the vocal cords* (Chapter 19) should also be considered in a worker with OA. Inducible laryngeal obstruction, an inappropriate, transient, reversible narrowing of the larynx in response to external triggers (63), may also potentially be seen in occupational contexts.

Research needs

It would be relevant to:

- assess the validity of surveillance programs in high-risk workplaces in relation to the nature of occupational agent and type of exposure;
- improve surveillance questionnaires for identifying the most relevant questions in terms of sensitivity/specificity;
- examine whether objective tests can be preferred to questionnaires; and
- obtain information on the level of knowledge and awareness of workers about the nature and risks of products.

Conclusion

While it may be difficult to distinguish work-exacerbated asthma from OA (Chapter 20), a combination of diagnostic tools will help the clinician to come to a proper diagnosis. Suspicion of the diagnosis can result from surveillance programs led by occupational nurses and physicians, and primary care providers. Referral to a specialized center is often necessary. Objective confirmation of asthma and WRA is essential as history is neither sensitive nor specific enough. SIC is still considered the reference standard although a combination of tests carried out in a stepwise approach may achieve a high diagnostic yield.

References

1. Nicholson PJ, Cullinan P, Burge S, et al. Concise guidance: diagnosis, management and prevention of occupational asthma. Clin Med. 2012;12:156–9.
2. Fishwick D, Barber CM, Bradshaw LM, et al. Standards of care for occupational asthma: an update. Thorax. 2012;67:278–80.
3. Dobashi K, Usami A, Yokozeki H, et al. Japanese guidelines for occupational allergic diseases 2020. Allergol Int. 2020;69(3):387–404.
4. Jeebhay MF, Quirce S. Occupational asthma in the developing and industrialised world: a review. Int J Tuberc Lung Dis. 2007;11:122–33.
5. de Bono J, Hudsmith L. Occupational asthma: a community based study. Occup Med. 1999;49:217–9.
6. Fishwick D, Forman S. Health surveillance for occupational asthma. Curr Opin Allergy Clin Immunol. 2018;18:80–6.
7. Nicholson PJ, Cullinan P, Newman Taylor AJ, et al. Evidence based guidelines for the prevention, identification, and management of occupational asthma. Occup Environ Med. 2005;62:290–9.
8. Szram J, Cullinan P. Medical surveillance for prevention of occupational asthma. Curr Opin Allergy Clin Immunol. 2013;13:138–44.
9. Brant A, Nightingale S, Berriman J, et al. Supermarket baker's asthma: how accurate is routine health surveillance? Occup Environ Med. 2005;62:395–9.
10. Lux H, Lenz K, Budnik LT, et al. Performance of specific immunoglobulin E tests for diagnosing occupational asthma: a systematic review and meta-analysis. Occup Environ Med. 2019;76:269–78.
11. Taghiakbari M, Pralong JA, Lemière C, et al. Novel clinical scores for occupational asthma due to exposure to high-molecular-weight agents. Occup Environ Med. 2019;76:495–501.
12. Malo JL, Cartier A, L'Archevêque J, et al. Prevalence of occupational asthma and immunologic sensitization to psyllium among health personnel in chronic care hospitals. Am Rev Respir Dis. 1990;142:1359–66.
13. Maghni K, Malo JL, L'Archevêque J, et al. Matrix metalloproteinases, IL-8 and glutathione in the prognosis of workers exposed to chlorine. Allergy. 2010;65:722–30.
14. Huang YC, Yang MC. Associations between occupational inhalation risks and FeNO levels in airway obstruction patients: results from the National Health and Nutrition Examination Survey, 2007-2012. Int J Chron Obstruct Pulmon Dis. 2017;12:3085–93.
15. Direction de santé publique. Agence de la santé et des services sociaux de Montréal, Juin 2013. Protocole et guide de pratique pour la surveillance médicale de la rhinite et de l'asthme professionnels avec période de latence. https://santemontreal.qc.ca/fileadmin/user_upload/Uploads/tx_asssmpublications/pdf/publications/978-2-89673-302-6.pdf (Accessed 22 June 2020). 2013.
16. Direction de santé publique. Agence de la santé et des services sociaux de Montréal. Protocole et guide de pratique pour la surveillance médicale de la rhinite et de l'asthme professionnels avec période de latence – Guide d'accompagnement, Juin 2013. https://santemontreal.qc.ca/fileadmin/user_upload/Uploads/tx_asssmpublications/pdf/publications/978-2-89673-302-6guide.pdf (Accessed 22 June 2020). 2013.
17. Cullinan P, Muñoz X, Suojalehto H, et al. Occupational lung diseases: from old and novel exposures to effective preventive strategies. Lancet Respir Med. 2017;5:445–55.
18. Moscato G, Vandenplas O, Van Wijk RG, et al. Occupational rhinitis. Allergy. 2008;63:969–80.
19. Labrecque M, Malo JL, Alaoui KM, et al. Medical surveillance programme for diisocyanate exposure. Occup Environ Med. 2011;68:302–7.
20. Pralong JA, Moullec G, Suarthana E, et al. Screening for occupational asthma by using a self-administered questionnaire in a clinical setting. J Occup Environ Med. 2013;55:527–31.
21. Baur X, Sigsgaard T, Aasen TB, et al. Guidelines for the management of work-related asthma. Eur Respir J. 2012;39:529–45.
22. Vandenplas O, Suojalehto H, Cullinan P. Diagnosing occupational asthma. Clin Exp Allergy. 2017;47:6–18.
23. Wilken D, Baur X, Barbinova L, et al. What are the benefits of medical screening and surveillance? Eur Respir Rev. 2012;21:105–11.
24. Moscato G, Vandenplas O, Van Wijk RG, et al. EAACI position paper on occupational rhinitis. Respir Res. 2009;10:16.
25. Suojalehto H, Karvala K, Haramo J, et al. Medical surveillance for occupational asthma-how are cases detected? Occup Med (Lond). 2017;67:159–62.
26. Burrows B, Martinez FD, Halonen M, et al. Association of asthma with serum IgE levels and skin-test reactivity to allergens. N Engl J Med. 1989;320:271–7.
27. Gautrin D, Infante-Rivard C, Dao TV, et al. Specific IgE-dependent sensitization, atopy and bronchial hyperresponsiveness in apprentices starting exposure to protein-derived agents. Am J Respir Crit Care Med. 1997;155:1841–7.
28. Blanc PD, Annesi-Maesano I, Balmes JR, et al. The Occupational Burden of Nonmalignant Respiratory Diseases. An Official American Thoracic Society and European Respiratory Society Statement. Am J Respir Crit Care Med. 2019;199:1312–34.
29. Henneberger PK, Redlich CA, Callahan DB, et al. An Official American Thoracic Society Statement: work-exacerbated asthma. Am J Respir Crit Care Med. 2011;184:368–78.

30. Mazurek JM, White GE, Moorman JE, et al. Patient-physician communication about work-related asthma: what we do and do not know. Ann Allergy Asthma Immunol. 2014;114:97–102.

31. Walters GI, McGrath EE, Ayres JG. Audit of the recording of occupational asthma in primary care. Occup Med (Lond). 2012;62:570–3.

32. Tarlo SM, Balmes J, Balkisssoon R, et al. ACCP consensus statement: diagnosis and management of work-related asthma. Chest. 2008;134:1S–41S.

33. Vandenplas O, Ghezzo H, Munoz X, et al. What are the questionnaire items most useful in identifying subjects with occupational asthma? Eur Respir J. 2005;26:1056–63.

34. Hull JH, Backer V, Gibson PG, et al. Laryngeal dysfunction: assessment and management for the clinician. Am J Respir Crit Care Med. 2016;194:1062–72.

35. Bernstein JA. Material safety data sheets: are they reliable in identifying human hazards? J Allergy Clin Immunol. 2002;110:35–8.

36. Rosenman KD, Beckett WS. Web based listing of agents associated with new onset work-related asthma. Respir Med. 2015;109:625–31.

37. Shao Z, Bernstein JA. Occupational rhinitis: classification, diagnosis, and therapeutics. Curr Allergy Asthma Rep. 2019;19:54.

38. Malo JL, Ghezzo H, D'Aquino C, et al. Natural history of occupational asthma: relevance of type of agent and other factors in the rate of development of symptoms in affected subjects. J Allergy Clin Immunol. 1992;90:937–44.

39. Siracusa A, Marabini A, Folletti I, et al. Smoking and occupational asthma. Clin Exper Allergy. 2006;36:577–84.

40. Zhou AY, Seed M, Carder M, et al. Sentinel approach to detect emerging causes of work-related respiratory diseases. Occup Med (Lond). 2020;70:52–9.

41. LindenSmith J, Morrison D, Deveau C, et al. Overdiagnosis of asthma in the community. Can Respir J. 2004;11:111–6.

42. Malo JL, Ghezzo H, L'Archevêque J, et al. Is the clinical history a satisfactory means of diagnosing occupational asthma? Am Rev Respir Dis. 1991;143:528–32.

43. Ginasthma.org. Global strategy for asthma management and prevention. Updated 2020. https://ginasthma.org/wp-content/uploads/2020/04/GINA-2020-full-report_-final-_wms.pdf.

44. Baur X, Huber H, Degens PO, et al. Relation between occupational asthma case history, bronchial methacholine challenge, and specific challenge test in patients with suspected occupational asthma. Am J Ind Med. 1998;33:114–22.

45. Cockcroft DW, Mink JT. Isocyanate-induced asthma in an automobile spray painter. CMA J. 1979;121:602–4.

46. Hargreave FE, Ramsdale EH, Pugsley SO. Occupational asthma without bronchial hyperresponsiveness. Am Rev Respir Dis. 1984;130:513–5.

47. Lemière C, Cartier A, Dolovich J, et al. Outcome of specific bronchial responsiveness to occupational agents after removal from exposure. Am J Respir Crit Care Med. 1996;154:329–33.

48. Anees W, Moore VC, Burge PS. FEV1 decline in occupational asthma. Thorax. 2006;61:751–5.

49. Graham BL, Steenbruggen I, Miller MR, et al. Standardization of spirometry 2019 update. An Official American Thoracic Society and European Respiratory Society Technical Statement. Am J Respir Crit Care Med. 2019;200(8):e70–e88.

50. Beretta C, Rifflart C, Evrard G, et al. Assessment of eosinophilic airway inflammation as a contribution to the diagnosis of occupational asthma. Allergy. 2018;73:206–13.

51. Talini D, Novelli F, Bacci E, et al. Sputum eosinophilia is a determinant of FEV1 decline in occupational asthma: results of an observational study. BMJ Open. 2015;5:e005748.

52. Moore V, Jaakkola M, Burge P. A systematic review of serial peak expiratory flow measurements in the diagnosis of occupational asthma. Ann Respir Med. 2010;1:31–40.

53. Pralong JA, Cartier A. Review of diagnostic challenges in occupational asthma. Curr Allergy Asthma Rep. 2017;17:1.

54. Cruz MJ, Munoz X. The current diagnostic role of the specific occupational laboratory challenge test. Curr Opin Allergy Clin Immunol. 2012;12:119–25.

55. Vandenplas O, Suojalehto H, Aasen TB, et al. Specific inhalation challenge in the diagnosis of occupational asthma: consensus statement. Eur Respir J. 2014;43:1573–87.

56. Tarlo SM. The role and interpretation of specific inhalation challenges in the diagnosis of occupational asthma. Can Respir J. 2015;22:322–3.

57. Rioux JP, Malo JL, L'Archevêque J, et al. Workplace specific challenges as a contribution to the diagnosis of occupational asthma. Eur Respir J. 2008;32:997–1003.

58. Suojalehto H, Suuronen K, Cullinan P. Specific challenge testing for occupational asthma: revised handbook. Eur Respir J. 2019;54(2):pii: 1901026.

59. Stenton SC, Avery AJ, Walters EH, et al. Statistical approaches to the identification of late asthmatic reactions. Eur Respir J. 1994;7:806–12.

60. Robertson W, Robertson AS, Burge CB, et al. Clinical investigation of an outbreak of alveolitis and asthma in a car engine manufacturing plant. Thorax. 2007;62:981–90.

61. Cordier JF, Cottin V, Lazor R, et al. Many faces of bronchiolitis and organizing pneumonia. Semin Respir Crit Care Med. 2016;37:421–40.

62. Greenberg MI, Vearrier D. Metal fume fever and polymer fume fever. Clin Toxicol (Phila). 2015;53:195–203.

63. Halvorsen T, Walsted ES, Bucca C, et al. Inducible laryngeal obstruction: an official joint European Respiratory Society and European Laryngological Society statement. Eur Respir J. 2017;50(3).

6

ASSESSMENT OF THE WORKPLACE

Gert Doekes,[1] Monika Raulf,[2] Dick Heederik,[3] and Carrie A. Redlich[4]
editors Susan M. Tarlo[5] and Jean-Luc Malo[6]
[1]Institute for Risk Assessment Sciences, Utrecht University, The Netherlands
[2]Department Allergology/Immunology of the Institute of Prevention and Occupational Medicine of the German
Social Accident Insurance; Institute of the Ruhr-University Bochum (IPA), Bochum, Germany
[3]Institute for Risk Assessment Sciences, Utrecht University, The Netherlands
[4]Pulmonary Section & Occupational and Environmental Medicine Program, Yale Occupational and
Environmental Medicine Program, Yale School of Medicine, New Haven, Connecticut, USA
[5]University Health Network and St Michael's Hospital, Toronto, Department of Medicine, University of Toronto, Ontario, Canada
[6]Hôpital du Sacré-Cœur de Montréal and Université de Montréal, Montréal, Québec, Canada

Contents

Introduction

Occupational asthma (OA) and work-related asthma (WRA) can be caused or aggravated by exposure to a wide range of chemical and biological agents. Exposure is defined as direct physical contact with an agent (1, 2) and since inhalation is obviously the most important route of exposure, this chapter mainly focuses on airborne agents. Dermal exposure will also be discussed briefly, since systemic allergic sensitization to some asthmagens can also occur after skin contact (3, 4).

Relevant questions include:

a. Which sensitizing, proinflammatory or irritant agents are present at the workplace: in handled materials, used equipment, the surrounding air, etc.?
b. What are the exposure levels: how much of each agent is inhaled by the worker?
c. When does exposure occur: which job tasks are associated with (high) airborne exposure?

d. How does exposure vary between and within workers with different tasks and over time?

Exposure assessment thus comprises much more than measuring allergens or irritants in samples from the workplace, although often an essential part of an investigation. This chapter therefore not only provides an overview of methods and equipment for measurement of chemical and biological agents, but also discusses strategy and design of exposure assessment surveys, which are of utmost importance to obtain accurate exposure estimates.

The first step is to clearly define the objectives of an exposure assessment study, which may be:

1. To compare air levels with existing exposure standards (*compliance sampling*), e.g. as part of systematic *surveillance* or *monitoring* programs;
2. Evaluation of *intervention* measures to lower exposure levels in a prevention program;
3. *Etiology* research, assessing relations between specific exposures and the risk of respiratory health effects;
4. As part of a *clinical evaluation,* for instance in specific inhalation challenge (SIC) testing in a challenge room or in the work environment (Chapters 5 and 8).

These objectives should be further qualified as in the following examples. Of note, most exposure standards for substances that can cause asthma were not established to prevent sensitization or are associated with a residual sensitization risk, and thus finding levels below occupational exposure limits (OELs) typically cannot be used to rule out a suspected occupational asthmagen in an individual patient. Measurement of asthmagens in the workplace as part of an individual patient diagnostic evaluation is usually not cost-effective or feasible, but may be informative in selected cases, such as asthma caused by a thus far unknown allergen, or a complex mixture that cannot be produced in a challenge test laboratory. The particular context for the exposure assessment thus should be taken into account, and its implications will be critically discussed in the final paragraph.

A measurement procedure usually consists of three steps:

a. Sampling at the workplace.
b. Storage and transport to a laboratory, where samples are further processed, including elution or extraction of analytes from the sampling device or matrix (filters, adsorbents, etc.), in some cases further chemical treatment, and often storage of eluates or extracts until further analysis.
c. Analysis of the contents of extracts using chemical, immunochemical, enzymatic, microbiological, or molecular biological methods.

Exceptions to this three-step procedure are direct real-time measurements of dusts, gases, and vapors, and so-called rapid tests in which dust samples are processed and directly semiquantitatively analyzed at the workplace (see section "Rapid Tests for Chemical and Biological Agents"). Measurement of viable micro-organisms (see section "Microbial Agents") requires microbial culture directly or soon after sampling, thus with minimal transport time, or culture done in an incubator close to the sampling site.

Measurement of airborne dust-associated agents (like many high-molecular-weight [HMW] allergens) is usually combined with gravimetric measurement of filters with the sampled dust, before further processing by extraction of specific agents from the dust and filter. Gravimetry should preferably be performed in a climate-controlled weighing room, and filters must have been preweighed before sampling under the same conditions (see section "Aerosols: Dust, Fumes, and Mists").

Each step from sampling until final analysis may show technical variations, which can impact measured findings. All field and laboratory work should therefore be done with standard operation procedures (SOPs), preferably in accordance with international or national standards for sampling and laboratory analysis (5). For many asthmagens—especially HMW allergens—no such standards are however available (6, 7); for others, such as diisocyanates, established standards may not protect against sensitization and asthma. It is therefore even more important that all sampling, sample processing, and analytic procedures are clearly defined and documented, and that exactly the same methods are used for all samples in a study that investigates variation in exposure between workers, job tasks, workplaces, or day-to-day variation in time.

Detailed explanatory guides to sampling and analysis were published in the corresponding chapter of the previous edition of this book (8) and on several websites:

- https://www.cdc.gov/niosh/nmam/5th_edition_web_book. html;
- http://www.irsst.qc.ca/media/documents/PubIRSST/T-15.pdf (9). These websites, among others, also give information about exposure standards.

Sampling

General considerations

The most accurate quantitative assessment of individual airborne exposures is achieved by active personal sampling from the worker's breathing zone as done with a portable air pump worn on the belt and connected to a sampling head close to the mouth and nose. Samples can be taken during a full work shift, or during specific job tasks in periods of minimally 15–20 minutes. The choice of the sampling time may also depend on the volume necessary for the analysis: a smaller sample volume means a higher detection limit, with a higher risk of nondetectable airborne levels and (possibly false) negative results. The sampling time thus should preferably be based on preliminary insight into exposure levels and patterns: for instance, whether the exposure is homogeneously distributed over time, short work cycles are frequently repeated, or when there are peaks of exposure followed by prolonged periods of nonexposure.

Stationary sampling from a fixed location in the workplace may approximate the personal exposure when the sampling site is close to the worker's actual position during most of the workday. Such "ambient air sampling" can monitor the average air quality at the workplace and is suitable for compliance with regulatory OELs. Personal and stationary airborne sampling can make use of the same calibrated pumps with well-known airflow; the product of the flow and the sampling time gives the exact volume of the sample, and airborne concentrations of inhalable dust can thus be expressed in weight units (micro- or milligrams) per m^3, and for specific molecular agents in traditional units like ppm (parts per million), or in molar or weight units per m^3.

Ambient air quality can also be measured with high-volume samplers using nonportable pumps with much higher flow rates, for instance to obtain more material for exploratory analyses, but the aerodynamic properties of aerosol particles collected at different airflows and with different sampling heads may differ from what exposed subjects actually inhale at the worksite (10, 11). Despite the described advantages of personal or ambient sampling, it should be noted that sampling only captures levels of exposure associated with the location and environmental conditions during the time of sampling, a limitation when the concern is cumulative exposure or when exposures are highly variable or sporadic. One should be aware about these limitations when extrapolation of measurements to prolonged periods of exposure is required (estimating cumulative exposure).

Passive personal sampling is a simpler and inexpensive, but less accurate, method to monitor average air quality during the workday or for more prolonged periods. Ambient airborne dust levels can be estimated with passive dust collectors of known surface area, on which deposited respirable-size dust particles are collected (see section "Passive Dust Sampling and Analysis of Dust Deposits"). Since the air volume from which measured agents are sampled is not known, however, results of passive sampling can only be given in units per sampler or surface area, and per hour or day of the sampling period.

An even more crude approach is the analysis of samples taken by dry or wet swiping from surfaces like desk or shelf tops, machinery, or other equipment, or of samples from materials handled by workers, like food or feed, manure or other waste, chemical products, or solvents used in the production process. Such procedures enable hazard identification but cannot be used to quantify levels of airborne exposures. Since skin exposure can be an effective route of sensitization with chemical sensitizers such as diisocyanates, wipe samples from surfaces that workers may handle can also identify surfaces to target for exposure reduction (12).

Gases and vapors

The term *gas* refers to substances that are in the gaseous state at 25°C and atmospheric pressure. *Vapors* are the volatile gaseous form of liquids, with which they are in equilibrium at atmospheric pressure and common temperature, but at many worksites may originate from heating of fluids—as part of the production process or due to dissipating heat from running equipment, inciting light, etc. Collection media for gases and vapors (Figure 6.1) are

bags, adsorbent tubes, or liquid impingers connected to a personal pump with a fixed flow rate.

Airborne chemical agents may be captured with specific adsorbents like charcoal, silica, or Tenax, through active or passive sampling, from which they can be eluted and analyzed in the laboratory, or with specific devices where a color reaction indicates that a threshold level has been exceeded. Passive sampling involves diffusion from the ambient air to an adsorbent medium at the bottom of a dosimeter or behind a membrane. The sampling rate (in mL/min) is a function of the substance and the dosimeter's geometric characteristics.

Individual analysis of each of the sections of the collection media verifies the adsorption efficiency of the collection medium and potential breakthrough. A sample is generally considered acceptable if less than 10% of the product is found in the second section. If it contains more than 25% of the product, the first section may have been overloaded, and measured values then underestimate the actual exposure. For certain gases, bags made of polymerized materials can be used for sampling. Diffusion through or adsorption on the surface of the bag can have an impact on the choice of materials for a given contaminant and the time that the sample can be kept.

Impingers, made of glass or polyethylene, are still commonly used to sample some inorganic acids and a few organic compounds, which are trapped in the collection fluid in the impinger through which sampled air is drawn (Figure 6.2). They have been used for sampling of isocyanates, which can be analyzed directly in the collection fluid, or indirectly, as a stable reaction product with a specific reagent in the collection fluid, like di-n-butylamine (DBA) (14). Spill-proof impingers, inserted in pockets, are also available for breathing zone sampling.

Aerosols: Dust, fumes, and mists

An aerosol is a suspension of airborne particles. Solid aerosols include dusts and fumes (very fine particles originating from condensation), while liquid aerosols are mists. Both may, as nonspecific irritants, aggravate asthma, but are also effective carriers of specific asthmagenic agents, like chemical or biological allergens or proinflammatory agents. The risk of adverse health effects of inhalation further depends on the average aerodynamic diameter of inhaled particles or droplets, and the ISO/CEN/ACGIH sampling conventions (15, 16) therefore distinguish well-defined specific—although partially overlapping—fractions that predominantly deposit in different regions of the respiratory tract (Figure 6.3):

- The *inhalable* fraction involves all particulates inhaled through the nose or mouth, thus targeting the entire respiratory tract.
- The *thoracic* fraction applies to particles with aerodynamic diameter of less than 10–15 μm, presenting a hazard for the lower airways and the gas exchange region.
- The *respirable* fraction includes particles smaller than 5–10 μm that present a hazard for the gas exchange region.

The thoracic fraction is generally considered most relevant for acute or chronic asthmatic inflammation. Common practice in occupational health studies however is to sample and analyze inhalable particles, thus aerosols that can be inhaled and deposit in any part of the respiratory tract, since (a) a comprehensive respiratory health risk assessment includes both upper and lower respiratory tract exposure and symptoms; (b) in case of allergies, work-related rhinitis may precede or indicate an enhanced risk

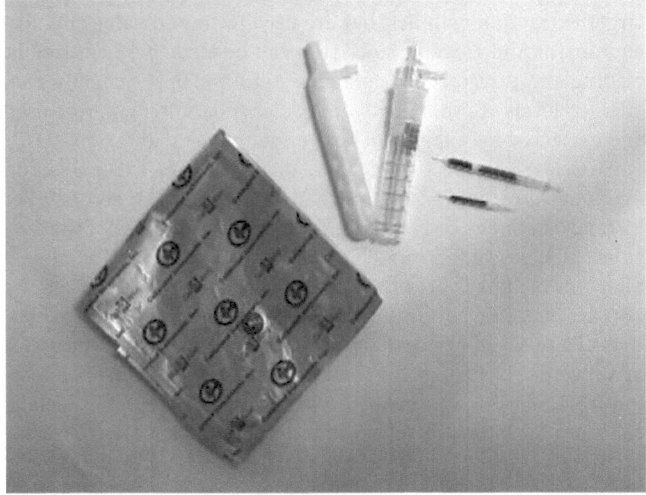

FIGURE 6.1 Collection media for gases and vapors (collection bag, miniimpingers, and adsorbent tubes). (From Reference [13].)

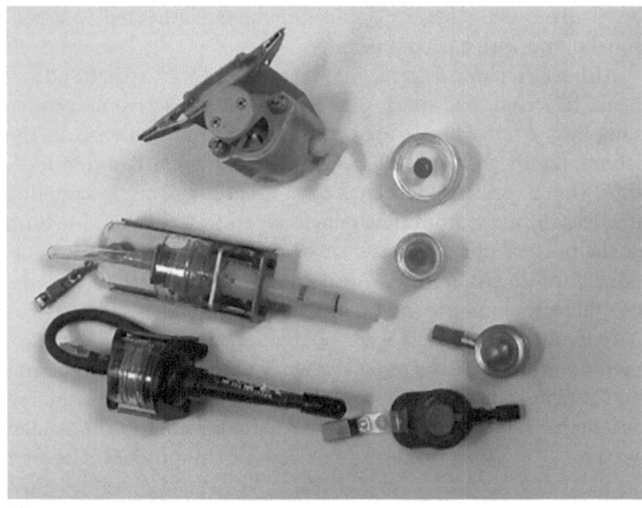

(A)

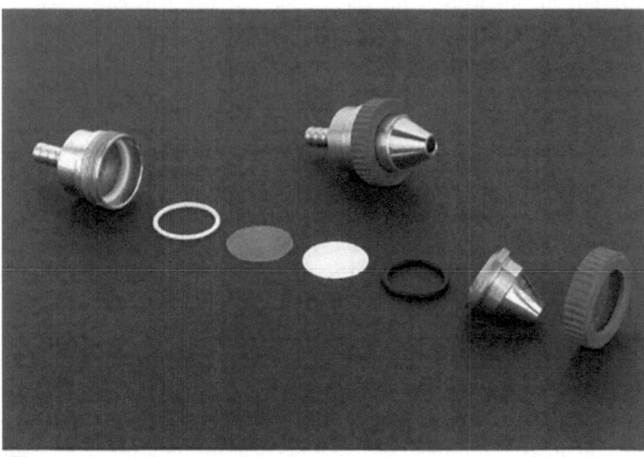

(B)

FIGURE 6.2 Collection media for aerosols. **(A)** Clockwise from left-hand corner: cyclone samplers (twice), multistage personal impactor, open-face samplers (twice), Button sampler, IOM sampler. **(B)** Open and closed PAS6 sampler. (From Reference [13].)

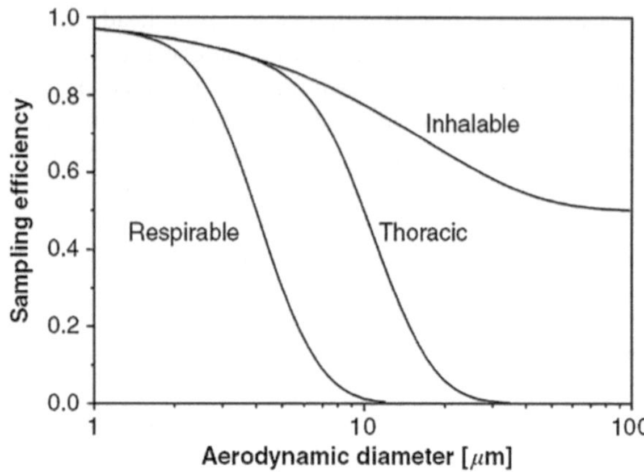

FIGURE 6.3 ISO/ACGIH/CEN sampling conventions. An ideal sampler has a sampling efficiency curve that matches one of these curves as closely as possible under all wind directions and velocities. The 50% cut points for the respirable and thoracic conventions are 4 and 10 μm, respectively. (From Reference [16] https://www.cdc.gov/niosh/nmam/pdf/NMAM_5thEd_EBook-508-final.pdf [public Domain].)

of developing OA (Chapter 22); (c) systemic allergic sensitization can also be induced by allergens via the nasal mucosa (17); (d) for many work-related dust aerosols, the thoracic fraction is roughly a constant percentage of the inhalable dust, although during peak exposures the proportion of large particles may be much higher, and the actual proportion may vary depending on the type of dust and workplace (18).

When exposure assessment is only focused on aerosol/dust levels, real-time measurements can be performed with techniques like particle counting based on light scatter/dispersion techniques. Various low-cost sensoring techniques have become available, allowing analysis of exposure patterns with high temporal resolution (seconds), but validation remains an issue (19). Furthermore, knowledge of specific allergens or microbial agents in an aerosol is of interest in most studies on asthmagenic exposures, and thus sampling methods like filtration or impaction that allow further processing and analysis of collected dust particles are needed.

Most aerosols are collected by filtration on a membrane in a plastic cassette (a so-called sampling head) that for personal sampling is carried in the breathing zone and connected to a pump

worn by the worker. Different types of sampling head are used to collect inhalable dusts, such as the IOM Sampler from the United Kingdom, the Button sampler from the United States, and in Europe the German GSP and Dutch PAS6 sampler (20). Most common flow rates are 2 L/min up to 3.5 L/min; the GSP sampler can also be used at a flow rate up to 10 L/min, but then also requires a much heavier pump carried by the worker (20, 21).

Careful pre- and postweighing of the filters in a conditioned weighing room allows gravimetric assessment of dust levels in the μg–mg range per filter, which nearly equals the concentration per m^3, when full (8-hour) work shift samples are taken at 2 L/min.

Filter membranes are available in various pore sizes and materials; the choice of the filter type (PTFE [Teflon], cellulose esters, polyvinyl chloride, glass fiber, silver, or other materials) depends on the analytes of interest. For measurement of high-molecular-weight (HMW) protein allergens Teflon filters are the first choice, since they allow a high recovery rate at low extraction volumes (22). Glass fiber filters retain, due to their porous structure, a much larger fraction of the extraction fluids, thus requiring larger extraction volumes, but are used for microbial agents like endotoxins and glucans, since they can be made pyrogen-free by heating and extracted at high temperature (23). When, however, allergen levels are sufficiently high, glass fiber filters may be used and extracted for analysis of both endotoxin and allergens (24).

Particle size selective devices placed before the collection medium allow analysis of specific fractions of the aerosol. For instance, cyclones can separate the respirable fraction of the dust at low airflows <1.7 L/min (25). Small particles are collected on a filter in the upper part of the cassette while the largest particles are carried to the bottom of the cyclone. A cascade impactor consists of a series of perforated plates, through which only particles of a specific size can pass. A filter placed after each plate collects the fractions in relation to the particle size. Mists are usually collected on filters, in tubes, or in impingers (see Figure 6.2 for examples).

Passive dust sampling and analysis of dust deposits

Airborne concentrations of HMW allergens are often in the pg–ng per m^3 range, around or just above the detection limits of most

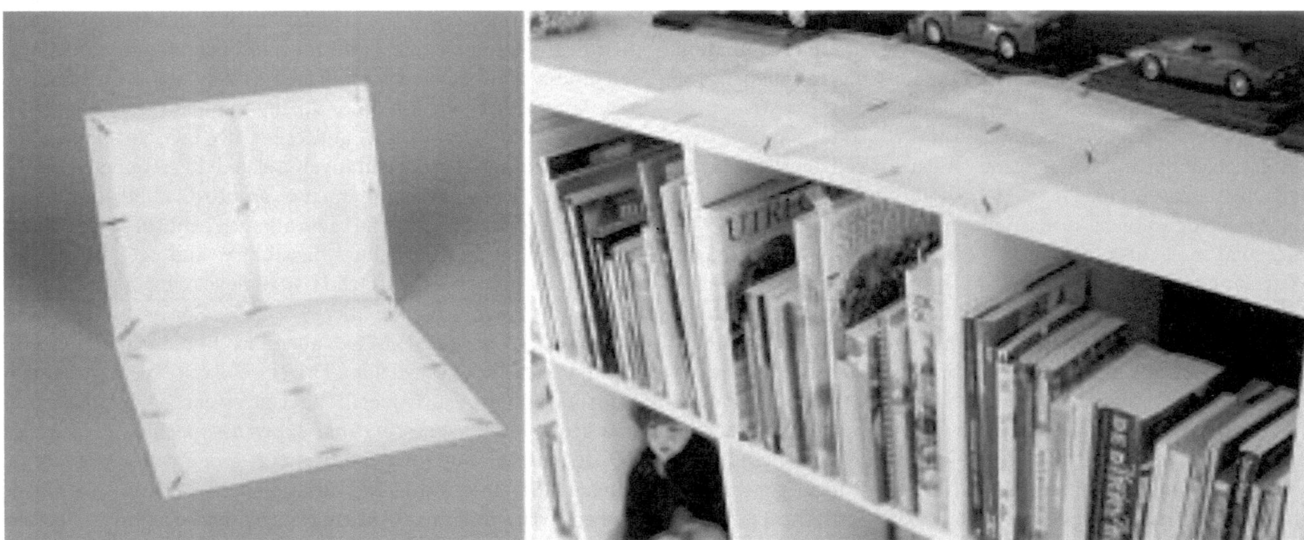

FIGURE 6.4   Passive airborne dust sampling with an electrostatic dust collector.

commonly used assays when combined with low-flow personal or ambient air dust samples, even at worksites with a well-known enhanced risk of occupational allergy (26). High-volume ambient air sampling may in principle be used, but requires specific equipment that is rarely available for simultaneous measurements at several locations, and the use of heavy pumps and associated noise preclude application at low-exposure sites like schools, offices, etc. Instead, low to moderate average airborne allergen levels may be estimated by analyzing dust deposited during a known period—days to weeks—on a quiet undisturbed surface at sufficient height, at least 1.5–2 m, to ensure that collected dust has been airborne and thus could have been inhaled. For more quantitative measurements, specifically designed "passive dust samplers" have been introduced of well-known surface size (Figure 6.4), consisting of a cardboard box with alum foil (a "pizza box") from which the contents after sampling can be collected by vacuuming (27), or an A5- or A4-sized frame in which simple electrostatic cleaning tissues ("Swiffer tissues") are mounted (28).

Both the "pizza box" method and especially the so-called electrostatic dust collectors (EDCs) have been used widely in environments with low to moderate levels of allergens and endotoxins like schools (29), day-care centers (30), veterinary clinics (24), and the home environment (31), but also as an attractive low-cost alternative for active workplace sampling in e.g. the farming environment (32) or laboratory animal facilities (33). Major advantages are the low costs, easy handling and transport, and versatility in use: extracts of tissues with sampled dust can be tested in assays for allergens or microbial agents, but also in qPCR for bacterial or fungal DNA and other methods to assess microbial exposures (34). Levels of measured analytes are expressed in units (e.g. ng allergen) per m^2 and per day or week, as proxy for, and presumably correlating with the actual average airborne concentrations during the sampling period (28, 34, 35). Analysis of passively sampled dust can be used to compare ambient air quality between worksites and homes (to assess carryover of allergens from the workplaces to the homes of the workers) or to compare air quality at the same worksite before and after introduction of intervention measures (32, 33, 36).

A less reliable crude method is analysis of dry or wet swipe samples from surfaces like desks, windowsills, lamp fixtures, etc.

When combined with a rapid test method (see section "Rapid Tests for Chemical and Biological Agents"), this can be useful to demonstrate directly a possible health hazard, e.g. during an occupational health survey of the workplace.

Analysis of floor dust, as commonly used in the home environment, is of limited use for industrial and agricultural workplaces: its contents can vary depending on work activities at the time of sampling, and often consist mainly of particles too large to become airborne and be inhaled by the worker.

Analysis of products and materials

A first inventory of hazards may focus on the presence and concentrations of toxic, allergenic, or proinflammatory agents in products and materials handled by workers, like allergenic feed and food proteins, enzymes, and other additives; mold spores and bacteria; or volatile chemicals in solvents. While an inventory does not specifically measure airborne contaminants, when combined with an occupational hygienist's estimate of the risks that dust or vapors from the handled materials are inhaled during specific job tasks, such analysis may be used to establish job exposure matrices with which workers and jobs are categorized as having a low, moderate, or high risk of work-related asthmagenic exposures (see section "Job Exposure Matrices").

Microbial agents

Airborne microbial agents can be whole intact bacteria, fungal spores, and hyphal fragments, but also microbial cell debris and toxic or proinflammatory cell wall or excreted molecules adsorbed to inorganic or organic dust particles (37). Inhalation may cause nonallergic asthma or asthma-like wheezing illness (see Chapters 19, 23, 24, and 26) or aggravate symptoms in existing asthma (Chapter 20), while some fungal allergens may act as type I sensitizers and be a primary cause of atopic asthma (38, 39) or as a type III sensitizer the cause of hypersensitivity pneumonitis (e.g. farmer's lung disease).

Viable airborne bacteria or fungal spores are measured either by direct sampling on culture substrates in petri dishes, such as with the Andersen sampler for ambient air sampling, or cultured after recovery from a sampling matrix or medium such as impinger fluid, which allows further stepwise dilution when concentrations are high. Culture methods are very sensitive but have various limitations and can lead to over- or underestimation of microbial exposures relevant for OA (40). Culture-independent microscopic methods detect morphologically distinct structures and thus distinguish between various microbial taxa, but neither detect molecular microbial agents as part of cell debris or other particulate matter (40, 41).

Personal or ambient dust samples on filters can be analyzed for microbial molecules for which specific assays are available like bacterial endotoxins, mold glucans, or other fungal antigens or allergens (37–40). Since airborne intact microorganisms behave as other airborne particulates of similar size, analysis of inhalable dust captures molecular microbial agents on both viable or nonviable solid or liquid particles in the sampled aerosol. Modern biological techniques have also allowed development of molecular techniques ranging from qPCR to shotgun sequencing with which DNA or RNA of specific bacterial or fungal genera and species of for instance specific (antimicrobial resistance) genes or even the whole microbiome and resistome can be quantified in small ambient or personal inhalable dust samples (34, 42).

Dermal exposure

Assessment of skin exposure is less developed than that of inhalation exposure (43). Sampling methods are not standardized, have undergone limited validation, and often are technically challenging (44, 45). Contamination on work surfaces such as tools, equipment, or desks may give an indication of *potential* dermal exposure. Simple screening techniques make use of a swab or filter impregnated with a detection reagent that shows an instantaneous visible color reaction with a specific substance on the screened surface. Such qualitative techniques are used mainly to detect heavy metals, amines, and isocyanates. Other methods make use of absorbent material on a defined section of the work surface. To obtain comparable samples, a template can be used. The adsorbent material is then sent to the laboratory for qualitative and quantitative analysis (44, 45).

Measurements on the skin have been considered mainly with regard to isocyanate exposure and some metals like beryllium. Techniques used to detect isocyanate skin exposure include pads (15), wipes, tape stripping, and analysis of contaminated gloves (46–48). Recovery of sampled isocyanates may be low due to their high reactivity, thus leading to underestimation of exposure. A Swedish study however showed that exposure to methylene diphenyl diisocyanate (MDI) can be quantified on workers' skin even if air levels are close to unquantifiable (49); the same research group also concluded that an only very small fraction of dermally applied MDI would penetrate the skin and lead to internal exposure (50).

Biomonitoring

Biological exposure monitoring, or shortly *biomonitoring*, is the measurement of xenobiotics or their metabolites in body fluids like blood, urine, or saliva, to assess the body load and internal exposure to these agents (51). It provides evidence of external exposure, and its dose or intensity, but not of the route of exposure, and neither about where and when exposure occurred, especially when toxicokinetics and dynamics are unknown. For OA it may be useful in studies on chemical substances like isocyanates, as exemplified in a study among isocyanate-exposed molders or spray-painters, in whom isocyanate diamine metabolites in urine were measured (49, 50, 52).

Biomonitoring of exposure to airborne allergenic proteins or microbial agents is not feasible, since most of these HMW molecules do not reach the circulation as intact molecules, and their degradation products (amino acids, partially modified carbohydrates) cannot be distinguished as xenobiotic metabolites. An indirect method of biomonitoring may be measurement of allergen-specific serum IgG, and especially IgG_4 antibodies, for which titres may be quantitatively related to frequency and/or intensity of work-related allergen exposure (53, 54). Individual IgG immune responses to the same allergen exposure levels show, however, wide interindividual variability, and IgG_4 responses may also be associated with the risk of developing a specific IgE response and symptomatic allergy (54, 55). For both HMW and low-molecular-weight (LMW) allergens like isocyanates (56, 57) and trimellitic anhydride (TMA) (58), associations between exposure and exposure-specific IgG titres can be demonstrated on a group level, suggesting that exposure-specific IgG, such as HDI-IgG or MDI-IgG may be useful as a biomarker to monitor exposure (56). Interindividual variation in titres within a group of workers with similar exposure may, however, be mainly reflecting differences in immune responsiveness rather than differences in exposure levels.

Sample analysis

Storage and transport

Sample analysis is usually done in specialized laboratories and specific attention must therefore be given to optimal and standardized storage and transport procedures. Since molecular properties of relevant analytic material vary, it is hard to define general requirements regarding optimal temperature (e.g. with or without freezing), humidity, maximum transport time, etc., and the reader is referred to specific protocols for each separate agent. Each procedure should be designed to avoid both contamination during handling and transport, and loss of analytes of interest to minimize the risk of false-positive or false-negative results, respectively, while leakage and spills of harmful agents should also be avoided to protect field and laboratory workers. Microbial contamination and growth in samples with a high organic content is of specific concern since it may decrease the contents of e.g. allergenic proteins by enzymatic breakdown, while considerably increasing levels of microbial agents. For such samples, storage and transport at low temperature and low humidity in airtight vials may in general be optimal.

Chemical (LMW) agents

For many chemical agents, OELs (like MAC values and other exposure limits) are set, and the documentation of these exposure standards also includes a clearly defined procedure for how to measure the agent (44, 59). Exposure standards to avoid allergic sensitization have however been poorly developed as yet. The list of (potential) chemical sensitizers is long and steadily increasing (Chapters 12–18), and for each agent another detailed analytical protocol may be needed. Many chemical sensitizers, such as isocyanates and anhydrides, are highly reactive with amino or hydroxy groups, and thus can covalently bind to and sometimes even cross-link proteins or other HMW compounds (60) (Chapter 14). This reactivity may be used during sampling to form stable conjugates with a known carrier molecule that can be more easily measured. The most commonly applied techniques for chemical analyses are gas chromatography (GC), very often combined with mass spectrometry (GC/MS), high-performance liquid chromatography (HPLC), atom absorption spectrometry (especially for metals), and UV, visible light, and infrared spectrometry to detect specific substances in an elution medium, while X-ray diffraction may be used to analyze solid particles in crystalline form, and microscopy is used to identify and count fibers.

Most chemical analyses require elution in organic solvents like methanol, acetone, or strongly denaturing agents like HCl, in contrast to HMW allergens that are commonly eluted in aqueous buffers (see section "Biological HMW Agents"). As a consequence, LMW chemical agents and biological agents like HMW proteins can rarely be measured in the same samples.

Biological (HMW) agents

Occupational HMW allergens, like feed and food proteins, animal-derived allergens, and enzymes used in washing powders or as food additives, are relatively stable water-soluble (glyco)proteins and can be easily eluted from dust, filters, EDC tissues, or other sample matrices, by agitation at room temperature in conventional physiological buffers, and measured in specific enzyme immunoassays (EIAs). Methods are less standardized than for chemicals, and most of the thus far used immunoassays are based on in-house produced polyclonal or monoclonal immune reagents, while units in which results are reported usually refer to the laboratory's own calibration standards. Collaborative studies have compared extraction and assay procedures, as summarized in position papers (26) with as main conclusions:

- Extraction yields may be far from 100% due to protein losses by adsorption to the filter, pipette tips, or the extraction vials, or to denaturing during sample processing. Although details for optimal extraction and storage procedures might differ per allergen, in most cases the yields can be strongly improved by addition of a mild detergent like Tween-20 (0.05%) to the medium (22, 61);
- For most occupational HMW allergens EIAs have been described and applied, but only few are commercially available. While some earlier procedures used as antibody source serum pools from sensitized workers and/or highly exposed workers with a high specific IgE or IgG_4 titre, most tests make use of specific polyclonal IgG antibodies from immunized rabbits (29, 32, 62), or specifically generated monoclonal antibodies (26, 33, 63–65).
- Since most laboratories use their own (semi-)purified allergen calibration standards, results are usually expressed in laboratory-dependent units, which complicates interlaboratory comparisons.
- Interlaboratory comparison studies with parallel samples taken simultaneously from the same worksite, or with duplicate aliquots from the dust sample extracts, have shown moderate to good correlations between results with different assays—but with systematic differences in reported concentrations, which could be largely ascribed to the use of different calibration standards (61, 64, 66, 67). This in principle allows for comparison of results of different assays and research groups with the use of conversion factors.
- Overall, sandwich EIAs have a much better sensitivity, with detection limits in the pg–ng/mL range, than inhibition assays with human or animal IgG, or human IgG_4 or IgE antibodies, with limits of detection (LOD) usually >10 ng/mL. Sandwich assays are therefore recommended for most occupational allergens, of which estimated 8-hour averaged airborne concentrations at the workplace rarely exceed levels >1–10 ng/m³.

Microbial agents

Extraction and assay procedures for molecular microbial agents like endotoxins and beta-glucans in dust samples are similar but with crucial differences. Since endotoxin is ubiquitous and the detection method very sensitive, all materials and media used during sampling, processing, and analysis must be pyrogen-free. Glass fiber filters and glassware therefore must be heated at >200°C before use.

Endotoxins are extracted at room temperature in pyrogen-free distilled water, and measured with the kinetic Limulus Amebocyte Lysate (LAL) assay, calibrated with an *E. coli* lipopolysaccharide (LPS) standard preparation. Results are expressed in endotoxin units (EU), with 1 EU corresponding to approximately 5–10 ng lipopolysaccharide (68, 69). A more recently introduced variant of the assay makes use of a more purified system with a recombinant version of the Limulus hemolymph factor C (rFC) (70), and produces comparable results (71), but has as yet not found widespread acceptance. Optimization studies have shown that addition of Tween-20 to the extraction medium markedly improves extraction yields, while the LAL assay shows optimal performance in pure pyrogen-free water (72–74).

Beta-(1, 3)- and -(1, 6)-glucans are insoluble microbial cell wall components, and extraction requires heating at >100°C, or incubation at high pH which partially hydrolyzes crossliked glucan polymers (75). Extracts can be tested in inhibition or sandwich EIAs or with a modified functional LAL assay (76–79). Beta-glucans vary widely in structural and functional reactivity (75, 80–82) and these structural differences and corresponding variation in antibodies may explain the large differences in concentrations found in different assays (76, 78, 79). Thus, reported concentrations in specific studies can only be interpreted with reference to the assay method with which they were produced.

A completely different approach is the measurement of bacterial or fungal DNA or RNA by quantitative PCR (qPCR) on filter or dust extracts or sequencing of specific genes (LTS for molds and 16S for bacteria) and bio-informatics analysis to obtain libraries of species from just one sample. Like colony-forming unit (CFU) measurements this allows identification and quantification of specific taxa at genus or species level, or even specific strains of e.g. antibiotic-resistant bacteria (40–42, 83–86). Although primarily of interest in risk assessment of infectious pathogen exposures, taxonomic identification of e.g. airborne fungal spores can also be important in studies on OA, hypersensitivity pneumonitis (Chapter 24), airway diseases due to exposure to organic dusts (Chapter 23), and sick building syndrome (Chapter 26), especially when sensitization to specific fungi may be involved.

Quality control

The two-step procedure with first extraction of samples, followed by analysis of the stored extracts, has major advantages. When high or low values are observed beyond the assay's range of quantification, a second stored aliquot may be tested at lower or higher dilutions. A subset of each sample series may be tested twice as part of a routine quality control procedure, to assess intra- and intertest repeatability. Parallel aliquots from the same extracts can also be used for intra- or interlaboratory comparison studies. Comparison of extraction procedures, however, requires parallel samples taken simultaneously at the same worksite; parallel sampling devices have been developed for such purposes (22, 23).

Rapid tests for chemical and biological agents
Direct reading instruments for chemical agents and dusts

Several portable direct-reading instruments are available, mainly for gas and vapor determination. These instruments provide a rapid and continuous reading in real time. Specificity, precision, accuracy, response time, and LOD should be considered. The operating principles of the instruments are electrochemistry (for nitrogen oxides, carbon monoxide, oxygen, sulfur dioxide, hydrogen sulfide, etc.), infrared spectrometry (for organic and inorganic compounds such as ammonia, formaldehyde, ethylene oxide, nitrous oxide), photo-ionization (for nonspecific organic vapors), and light scattering (for particulates).

The colorimetric technique is simple, rapid, and inexpensive. It is based on the color of the reaction product of the measured airborne substance with a specific reaction in sampling devices like tubes or plates consisting of capillary tubes, through which air passively diffuses or is actively pumped. The color intensity can be visually read or measured objectively with an optical reader and is proportional to the measured substance's concentration. Limitations are however a lack of specificity and low accuracy.

Laminar flow immunoassays: Direct tests for allergens

Direct demonstration of some allergens at the workplace can be done with laminar flow immunoassays (LFIAs), using allergen-specific antibodies fixed on a paper or nitrocellulose strip. A droplet of extract fluid is mixed with gold- or carbon-conjugated secondary antibodies and complexes of the antibodies with allergen molecules in the extract move by capillary flow through the strip up to the line of trapping antibodies where a sharp colored line will appear within 10–15 minutes. LFIAs have been developed for enzyme and laboratory animal allergens (87, 88), and have a sensitivity in the range of 1–10 ng/mL of allergenic proteins. LFIAs may be particularly useful to quickly assess the presence of allergens in surface dust or samples taken at the worksite. They may be particularly useful to detect allergens in e.g. surface dust, swipe of product samples, and when provided as a test kit together with simple means for quick extraction, the whole procedure can be completed within 30–60 minutes.

Exposure assessment strategies

General considerations

The use of sensitive, precise, and specific sampling and analytic procedures is only one prerequisite to achieve reliable exposure assessment data (Table 6.1). Exposure at the workplace varies in time and space, and especially personal exposure often shows large inter- and intraindividual variation. Personal measurements are in general more accurate to assess risks of OA than ambient air sampling, but require more effort—equipment, collaboration, and compliance of workers as well as larger series of samples to be analyzed. Ideally, each worker and work situation should be evaluated over weeks or even months, which would involve unrealistic amounts of resources. Sampling strategies based on statistical sampling theory and homogeneous exposure groups can be used to address this problem. The reader is referred to more specialized literature on exposure analysis (89–91). Only a few major issues are discussed briefly in the following paragraphs (see section "Variation in Exposure Levels").

Variation in exposure levels

To define the extent and the variability in the exposures of individual workers or a homogeneous exposure group, its distribution must be studied. Most exposures show a right-skewed, approximately lognormal distribution, and measurement series are therefore commonly reported with both arithmetic means (AM) and geometric means (GM), and the geometric standard deviation (GSD) as measure of dispersion, while the median, percentile values, and minimum and maximum may be added to further document the distribution, and the occurrence of extreme peak exposures. The data can be compared with exposure limits (89–91). However, since only a subset of values of a complete exposure profile (a few days instead of all the days in a year) is measured, uncertainty results from any sampling strategy and can only be reduced by increasing the number of measurements. The uncertainty is quantified by giving confidence intervals associated with reported values.

Occupational exposures to HMW allergens are typical examples with a wide between-worker and day-to-day variation, as shown by high GSD values; also, within the workday, strong variations can be observed, due to some specific tasks of short (15–20 minutes) duration but very high exposure, like cage cleaning (92–95) or addition of an enzyme preparation to flour batches (96, 97). Exposure-response analyses have revealed that these allergens, and also some LMW sensitizers like metals and isocyanates, might cause sensitization at very low average levels, in the high pg/m^3 or ng/m^3 range (92, 98). Exposure however occurs in the form of particulates, of which the allergen content in some cases may be estimated in the 10–100 pg range per particle (99), which implies that the average exposure during a workday may exist of no more than inhalation of a relatively small number (<100) of allergen-carrying particles. Most of this exposure occurs during short activities that are only incidentally (i.e. not daily) performed, while during most of the time the exposure may be practically zero, or at least below the detection limits of even the most sensitive methods. As a consequence, exposure may be missed when the exposure assessment strategy does not cover all relevant activities. Use of more sensitive assays will not solve the issue; this is merely a matter that needs to be dealt with in the analysis by considering alternative methods to describe the exposure like a β-Poisson distribution (100). These observations may also be of etiologic relevance, since they allow an alternative interpretation of dose-response relations: it might not be the average (remarkably low) full-shift exposure levels *per se* that determine the risk of sensitization, but the combination with a large GSD, thus the risk that incidentally (e.g. on some days or even only hours) 10- to 100-fold higher concentrations of allergenic particles are inhaled, and that this is the actual sensitizing event. These considerations underscore the importance of considering the distribution of exposure levels in groups of workers.

Additional data from the workplace

A careful and detailed documentation of the work environment, products made, implementation of new substances in the work processes used, the physical organization, ventilation, and emission sources is essential in evaluating WRA. Similarly, task-associated exposures must be recorded, and preferably supported with task-specific measurements, and a description of duration, the number of workers simultaneously performing these tasks, procedures, work habits, safety procedures, as well as use of protective equipment. When planning a measurement series, a preliminary inventory of reported health problems and accidents

TABLE 6.1 Different Approaches Used for Exposure Assessment

Method	Indication	Advantages/Disadvantages
Occupational history	Clinical evaluation of individual workers	Useful information on jobs exposure for clinician
Questionnaires, job history, self-reported exposures	Epidemiological studies	For some studies, may be available information
	Medical surveillance of workers	Qualitative information
		Potential biases such as recall bias
Qualitative documentation of the work environment and task-associated exposure	First step of epidemiological studies, surveillance programs	Preliminary information in epidemiological studies and surveillance programs
	Description of workplace in workers with possible OA by industrial hygienists	Useful information for clinicians investigating workers with possible OA
Quantitative air sampling	Epidemiological studies	Captures levels of exposure associated with the location and environmental conditions during the time of sampling
Active personal sampling or ambient air sampling	Surveillance programs	
Passive ambient air sampling		Allows for exposure-response studies
		Personal sampling: most accurate, requires more efforts
		Passive ambient air sampling: less expensive
Sampling by dry or wet swiping of surfaces	Epidemiological studies	Enables hazard identification
	Surveillance programs	Does not quantify levels
Skin exposure	Epidemiological studies	Not standardized
		Limited validation
		Technically challenging
Biomonitoring	Epidemiological studies	Evidence of exposure and its intensity but not the route of exposure nor where and when exposure occur; collection of blood, urine, etc. if necessary
	Surveillance programs for LMW agents	
Job-exposure matrices	Epidemiological studies in the general population to assess risks of asthma associated with specific jobs	Qualitative (possibly semiquantitative)

can help identify the main contaminants and risks and to determine which work situations need to be evaluated.

Homogeneous exposure groups

Effort can be reduced by sampling from so-called homogeneous exposure groups, in which workers share the same exposure profile due to the similarity of the exposure determinants, such as jobs or tasks in the same department, working in the same processes and with the same materials. Homogeneous exposure groups can be established by observation or by statistical inference. The first requires examination of activities in a workforce and an occupational hygienist's professional judgment about their similarity with respect to exposure. The statistical approach requires a series of repeated measurements to quantify inter- and intraworker variation. The population is then grouped and categorized such that within each category (=group) the between-worker variance is minimalized.

For compliance testing, criteria are sometimes given for the homogeneity of a population, although these are arbitrary (101, 102). For surveys, only the contrast between exposure categories relative to the intragroup differences is relevant (102). In exposure-response studies, the population is most often categorized in homogeneous groups and repeated samples are taken from the different exposure groups. The number of samples taken from each group is ideally based on the group size and the (expected) within-group variation.

The American Industrial Hygiene Association recommends that six to ten measurements be performed per homogeneous exposure group, spread out over several days to cover the fluctuations in exposure (102), but in many situations variability in exposure requires a larger number of measurements. When results are ambiguous, more than ten measurements are needed per exposure group to refine the determination of the distribution. Power calculations may guide the decision on the number of samples that needs to be taken to obtain meaningful results with acceptable confidence limits.

Compliance strategies

Exposure assessment can be used to compare airborne concentrations of hazardous substances with occupational exposure limits, like Threshold Limit Values (TLV) or Maximum Allowable Concentration (MAC) values (15). Compliance sampling usually focuses on workers with the highest exposure ("worst-case sampling"), but other approaches exist and more details can be found in the literature (103).

Few exposure standards have been developed for allergens and those available are not always health based. Standards based on animal experiments are often insufficient to prevent sensitization or OA in humans, where individual susceptibility plays an important role in the sensitization process. Moreover, average low levels with high GSDs are often associated with incidental but regularly occurring peak exposures at 10- to 100-fold higher levels therefore with a high risk of sensitization (6, 98, 104–106). The thresholds that would protect all workers from developing OA are difficult to quantify, but approaches to derive standards have been given (6, 7, 107). In addition, already sensitized or asthmatic workers will react to concentrations much lower than those established for healthy workers. In dealing with the agents causing OA, emphasis must be on their identification and detection, at the lowest concentrations possible. In some cases, there is a need to ensure the absolute absence of a causal substance in the workplace.

Exposure modeling in exposure-response studies

Exposure-response studies for occupational allergy have become possible since the development of sensitive immunoassays measuring sensitizing proteins at <1 ng/mL levels in personal airborne dust samples taken during a work shift, or even job tasks of only 30–60 minutes. Identification of determinants like job tasks, building and ventilation characteristics, etc. ("exposure analysis"), has been essential for dose-response studies based on "exposure modeling" (97, 104, 105). The exposure of each study participant is not the allergen concentration measured for that individual, but a predicted exposure for that worker based on a statistical model with significant work-related and individual characteristics as input variables (2). Modeling can result in more accurate estimates of exposure by reducing the impact of intra-individual, day-to-day variation in exposure for each individual (108). Another benefit is the efficiency in sampling, as fewer samples are needed. Moreover, as long as the worksite and work conditions do not significantly change, a well-validated exposure model may be applied in new studies with only limited assessment by new measurements.

Intervention studies

Hygiene approaches have been used in intervention studies, such as in the baking industry (109, 110), to evaluate changes in exposure across sectors of industry. However, such studies require considerable numbers of measurements, and detailed ancillary information (technology of the process, job title and tasks performed, etc.). Moreover, just like other intervention studies in preventive medicine, the evaluation of specific measures may be complicated by inadvertent simultaneous changes in exposures due to use of new equipment, change in materials and products handled, and changing work practices and newly hired personnel.

Job-exposure matrices

Epidemiological studies in the general population may focus on the risks of asthma associated with specific jobs without having resources to perform detailed exposure measurements of each job. Exposure is then often estimated with so-called job-exposure matrices (JEM): expert systems that translate a job title in a series of likely exposures (111–113). An improved version of the initially proposed JEM with application to 30 sensitizers, use of semi-quantitative metrics, and evaluated by three experts has been developed (114). JEM estimated exposures have been shown to be significantly associated with the risk of development of sensitization to HMW agents by using data obtained from a cohort of apprentices (115). In general population studies the prevalence of specific job-related exposures is low, and when the job-based exposure assignment is not sufficiently specific, non-exposed can be classified as exposed, leading to a strong underestimation of exposure-response associations. Because many researchers are aware of this phenomenon, some JEMs like the asthma-specific JEM include an evaluation step by a panel of hygienists after the initial assignment to improve the quality of the exposure estimation process and optimize performance of the matrix in a specific context. A matrix using occupation coding that prevails in the United States has shown that 43% of workers had probable exposure to at least one type of OA agent (116).

Allergen exposure measurements in the diagnosis of individual patients

The most helpful way to assess whether work exposures contribute to an individual patient's asthma is through a careful occupational and medical history, discussed further in Chapter 5. This history, which should focus on the period of time when the asthmatic symptoms started and/or worsened, is also important to inform the workplace sampling strategy. Briefly, clinicians can gain substantial information about both specific work exposures and also the magnitude and duration of exposures from the patient. Information on specific work exposures can be obtained by asking the patient about the type of work, substances, activities or processes at the workplace of concern, and review of safety data sheets (SDSs) on products with which the patient works. In addition, the occupational history can provide useful qualitative information about the magnitude, frequency, and duration of work exposures. Questions about work processes or tasks (e.g. spraying, heating, machining), the size or scale of the operation, duration of at-risk activities, the presence of industrial hygiene controls and ventilation, and use of personal protective equipment can be more informative than quantitative workplace sampling. This is especially the case with sensitizers, where levels below regulatory limits do not rule out causative exposures. In addition, intermittent acute exposure events and skin exposure, which both may contribute to the development of OA, are particularly challenging to measure quantitatively, but can be assessed qualitatively by history and questionnaire.

Allergen measurements may be part of an individual diagnostic evaluation if the anamnesis and SPT or IgE tests point to a work-related allergic disease. This may be particularly useful when the patient's worksite is not a priori recognized as a "high risk" environment, like the canteen of a flour mill or enzyme producing factory, or the offices of a laboratory animal facility. Although exposures at such locations are usually much lower than primary production sites, dispersion through the air and unintentional transfer of allergen-carrying particles within a building may lead to clinically relevant exposure. Several studies have demonstrated transfer of common or occupational allergens to "nonsuspected" sites, like schools where pet allergens carried by cat or dog owners may affect the respiratory health of schoolchildren and teachers (117, 118).

Conclusion and research needs

Exposure assessment at the workplace has traditionally been focused on exposure to toxic chemicals and physical factors, for which methods and strategies have undergone gradual improvement. In the last decades the scope has widened to also include exposure to biological agents, such as viable microorganisms, microbial toxins and allergens, which are responsible for many cases of OA and WRA-like symptoms. Development of sensitive immunoassays for HMW allergens has allowed large-scale exposure studies, which, combined with well-designed exposure modeling, led to establishment of exposure-response relations for various occupational allergens.

In addition to "classical" occupational allergy due to allergic sensitization to proteins or LMW chemical agents, the importance of work-related microbial exposures—as causes of non-allergic asthma-like illness, and aggravating factors of asthma morbidity—has become more and more recognized, and included in many occupational respiratory health surveys.

JEMs can be used in general population studies to categorize study participants in groups with low, moderate, or high exposure to asthma-relevant agents, and to assess the contribution of work-related exposures to the risk of asthma. These approaches and also the evaluations of intervention studies should be based on up-to-date measurements in the respective workplaces.

The specific objectives of monitoring exposure in the workplace must be taken into account when planning a series of measurements, and a well-designed sampling strategy is of utmost importance to achieve meaningful data. The importance of exposure assessment in the field of asthma and allergy is underpinned by evidence-based-medicine type of approach documents from a Taskforce of the European Respiratory Society, especially in the documents on primary and secondary prevention (119, 120). These documents illustrate that exposure assessment has matured and found its place in evaluation and management of allergy and asthma risks in the environment.

References

1. Zartarian VG, Ott WR, Duan N. A quantitative definition of exposure and related concepts. J Expo Anal Environ Epidemiol. 1997;7:411–37.
2. Nieuwenhuijsen MJ. Introduction to exposure assessment. Exposure assessment in occupational and environmental epidemiology. Ch. 1. Oxford Scholarship Online; 2009. doi:101093/acprof:oso/9780198528616001000.
3. Redlich CA, Herrick CA. Lung/skin connections in occupational lung disease. Curr Opin Allergy Clin Immunol. 2008;8:115–9.
4. Tsui HC, Ronsmans S, De Sadeleer LJ, et al. Skin exposure contributes to chemical-induced asthma: what is the evidence? a systematic review of animal models. Allergy Asthma Immunol Res. 2020;12(4):579–98.
5. (ACGIH®) American Conference of Governmental Industrial Hygienists. TLV® and BEIs® Based on the Documentation of the Threshold Limit Values for Chemical Substances and Physical Agents & Biological Exposure. Cincinnati, OH: Signature Publications; 2012.
6. Heederik D, Thorne PS, Doekes G. Health-based occupational exposure limits for high molecular weight sensitizers: How long is the road we must travel? Ann Occup Hyg. 2002;46:439–46.
7. Nielsen GD, Larsen ST, Hansen JS, et al. Experiences from occupational exposure limits set on aerosols containing allergenic proteins. Ann Occup Hyg. 2012;56(8):888–900.
8. Heederik D, Houba R, Liss GM, et al. Protecting the worker and modifying the work environment. In: Asthma in the Workplace, 4th ed. CRC Press; 2013: Chapter 11, 138–49.
9. Drolet D, Beauchamp G. Sampling guide for air contaminants in the workplace, 8th ed. IRRST; 2013: version 81 updated. http://www.irsst.qc.ca/media/documents/PubIRSST/T-15.pdf.
10. Görner P, Simon X, Boivin A, et al. Sampling efficiency and performance of selected thoracic aerosol samplers. Ann Work Expo Health. 2017;61(7):784–96.
11. Stacey P, Thorpe A, Echt A. Performance of high flow rate personal respirable samplers when challenged with mineral aerosols of different particle size distributions. Ann Occup Hyg. 2016;60(4):479–92.
12. Liu Y, Sparer J, Woskie SR, et al. Qualitative assessment of isocyanate skin exposure in auto body shops: a pilot study. Am J Ind Med. 2000;37:265–74.
13. Heederik D, Budnik L, Roberge B, et al. Assessment of the workplace. In: Malo JL, Chan-Yeung M, Bernstein DI, eds. Asthma in the Workplace. 4th ed. CRC Press; 2013:85–98.
14. Pronk A, Tielemans E, Skarping G, et al. Inhalation exposure to isocyanates of car body repair shop workers and industrial spray painters. Ann Occup Hyg. 2006;50:1–14.
15. Perkins LP. Modern industrial hygiene, recognition and evaluation of chemical agents. Volume 1 American Conference of Governmental Industrial Hygienists. Cincinnati, OH: John Wiley & Sons; 2008: Publication #9833.
16. NIOSH. Manual of Analytical Methods. 5th ed.; 2020: https://www.cdc.gov/niosh/nmam/pdf/NMAM_5thEd_EBook-508-final.pdf.
17. Braunstahl GJ, Fokkens W. Nasal involvement in allergic asthma. Allergy. 2003;58(12):1235–43.
18. Wippich C, Rissler J, Koppisch D, et al. Estimating respirable dust exposure from inhalable dust exposure. Ann Work Expo Health. 2020;64(4):430–44.
19. Li Z, Che W, Lau AKH, et al. A feasible experimental framework for field calibration of portable light-scattering aerosol monitors: case of TSI DustTrak. Environ Pollut. 2019;255(Pt 1):113136.
20. Sleeth DK, Vincent JH. Performance study of personal inhalable aerosol samplers at ultra-low wind speeds. Ann Occup Hyg. 2012;56:207–20. Available from: http://annhyg.oxfordjournals.org/content/early/2011/10/10/annhyg.mer089.full.pdf+html.
21. Anthony TR, Cai C, Mehaffy J, et al. Performance of prototype high-flow inhalable dust sampler in a livestock production facility. J Occup Environ Hyg. 2017;14(5):313–22.
22. Bogdanovic J, Wouters IM, Sander I, et al. Airborne exposure to wheat allergens: optimised elution for airborne dust samples. J Environ Monit. 2006;8:1043–8.
23. Spaan S, Heederik DJ, Thorne PS, et al. Optimization of airborne endotoxin exposure assessment: effects of filter type, transport conditions, extraction solutions, and storage of samples and extracts. Appl Environ Microbiol. 2007;73(19):6134–43.
24. Samadi S, Heederik DJ, Krop EJ, et al. Allergen and endotoxin exposure in a companion animal hospital. Occup Environ Med. 2010;67:486–92.
25. Cao G, Noti JD, Blachere FM, et al. Development of an improved methodology to detect infectious airborne influenza virus using the NIOSH bioaerosol sampler. J Environ Monit. 2011;13(12):3321–8.
26. Raulf M, Buters J, Chapman M, et al. Monitoring of occupational and environmental aeroallergens—EAACI Position Paper. Concerted action of the EAACI IG Occupational Allergy and Aerobiology & Air Pollution. Allergy. 2014;69(10):1280–99.
27. Würtz H, Sigsgaard T, Valbjørn O, et al. The dustfall collector–a simple passive tool for long-term collection of airborne dust: a project under the Danish Mould in Buildings program (DAMIB). Indoor Air. 2005;15(Suppl 9):33–40.
28. Noss I, Wouters IM, Visser M, et al. Evaluation of a low-cost electrostatic dust fall collector for indoor air endotoxin exposure assessment. Appl Environ Microbiol. 2008;74(18):5621–7.
29. Krop EJ, Jacobs JH, Sander I, et al. Allergens and β-glucans in Dutch homes and schools: characterizing airborne levels. PLOS ONE. 2014;9(2):e88871.
30. Sander I, Lotz A, Neumann HD, et al. Indoor allergen levels in settled airborne dust are higher in day-care centers than at home. Allergy. 2018;73(6):1263–75.
31. Kilburg-Basnyat B, Metwali N, Thorne PS. Performance of electrostatic dust collectors (EDCs) for endotoxin assessment in homes: effect of mailing, placement, heating, and electrostatic charge. J Occup Environ Hyg. 2016;13(2):85–93.
32. Zahradnik E, Sander I, Kendzia B, et al. Passive airborne dust sampling to assess mite antigen exposure in farming environments. J Environ Monit. 2011;13(9):2638–44.
33. Feistenauer S, Sander I, Schmidt J, et al. Influence of 5 different caging types and the use of cage-changing stations on mouse allergen exposure. J Am Assoc Lab Anim Sci. 2014;53(4):356–63.
34. Leppänen HK, Täubel M, Jayaprakash B, et al. Quantitative assessment of microbes from samples of indoor air and dust. J Expo Sci Environ Epidemiol. 2018;28(3):231–41.
35. Normand AC, Ranque S, Cassagne C, et al. Comparison of air impaction and electrostatic dust collector sampling methods to assess airborne fungal contamination in public buildings. Ann Occup Hyg. 2016;60(2):161–75.
36. Zahradnik E, Raulf M. Animal allergens and their presence in the environment. Front Immunol. 2014;5:76.
37. Walser SM, Gerstner DG, Brenner B, et al. Evaluation of exposure-response relationships for health effects of microbial bioaerosols—a systematic review. Int J Hyg Environ Health. 2015;218(7):577–89.
38. Rick EM, Woolnough K, Pashley CH, et al. Allergic fungal airway disease. J Investig Allergol Clin Immunol. 2016;26(6):344–54.
39. Caillaud D, Leynaert B, Keirsbulck M, et al. Indoor mould exposure, asthma and rhinitis: findings from systematic reviews and recent longitudinal studies. Eur Respir Rev. 2018;27(148):170137.
40. Eduard W, Heederik D, Duchaine C, et al. Bioaerosol exposure assessment in the workplace: the past, present and recent advances. J Environ Monit. 2012;14(2):334–9.
41. Afanou AK, Straumfors A, Eduard W. Fungal aerosol composition in moldy basements. Indoor Air. 2019;29(5):780–90.
42. Cox J, Indugula R, Vesper S, et al. Comparison of indoor air sampling and dust collection methods for fungal exposure assessment using quantitative PCR. Environ Sci Process Impacts. 2017;19(10):1312–9.
43. Redlich CA. Skin exposure and asthma: is there a connection? Proc Am Thorac Soc. 2010;2:134–7.
44. OSHA. Regulations (Standards-29 CFR). 2020: https://www.osha.gov/laws-regs/regulations/standardnumber.
45. Ostiguy C, Gagné S, Lesage J, et al. Développement d'une méthode d'analyse d'isocyanates à très haute sensibilité. Études et recherches/Rapport R-419. Montréal, Canada: IRSST; 2005:43. Available from: http://www.irsstqcca/media/documents/PubIRSST/R-419.pdf.
46. Bello D, Redlich CA, Stowe MH, et al. Skin exposure to aliphatic polyisocyanates in the auto body repair and refinishing industry: II. A quantitative assessment. Ann Occup Hyg. 2008;52(2):117–24.

47. Fent KW, Jayaraj K, Ball LM, et al. Quantitative monitoring of dermal and inhalation exposure to 1,6-hexamethylene diisocyanate monomer and oligomers. J Environ Monit. 2008;10:500–7.

48. Harari H, Bello D, Woskie S, et al. Development of an interception glove sampler for skin exposures to aromatic isocyanates. Ann Occup Hyg. 2016;60(9):1092–103.

49. Liljelind I, Norberg C, Egelrud L, et al. Dermal and inhalation exposure to methylene bisphenyl isocyanate (MDI) in iron foundry workers. Ann Occup Hyg. 2010;54(1):31–40.

50. Hamada H, Liljelind I, Bruze M, et al. Assessment of dermal uptake of diphenylmethane-4,4'-diisocyanate using tape stripping and biological monitoring. Eur J Dermatol. 2018;28(2):143–8.

51. Louro H, Heinälä M, Bessems J, et al. Human biomonitoring in health risk assessment in Europe: current practices and recommendations for the future. Int J Hyg Environ Health. 2019;222(5):727–37.

52. Scholten B, Kenny L, Duca RC, et al. Biomonitoring for occupational exposure to diisocyanates: a systematic review. Ann Work Expo Health. 2020;64:569–85.

53. Krop EJ, Doekes G, Heederik DJ, et al. IgG4 antibodies against rodents in laboratory animal workers do not protect against allergic sensitization. Allergy. 2011;66:517–22.

54. Gautrin D, Malo JL. Risk factors, predictors, and markers for work-related asthma and rhinitis. Curr Allergy Asthma Rep. 2010;10:365–72.

55. Portengen L, De Meer G, Doekes G, et al. Immunoglobulin G4 antibodies to rat urinary allergens, sensitization and symptomatic allergy in laboratory animal workers. Clin Exp Allergy. 2004;34:1243–50.

56. Wisnewski AV, Stowe MH, Nerlinger A, et al. Biomonitoring hexamethylene diisocyanate (HDI) exposure based on serum levels of HDI-specific IgG. Ann Occup Hyg. 2012;56:901–10.

57. Tsuji M, Ishihara Y, Isse T, et al. Evaluation of chemical-specific IgG antibodies in male workers from a urethane foam factory. Environ Health Prev Med. 2018;23(1):24.

58. Dominguez-Ortega J, Barranco P, Rodríguez-Pérez R, et al. Biomarkers in occupational asthma. Curr Allergy Asthma Rep. 2016;16(9):63.

59. EU-OSHA. 2020. https://osha.europa.eu/en

60. Wisnewski AV, Kanyo J, Asher J, et al. Reaction products of hexamethylene diisocyanate vapors with "self" molecules in the airways of rabbits exposed via tracheostomy. Xenobiotica. 2018;48(5):488–97.

61. Hollander A, Gordon S, A Renstrom, et al. Comparison of methods to assess airborne rat or mouse allergen levels. I. Analysis of air samples. Allergy. 1999;54:142–49.

62. Bogdanovic J, Wouters IM, Sander I, et al. Airborne exposure to wheat allergens: measurement by human immunoglobulin G4 and rabbit immunoglobulin G immunoassays. Clin Exp Allergy. 2006;36(9):1168–75.

63. Gómez-Ollés S, Cruz MJ, Renström A, et al. An amplified sandwich EIA for the measurement of soy aeroallergens. Clin Exp Allergy. 2006;36(9):1176–83.

64. Gómez-Ollés S, Cruz MJ, Bogdanovic J, et al. Assessment of soy aeroallergen levels in different work environments. Clin Exp Allergy. 2007;37:1863–72.

65. King EM, Filep S, Smith B, et al. A multi-center ring trial of allergen analysis using fluorescent multiplex array technology. J Immunol Methods. 2013;387(1-2):89–95.

66. Renstrom A, Gordon S, Hollander A, et al. Comparison of methods to assess rat or mouse allergen levels. II. Factors influencing antigen detection. Allergy. 1999;54:150–7.

67. Sander I, Zahradnik E, Bogdanovic J, et al. Optimized methods for fungal alpha-amylase airborne exposure assessment in bakeries and mills. Clin Exp Allergy. 2007;37(8):1229–38.

68. Park JH, Szponar B, Larsson L, et al. Characterization of lipopolysaccharides present in settled house dust. Appl Environ Microbiol. 2004;70(1):262–7.

69. Findlay L, Desai T, Heath A, et al. Collaborative study for the establishment of the WHO 3(rd) International Standard for Endotoxin, the Ph. Eur. endotoxin biological reference preparation batch 5 and the USP Reference Standard for Endotoxin Lot H0K354. Pharmeur Bio Sci Notes. 2015;73–98.

70. Alwis KU, Milton DK. Recombinant factor C assay for measuring endotoxin in house dust: comparison with LAL, and (1 -> 3)-beta-D-glucans. Am J Ind Med. 2006;49(4):296–300.

71. Thorne PS, Perry SS, Saito R, et al. Evaluation of the Limulus amebocyte lysate and recombinant factor C assays for assessment of airborne endotoxin. Appl Environ Microbiol. 2010;76(15):4988–95.

72. Liebers V, Raulf-Heimsoth M, Linsel G, et al. Evaluation of quantification methods of occupational endotoxin exposure. J Toxicol Environ Health A. 2007;70(21):1798–805.

73. Spaan S, Doekes G, Heederik D, et al. Effect of extraction and assay media on analysis of airborne endotoxin. Appl Environ Microbiol. 2008;74(12):3804–11.

74. McKenzie JH, Alwis KU, Sordillo JE, et al. Evaluation of lot-to-lot repeatability and effect of assay media choice in the recombinant Factor C assay. J Environ Monit. 2011;13(6):1739–45.

75. Stone BA, Clarke AE. Chemistry and biology of (1-3) beta-glucans. Bundora, Australia: La Trobe University Press; 1992:803.

76. Milton DK, Alwis KU, Fisette L, et al. Enzyme-linked immunosorbent assay specific for (1->6) branched, (1->3)-beta-D-glucan detection in environmental samples. Appl Environ Microbiol. 2001;67(12):5420–4.

77. Noss I, Wouters IM, Bezemer G, et al. beta-(1,3)-Glucan exposure assessment by passive airborne dust sampling and new sensitive immunoassays. Appl Environ Microbiol. 2010;76(4):1158–67.

78. Cherid H, Foto M, Miller JD. Performance of two different Limulus amebocyte lysate assays for the quantitation of fungal glucan. J Occup Environ Hyg. 2011;8(9):540–3.

79. Brooks CR, Siebers R, Crane J, et al. Measurement of β-(1,3)-glucan in household dust samples using Limulus amebocyte assay and enzyme immunoassays: an inter-laboratory comparison. Environ Sci Process Impacts. 2013;15(2):405–11.

80. Douwes J. (1->3)-Beta-D-glucans and respiratory health: a review of the scientific evidence. Indoor Air. 2005;15(3):160–9.

81. Noss I, Doekes G, Thorne PS, et al. Comparison of the potency of a variety of β-glucans to induce cytokine production in human whole blood. Innate Immun. 2013;19(1):10–9.

82. Han B, Baruah K, Cox E, et al. Structure-functional activity relationship of β-glucans from the perspective of immunomodulation: a mini-review. Front Immunol. 2020;11:658.

83. Hong PY, Li X, Yang X, et al. Monitoring airborne biotic contaminants in the indoor environment of pig and poultry confinement buildings. Environ Microbiol. 2012;14(6):1420–31.

84. Unterwurzacher V, Pogner C, Berger H, et al. Validation of a quantitative PCR based detection system for indoor mold exposure assessment in bioaerosols. Environ Sci Process Impacts. 2018;20(10):1454–68.

85. Cox J, Mbareche H, Lindsley WG, et al. Field sampling of indoor bioaerosols. Aerosol Sci Technol. 2020;54(5):572–84.

86. Gao M, Jia R, Qiu T, et al. Size-related bacterial diversity and tetracycline resistance gene abundance in the air of concentrated poultry feeding operations. Environ Pollut. 2017;220(Pt B):1342–8.

87. Bogdanovic J, Koets M, Sander I, et al. Rapid detection of fungal alpha-amylase in the work environment with a lateral flow immunoassay. J Allergy Clin Immunol. 2006;118:1157–63.

88. Koets M, Renström A, Zahradnik E, et al. Rapid one-step assays for on-site monitoring of mouse and rat urinary allergens. J Environ Monit. 2011;13(12):3475–80.

89. Jahn SD, Bullock WH, Ignacio JS (eds.). A strategy for assessing and managing occupational exposures, 4th ed. AIHA; 2015.

90. Leidel NA, Busch KA, Lynch JR. Occupational exposure sampling strategy manual. Cincinnati, OH: National Institute for Occupational Safety and Health; 1977.

91. Clerc F, Vincent R. Assessment of occupational exposure to chemicals by air sampling for comparison with limit values: the influence of sampling strategy. Ann Occup Hyg. 2014;58(4):437–9.

92. Heederik D, Venables KM, Malmberg P, et al. Exposure-response relationships for work-related sensitization in workers exposed to rat urinary allergens: results from a pooled study. J Allergy Clin Immunol. 1999;103:678–84.

93. Hollander A, Heederik D, Doekes G, et al. Determinants of airborne rat and mouse urinary allergen exposure. Scand J Work Environ Health. 1998;24:228–35.

94. Pacheco KA, McCammon C, Thorne PS, et al. Characterization of endotoxin and mouse allergen exposures in mouse facilities and research laboratories. Ann Occup Hyg. 2006;50:563–72.

95. Straumfors A, Eduard W, Andresen K, et al. Predictors for increased and reduced rat and mouse allergen exposure in laboratory animal facilities. Ann Work Expo Health. 2018;62(8):953–65.

96. Houba R, van Run P, Doekes G, et al. Airborne levels of alpha-amylase allergens in bakeries. J Allergy Clin Immunol. 1997;99:286–92.

97. Elms J, Robinson E, Mason H, et al. Enzyme exposure in the British baking industry. Ann Occup Hyg. 2006;50:379–84.

98. Houba R, Heederik DJJ, Doekes G, et al. Exposure-sensitization relationship for a-amylase allergens in the baking industry. Am J Respir Crit Care Med. 1996;154:130–6.

99. Tovey ER, Chapman MD, Platts-Mills TA. Mite faeces are a major source of house dust allergens. Nature. 1981;289:592–3.

100. Teunis PF, Havelaar AH. The Beta Poisson dose–response model is not a single-hit model. Risk Anal. 2000;20:513–20.

101. CEN. Workplace Atmospheres—Guidance for the Assessment of Exposure by Inhalation to Chemical Agents for Comparison with Limit Values and Measurement Strategy. EN 689 Brussels: CEN, European Committee for Standardization; 1995.

102. Ignacio JS, Bullock WH. A Strategy for Assessing and Managing Occupational Exposures. American Industrial Hygiene Association Exposure Assessment Strategies Committee. In: Gardiner K, Harrington JM, Kromhout H, van Tongeren M, Burstyn I. Design of exposure measurement surveys and their statistical analyses. In: Gardiner K, Harrington JM, eds. *Chapter 3 of occupational hygiene*. Fairfax, VA, USA, 2006, 3rd ed. Oxford: Blackwell Publishing; 2005.

103. Ogden T. Proposed British–Dutch guidance on measuring compliance with occupational exposure limits. Ann Occup Hyg. 2009;53:775–7.

104. Nieuwenhuijsen MJ, Heederik D, Doekes G, et al. Exposure-response relations to alpha-amylase sensitisation in British bakeries and flour mills. Occup Env Med. 1999;56:197–201.

105. Hollander A, Heederik D, Doekes G. Respiratory allergy to rats: exposure-response relationships in laboratory animal workers. Am J Respir Crit Care Med. 1997;155:562–7.

106. Matsui EC, Krop EJ, Diette GB, et al. Mouse allergen exposure and immunologic responses: IgE-mediated mouse sensitization and mouse specific IgG and IgG4 levels. Ann Allergy Asthma Immunol. 2004;93(2):171–8.

107. Rijnkels JM, Smid T, Van den Aker EC, et al. Prevention of work-related airway allergies; summary of the advice from the Health Council of the Netherlands. Allergy. 2008;63:1593–6.

108. Peretz C, de Pater N, de Monchy J, et al. Assessment of exposure to wheat flour and the shape of its relationship with specific sensitization. Scand J Work Environ Health. 2005;31:65–74.

109. Baatjies R, Meijster T, Lopata A, et al. Exposure to flour dust in South African supermarket bakeries: modeling of baseline measurements of an intervention study. Ann Occup Hyg. 2010;54:309–18.

110. Meijster T, Tielemans E, Heederik D. Effect of an intervention aimed at reducing the risk of allergic respiratory disease in bakers: change in flour dust and fungal alpha-amylase levels. Occup Environ Med. 2009;66:543–9.

111. Kennedy SM, Le Moual N, Choudat D, et al. Development of an asthma specific job exposure matrix and its application in the epidemiological study of genetics and environment in asthma (EGEA). Occup Environ Med. 2000;57:635–41.

112. deVocht F, Zock JP, Kromhout H, et al. Comparison of self-reported occupational exposure with a job exposure matrix in an international community-based study on asthma. Am J Ind Med. 2005;47:434–42.

113. Kogevinas M, Zock JP, Jarvis D, et al. Exposure to substances in the workplace and new-onset asthma: an international prospective population-based study (ECRHS-II). Lancet. 2007;370:336–41.

114. Le Moual N, Zock JP, Dumas O, et al. Update of an occupational asthma-specific job exposure matrix to assess exposure to 30 specific agents. Occup Environ Med. 2018;75:507–14.

115. Suarthana E, Heederik D, Ghezzo H, et al. Risks for the development of outcomes related to occupational allergies: an application of the asthma-specific job exposure matrix compared with self-reports and investigator scores on job-training-related exposure. Occup Environ Med. 2009;66:256–63.

116. Henneberger PK, Kurth LM, Doney B, et al. Development of an asthma-specific job exposure matrix for use in the United States. Ann Work Expo Health. 2020;64(1):82–95.

117. Kielb C, Lin S, Muscatiello N, et al. Building-related health symptoms and classroom indoor air quality: a survey of school teachers in New York State. Indoor Air. 2015;25(4):371–80.

118. Esty B, Permaul P, DeLoreto K, et al. Asthma and allergies in the school environment. Clin Rev Allergy Immunol. 2019;57(3):415–26.

119. Vandenplas O, Dressel H, Nowak D, et al. ERS task force on the management of work-related asthma. What is the optimal management option for occupational asthma? Eur Respir Rev. 2012;21:97–104.

120. Heederik D, Henneberger PK, Redlich CA. ERS task force on the management of work-related asthma. Primary prevention: exposure reduction, skin exposure and respiratory protection. Eur Respir Rev. 2012;21:112–24.

7

IMMUNOLOGICAL AND INFLAMMATORY ASSESSMENTS

Catherine Lemière,[1] Joaquin Sastre,[2] Monika Raulf,[3] Piero Maestrelli,[4] and Olivier Vandenplas[5]

[1]CIUSSS du Nord de l'île de Montréal, Hôpital du Sacré-Coeur de Montréal and Université de Montréal, Montréal, Québec, Canada
[2]Allergology Department. Fundacion Jimenez Diaz, Facultad de Medicina, Universidad Autonoma de Madrid, Madrid, Spain
[3]Department of Allergology/Immunology of the Institute of Prevention and Occupational Medicine of the
German Social Accident Insurance; Institute of the Ruhr-University Bochum (IPA), Bochum, Germany
[4]University of Padova, Padova, Italy
[5]Department of Chest Medicine, Centre hospitalier Universitaire UCL Namur, Université Catholique de Louvain, Yvoir, Belgium

Contents

CASE HISTORY

MEDICAL AND OCCUPATIONAL HISTORY

A 30-year-old man has been employed for 5 years in a platinum refinery. After 2 years in his new employment, he noticed that 1 hour after arriving at his workplace, symptoms of shortness of breath, chest tightness, wheezing, a persistent dry cough, a runny and stuffy nose, and sneezing usually started. These symptoms would substantially improve on weekends. On initial presentation, both physical examination and chest radiograph were normal. The provided treatment consisted of as needed low-dose corticosteroid and formoterol, as well as a budesonide nasal spray. After 3 weeks away from his workplace, he had become free of all respiratory symptoms. During the initial evaluation, the spirometry testing showed an $FEV_1/FVC = 4.56/5.63$ L (pred. = 4.14/4.99 L).

IMMUNOLOGIC EVALUATION

Skin-prick test (SPT) results using 19 common aeroallergens were negative. Respiratory function tests had not been performed while he was at the workplace. SPT to a dilute solution of sodium hexachloroplatinate (10^{-6} dilution) was positive (7 mm wheal/13 mm flare response).

The following section of this chapter discusses the immunological testing that can be performed in subjects suspected of occupational asthma (OA).

Introduction

An objective diagnosis of OA relies on the demonstration of clinically significant changes in forced expiratory volume in 1 second (FEV_1) (15% to 20%) or serial peak-expiratory flow (PEF) monitoring related to the exposure to a specific agent at the workplace. The performance of specific inhalation challenges (SICs) or serial PEF monitoring at work and off work usually allows for an accurate diagnosis of OA. However, when it is not possible to perform such tests, the diagnosis of OA can become challenging.

Additional methods for assessing sensitization to an occupational agent or demonstrating inflammatory changes in response to exposure to occupational agents can be very helpful by bringing additional elements in favor of or against a diagnosis of OA.

This chapter addresses the methods of immunological assessment using skin testing and serological assays. It also describes the role of the noninvasive assessment of airway inflammation in the investigation of OA.

Immunological testing

Immunological assessment by skin-prick and intradermal tests

History

The immunological assessment of individuals with suspected OA by skin testing is an essential tool in the diagnosis of OA. The first skin test technique was developed by Blackley (1) in 1865 and involved scratching the surface of the skin and applying grass pollen grains. The skin test underwent several modifications. In 1975, Pepys (2) introduced a modified SPT technique, which has become the reference method in clinical practice. The classic work of Pepys (3, 4) demonstrated the usefulness of SPT in the diagnosis of OA among workers exposed to industrial enzymes in the detergent industry and those handling platinum salts in the refining industry.

Skin-prick tests

SPTs should be carried out according to international recommendations (5). Unfortunately, very few extracts of occupational agents are well standardized, which is the major limitation for SPT use. Sometimes allergen extracts have to be prepared in the laboratory due to a lack of commercial availability. Prick-prick technique may also solve the lack of commercial standardized allergenic extracts. In this case, the lancet is pricked on the substance to test and then pricked on the skin.

High-molecular-weight agents

There can be significant variation in the allergenic potency of nonstandardized extracts among the same and between different manufacturers (6). The trend is to standardize the allergenic potency of the commercial diagnostic and therapeutic allergen extracts with reference antigens and introduce the biological equivalency to the allergen materials (6). Although allergen solutions with a higher protein content seem to have a greater potency in vivo, the determination of protein content alone is not a reliable predictive marker for the quality of a SPT solution. Recombinant allergens are being developed and are highly specific, but may be less sensitive than the natural extract (7), depending upon the representation of major allergens in recombinant products. Therefore, this should still be considered as an experimental tool. In workers with baker's asthma, the main determinant of bronchial responsiveness to an allergen is the degree of sensitization to occupational allergens as determined by skin reactivity, this being modulated to a lesser extent by nonspecific bronchial hyperresponsiveness (8). Other models of OA due to high-molecular-weight (HMW) agents also have demonstrated that allergy testing together with pulmonary function tests help predict the bronchial response to a specific allergen (9).

Low-molecular-weight agents

Low-molecular-weight (LMW) agents are chemical allergens that require conjugation to an appropriate carrier protein for initiating the process of sensitization. Such antigens are not commercially available and have to be prepared and characterized in specialized laboratories. Chemical protein conjugates are chemically characterized for ligand-protein binding ratio (e.g.

via mass spectroscopy) and specific immunoglobulin E (IgE) and/or immunoglobulin G (IgG) binding (e.g. via enzyme-linked immunosorbent assay [ELISA] using both negative and positive reference sera from exposed workers). The acid anhydrides (e.g. phthalic anhydride [PA]) are prototypic occupational haptens and form in vitro adducts with endogenous proteins (e.g. hemoglobin) (10) and serum albumin (HSA) (11). SPTs to acid anhydride conjugates are biologically relevant as it has been demonstrated that the binding pattern of specific IgE to adducts found in the nasal lavage (12) is similar to conjugates formed spontaneously in vitro.

Diisocyanates have also been shown to form adducts with endogenous human serum albumin (HSA) (13). However, diisocyanate–albumin conjugates, which form in vivo in exposed workers, remain largely uncharacterized. Diisocyanate-albumin conjugates produced in the laboratory are extremely diverse, and their antigenicity may differ significantly depending on the in vitro reaction conditions (e.g. reaction time) under which they are formed (14). The lack of conjugates, which mimic in vivo adduct formation, could explain why diisocyanate–albumin-specific IgE antibodies are detected in only a minority of affected workers with isocyanate-induced asthma (15, 16). Further biochemical techniques, such as tandem mass spectroscopy, are currently being used to characterize diisocyanate–albumin conjugates, which should lead to an improved allergen in the determination of sensitization in exposed workers (17). Positive skin tests with LMW agents have been described in cases of OA to Chloramine T, chlorhexidine, persulphate salts, and metallic salts (18). Nevertheless, these results should be carefully interpreted and related to clinical symptoms and other diagnostic tests as a potential irritant effect of LMW on the skin cannot be discarded. Table 7.1 summarizes the sensitivities, specificities, and predictive values of SPTs to a variety of occupational sensitizers in regards to the presence or absence of OA as confirmed by objective testing.

Patch tests in occupational asthma

In the workplace, workers are exposed to chemicals that may cause both occupational contact dermatitis (irritant or allergic) (OCD) and OA. Up to 20% of patients with OA have associated OCD (19). In addition, there is an emerging body of research that examines whether each route (e.g. dermal and inhalation) of exposure is capable of inducing sensitization and response in the other system. It has been shown in animal models that dermal exposure can cause sensitization, which upon the first inhalation exposure (in a naïve animal) results in an asthma-like response (19). The most frequent agents causing responses in both systems are epoxy resins, nickel sulfate, cobalt chloride, potassium dichromate, p-phenylenediamine, formaldehyde, glutaraldehyde, colophony, and metalworking fluids. This highlights the importance of considering both a dermal and respiratory work-related allergic disease in the same patient.

Immunological assessment by serological assays

Total IgE assays

The total IgE value alone is not sufficient to diagnose an IgE-mediated allergy or atopy. However, the total IgE level is important in the evaluation and classification of specific IgE (sIgE) test results. Therefore, the measurement of total IgE is always recommended within the context of sIgE measurements (20). The determination of total IgE facilitates the assessment of sIgE values but can never exclude or detect specific sensitization, and thus, plays only a minor role in the diagnosis of OA.

TABLE 7.1 Predictive Values of Skin-Prick Tests to Occupational Sensitizers in Regards to Confirmed Diagnosis of OA

SPT Extract	Sensitivity, %	Specificity, %	PPV, %	NPV, %
Wheat flour*	38–58	89–93	88–92	49–58
Rye flour*	21–81	88–98	89–97	40–72
Soy*	33–44	82–85	36–48	80–84
Cow*	50–92	90–97	83–93	77–89
Natural rubber latex*	67–89	92–96	75–89	88–96
Enzymes**	95–98	50–80	—	—
Persulphate salts***	0–80	60		
Chloramine***	50	70		
Isocyanates (HSA conjugate)***	0–30	95		

Abbreviations: HSA: human serum albumin; NPV: negative predictive value; PPV: positive predictive value; SPT: skin-prick test.

*van Kampen V, et al. EAACI position paper: skin prick testing in the diagnosis of occupational type I allergies. *Allergy*. 2013;68:580–4.

**Cullinan P, et al. An outbreak of asthma in a modern detergent factory. *Lancet*. 2000;356:1899–1900.

***Helaskoski E, et al. Prick testing with chemicals in the diagnosis of occupational contact urticaria and respiratory diseases. *Contact Dermatitis*. 2015;72:20–32.

Allergen-specific IgE assays

Specific IgE solid-phase immunoassays have been available since the early 1970s. Currently, radioallergosorbent-based assays (RAST) consisting of allergens that are bound to new solid-phase matrix materials with higher binding capacities of the allergenic molecules were developed. The modern sIgE antibody immunoassays allow for the interpolation of IgE antibody results from a quantification limit of 0.1 kU_A/l to 100 kU_A/l, but in most clinical cases, 0.35 kU_A/l is used as the lower threshold limit.

IgE antibody tests are run as singleplex (one), multiallergen (<10), and multiplex (>100 allergen specificities) assays, all with particular design and performance features.

Allergen-specific IgE assays have two well-known limitations: (1) a false-positive test may occur in patients with a high total IgE due to a nonspecific binding of IgE resulting in an overestimation of the amount of specific IgE; and (2) false-negative tests may occur in patients with high levels of an allergen-specific antibody for other isotypes, such as specific IgG. In these cases, the binding of specific IgE may be inhibited, resulting in an underestimation of the quantity of the specific IgE (21).

Developments in the analysis of specific IgE component-resolved diagnosis

In the past few years, rapid developments have been made in molecular allergy diagnosis or component-resolved diagnosis (CRD), which is based upon the detection and quantification of specific IgE antibodies to recombinant allergen protein components. The CRD is based on specific IgE testing with single allergenic components and not with crude extract preparations from native allergen material. As such, it offers the possibility of establishing personalized sensitization patterns to discriminate between a genuine allergy and merely sensitization as well as assessing the individual allergy's risk of severity (22). Only a few of the 400 agents identified as occupational sensitizers are both biochemically and molecularly characterized and produced in recombinant form. Given the current lack of knowledge of the allergen components and their allergenicity, only a limited number of recombinant or native occupational relevant allergens are commercially available for the in vitro diagnosis for singleplex or for multiplex chip-based analysis.

A CRD with single recombinant allergens is a reliable tool for diagnosing natural rubber latex allergy. Currently, 15 allergens identified from natural rubber latex (NRL) *Hevea brasiliensis* have been included in the nomenclature list of the International Nomenclature Committee of Allergens (part of the World Health Organization [WHO]/International Union of Immunological Societies [IUIS]) and assigned official numbers (Hev b 1-15; http://www.allergen.org) (23). Most of the allergens are available in recombinant form and commercially coupled to ImmunoCAP (rHev b 1, 3, 5, 6.01, 6.02, 5, 8, 9, and 11) while five of them are (rHev 1, 3, 5, 6.01 and 8) on the Immuno Solid-Phase Allergen Chip (ISAC*, ThermoFischer Scientific). The specific IgE measurement with NRL extract, an important method to diagnose latex sensitization, has been significantly improved by the addition ("spiking") of the major allergen rHev b 5 as a stable recombinant protein to the NRL extract preparation (24). In the case of healthcare workers suffering from occupational latex allergy, the most important NRL allergens are Hev b 5 and Hev 6.01 or Hev b 6.02. If there are false-positive NRL-specific IgE results in subjects without clinical symptoms to latex and/or exposure that arise, inhibition studies with "cross-reactive carbohydrate determinants" can be performed to clarify the origin of the IgE-binding to latex (protein epitopes versus glycol-peptides) (23). The serological work-up with the starting point of the improved ImmunoCAP test with the Hev b 5-amplified latex extract (k82 "spiked" with rHev b 5) followed by the inclusion of at least one CRD screening tool and the recombinant allergens rHev b 1, rHev b 3, rHev b 5, and rHev b 6.01 is highly recommended and might support the proper diagnosis in patients with suspected type I allergy to NRL (25). Despite the many efforts to characterize the occupationally relevant wheat allergens for baker's asthma (*Triticum aestivum* [Tri a] allergens are listed in the WHO/IUIS allergen nomenclature database [available at www.allergen.org]), the results remain highly variable (26). Wheat sensitization profiles of bakers showed great interindividual variability, and no wheat allergen could be classified as major allergens. A whole-wheat extract is still the best option for identifying specific IgE in the investigation of baker's asthma. However, single wheat allergens might help to discriminate between wheat-induced food allergy, grass pollen allergy, and baker's asthma.

Workplace-related allergens such as coffee, wood, soybean, seafood, and mold allergens have been characterized, but very few are currently available. Their relevance for occupational sensitization routes should be validated in further studies.

High-molecular-weight allergens

In general, either a skin test or a serological assay are useful diagnostic tools to detect specific IgE directed against the putative HMW agent causing OA (27). However, the relevance of the positive allergen-specific tests can only be interpreted within the clinical context. Table 7.2 summarizes the sensitivity, specificity, and predictive values of specific IgE to NRL (28), flour, (29), bovine protein (30), and mouse allergens (31) in regards to the diagnosis of OA made by objective testing.

Low-molecular-weight allergens

Many occupational allergens are LMW compounds that are not complete antigens (e.g. diisocyanates, anhydrides) (32–34). In vivo, their first interaction is with a native human macromolecule, such as albumin, leading to recognizable epitopes, either on the hapten-protein conjugate or through interaction of the hapten with the constitutive macromolecule leading to the formation of new antigenic determinants. Care must be taken when synthesizing these hapten-protein conjugates for in vitro serologic testing, as the synthesized hapten-protein conjugates may not be equivalent to those formed in vivo.

An IgE-mediated mechanism has been documented for a few LMW agents such as anhydride acids—used as hardeners in epoxy resins in chemical plants and in powder paints, complex platinum salts—used in platinum refineries or the production of catalysts, and reactive dyes—used in textile manufactures. It is generally assumed that the allergenicity of these LMW or their metabolites results from a mostly covalent interaction with some carrier proteins to build a hapten-carrier complex, because most have highly reactive functional groups (35). In the case of diisocyanates, characterized by highly reactive NCO groups (36) including hexamethylene diisocyanate (HDI) and toluene diisocyanate (TDI), specific IgE are identified in only 21%–55% of subjects with OA, confirmed by a positive specific bronchial inhalation challenge test (37). Therefore, elevated serum specific IgE against diisocyanates, if present, is strongly supportive of the diagnosis (38). However, their absence does not exclude diisocyanate-induced asthma as the sensitivity of the test is low.

The predictive value of the presence of specific IgE antibodies to trimellitic anhydride using ELISA methods has been assessed in a study that included 16 exposed workers, nine of whom with specific IgE, either with OA or developing it within 5 years of follow-up, compared with 1 in 165 workers without these antibodies (32).

Limitations of commercially available specific IgE assays in the diagnosis of occupational asthma

Serological assays used in the diagnosis of OA are hampered by the lack of commercially available standardized allergen reagents (39). This is actually a problem for most allergenic products or extracts. The development of certified reference material for allergenic products and validation of methods for their quantification have been performed for only a few nonoccupational allergens. The presence of cross-reactive carbohydrate determinants (CCDs) can negatively influence the specificity of the in vitro diagnostic tests, especially in the case of plant allergens (40) (e.g. wood dust and NRL). Therefore, it is necessary to exclude glyco-epitopes with low clinical relevance, which are responsible for IgE-binding.

Inflammatory biomarkers

Blood eosinophil counts

A large European cohort of patients with OA due to HMW and LMW agents showed a slightly higher blood eosinophil count at baseline in subjects with OA caused by HMW compared with LMW (41). However, this finding is unlikely to be helpful in clinical practice for a specific patient. Blood eosinophil counts measured before and after exposure in subjects with and without OA showed a low diagnostic accuracy to predict the diagnosis of OA (42). Although blood eosinophil counts are easy to obtain in clinical practice, their usefulness to support a diagnosis of OA is limited.

TABLE 7.2 Predictive Values of Immunological Tests in Regards to Confirmed Diagnosis of Occupational Asthma

Allergen	Test	Sensitivity, %	Specificity, %	PPV, %	NPV, %	References
Natural rubber latex	sIgE to rHev b 5, 6.01 or 6.02 (≥1.46 kUA/l)	79 (69–98)	88 (69–98)	96 (88–99)	56 (40–72)	*1. Vandenplas, 2016*
Flour	sIgE (ImmunoCap)	51	100	100	65	*2. van Kampen, 2008*
	sIgE to wheat flour ≥2.32 kUA/l	30	100	100	42	
	sIgE to rye flour ≥9.64 kUA/l					
Bovine proteins	Fluoro-enzymatic immunoassay Bovine-specific IgE ≥5UI/l	82	100	100	93	*3. Koskela, 2003*
Mouse allergen	Mouse urine ImmunoCAP sIgE to mouse ≥0.35 kU/l	47	91	70	79	*4. Sharma, 2008*

Abbreviations: NPV: negative predictive value; PPV: positive predictive value.

References: *1. Vandenplas O, et al. The role of allergen components for the diagnosis of latex-induced occupational asthma. Allergy. 2016;71:840–9; 2. Kampen V, et al. Prediction of challenge test results for flour-specific IgE and skin prick test in symptomatic bakers. Allergy. 2008;63:897–902; 3. Koskela H, et al. Inhalation challenge with bovine dander allergens: who needs it? Chest. 2003;124:383–91; 4. Sharma HP, et al. A comparison of skin prick tests, intradermal skin tests, and specific IgE in the diagnosis of mouse allergy. J Allergy Clin Immunol. 2008;121:933–9.*

CASE HISTORY (CONTINUED)

An investigation at and away from work was performed using serial peak expiratory flow (PEF) monitoring, PC20 monitoring, as well as performance of sputum cell counts after periods at and away from work. Serial PEF monitoring was not interpretable because of the patient's poor adherence to the test. Methacholine PC20 was 2 mg/ml after 2 weeks at work and 3 mg/ml after 3 weeks away from work. After 2 weeks at work, induced sputum cell counts showed eosinophilic inflammation (sputum eosinophils: 10%) that decreased after 2 weeks away from work (sputum eosinophils: 1%). The following sections discuss how noninvasive measures of airway inflammation may be used in the investigation to support the diagnosis of OA.

Sputum cell counts
Sputum eosinophil counts

The early observation that sputum eosinophil counts increase in subjects with OA who are exposed to their offending agents and decrease when they are removed from the exposure (43), has led to a number of studies trying to establish the place of the sputum eosinophil count in the investigation of OA.

Sputum eosinophil counts achieve the best diagnostic accuracy when performed serially during periods at and away from work or before and after exposure to an offending agent during SICs (44). Sputum eosinophil counts show an increase of at least 3% in approximately 70% of patients with OA after exposure to the offending agent, showing a 90% specificity (42).

Sputum eosinophil counts are also useful when combined with other tests; for example, when added to serial peak flow monitoring at and away from work, sputum eosinophil counts can improve the specificity of this test by 18% to 27% depending on the chosen eosinophil cut-off (45). Combining the results of nonspecific bronchial provocation tests to sputum eosinophil counts has a high negative predictive value (91%) for the diagnosis of OA (42).

There is also a number of examples where sputum eosinophil counts prove to be helpful in the investigation of OA. An early increase in sputum eosinophils can precede the occurrence of changes in FEV_1 during SIC (46). In contrast, negative challenges do not usually induce an eosinophilic inflammation (47). However, the lack of increase in sputum eosinophil counts after exposure to occupational agents should not discard the diagnosis of OA. Indeed, some subjects can experience a 20% fall in FEV_1 without showing sputum eosinophilia (48), whereas others can experience a 20% fall in FEV_1 accompanied by an important increase in airway inflammation without airway hyperresponsiveness (49). Interfering factors that can modify the sputum cell response such as oral or inhaled corticosteroid treatment should be considered in the interpretation.

Several studies have assessed the outcome of airway eosinophilic inflammation at different time points after removal from exposure to the offending agents in subjects with OA. In most cases, the eosinophilic inflammation decreases rapidly within 2 weeks following the removal from exposure (50). However, it can persist in some subjects. The persistence of eosinophilic inflammation seems more frequent in subjects who had little improvement in their airway hyperresponsiveness after removal from exposure (51). The persistence of eosinophilic airway inflammation seems to be associated with the magnitude of impairment of the respiratory function tests in workers who have or have not been removed from their workplace (52).

Sputum neutrophil counts

A neutrophilic airway inflammation has also been reported after exposure to isocyanates in subjects with isocyanate-induced OA (53) as well as in a subject reporting chronic cough related to isocyanate exposure suggesting a diagnosis of neutrophilic bronchitis (54). However, the interpretation of a neutrophilic inflammation following exposure to LMW is difficult as an increase in the sputum neutrophil count has also been observed in patients exposed to LMW without OA.

Using sputum differential cell counts during the investigation of OA can improve its diagnosis by bringing an additional objective measure to this investigation. Although the reliability of FEV_1 and PC20 can be affected by inadequate spirometric maneuvers, the presence or the absence of airway inflammation cannot be falsified.

Fractional exhaled nitric oxide

The measurement of a fractional nitric oxide (NO) concentration in exhaled breath (FeNO) is a quantitative, noninvasive, simple, and safe method of detecting eosinophilic airway inflammation. There are recommendations for standardized procedures and interpretation of this tool in airway diseases, including asthma (55).

Initial studies that assessed the usefulness of FeNO in the investigation of OA provided inconsistent results (45). These conflicting results might be explained by several factors: (1) the insufficient duration of monitoring of patients after the acute exposure—the level of exhaled NO tends to increase only 24–48 hours after exposure (56); (2) glucocorticosteroids inhibit the induction of NO synthase, and FeNO falls after treatment with oral or inhaled corticosteroids in subjects with asthma (57)—FeNO response might have been blunted in studies, which included patients on steroid treatment at the time of the test; and (3) an increase of NO production in the presence of bronchoconstriction might have been underestimated (58).

Changes in FeNO 24 hours after exposure to occupational agents during SICs were shown to correlate with the increase in sputum eosinophil counts in subjects with OA (56, 59). However, this relationship was generally weak. A reason may be the different kinetics of changes in sputum eosinophil and FeNO after exposure to a sensitizer. In addition, different levels of the bronchial tree are examined by the two tools: sputum is cleared by cough from central airways, whereas FeNO concentration reflects changes in more peripheral airways (60).

More recent investigations established that subjects with OA caused by HMW agents showed a greater increase in post-SIC FeNO as compared to subjects with OA due to LMW agents (41, 61–63). Among the latter agents, a large European, multicenter, retrospective cohort of subjects with OA (n = 473) showed that the postchallenge FeNO increase was higher in acrylate-induced OA than in OA induced by other LMW agents (64). A postchallenge increase in FeNO ≥13–17.5 ppb or >41% over baseline value showed a high specificity (90%–95%), but a low sensitivity (45%–50%) in predicting a positive SIC (61, 65, 66). Indeed, there was a consensus by the ERS Task Force on Specific Inhalation Challenges with Occupational Agents that the assessment of the FeNO level during SIC may be useful in subjects who fail to provide suitable sputum samples, although changes in FeNO were less discriminant than those in sputum eosinophils (59). In cases where the changes in FEV_1 are equivocal, an increase in FeNO 24 hours after the challenge would support a positive SIC response (67).

Baseline FeNO measurements alone cannot be considered a useful screening test in diagnosing OA since it has less sensitivity than nonspecific bronchial hyperresponsiveness (NSBHR) (68). However, combining a FeNO ≥25 ppb to the presence of NSBHR increased the sensitivity from 87% to 91% in predicting a positive SIC (69).

The diagnostic value of serial measurements of FeNO at and away from work in predicting OA has not been sufficiently investigated, although some reports suggest that they may give some complementary information (70–72).

Exhaled breath condensate

Exhaled breath condensate (EBC), obtained by cooling exhaled breath, has been proposed to monitor airway inflammation and oxidative stress. A wide range of volatile substances in gas phase and nonvolatile compounds from the respiratory tract can be collected in condensed water. A major issue is the standardization of the sample collection and the evaluation of different analytic approaches, since there is an absence of a valid method to assess the dilution factor and many biomarkers have been detected near the lower limit of the assay. There was a consensus that efficacy of the collection should be assessed by reporting the volume of exhaled breath, the volume of the condensate, and the time of collection (73).

A few studies have used exhaled breath condensate to assess the inflammatory markers in workers with OA. Ferrazzoni et al. measured EBC pH in subjects with positive SICs to isocyanates (56). They did not find any association between positive asthmatic reaction to isocyanates and EBC pH. Klusackova et al. measured leukotrienes and 8-isoprostane in EBC in subjects with suspected OA. There was no significant change in those markers before and after the occurrence of the asthmatic reaction (74). Do et al. assessed the biomarkers of airway acidity (pH, $NH_4{}^+$) and oxidative stress (8-isoprostane) in 75 grain elevator workers (75). They found an association between smoking and obesity with decreased pH and $NH_4{}^+$, whereas grain dust and endotoxin exposure were associated with increased 8-isoprostane. Tafuro et al. performed an observational study with the aim of validating biomarkers of airway inflammation in laboratory animal workers (76). The conclusion of the authors is that EBC hydrogen peroxide levels do not seem to be a useful marker in laboratory animal allergy.

Although EBC might be an interesting additional tool in the investigation or the screening of subjects with airway disease, further research is needed to assess whether some EBC pH or mediators are useful in the investigation of OA.

Directions of future research

* The standardization of occupational allergens needs to be improved in order to increase the diagnostic accuracy of SPT and serological testing. Extracts of an occupational allergen for SPT should be made more easily available.
* The development of serological testing to LMW agents would improve the screening and the diagnosis of OA caused by this type of agent.
* Studies assessing the diagnostic probability of combined indices such as airway hyperresponsiveness, allergen sensitization, and inflammatory markers may allow the development of alternative methods to diagnose OA.

References

1. Blackley C. *Experimental researchers on the causes and nature of Catarrhus aestivus (hay fever or hay asthma).* Cox BT, ed. London. 1873.
2. Pepys J. Skin testing. *Br J Hosp Med.* 1975;14:412–5.
3. Murdoch RD, Pepys J, Hughes EG. IgE antibody responses to platinum group metals: a large scale refinery survey. *Br J Ind Med.* 1986;43(1):37–43.
4. Pepys J. Allergic asthma to Bacillus subtilis enzyme: a model for the effects of inhalable proteins. *Am J Ind Med.* 1992;21:587–93.
5. Bousquet J, Heinzerling L, Bachert C, et al. Practical guide to skin prick tests in allergy to aeroallergens. *Allergy.* 2012;67(1):18–24.
6. van Kampen V, de Blay F, Folletti I, et al. Evaluation of commercial skin prick test solutions for selected occupational allergens. *Allergy.* 2013;68(5):651–8.
7. Schmid-Grendelmeier P, Crameri R. Recombinant allergens for skin testing. *Int Arch Allergy Immunol.* 2001;125(2):96–111.
8. Quirce S, Fernandez-Nieto M, Escudero C, et al. Bronchial responsiveness to bakery-derived allergens is strongly dependent on specific skin sensitivity. *Allergy.* 2006;61:1202–8.
9. Taghiakbari M, Pralong JA, Lemiere C, et al. Novel clinical scores for occupational asthma due to exposure to high-molecular-weight agents. *Occup Environ Med.* 2019;76(7):495–501.
10. Lindh CH, Jonsson BA. Quantification method of human hemoglobin adducts from hexahydrophthalic anhydride and methylhexahydrophthalic anhydride. *J Chromatogr B Biomed Sci Appl.* 1998;710(1-2):81–90.

DISCUSSION ON ILLUSTRATIVE CASE HISTORY

The clinical case presented at the beginning of this chapter summarizes the case of a worker who is sensitized to platinum salts, has asthma confirmed by the combination of respiratory symptoms suggestive of asthma, and a positive methacholine challenge. The causality between the onset of asthma and the sensitization to platinum salts cannot be confirmed by objective measures as PEF/methacholine challenge monitoring was not contributive.

This case illustrates the benefit of additional tools for assessing the causality between asthma symptoms and exposures at the workplace, especially when respiratory function tests cannot be performed or are unreliable. Sensitization to platinum salts can be assessed by SPTs, which are the most sensitive tests to detect the sensitization to an allergen. However, there are situations where SPT cannot be performed. Indeed, there are no allergenic extracts available for testing the majority of LMW agents. In the present case, OA due to platinum salts is clearly IgE dependent and allergenic extracts for platinum salts are available. However, SPT cannot be interpreted reliably when subjects are taking antihistamines or are experiencing dermographism. In the present case, the positivity of SPT to platinum salts confirms the sensitization to this agent but does not confirm the diagnosis of OA to platinum salts.

Serum-specific IgE antibodies to HMW allergens and some LMW allergens could be useful for predicting the phenotype of OA or identifying asymptomatic exposed workers. Serum-specific IgG does not appear to have a pathological role, but does indicate exposure. More efforts should be focused on developing more sensitive early diagnostic biomarkers. Finally, a large increase in the eosinophil count when at work along with a compatible history of asthma confirmed by pulmonary function tests supports the diagnosis of OA.

11. Rosqvist S, Johannesson G, Lindh CH, Jonsson BA. Quantification of protein adducts of hexahydrophthalic anhydride and methylhexahydrophthalic anhydride in human plasma. *J Environ Monit.* 2000;2(2):155–60.

12. Kristiansson MH, Lindh CH, Jonsson BA. Determination of hexahydrophthalic anhydride adducts to human serum albumin. *Biomarkers.* 2003;8(5):343–59.

13. Wisnewski AV, Srivastava R, Herick C, Xu L, et al. Identification of human lung and skin proteins conjugated with hexamethylene diisocyanate in vitro and in vivo. *Am J Respir Crit Care Med.* 2000;162(6):2330–6.

14. Campo P, Wisnewski A, Lummus Z, et al. Diisocyanate conjugate and immunoassay characteristics influence detection of specific antibodies in HDI-exposed workers. *Clin Exp Allergy.* 2007;37:1095–102.

15. Cartier A, Grammer L, Malo JL, et al. Specific serum antibodies against isocyanates: association with occupational asthma. *J Allergy Clin Immunol.* 1989;84:507–14.

16. Tee RD, Cullinan P, Welch J, et al. Specific IgE to isocyanates: a useful diagnostic role in occupational asthma. *J Allergy Clin Immunol.* 1998;101(5):709–15.

17. Hettick JM, Siegel PD, Green BJ, et al. Vapor conjugation of toluene diisocyanate to specific lysines of human albumin. *Anal Biochem.* 2012;421(2):706–11.

18. Helaskoski E, Suojalehto H, Kuuliala O, Aalto-Korte K. Prick testing with chemicals in the diagnosis of occupational contact urticaria and respiratory diseases. *Contact Dermatitis.* 2015;72(1):20–32.

19. Arrandale VH, Liss GM, Tarlo SM, et al. Occupational contact allergens: are they also associated with occupational asthma? *Am J Ind Med.* 2012;55(4):353–60.

20. Hamilton RG. Proficiency survey-based evaluation of clinical total and allergen-specific IgE assay performance. *Arch Pathol Lab Med.* 2010;134(7):975–82.

21. Reid MJ, Kwasnicki JM, Moss RB, Cheung NK. Underestimation of specific immunoglobulin E by microtiter plate enzyme-linked immunosorbent assays. *J Allergy Clin Immunol.* 1985;76(2 Pt 1):172–6.

22. Raulf M. Allergen component analysis as a tool in the diagnosis and management of occupational allergy. *Mol Immunol.* 2018;100:21–7.

23. Raulf M. The latex story. *Chem Immunol Allergy.* 2014;100:248–55.

24. Lundberg M, Chen Z, Rihs HP, Wrangsjo K. Recombinant spiked allergen extract. *Allergy.* 2001;56(8):794–5.

25. Raulf M, Rihs H. Latex allergens: source of sensitization and single allergens. In: Kleine-Tebbe J, Jalob T, eds. *Molecular Allergy Diagnostics.* 2017;459–70.

26. Sander I, Rihs HP, Doekes G, et al. Component-resolved diagnosis of baker's allergy based on specific IgE to recombinant wheat flour proteins. *J Allergy Clin Immunol.* 2015;135(6):1529–37.

27. Moscato G, Pala G, Barnig C, et al. EAACI consensus statement for investigation of work-related asthma in non-specialized centres. *Allergy.* 2012;67(4):491–501.

28. Vandenplas O, Froidure A, Meurer U, et al. The role of allergen components for the diagnosis of latex-induced occupational asthma. *Allergy.* 2016;71(6):840–9.

29. van Kampen V, Rabstein S, Sander I, et al. Prediction of challenge test results by flour-specific IgE and skin prick test in symptomatic bakers. *Allergy.* 2008;63(7):897–902.

30. Koskela H, Taivainen A, Tukiainen H, Chan H. Inhalation challenge with bovine dander allergens: who needs it? *Chest.* 2003;124:383–91.

31. Sharma HP, Wood RA, Bravo AR, Matsui EC. A comparison of skin prick tests, intradermal skin tests, and specific IgE in the diagnosis of mouse allergy. *J Allergy Clin Immunol.* 2008;121(4):933–9.

32. Grammer L, Shaughnessy M, Kenamore B. Utility of antibody in identifying individuals who have or will develop anhydride-induced respiratory disease. *Chest.* 1998;114:1199–202.

33. Bernstein D, Jolly A. Current diagnostic methods for diisocyanate induced occupational asthma. *Am J Ind Med.* 1999;36:459–68.

34. Wisnewski A. Developments in laboratory diagnostics for isocyanate asthma. *Curr Opin Allergy Clin Immunol.* 2007;7:138–45.

35. Enoch SJ, Seed MJ, Roberts DW, et al. Development of mechanism-based structural alerts for respiratory sensitization hazard identification. *Chem Res Toxicol.* 2012;25(11):2490–8.

36. Pronk A, Preller L, Raulf-Heimsoth M, et al. Respiratory symptoms, sensitization, and exposure response relationships in spray painters exposed to isocyanates. *Am J Respir Crit Care Med.* 2007;176(11):1090–7.

37. Tarlo SM, Balmes J, Balkissoon R, et al. Diagnosis and management of work-related asthma: American College Of Chest Physicians Consensus Statement. *Chest.* 2008;134(3 Suppl):1S–41S.

38. Redlich CA, Karol MH. Diisocyanate asthma: clinical aspects and immunopathogenesis. *Int Immunopharmacol.* 2002;2(2-3):213–24.

39. Nicholson PJ, Cullinan P, Newman-Taylor AJ, et al. Evidence based guidelines for the prevention, identification, and management of occupational asthma. *Occup Environ Med.* 2005;62(5):290–9.

40. Kespohl S, Schlunssen V, Jacobsen G, et al. Impact of cross-reactive carbohydrate determinants on wood dust sensitization. *Clin Exp Allergy.* 2010;40(7):1099–106.

41. Vandenplas O, Godet J, Hurdubaea L, et al. Are high- and low-molecular-weight sensitizing agents associated with different clinical phenotypes of occupational asthma? *Allergy.* 2019;74(2):261–72.

42. Racine G, Castano R, Cartier A, Lemiere C. Diagnostic accuracy of inflammatory markers for diagnosing occupational asthma. *J Allergy Clin Immunol Pract.* 2017;5(5):1371–7 e1.

43. Lemière C, Pizzichini M, Balkissoon R, et al. Diagnosing occupational asthma: use of induced sputum. *Eur Respir J.* 1999;13:482–8.

44. Lemiere C, Boulet LP, Chaboillez S, et al. Work-exacerbated asthma and occupational asthma: do they really differ? *J Allergy Clin Immunol.* 2013;131(3):704–10.

45. Quirce S, Lemiere C, de Blay F, et al. Noninvasive methods for assessment of airway inflammation in occupational settings. *Allergy.* 2010;65(4):445–58.

46. Vandenplas O, D'Alpaos V, Heymans J, et al. Sputum eosinophilia: an early marker of bronchial response to occupational agents. *Allergy.* 2009;64(5):754–61.

47. Lemière C, Chaboillez S, Malo JL, Cartier A. Changes in sputum cell counts after exposure to occupational agents: what do they mean? *J Allergy Clin Immunol.* 2001;107:1063–8.

48. Obata H, Dittick M, Chan H, Chan-Yeung M. Sputum eosinophils and exhaled nitric oxide during late asthmatic reaction in patients with Western red cedar asthma. *Eur Respir J.* 1999;13:489–95.

49. Lemière C, Weytjens K, Cartier A, Malo JL. Late asthmatic reaction with airway inflammation but without airway hyperresponsiveness. *Clin Exp Allergy.* 2000;30:415–7.

50. Lemiere C, Chaboillez S, Welman M, Maghni K. Outcome of occupational asthma after removal from exposure: a follow-up study. *Can Respir J.* 2010;17(2):61–6.

51. Maghni K, Lemiere C, Ghezzo H, et al. Airway inflammation after cessation of exposure to agents causing occupational asthma. *Am J Respir Crit Care Med.* 2004;169(3):367–72.

52. Chan-Yeung M, Obata H, Dittrick M, et al. Airway inflammation, exhaled nitric oxide, and severity of asthma in patients with Western red cedar asthma. *Am J Respir Crit Care Med.* 1999;159:1434–8.

53. Lemière C, Romeo P, Chaboillez S, et al. Airway inflammation and functional changes after exposure to different concentrations of isocyanates. *J Allergy Clin Immunol.* 2002;110:641–6.

54. Pala G, Pignatti P, Moscato G. Occupational exposure to toluene diisocyanate and neutrophilic bronchitis without asthma. *Clin Toxicol (Phila).* 2011;49(6):506–7.

55. Dweik RA, Boggs PB, Erzurum SC, et al. An official ATS clinical practice guideline: interpretation of exhaled nitric oxide levels (FENO) for clinical applications. *Am J Respir Crit Care Med.* 2011;184(5):602–15.

56. Ferrazzoni S, Scarpa MC, Guarnieri G, et al. Exhaled nitric oxide and breath condensate pH in asthmatic reactions induced by isocyanates. *Chest.* 2009;136(1):155–62.

57. Massaro A, Gaston B, Kita D, et al. Expired nitric oxide levels during treatment of acute asthma. *Am J Respir Crit Care Med.* 1995;152:800–3.

58. Mason P, Scarpa MC, Guarnieri G, et al. Exhaled nitric oxide dynamics in asthmatic reactions induced by diisocyanates. *Clin Exp Allergy.* 2016;46(12):1531–9.

59. Lemiere C, D'Alpaos V, Chaboillez S, et al. Investigation of occupational asthma: sputum cell counts or exhaled nitric oxide? *Chest.* 2010;137(3):617–22.

60. Cattoni I, Guarnieri G, Tosetto A, et al. Mechanisms of decrease in fractional exhaled nitric oxide during acute bronchoconstriction. *Chest.* 2013;143(5):1269–76.

61. Lemiere C, Nguyen S, Sava F, et al. Occupational asthma phenotypes identified by increased fractional exhaled nitric oxide after exposure to causal agents. *J Allergy Clin Immunol.* 2014;134(5):1063–7.

62. Sastre J, Costa C, del Garcia Potro M, et al. Changes in exhaled nitric oxide after inhalation challenge with occupational agents. *J Investig Allergol Clin Immunol.* 2013;23(6):421–7.

63. Walters GI, Moore VC, McGrath EE, Burge S. Fractional exhaled nitric oxide in the interpretation of specific inhalational challenge tests for occupational asthma. *Lung.* 2014;192(1):119–24.

64. Suojalehto H, Suuronen K, Cullinan P, et al. Phenotyping occupational asthma caused by acrylates in a multicenter cohort study. *J Allergy Clin Immunol Pract.* 2020;8(3):971-9 e1.

65. Engel J, van Kampen V, Lotz A, et al. An increase of fractional exhaled nitric oxide after specific inhalation challenge is highly predictive of occupational asthma. *Int Arch Occup Environ Health*. 2018;91(7):799–809.

66. Engel J, van Kampen V, Gering V, et al. Non-invasive tools beyond lung function before and after specific inhalation challenges for diagnosing occupational asthma. *Int Arch Occup Environ Health*. 2019;92(7):1067–76.

67. Vandenplas O, Suojalehto H, Aasen TB, et al. Specific inhalation challenge in the diagnosis of occupational asthma: consensus statement. *Eur Respir J*. 2014;43(6):1573–87.

68. Florentin A, Acouetey DS, Remen T, et al. Exhaled nitric oxide and screening for occupational asthma in two at-risk sectors: bakery and hairdressing. *Int J Tuberc Lung Dis*. 2014;18(6):744–50.

69. Beretta C, Rifflart C, Evrard G, et al. Assessment of eosinophilic airway inflammation as a contribution to the diagnosis of occupational asthma. *Allergy*. 2018;73(1):206–13.

70. van Kampen V, Bruning T, Merget R. Serial fractional exhaled nitric oxide measurements off and at work in the diagnosis of occupational asthma. *Am J Ind Med*. 2019;62(8):663–71.

71. Hewitt RS, Smith AD, Cowan JO, et al. Serial exhaled nitric oxide measurements in the assessment of laboratory animal allergy. *J Asthma*. 2008;45(2):101–7.

72. Merget R, Sander I, van Kampen V, et al. Serial measurements of exhaled nitric oxide at work and at home: a new tool for the diagnosis of occupational asthma. *Adv Exp Med Biol*. 2015;834:49–52.

73. Horvath I, Barnes PJ, Loukides S, et al. A European Respiratory Society technical standard: exhaled biomarkers in lung disease. *Eur Respir J*. 2017;49(4).

74. Klusackova P, Lebedova J, Kacer P, et al. Leukotrienes and 8-isoprostane in exhaled breath condensate in bronchoprovocation tests with occupational allergens. *Prostaglandins Leukot Essent Fatty Acids*. 2008;78(4-5):281–92.

75. Do R, Bartlett KH, Dimich-Ward H et al. Biomarkers of airway acidity and oxidative stress in exhaled breath condensate from grain workers. *Am J Respir Crit Care Med*. 2008;178(10):1048–54.

76. Tafuro F, Selis L, Goldoni M, et al. Biomarkers of respiratory allergy in laboratory animal care workers: an observational study. *Int Arch Occup Environ Health*. 2018;91(6):735–44.

8

FUNCTIONAL ASSESSMENT

Hille Suojalehto,[1] Vicky C. Moore,[2] Gianna Moscato,[3] P. Sherwood Burge,[4] Jean-Luc Malo,[5] and Olivier Vandenplas[6]

[1]*Finnish Institute of Occupational Health, University of Helsinki, Helsinki, Finland*
[2]*Department of Respiratory Medicine, University Hospitals Birmingham NHS Foundation Trust, Birmingham, UK*
[3]*Specialization School in Occupational Medicine, University of Pavia, Pavia, Italy*
[4]*University of Birmingham Hospital and Birmingham University, Birmingham, UK*
[5]*Hôpital du Sacré-Cœur de Montréal and Université de Montréal, Montréal, Canada*
[6]*Department of Chest Medicine, Centre Hospitalier Universitaire UCL Namur, Université Catholique de Louvain, Yvoir, Belgium*

Contents

Introduction

The diagnosis of occupational asthma (OA) needs objective confirmation as the history lacks sufficient specificity. Available tests include the following:

- Measurement of lung function parameters, including forced expiratory volume in 1 second (FEV_1) and/or peak expiratory flow (PEF), during periods at work and away from work.
- Assessment of nonspecific bronchial hyperresponsiveness (NSBH) when the subject is at work and symptomatic. Specific inhalation challenges (SICs) in the laboratory or at the workplace.

Measurements of lung function

If OA exists, exposure to usual exposures of the causative agent must result in measurable increases in airflow obstruction, measured with PEF or FEV_1.

Diurnal variation in airways caliber

There is a spontaneous diurnal rhythm of airway caliber that can be demonstrated in the majority of the normal population but is exaggerated in asthmatics (1). The lowest readings are usually around the time of waking; there is then an improvement for 6–8 hours followed by a subsequent decline until sleeping, with a further decline overnight. Any reaction at work will be superimposed on this diurnal variation. The relationship between work and sleep can be substantially altered by shift work. Most day workers and workers on early shifts wake shortly before going to work. The first few hours at work will therefore coincide with the period of improving lung function. The effects of an immediate reaction may then be to blunt the rise in peak flow rather than to

cause any fall (2). Workers on afternoon shifts usually wake some time before going to work and go to sleep shortly after returning from work. This results in the occupational exposure, coinciding with the declining phase of lung function. Immediate reactions are usually more obvious on such shifts. The patterns of sleep in night workers are highly variable and usually change between the days at work and the days away from work (3). The patterns of reaction can then be complex.

Before- and after-shift measurements

Before- and after-shift measurements are an unreliable method of separating those with and without OA (4). In a study of electronics workers exposed to colophony, FEV_1 fell by more than 10% in only 16 out of 48 workers having symptoms of OA, but also in 2 out of 43 asymptomatic workers (5). A study comparing mean changes in pre- and postshift PEF over several days found that a cross-shift decrease in PEF of 5 L/min achieved a specificity of 91% (similar with OASYS) and a sensitivity of 50% (83% with OASYS) in those working morning or day shifts (6).

Serial measurements of PEF and FEV_1
Plotting of serial records

PEF records are commonly plotted serially, predominantly to document the response to treatment, that is, to look for progressive change over time (Figure 8.1). Occupational records plotted in this way are difficult to interpret, unless the changes are obvious. The differences related to work exposure can be seen more easily by plotting the daily maximum, mean, and minimum peak flow, as illustrated for the same data in Figure 8.2. Days at work are differentiated from days away from work by background shading. To maximize the difference between the days at and the days away from work, the workday starts with the first reading at work and finishes with the last reading before work the following day. In this way, the morning dip is included with the previous day's

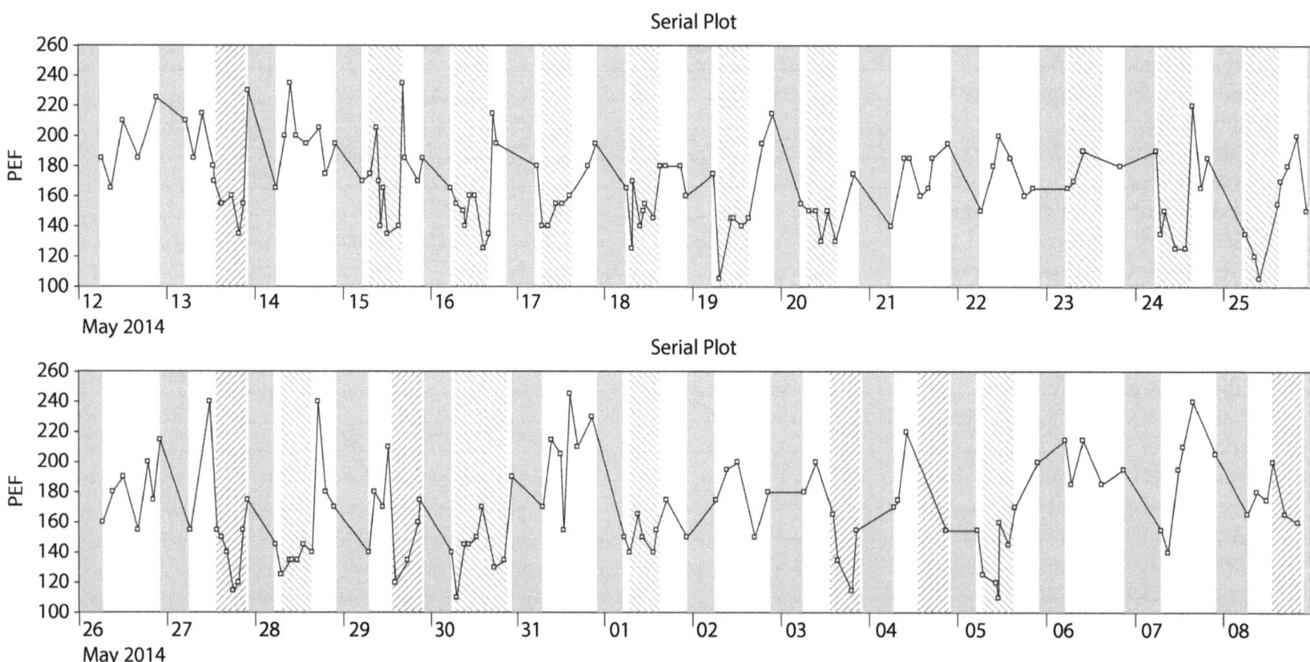

FIGURE 8.1   Serial PEF plot. The grey shaded areas are sleep times, times at work on morning shifts have backward sloping hatching, and times at work on afternoon shifts have forward sloping hatching.
Abbreviation: PEF, peak expiratory flow.

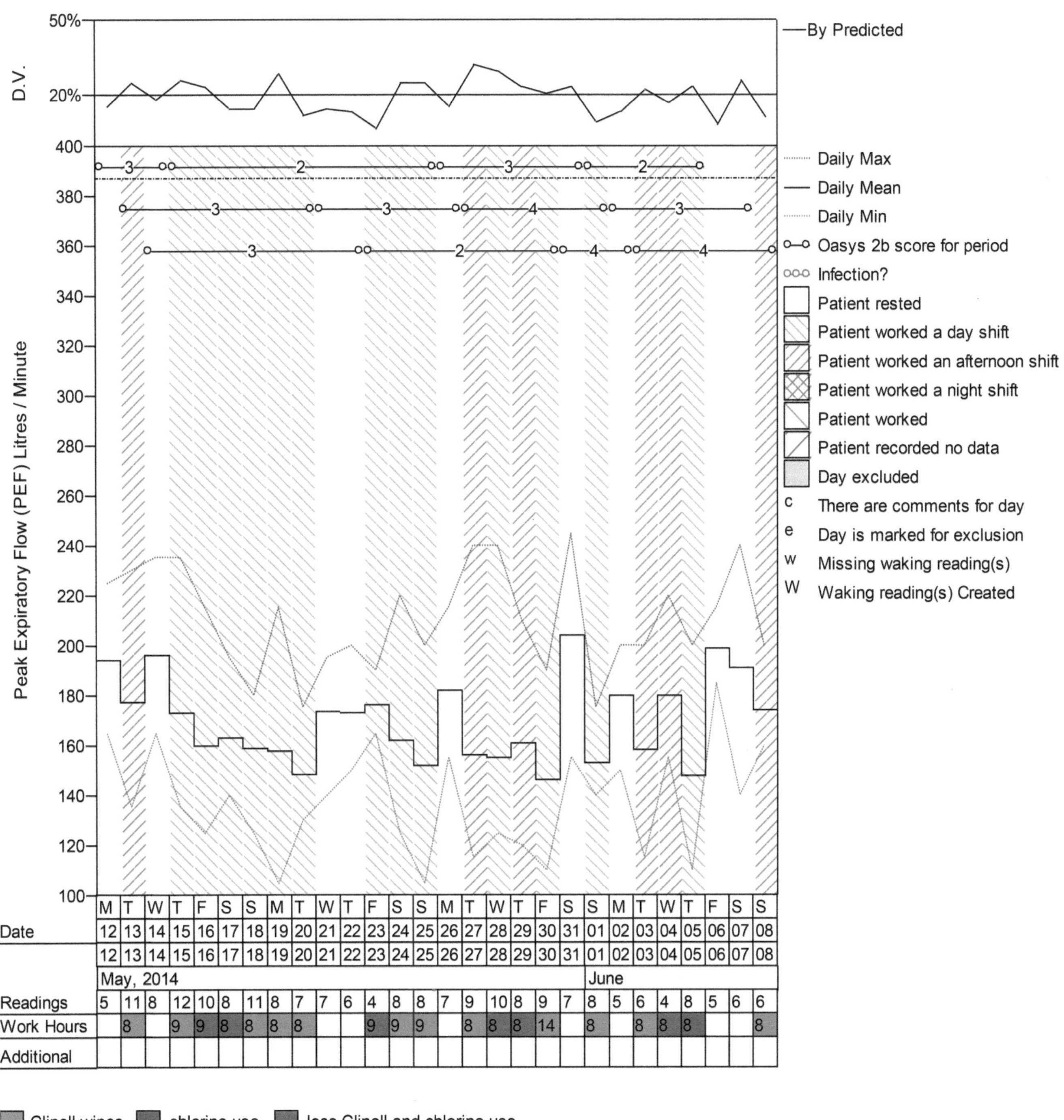

Date	M	T	W	T	F	S	S	M	T	W	T	F	S	S	M	T	W	T	F	S	S	M	T	W	T	F	S	S
	12	13	14	15	16	17	18	19	20	21	22	23	24	25	26	27	28	29	30	31	01	02	03	04	05	06	07	08
	12	13	14	15	16	17	18	19	20	21	22	23	24	25	26	27	28	29	30	31	01	02	03	04	05	06	07	08
	May, 2014																				June							
Readings	5	11	8	12	10	8	11	8	7	7	6	4	8	8	7	9	10	8	9	7	8	5	6	4	8	5	6	6
Work Hours		8		9	9	8	8	8	8			9	9	9		8	8	8	14		8		8	8	8			8
Additional																												

FIGURE 8.2 OASYS plot of data in Figure 8.1. The top panel shows the diurnal variation on each day (% predicted). The center panel shows the daily maximum PEF (grey upper line), mean (black line), and minimum (grey lower line). Days at work on morning shifts have backward sloping hatching, days at work on afternoon shifts have forward sloping hatching, and days off work have a clear background. The predicted PEF (385 L/min) is shown at the top of the central panel. The horizontal bars show the scores from the OASYS discriminant analysis for each complex. The bottom panel shows the day, the date, the number of readings on each day, and the hours worked on each day. Chlorine use occurred on June 5, Clinell wipes were used on the other days identified by grey squares, except for May 16, 17, 23, 28, and 29 and June 4 when there were fewer Clinell wipes and less chlorine used. Visually, there is improvement in each period off work and deterioration in each period at work. There are some workdays with no deterioration (May 23, June 4). The clue to the cause may be found by identifying exposures not present on these days. The OASYS score is 3.20 (definite OA). The overall ABC score is 26 L/min/hour (definite OA), the mean diurnal variation on workdays is 20%, and that on rest days is 16%. The subject had a positive specific challenge to chloramines.

Abbreviations: ABC, area between curves; PEF, peak expiratory flow.

measurements. It is very important to include a waking value in each day's plot and to make sure that records are made on waking on days away from work, because a delay after waking can increase the peak flow and occasionally produce artificial improvement on rest days. Taking readings in workers changing shifts is more complicated. The "day interpreter" in the OASYS program (available free of charge at www.occupationalasthma.com) automatically adjusts readings to the appropriate "day," including changes from night to day work.

Plots of the mean PEF in 2-hour time blocks provide graphs that resemble the results of specific challenge testing and may be easier to understand. Days with different exposures can be separated, and compared with days with no exposure. Plots can be from clock time, or for shift workers as hours from waking, so that the effects of different shift patterns can be amalgamated. There is a good correlation between the time-course of the change in PEF related to work exposures and the pattern of response during SIC (7). Changes in FEV_1 and PEF are not specific for asthma but may also be seen in hypersensitivity pneumonitis (8).

Interpretation of serial PEF plots

The main choice is between an expert opinion and a quantitative or statistical analysis of the record. Original methods utilized expert opinion; the best had high sensitivity and specificity. Analytical methods have now developed to an extent where they are the best method for general use. Expert opinion is still likely to detect subtle changes missed by analytical systems and can supplement them.

Visual analysis

In a study of 25 workers exposed to plicatic acid, a sensitivity of 87% and specificity of 90% compared to SIC was achieved when there was agreement between two out of three physicians (9). Interobserver agreement using this method is generally satisfactory. In one study comparing seven experts from different centers, kappa values for diagnosing OA with increasing likelihood were 0.62 (10). Agreement between three experts from the same institution was 78% in one study (11), 69% between all four observers

in another study, as well as 69% (12) and 71% (13) between three observers in two other studies.

Analytical methods

Plots of serial measurements of PEF identify differences between workdays and rest days. There is no general agreement as to how big the changes in mean PEF or diurnal variation have to be to diagnose OA. Studies of healthy dockers and farmers exposed to high levels of grain dust showed that the upper 95% confidence interval (CI) for mean differences in PEF between work and rest days was 16 L/min (14). Only about one-third of asthmatics have high (20% or more) diurnal variations (15). In our experience, workers with positive SIC may have diurnal variations in PEF below 10% and mean rest-work PEF differences not exceeding 15 L/min and still have positive SIC.

There are several independently validated methods for the analysis of serial PEF measurements, each with their own minimum quality standards (Table 8.1). The sensitivity and specificity for a diagnosis of OA using independent records is shown in Table 8.2. There is a trade-off between frequent measurements over a shorter period of time and less frequent measurements for longer periods. The OASYS score is based on pattern recognition and uses a discriminant analysis to mimic expert opinion. It compares a period at work (at least 3 consecutive days) with the two adjacent periods off work (a rest-work-rest complex) or its counterpart (a work-rest-work complex) to identify deterioration on periods of consecutive workdays or improvement on consecutive periods off work. It scores each complex from 1 (no occupational effect) to 4 (definite occupational effect). It then sums all the scores, gives double weight to scores of 1 and 4, and produces a mean score. It requires the least regular measurements of the validated methods, but requires about 3 weeks of consecutive measurement. A score >2.5 has a high sensitivity and specificity for OA (Table 8.2).

The area between curves (ABC) score compares the mean PEF in two hourly blocks over the 24 hours between days at work and days off work. It calculates the area between the two lines and divides this by the time for which there are at least three readings at the same time on workdays and rest days to give a value in

TABLE 8.1 Requirements for Different Validated Methods for Analysis of Serial Measurements of PEF in the Diagnosis of Occupational Asthma

Analytic Method	Minimum Readings/Day	Minimal Workdays ≥3 Complexes	Minimum Rest Days	Other Requirements
OASYS score	4	˜3 weeks of data		≥3 workdays in any work period
1. Gannon, 1996				
2. Anees, 2004				
Area between curves (ABC)	8	**8** (longer records for less frequent measurements)	**3** (longer period for less frequent measurements)	Further improved with additional 7 days off work
3. Moore, 2009				
4. Moore, 2009				
Time point	4 (at same time on workdays and rest days)	**3**	3	Mode waking times within 2 hours on workdays and rest days
5. Burge, 2009				
Diurnal variation	4	4	4	Evenly spaced including a waking reading
6. Burge, 2009				

References:　1. Gannon PFG, et al. Thorax. 1996;51:484–9. 2. Anees W, et al. Eur Respir J. 2004;23:730–4; 3. Moore VC, et al. Chest. 2009;135:307–14; 4. Moore VC, et al. Occup Med. 2009;59:413–7; 5. Burge C, et al. Thorax. 2009;64:1032–6; 6. Moore V, et al. Eur Respir J. 2011;38:902s.

TABLE 8.2 Diagnostic Sensitivity and Specificity for Different Validated Methods of Analysis of Serial Measurements of PEF in the Diagnosis of Occupational Asthma

Analytical Method	Upper 95% CI Nonoccupational Asthma	Sensitivity (%)	Specificity (%)	Comments
OASYS score	2.5	78	92	Sensitivity 82% and specificity 94% with 6 complexes
1. Anees, 2004				
ABC rest days/workdays (L/min/hr)	<15	72	100	Sensitivity 80% and specificity 96% with additional 7 days off work
2. Moore, 2009, 3. Moore, 2010				
Time point	1 nonwaking time point	77	93	Sensitivity 67% and specificity 99% with 2 or more positive time points
4. Burge, 2009				
Diurnal variation workdays/rest days	<3.4%	44	95	Sensitivity 63% and specificity 83% for a difference 1.4% or more
5. Moore, 2011				

Abbreviations: ABC: area between curves; CI: confidence interval.

References: 1. Anees W, et al. Eur Respir J. 2004;23:730–4; 2. Moore VC, et al. Chest. 2009;135:307–14; 3. Moore VC, et al. Occup Environ Med. 2010;67:562–7; 4. Burge CB, et al. Thorax. 2009;64:1032–6; 5. Moore V, et al. Eur Respir J. 2011;38:902s.

liters/minute/hour. A value ≥15 L/min/hr is required for a diagnosis of OA. For two hourly readings, it needs only 8 workdays, which need not be consecutive, and 3 rest days to have high specificity. A further 7 days away from work increases the sensitivity to 73%–80% (Table 8.2).

Time-point analysis is a statistical method developed from methods used to identify late asthmatic reactions following SICs (16). It uses the same hourly plots used in the ABC score, calculates the pooled 95% CI for rest days, and identifies workdays with mean PEF values below this. It is dependent in practice on stable readings on days away from work, as this reduces the magnitude of deterioration required to identify significant deterioration on workdays (Table 8.2).

Differences in diurnal variation between workdays and rest days have been used to diagnose OA. This analysis has been added to the OASYS program but has poor sensitivity compared with other methods and no particular advantages (Table 8.2). Workers with immediate reactions at work and rapid recovery away from work usually have higher diurnal variations in PEF on workdays and are identified using this analysis. There are many workers with OA where the work exposure blunts the normal circadian rise in PEF during the day, resulting in lower PEF diurnal variations on workdays compared with rest days contributing to the lack of sensitivity of this method.

Other methods of analysis

Several other methods of serial PEF analysis have been suggested. Coté et al. compared 25 workers exposed to plicatic acid with 15 nonoccupational asthmatics; the difference between the maximum PEF on rest days and the minimum PEF on workdays was the only one to have a slightly higher sensitivity (93%) than qualitative methods with similar specificity (9). Of all the quantitative methods analyzed, Perrin et al. found a lower sensitivity (81%) and specificity (74%) using qualitative methods in 61 workers referred for possible OA (11).

Ricciardi et al. analyzed differences in mean PEF at work with iroko dust, with other woods, and away from work in 19 woodworkers. They showed a significant decrease in mean PEF in workers who had a positive SIC (17).

Hayati et al. investigated the use of Shewhart control charts to detect OA (18). The lower control limit at work control chart (LCL(W)) was compared to each subject's personal best value. LCL(W) <60% of the personal best value had a sensitivity of 86% and specificity of 88% compared to SIC. Using the same method, this group further showed that a ratio of the average daily PEF diurnal variation at work to the baseline average diurnal variation greater than 15% had a sensitivity of 94% and a specificity of 61% (19).

Validity and limitations of PEF monitoring

A meta-analysis and evidence-based review showed that the pooled sensitivity of serial PEF fulfilling minimum data quantity requirements for a diagnosis of OA was 82% (95% CI 76%–90%) and the pooled specificity was 88% (95% CI 80%–95%) (20). PEF monitoring cannot usually identify the precise cause nor the mechanism for the asthma. Positive records can be obtained when the cause is unrelated to IgE sensitization, or when the agent is likely to be acting as a low-dose irritant (21). Initial validation involved readings reported from mechanical peak flow meters, with workers writing down their measurements. The introduction of data logging meters has overcome some of the problems of data validity, identifying an average 20% of readings documented by the worker and absent from the logging meter download (22). The specificity of 88% from the meta-analysis includes any prefabricated readings. There are many reasons also related to software specifications in the meters, discrepancies of 6% to 15% being documented between hand-recorded and logged readings when testing a variety of meters (23).

PEF records for the investigation of OA should be carried out when the worker is in their usual job and is due to have usual days away from work; a consecutive period of >7 days off work improves the sensitivity of the ABC score. Any treatment should be kept constant. Many feel that workers will not make measurements more than four times a day. Most workers with encouragement are able to keep records about eight times daily, particularly if these are timed for events rather than clock time (for instance, on waking, arriving at work, during each work break, on leaving work, mid-evening, and bedtime), with most importantly similar timed readings on days off work. At Birmingham Heartlands Hospital (Birmingham, United Kingdom), a hospital-based service sends a meter and instructions by post following referral. Fifty-six percent of the patients arrive in the clinic with adequate records, increasing to 85% at a second visit after personal instruction. The meta-analysis of all published papers showed that the mean return rate was 85% during workplace studies and 78% for clinic referrals, with 61% meeting the quality standards for the diagnostic method used (23).

Selecting a pocketable logging meter helps, particularly if it is single-patient use or sufficiently cheap, to remove worries about unreturned meters. The Vitalograph asma-1 (Vitalograph, Buckingham, UK) meter downloads directly into the OASYS program. Some portable instruments measure FEV_1 as well as PEF. It is easier to apply quality control to FEV_1 than PEF, but harder to get reproducible readings in practice. The percentage changes in PEF and FEV_1 are very similar; although 2-hour assessment of FEV_1 is possible, at present, there is no advantage in terms of diagnostic precision for measuring FEV_1 rather than PEF (24).

Obtaining records that are suitable for analysis involves repeated and usually unsupervised exposures to a work environment that may be causing OA. Records should be made before relocation or discharge from work, and preferably before treatment for asthma is increased, although in practice most records are now completed in workers taking regular asthma medication. The method is clearly not suitable for workers with severe asthmatic reactions, for whom carefully controlled SIC is more appropriate. The OASYS score performs poorly when workdays are intermittent, such as in part-time cleaners, or when used to analyze records with 2 weeks at work and 2 weeks (not necessarily consecutive) away from work. The ABC and time-point analyses should work better in these circumstances.

Measurement of nonspecific bronchial hyperresponsiveness (NSBH)

Methods of measurement of NSBH

In the 1970s, standardizations were proposed using two different methodologies for assessing NSBH: the deep inspiration method and the tidal volume breathing method, which led to consensus and clinical guideline documents (25, 26). NSBH can be evaluated using a number of stimuli, direct (pharmacological) or indirect (exercise, hyperventilation, mannitol). Methacholine is the most common agent employed. When carried out by proposed well-standardized methodologies, methacholine test is very safe and does not cause side effects, even when using concentrations of methacholine up to 128 mg/mL. It can be also used in epidemiological studies. The occurrence of major bronchoconstrictive events not responsive to bronchodilator is rare. The response is usually measured as the percentage change in the FEV_1 from baseline. The result is usually reported as the dose or concentration that causes a 20% fall in FEV_1, i.e. the provocative dose of methacholine/histamine inducing a 20% fall in FEV_1 (PD20) recently favored by some (27) or the provocative concentration of methacholine/histamine inducing a 20% fall in FEV_1 (PC20). Values for PC20 are reproducible to within 1.5–2 doubling doses. Abnormal bronchial responsiveness corresponds to PC20 values ≤8–16 mg/m and PD20 values ≤0.4 mg.

NSBH is present in almost all subjects with current symptomatic asthma. Mild degrees of NSBH can be found in some subjects with rhinitis but without chest symptoms and in some asymptomatic individuals and in other conditions (COPD). The absence of NSBH excludes the diagnosis of asthma in most subjects with current respiratory symptoms (provided there is no other reason such as the use of inhaled steroids). However, some symptomatic subjects may not have NSBH within the usual asthmatic range but, on exposure to the offending agent, develop reduction in lung function and increase in symptoms. In subjects with a predominant symptom of coughing, and a normal level of bronchial responsiveness assessing induced sputum may help to exclude eosinophilic bronchitis (28).

Technical factors may influence measurement of NSBH; the most important is nebulizer output, which should be calibrated regularly. Several individual factors also influence measurement of NSBH, the most important being the prechallenge airway caliber. Other factors include recent exposure to ubiquitous allergens or occupational sensitizers (29), recent respiratory infections, acute exacerbations of asthma, and medication (30).

Besides methacholine and histamine, many other physical and pharmacological agents may induce NSBH (31). Challenge tests with chemical agents, such as mannitol and adenosine, are more specific than sensitive for the diagnosis of asthma.

The role of measurement of NSBH in the management of OA

The assessment of NSBH is potentially useful in several steps of the management of OA.

Diagnosis of asthma

Patients with OA may be asymptomatic and have normal pulmonary function when they are not exposed to the causative occupational agent. The measurement of NSBH can help in diagnosing asthma (32, 33). However, the absence of NSBH does not exclude the diagnosis of OA, particularly when subjects are tested after they have been away from work since NSBH may improve and even return to normal after cessation of exposure to the culprit agent. Several studies have shown that NSBH may be normal in 5%–40% of patients with positive SICs. Conversely, NSBH may recur or increase on re-exposure to the offending agent. Therefore, the level of NSBH should preferably be assessed when the worker is currently exposed (32, 33). Nevertheless, there have been reports of normal NSBH both before and after a positive SIC in a substantial fraction of subjects with OA (34, 35).

Assessment of the work-relatedness of asthma

Serial measurements of NSBH at work and away from work can enhance the sensitivity of PEF monitoring in investigating the work-relatedness of asthma (36). During SIC in the laboratory, a postchallenge increase in NSBH is an early marker of a specific bronchial response to occupational agents, especially in subjects removed from workplace exposure for a long time. In the absence of significant changes in FEV_1, a significant postchallenge increase in NSBH means that the challenge exposure should be repeated before ruling out the possibility of OA (37, 38).

The degree of specific responsiveness to an occupational agent during SIC is correlated with the degree of baseline NSBH. When the latter is high, inhalation should be started using a very low dose of the specific agent (39).

Diagnosis of irritant-induced OA

The presence of NSBH is crucial to the diagnosis of reactive airways dysfunction syndrome (RADS), which develops after a single high-level exposure to irritants and of other types of delayed-onset irritant-induced OA (39).

Assessment of impairment for OA

Airway caliber and NSBH as well as medication required to control asthma are key items for assessing impairment for OA (see Chapter 11A).

Validity of NSBH measurements

Lau and Tarlo reported an overall relatively high sensitivity (87%) and a low specificity (36%) for methacholine testing, as expected from a test that reflects all forms of asthma (40). Adding skin-prick tests (SPTs), or specific IgE measurement, can enhance sensitivity and specificity, and may be a suitable alternative to SIC in diagnosing OA when SIC is not available (41). In a retrospective analysis of all subjects who underwent SIC in the investigation of OA in Montreal, the presence of NSBH to methacholine yielded a low (35%) positive predictive value for OA, but coupling information on the level of eosinophils in induced sputum to NSBH increased positive predictive values for OA from 39% to 69%, depending on the thresholds used (42). Pralong and coworkers concluded that a normal methacholine test excludes OA in patients currently exposed to a causative agent because of its high sensitivity and negative predictive value, 98.1% and 97.7%, respectively, whereas in patients currently unexposed, overall sensitivity and negative predictive value are lower (67% and 82%, respectively) (34).

Occupational challenge tests

In 1970, Professor Pepys suggested the use of SIC in the investigation of OA. Originally, these tests were carried out in the corridors of the Brompton Hospital. A well-ventilated cubicle in a room was later made available. A series of reports were published beginning in 1972, dealing with agents in various forms (43). Subjects were asked to reproduce their usual work under supervision and with functional assessment. Different groups have since improved the methodology and safety of SIC (39, 44, 45).

Purpose and justification for the tests

The purpose of SIC is to explore the causal relationship between exposure to occupational agents and the onset of immunological OA. The documented reaction should "induce" the characteristic features of variable airflow limitation, NSBH, and airway inflammation and not trigger asthma as "inciters" or triggers do (46). The major rationale for performing challenges with occupational agents is that this approach remains the most reliable procedure to document organ-specific responsiveness.

Diagnosing OA requires the highest level of reliability, as it is associated with considerable health and socioeconomic consequences. The accurate identification of an index case of OA and its etiology is also important for implementing preventive measures for other exposed workers. Diagnosing OA cannot be based solely on the presence of asthma and workplace exposure to agents known to cause asthma, because both are common occurrences. A number of procedures can be used for investigating work-related symptoms, including the clinical history, spirometry, and assessment of NSBH, inflammatory, and immunological tests. None of these tests taken alone allows for diagnosing OA with a sufficient level of confidence, although a combination in a stepwise approach can make the diagnosis of OA likely or very likely (47), especially for HMW agents (41).

A European Respiratory Society Task Force (38) agreed that the indications for performing SIC should include: (1) confirmation of the diagnosis or (2) identification of the cause of OA when other objective methods do not bring definitive results; (3) identification of a not formerly described cause of OA; and (4) research into the mechanisms.

Methodology of SIC

General safety requirements

SICs should only be carried out in hospital-based specialized centers (39, 45). SIC should be supervised by physicians with expertise in the field. The centers should do a sufficient number of tests each year.

SIC should be performed in rooms equipped with adequate exhaust ventilation or using closed-circuit devices in order to prevent inadvertent exposure of the technicians and the tested worker after discontinuation of the challenge. Subjects who undergo SIC should receive detailed information, including for women that SIC is not advised during pregnancy.

Subjects should be monitored for 6–8 hours after the end of the exposure to detect late asthmatic reactions. SICs can be performed on an outpatient basis, but subjects should be allowed to leave only when airway caliber is near baseline value. They should be instructed on how to record their FEV_1/PEFs using portable instruments and how to treat bronchoconstriction. If the response to bronchodilators at the end of the day is insufficient, the subject should be kept in hospital and the asthmatic reaction treated accordingly. Subjects who develop marked late and atypical progressive reactions should be treated with inhaled/oral corticosteroids after the challenge.

Absolute contraindications for performing SIC include pregnancy and recent (<3 months) or unstable cardiovascular diseases. SICs are contraindicated in subjects with severe airway obstruction. It has been recommended that the SIC should not be performed when the FEV_1 <2 L or below predicted value minus 1.5 L in males and below predicted value minus 1.2 L in females (24) or <60% predicted or <1.5 L (48). Airway caliber should be monitored on a control day with no exposure to occupational agents to ensure stability of asthma (39).

Medications

Prior to the SIC, inhaled bronchodilators, theophylline, leukotriene receptor antagonists, and antihistamines should be withdrawn according to their duration of action. Inhaled corticosteroids should be withheld 72 hours before the tests, but the daily dose can be administered at the end of each challenge day for maintaining asthma control. Inhaled and oral corticosteroids attenuate the bronchial response to allergens, especially the late phase component, but they do not completely inhibit the bronchial response (39).

Assessment of bronchial response

The main methodological procedure for SIC is summarized in Table 8.3.

Airway obstruction

The FEV_1 is the reference parameter for assessing airway caliber. However, it is effort-dependent and requires a satisfactory collaboration from the subject. It is also influenced by volume history (i.e. the inspiratory maneuver), which can provoke bronchodilatation, whereas forced expiratory maneuvers can cause bronchoconstriction in asthmatic subjects.

TABLE 8.3 Scheme for Performing Specific Inhalation Challenges with Occupational Agents*

Procedures	Aims
	Control Day
Baseline spirometry, oral temperature, and DL_{CO}	
Exposure to a control agent (e.g. lactose if the causal agent is flour, control wood dust, diluent of diisocyanates)	Absence of contraindication
	Satisfactory airway caliber and no significant fluctuations
	Make sure subjects do not react to a control agent (nonspecific irritant response)
Monitoring of FEV_1, frequent in the first and second hours and hourly for 6–8 hours	Assessment of "baseline" values
	Identify late reactions
Assessment of PC20, DL_{CO}, induced sputum, and/or FeNO at the end of the day	
PEF monitoring in the evening at home	
Active Challenge Day(s)	
Assessment of spirometry, oral temperature, DL_{CO}	
Progressive exposure to relevant occupational agent	
HMW agent, IgE-mediated mechanism	
Tipping or dusting powder	
Mimicking procedure of the workplace	
Using closed-circuit generation equipment	
Aqueous extract: initial concentration based on results of skin-prick test and PC20; assess protein concentration if extract prepared in the local unit	
LMW agent	
Generation by heating, spraying, mimicking workplace procedure, use of closed-circuit generation equipment	
Level of exposure continuously monitored with online devices and keeping concentration between 5 to 20 ppb	
Other agents	
Mimicking work tasks, monitoring concentrations of agent if feasible	
Assess FEV_1 immediately and 10–15 min after each exposure period; if changes <10%, continue with the proposed protocol; if changes >10%, repeat a similar period of exposure as the previous one; if changes ≥20%, stop exposure	
Monitoring of FEV_1 and oral temperature as for the control day as well as PC20, DL_{CO}, induced sputum, and/or FeNO at the end of the day	Verify if subjects show a significant reaction after exposure to the suspected agent and identify hypersensitivity-like reactions
	Administer SABA before discharge
	At the end of the day, if FEV_1 back to ± 10% baseline 20 min later, discharge with advice to subject that the SABA agent may be required in the evening or night; if FEV_1 is not back to baseline after SABA, administer oral steroids; see the subject on the following day to make sure FEV_1 is back to baseline
If absence of changes in FEV_1, reassess PC20, sputum and/or FeNO, at the end of the day; if no significant change, no further exposure; if significant changes in PC20 (2- to 3-fold difference from baseline) or increase in sputum eosinophils (>3%) or FeNo (>17.5 ppb) compared to baseline, repeat exposure to a maximum of 4 hours to the suspected agent on the following day	Assess the need for increasing duration of exposure to the suspected agent
PEF monitoring in the evening at home	Identify late reactions

* See for detailed suggestion of procedures, in particular for progressive durations of exposure to the suspected agent: European Guidelines (Vandenplas O, Suojalehto H, Aasen TB, et al. Specific inhalation challenge in the diagnosis of occupational asthma: consensus statement. *Eur Respir J.* 2014;43:1573–1587) and Handbook (Suojalehto H, Suuronen K, Cullin P. Specific challenge testing for occupational asthma: revised handbook. *Eur Respir J.* 2019;54:pli1901026).

Abbreviations: DL_{CO}, lung diffusion capacity for carbon monoxide; FEV_1, forced expiratory volume in 1 second; HMW, high-molecular-weight; LMW, low-molecular-weight; PC20, provocative concentration of methacholine/histamine inducing a 20% fall in FEV_1; SABA, inhaled short-acting beta-2 agonist.

Other functional indices have been proposed. PEF has a reproducibility that is little less than FEV_1. PEF is more effort-dependent than the FEV_1 and has no benefit over FEV_1 for supervised measurements in hospital. Measurements of airway resistance or conductance by body plethysmography and respiratory resistance by the forced oscillation technique are not affected by inspiratory maneuvers and are not effort-dependent, but they are less reproducible and require more expensive equipment. They may be useful in subjects who are not able to perform reproducible spirometric maneuvers and if changes in FEV_1 are equivocal (49).

Parameters of airway caliber should be measured serially after each exposure (Table 8.3) (39). Assessment of FEV_1 24 hours after challenge exposure may disclose a "day-to-day" pattern of reaction.

Nonspecific bronchial hyperresponsiveness

A baseline assessment of NSBH to pharmacological agents such as histamine or methacholine should be carried out at the end of the control day (Table 8.3). The level of NSBH before the test is one of the predictors of a response to a specific agent (50). However, the absence of baseline NSBH does not exclude the possibility of a positive response as workers may have ended the exposure to the agent a long time before (34, 35). Most workers will show an increase in NSBH after a positive SIC response but in 6% to 10% of subjects with OA, the level of NSBH remains within the nonasthmatic range although an asthmatic reaction has occurred (34, 35).

The level of NSBH should also be reassessed after the SIC, especially when there have been no significant changes in airway caliber. An increase in NSBH may precede the changes in FEV_1 and should be considered as an early marker of a bronchial response. A significant increase in postchallenge NSBH means that the subject should be further challenged before excluding the diagnosis of OA, nearly 20% of subjects with a negative SIC who had shown changes in NSBH developing an asthmatic reaction on subsequent SIC (37).

Airway inflammation

Noninvasive assessment of airway inflammation through induced sputum cell analysis and measurement of fractional exhaled nitric oxide (FeNO) represent complementary tools to lung function tests in the diagnosis of asthma and OA (Chapter 7).

Induced sputum cells   It is useful to evaluate sputum eosinophil counts at baseline and after SIC, especially when the exposure does not elicit significant changes in FEV_1. A postchallenge increase in sputum eosinophils is an early marker of specific bronchial reactivity to occupational agents and, as for changes in NSBH, may identify subjects who are likely to develop an asthmatic reaction after repeated exposure (51). The change in sputum eosinophil counts induced by exposure to the offending agent has the highest diagnostic accuracy for identifying a positive SIC compared with changes in NSBH and blood eosinophil counts (51). The assessment of sputum eosinophil count before and after an SIC procedure is also crucial for the identification of occupational eosinophilic bronchitis (Chapter 21).

A postchallenge increase in sputum neutrophil count has also been documented especially after exposure to LMW agents (52). However, the interpretation of changes in sputum neutrophil counts has not yet been validated.

Fractional exhaled nitric oxide   Assessment of changes in FeNO level may be useful in subjects who fail to provide suitable sputum samples (Chapter 7). A significant increase in FeNO level after a positive challenge occurs later (24 hr) than the increase in sputum eosinophils, which is already observed 7 hours postchallenge (53). A postchallenge increase in FeNO ≥17.5 ppb shows a specificity of 90% and a sensitivity of 45% in identifying a positive SIC result and occurred more consistently in subjects with OA caused by HMW than by LMW agents (54).

Other assessments

Body temperature, forced vital capacity, and carbon monoxide diffusion indices should be assessed during SIC in order to identify hypersensitivity pneumonitis-like reactions (Chapter 24).

Assessment of nasal response during SIC may be useful for confirming associated occupational rhinitis. Symptom scores should be combined with objective measurements of nasal patency and/or nasal inflammation (Chapter 22).

Schedule of exposure
Control challenge

Prior to the challenge with the suspected occupational agent, a "control" (i.e. sham or placebo) challenge should be performed on a separate day by exposing the worker to a nonsensitizing substance, usually for 30–60 minutes, with functional monitoring as after exposure to the suspected occupational agent (39). The control substance is selected with reference to the nature of the suspected occupational agent. Ideally the control substance is equally irritant and has the same physical appearance as the tested occupational agent. The most common control substances are lactose powder for agents in powder form (flours, enzymes, drugs), a control wood dust, saline for aqueous extracts, and solvents for coatings, glues, and related resinous products (45) (Table 8.3).

Duration of exposure

The duration of exposure to occupational agents should be gradually increased (Table 8.3). This is most relevant when the subject reports a history of severe acute reactions at work or has marked NSBH and when the challenge involves a LMW agent (55), an agent with a high allergenic potential (e.g. enzymes) or previously unknown sensitizing agent. For HMW agents, the duration of exposure can be increased progressively on the same day until an immediate reaction occurs or until the maximum duration of exposure (for example 60–120 min) is reached. For LMW agents that are more likely to cause isolated late and atypical reactions, the duration of exposure should be increased from one day to the next, with, for instance, a cumulative exposure limited to less than 30 minutes on the first challenge day (39). An alternative approach is to increase the concentration of the agent (56). The initial concentration/dilution of the delivered agent can be guided by the level of specific IgE sensitization in case of agents acting through an IgE-mediated mechanism.

It is unclear how long a subject should be exposed to the suspected agent before the test can be considered negative. A retrospective review of 335 positive SICs showed that 25% of the subjects required a cumulative duration of challenge exposure of more than 2 hours to develop an asthmatic reaction (57).

Delivery of occupational agents

The method for delivering occupational agents during SICs should be adapted to the chemical (e.g. monomer vs. polymer) and physical (i.e. gas, liquid, particles, or aerosol) properties as well as the mode of usage of the agent.

The air concentration of the occupational agent during SIC should be based on the estimated level in the workplace but should not exceed relevant occupational exposure limits (OEL) to avoid irritant responses and severe asthmatic reactions (39). It is recommended to monitor the air concentration during SIC when a feasible method is available, especially for LMW agents with a potential for inducing severe reactions.

Methodology of exposure

A scheme of procedure of SIC is summarized in Table 8.3. A detailed methodological handbook has been prepared by the European Task Force on SIC (45) as a complement to the full report (39). This document covers practical issues that represent the experience of twelve European centers familiar with the SIC procedure: aspects related to the type of agent (powder or dust, aqueous allergen extracts, polyisocyanates, and LMW agents), the agent suggested for exposure on the control day, the method of delivery, the amount and dilution of the agent, and the duration of the challenge, with comments and references. The interested reader is therefore referred to this important handbook for all issues related to the exposure methodology.

Workplace challenges

Supervised workplace challenges are theoretically the most appropriate defining test for OA. The exposures should be representative of usual exposure, but the planned arrival of a medical team is often preceded by a clean-up and the nonworking of more problematical processes. Workplace challenges can be performed if more than one potential sensitizing agent is present and if the worker's history is highly suggestive of OA (58).

Interpretation of SIC results

An SIC is generally considered positive when there is a sustained (i.e. recorded on two consecutive assessments) fall in FEV_1 of at least 15%–20% from prechallenge value, provided that fluctuations in FEV_1 are <10% on a control day (39). This threshold value is arbitrary and a more rational approach would be to examine the subject's variability in FEV_1 when not exposed to the suspected agent, a method more likely to be sensitive but requiring several (at least three) unexposed days to obtain the daily variance.

In cases where the changes in FEV_1 are equivocal, a significant postchallenge increase in the level of NSBH (2- to 3-fold) or in sputum eosinophils (>3%) or in FeNO level (>17.5 ppb) compared to baseline values would support a positive SIC response and lead to conduct additional exposure(s) on the following day(s) in the laboratory or at the workplace.

Temporal patterns of response

SICs can induce different patterns of bronchial response. The typical patterns (43) are illustrated in Figure 8.3. The immediate reaction is characterized by a brisk onset at a maximum of 10 minutes (HMW agents) to 20 minutes (LMW agents) (59) after exposure ends and lasting for 1 to 2 hours. These reactions can actually be the most dangerous because they can be unpredictable. The fall in FEV_1 is generally more marked after immediate than late reactions (50). Late reactions develop slowly and progressively either 1 to 2 hours ("early late") or 4 to 8 hours (late) after exposure. Dual reactions are a combination of immediate and late reactions. Atypical reactions occurring principally after exposure to polyisocyanates have been reported (11) (Figure 8.4). Immediate reactions are more common after exposure to HMW agents and late reactions, for LMW agents (60).

Validity of SIC

The major challenge in diagnosing OA is the lack of a widely acknowledged "gold standard" test. Nevertheless, the evidence-based guidelines issued in 2005 by the British Occupational Health Research Foundation (BOHRF) acknowledged that: "A carefully controlled SIC comes closest to a gold standard test for some agents causing OA," but "a negative test in a worker with

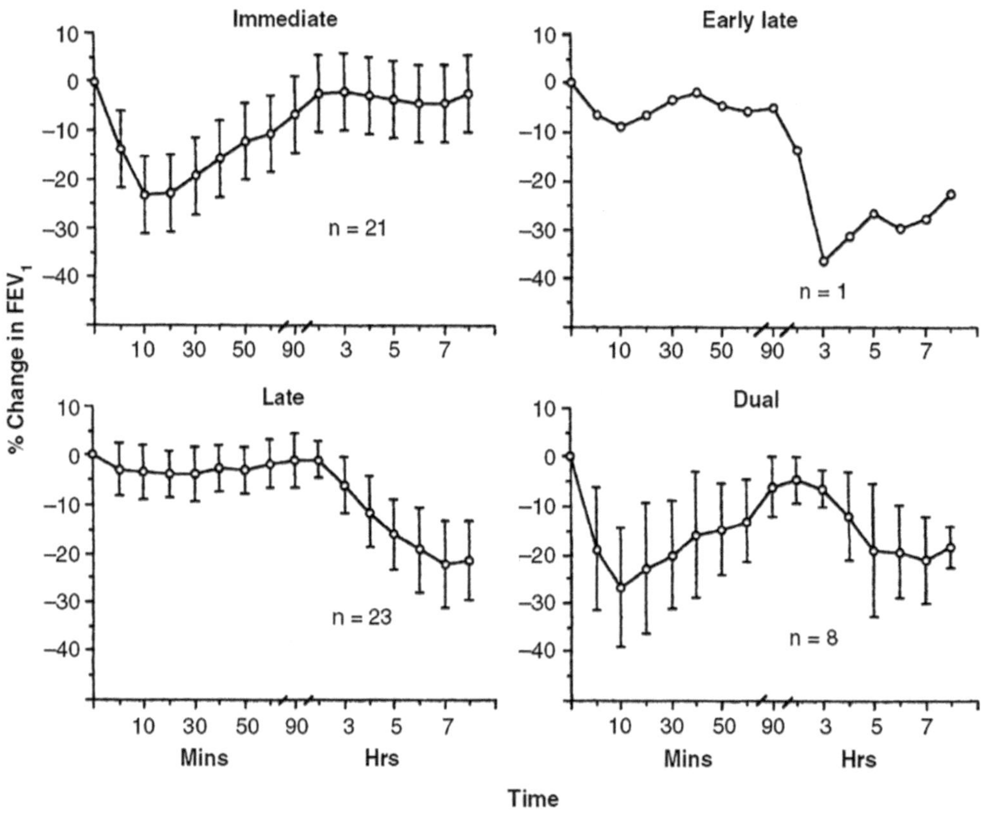

FIGURE 8.3 Typical patterns of bronchial response to specific inhalation challenges. Mean ± SD or individual values of the percentage change in FEV_1 (on the ordinate) as a function of time since exposure (on the abscissa) for the four typical patterns of reactions (see text for definitions). The number of subjects for each pattern is shown.

Abbreviations: FEV_1, forced expiratory volume in 1 second; SD, standard deviation. (From Vandenplas O, Burge PS, Moscato G, Malo JL. Functional assessment. In: Malo JL, Chan-Yeung M, Bernstein DI. *Asthma in the Workplace.* 4th ed. Boca Raton, FL: CRC Press; 2013:125. Perrin B, et al. *J Allergy Clin Immunol.* 1991;87:630–9. By permission.)

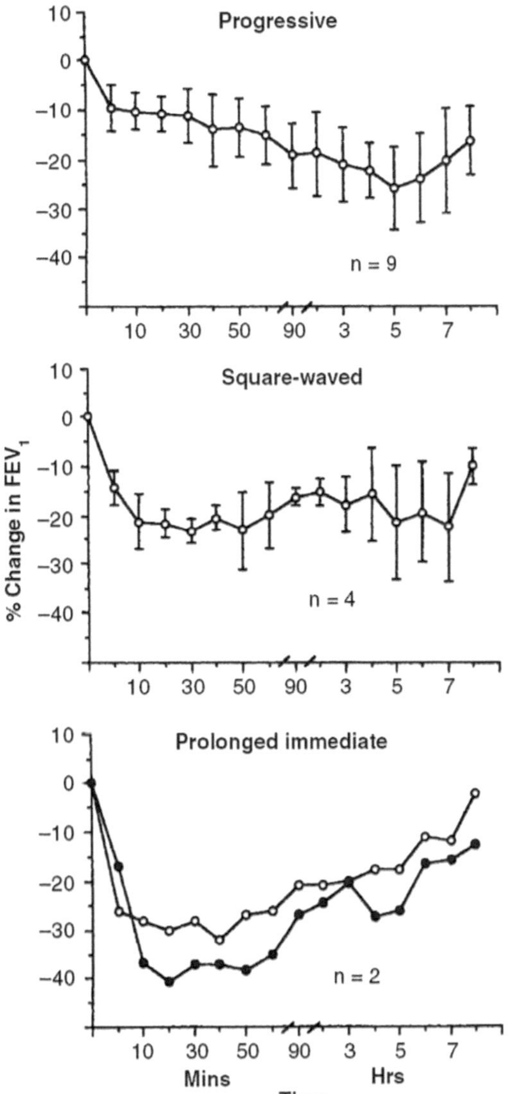

FIGURE 8.4 Atypical patterns of bronchial response to specific inhalation challenges. Mean ± SD or individual values of the percentage change in FEV$_1$ (on the ordinate) as a function of time since exposure (on the abscissa) for the three atypical patterns of reactions (see text for definitions). The number of subjects for each pattern is shown. (From Vandenplas O, Burge PS, Moscato G, Malo JL. Functional assessment. In: Malo JL, Chan-Yeung M, Bernstein DI. *Asthma in the Workplace.* 4th ed. Boca Raton, FL: CRC Press; 2013:126. Perrin B, et al. *J Allergy Clin Immunol.* 1991; 87:630–9. By permission.)
Abbreviations: FEV$_1$, forced expiratory volume in 1 second; SD, standard deviation.

otherwise good evidence of OA is not sufficient to exclude the diagnosis" (61). However, the updated version of these guidelines stated that: "Specific inhalation testing, the gold standard, is available in a few specialist centers only and the diagnosis of occupational asthma can usually be made without this test" (62). A systematic review conducted by the Agency for Healthcare Research and Quality (AHRQ) concluded that "none of the diagnostic tests used alone yields a sufficiently high combination of sensitivity and specificity for replacing SIC. Other combinations

of tests have not been evaluated in sufficient detail to provide recommendations" (63). In the case of HMW agents, a combination of other tests reaches a high degree of sensitivity and specificity (40). Although the BOHRF guidelines and the AHRQ systematic review concluded that SIC should be considered as the "reference standard" test for diagnosing OA, the procedure is infrequently completed in subjects evaluated for OA (64). Potential barriers for performing SICs include concerns about false-positive and false-negative results, the risk of adverse events, the lack of availability of appropriate facilities, the time and expertise required, and the cost of the procedure.

Limitations of SIC
False-negative results
A false-negative SIC result may occur when the subject has not been challenged with the agent that caused their asthma at work or with the appropriate physical or chemical form of the product (e.g. monomers instead of polymers). This issue can be minimized by collecting detailed information from safety data sheets (SDSs) and obtaining a job analysis by hygienists (Chapter 6). False-negative results may also be related to a decrease in specific bronchial reactivity. Complete loss of specific bronchial reactivity is a rare occurrence after cessation of exposure, although the duration of exposure required to elicit a positive SIC response significantly increases (65). Such false-negative SIC results can be markedly reduced by assessing the level of NSBH and/or sputum eosinophils and/or FeNO after SICs that do not induce a significant fall in FEV$_1$; significant postchallenge changes in these markers should lead to further challenge. When an SIC is negative in the laboratory, provisions should be made to return the subject to their normal workplace while serial monitoring of PEF is done. As soon as changes in PEF are demonstrated, SIC should be repeated in the laboratory or at the workplace.

False-positive results
A false-positive bronchial reaction may result from a nonspecific irritant bronchoconstriction, which does not fit the definition of OA. Immediate bronchial responses elicited by irritant stimuli cannot be easily distinguished from those caused by sensitizing agents. However, such irritant reactions are brisker and briefer than immediate reactions due to OA (maximum reaction at 10–20 min with 1 hour for recovery). Such false-positive SIC results can be reduced by exposure to a control substance and keeping concentrations of the suspected agent below the OEL. Most controlled experiments in asthmatic volunteers have failed to demonstrate a physiological effect of exposure to irritant substances at permissible levels. However, maintaining the level of exposure below the OEL would imply monitoring the concentrations of a wide variety of compounds during SICs, which is generally not feasible. Development of devices that allow continuous concentration measurement and regulation of the products generated could be helpful in reducing nonspecific reactions.

Adverse effects
The experience of specialized centers indicates that SIC are associated with only minimal risk of inducing severe asthmatic reactions provided that safety requirements are stringently respected, risk factors are taken into account, exposure to occupational agents is progressively increased, and bronchial responses are carefully monitored. Among 335 positive SICs performed using realistic methods of exposure, 12% of the subjects required

repeated administration of an inhaled short-acting bronchodilator, while few (3%, 95% CI: 1%–5%) required additional oral or intravenous corticosteroids (55).

It is recommended to increase or initiate inhaled corticosteroids for a few days in subjects who develop marked late reactions to minimize the associated increase in inflammatory processes and NSBH.

Urticarial and anaphylactic reactions have rarely been reported during SICs (55). Skin contact with occupational agents should be reduced during SIC by using protective clothes. Fever and leukocytosis may occur in about 5% of subjects with a positive SIC (66).

The possibility of inducing or increasing sensitization to occupational agents in workers through the SIC procedure has been raised as an ethical issue although this concern is highly theoretical. The usual workplace exposure is much more prolonged than that produced in the context of SIC.

Practical limitations

There are very few data on the relative cost and effectiveness of available diagnostic procedures. Kennedy and coworkers found that the SIC, used as the reference test with an assumed 100% accuracy, was the most expensive technique, but correctly diagnosed 28% more OA subjects than other diagnostic means (67). The cost of SIC is likely to outweigh the financial consequences of falsely negative and falsely positive diagnoses of OA for the workers, employers, healthcare insurance organizations, and society.

Conclusion and research needs

There are currently at least two options to confirm OA: (1) SICs, considered for long as the reference standard, though expensive and time consuming, and (2) a combination of simpler, readily available, and less expensive diagnostic tools (assessment of NSBH, monitoring of PEF, immunological testing) that can be applied in combination and sequentially to achieve a high diagnostic accuracy.

Research avenues can include:

* Improvement in the methodology of SICs with more accurate assessment of the dose administered
* Identify and correct difficulties in persuading centers investigating work-related asthma to use PEF recording
* Compare PEF tracings in OA and work-exacerbated asthma
* Cost-effectiveness evaluation of diagnostic tests used solely or in combination

References

1. Hetzel MR, Clark TJH. Comparison of normal and asthmatic circadian rhythms in peak expiratory flow rate. Thorax. 1980;35:732–8.
2. Randem B, Smolensky MH, Hsi B, et al. Field survey of circadian rhythm in PEF of electronics workers suffering from colophony-induced asthma. Chronobiology International. 1987;4:263–71.
3. Moore VC, Jaakkola MS, Burge CB, et al. Shift work effects on serial PEF measurements for occupational asthma. Occup Med (Lond). 2012;62:525–32.
4. Nicholson PJ, Cullinan P, Burge PS, et al. Occupational Asthma, Prevention, Identification & Management: Systematic Review & Recommendations. London: British Occupational Health Foundation. 2010.
5. Burge PS, Perks WH, O'Brien IM, et al. Occupational asthma in an electronics factory: a case control study to evaluate aetiological factors. Thorax. 1979;34:300–7.
6. Park D, Moore VC, Burge CB, et al. Serial PEF measurement is superior to cross-shift change in diagnosing occupational asthma. Eur Respir J. 2009;34:574–8.
7. Burge PS, Moore VC, Robertson AS, et al. Do laboratory challenge tests for occupational asthma represent what happens in the workplace? Eur Respir J. 2018;51.
8. Burge PS, Moore VC, Burge CB, et al. Can serial PEF measurements separate occupational asthma from allergic alveolitis? Occup Med (Lond). 2015;65:251–5.
9. Côté J, Kennedy S, Chan-Yeung M. Quantitative versus qualitative analysis of peak expiratory flow in occupational asthma. Thorax. 1993;48:48–51.
10. Baldwin DR, Gannon P, Bright P, et al. Interpretation of occupational peak flow records: level of agreement between expert clinicians and Oasys-2. Thorax. 2002;57:860–4.
11. Perrin B, Cartier A, Ghezzo H, et al. Reassessment of the temporal patterns of bronchial obstruction after exposure to occupational sensitizing agents. J Allergy Clin Immunol. 1991;87:630–9.
12. Venables KM, Burge PS, Davison AG, et al. Peak flow rate records in surveys: reproducibility of observers' reports. Thorax. 1984;39:828–32.
13. Winck JC, Delgado L, Vanzeller M, et al. Monitoring of peak expiratory flow rates in cork workers' occupational asthma. J Asthma. 2001;38:357–62.
14. Anees W, Blainey D, Moore VC, et al. Differentiating occupational asthmatics from non-occupational asthmatics and irritant-exposed workers. Occup Med (Lond). 2011;61:190–5.
15. Higgins BG, Britton JR, Chinn S, et al. Comparison of bronchial reactivity and peak expiratory flow variability measurements for epidemiologic studies. Am Rev Respir Dis. 1992;145:588–93.
16. Stenton SC, Avery AJ, Walters EH, et al. Statistical approaches to the identification of late asthmatic reactions. Eur Respir J. 1994;7:806–12.
17. Ricciardi L, Fedele R, Saitta S, et al. Occupational asthma due to exposure to iroko wood dust. Ann Allergy Asthma Immunol. 2003;91:393–7.
18. Hayati F, Maghsoodloo S, Devivo MJ, et al. Control chart for monitoring occupational asthma. J Safety Res. 2006;37:17–26.
19. Hayati F, Maghsoodloo S, Devivo MJ, et al. Quality control chart method for analyzing PEF variability in occupational asthma. Am J Ind Med. 2008;51:223–8.
20. Moore V, Jaakkola M, Burge PS. A systematic review of serial peak expiratory flow measurements in the diagnosis of occupational asthma. Ann Respir Med. 2010;1:31–40.
21. Burge PS, Moore VC, Robertson AS. Sensitization and irritant-induced occupational asthma with latency are clinically indistinguishable. Occup Med. 2012;62:129–33.
22. Malo JL, Cartier A, Ghezzo H, et al. Compliance with peak expiratory flow readings affects the within- and between-reader reproducibility of interpretation of graphs in subjects investigated for occupational asthma. J Allergy Clin Immunol. 1996;98:1132–4.
23. Anees W, Robertson AS, Burge PS. Glutaraldehyde induced asthma in endoscopy nursing staff. Occup Environ Med. 2001;58:544–5.
24. Parkes ED, Moore, VC, Walters GI, Burge PS. Diagnosis of occupational asthma from serial measurements of forced expiratory volume in 1 s (FEV1) using the area between curves (ABC) score from the Oasys plotter. Occup Environ Med. 2020;77:801–5.
25. Sterk PJ, Fabbri LM, Quanjer PH, et al. Airway responsiveness. Standardized challenge testing with pharmacological, physical and sensitizing stimuli in adults. Report working party standardization of lung function tests European Community for Steel and Coal. Official statement of the European Respiratory Society. Eur Respir J. 1993;6(Suppl 16):53–83.
26. American Thoracic Society. Guidelines for methacholine and exercise challenge testing. Am J Respir Crit Care Med. 2000;161:309–29.
27. Dell SD, Bola SS, Foty RG, et al. Provocative dose of methacholine causing a 20% drop in FEV1 should be used to interpret methacholine challenge tests with modern nebulizers. Ann Am Thorac Soc. 2015;12:357–63.
28. Moscato G, Pala G, Cullinan P, et al. EAACI Position Paper on assessment of cough in the workplace. Allergy. 2014;69:292–304.
29. Cartier A, L'Archevêque J, Malo JL. Exposure to a sensitizing occupational agent can cause a long-lasting increase in bronchial responsiveness to histamine in the absence of significant changes in airway caliber. J Allergy Clin Immunol. 1986;78:1185–9.
30. Coates AL, Wanger J, Cockcroft DW, et al. ERS technical standard on bronchial challenge testing: general considerations and performance of methacholine challenge tests. Eur Respir J. 2017;49(5):pii:1601526.
31. Nair P, Martin JG, Cockcroft DC, et al. Airway hyperresponsiveness in asthma: measurement and clinical relevance. J Allergy Clin Immunol Pract. 2017;5:649–59.
32. Tarlo SM, Balmes J, Balkissoon R, et al. Diagnosis and management of work-related asthma: American College of Chest Physicians Consensus Statement. Chest. 2008;134:1S–41S.

33. Moscato G, Pala G, Barnig C, et al. EAACI consensus statement for investigation of work-related asthma in non-specialized centres. Allergy. 2012;67:491–501.

34. Pralong JA, Lemière C, Rochat T, et al. Predictive value of nonspecific bronchial responsiveness in occupational asthma. J Allergy Clin Immunol. 2016;137:412–6.

35. Beretta C, Rifflart C, Evrard G, et al. Assessment of eosinophilic airway inflammation as a contribution to the diagnosis of occupational asthma. Allergy. 2018;73:206–13.

36. Perrin B, Lagier F, L'Archevêque J, et al. Occupational asthma: validity of monitoring of peak expiratory flow rates and non-allergic bronchial responsiveness as compared to specific inhalation challenge. Eur Respir J. 1992;5:40–8.

37. Vandenplas O, Delwiche JP, Jamart J, et al. Increase in non-specific bronchial hyperresponsiveness as an early marker of bronchial response to occupational agents during specific inhalation challenges. Thorax. 1996;51:472–8.

38. Sastre J, Fernandez-Nieto M, Novalbos A, et al. Need for monitoring non-specific bronchial hyperresponsiveness before and after isocyanate inhalation challenge. Chest. 2003;123:1276–9.

39. Vandenplas O, Suojalehto H, Aasen TB, et al. Specific inhalation challenge in the diagnosis of occupational asthma: consensus statement. Eur Respir J. 2014;43:1573–87.

40. Lau A, Tarlo SM. Update on the management of occupational asthma and work-exacerbated asthma. Allergy Asthma Immunol Res. 2019;11:188–200.

41. Taghiakbari M, Pralong JA, Lemière C, et al. Novel clinical scores for occupational asthma due to exposure to high-molecular-weight agents. Occup Environ Med. 2019;76:495–501.

42. Malo JL, Cardinal S, Ghezzo H, et al. Association of bronchial reactivity to occupational agents with methacholine reactivity, sputum cells and immunoglobulin E-mediated reactivity. Clin Exp Allergy. 2011;41:497–504.

43. Pepys J, Hutchcroft BJ. Bronchial provocation tests in etiologic diagnosis and analysis of asthma. Am Rev Respir Dis. 1975;112:829–59.

44. Cloutier Y, Malo JL. Update on an exposure system for particles in the diagnosis of occupational asthma. Eur Respir J. 1992;5:887–90.

45. Suojalehto H, Suuronen K, Cullinan P. Specific challenge testing for occupational asthma: revised handbook. Eur Respir J. 2019;54(2):pii:1901026.

46. Dolovich J, Hargreave FE. The asthma syndrome: inciters, inducers, and host characteristics. Thorax. 1981;36:641–4.

47. Vandenplas O, Suojalehto H, Cullinan P. Diagnosing occupational asthma. Clin Exp Allergy. 2017;47:6–18.

48. Crapo RO, Casaburi R, Coates AL, et al. Guidelines for methacholine and exercise challenge testing-1999. This official statement of the American Thoracic Society was adopted by the ATS Board of Directors, July 1999. Am J Respir Crit Care Med. 2000;161:309–29.

49. Larbanois A, Delwiche JP, Jamart J, et al. Comparison of FEV1 and specific airway conductance in assessing airway response to occupational agents. Allergy. 2003;58:1256–60.

50. Hu C, Cruz MJ, Ojanguren I, et al. Specific inhalation challenge: the relationship between response, clinical variables and lung function. Occup Environ Med. 2017;74:586–91.

51. Vandenplas O, D'Alpaos V, Heymans J, et al. Sputum eosinophilia: an early marker of bronchial response to occupational agents. Allergy. 2009;64:754–61.

52. Lemière C, Romeo P, Chaboillez S, et al. Airway inflammation and functional changes after exposure to different concentrations of isocyanates. J Allergy Clin Immunol. 2002;110:641–6.

53. Lemière C, D'Alpaos V, Chaboillez S, et al. Investigation of occupational asthma: sputum cell counts or exhaled nitric oxide? Chest. 2010;137:617–22.

54. Lemiere C, Nguyen S, Sava F, et al. Occupational asthma phenotypes identified by increased fractional exhaled nitric oxide after exposure to causal agents. J Allergy Clin Immunol. 2014;134:1063–7.

55. Vandenplas O, D'Alpaos V, Evrard G, et al. Incidence of severe asthmatic reactions after challenge exposure to occupational agents. Chest. 2013;143:1261–8.

56. Scheidler L, Sucker K, Taeger D, et al. Evaluation of a 4-steps-1-day whole body challenge protocol for the diagnosis of occupational asthma due to diisocyanates. Adv Exp Med Biol. 2013;788:301–11.

57. D'Alpaos V, Vandenplas O, Evrard G, et al. Inhalation challenges with occupational agents: threshold duration of exposure. Respir Med. 2013;107:739–44.

58. Rioux JP, Malo JL, L'Archevêque J, et al. Workplace specific challenges as a contribution to the diagnosis of occupational asthma. Eur Respir J. 2008;32:997–1003.

59. Malo JL, Ghezzo H, L'Archevêque J. Distinct temporal patterns of immediate asthmatic reactions due to high- and low-molecular-weight agents. Clin Exp Allergy. 2012;42:1021–7.

60. Lipinska-Ojrzanowska A, Nowakowska-Swirta E, Wiszniewska M, et al. Bronchial response to high and low molecular weight occupational inhalant allergens. Allergy Asthma Immunol Res. 2020;12:164–70.

61. Nicholson PJ, Cullinan P, Newman Taylor AJ, et al. Evidence based guidelines for the prevention, identification, and management of occupational asthma. Occup Environ Med. 2005;62:290–9.

62. Nicholson PJ, Cullinan P, Burge S, et al. Concise guidance: diagnosis, management and prevention of occupational asthma. Clin Med. 2012;12:156–9.

63. Beach J, Russell K, Blitz S, et al. A systematic review of the diagnosis of occupational asthma. Chest. 2007;131:569–78.

64. Suojalehto H, Cullinan P. Specific inhalation challenge tests for occupational asthma in Europe: a survey. Eur Respir Rev. 2014;23:266–70.

65. Lemière C, Cartier A, Malo JL, et al. Persistent specific bronchial reactivity to occupational agents in workers with normal nonspecific bronchial reactivity. Am J Respir Crit Care Med. 2000;162:976–80.

66. Lemiere C, Gautrin D, Trudeau C, et al. Fever and leucocytosis accompanying asthmatic reactions due to occupational agents: frequency and associated factors. Eur Respir J. 1996;9:517–23.

67. Kennedy WA, Girard F, Chaboillez S, et al. Cost-effectiveness of various diagnostic approaches for occupational asthma. Can Respir J. 2007;14:276–80.

Part III
Management

9

MANAGEMENT OF THE WORKER

David N. Weissman,[1] Santiago Quirce,[2] André Cartier,[3] and Jean-Luc Malo[4]
[1]Respiratory Health Division, CDC-NIOSH, Morgantown, West Virginia, USA
[2]Department of Allergy, La Paz University Hospital, IdiPAZ, and Universidad Autonoma de Madrid, Madrid, Spain
[3]University of Montreal, Montreal, Quebec, Canada
[4]Hôpital du Sacré-Cœur de Montréal and Université de Montréal, Montréal, Québec, Canada

Contents

CASE HISTORY

A 25-year-old worker has been employed for 5 years in a small family-owned bakery that employs three other bakers and two helpers.

1. During his apprenticeship course, the worker received information on possible allergies to cereals, enzymes, and other products in flour.
2. He started sneezing at work 1 year before being seen at the clinic, and his wife noticed that he had some wheezy breathing at home in the evening for the past few months.
3. The local health department had started a surveillance program in bakeries in the area. After some hesitation, the employer allowed an industrial hygienist from that department to visit the workplace and a nurse to meet with the workers.
4. An informative session was offered and short self-administered questionnaires were completed by all attending workers.
5. Because the worker had positive responses on the self-administered questionnaires, he met with the occupational nurse, who inquired about the details of his symptoms with more detailed medical questionnaires. The results of these questionnaires indicated that the worker had symptoms consistent with work-related rhinitis and asthma.
6. The worker was seen by the occupational physician of the local health department. Skin-prick tests (SPTs) to various cereals and enzymes showed positive immediate skin reactions to wheat and soya flours allergens. He was given inhaled formoterol on demand.
7. The nurse and physician suggested that the worker make an appointment at a specialized center for further testing.
8. The worker, a recent immigrant with two children, feared losing his job but followed the advice and scheduled an appointment.
9. Monitoring of peak expiratory flows (PEFs) and nonspecific bronchial responsiveness (NSBR), at work and off work, suggested the diagnosis of OA to flour.
10. A claim was filed to the workers' compensation board and the worker was removed from work.
11. Following the diagnosis of OA, he was given the opportunity to follow a course on truck driving and was able to find a new job.
12. Two years later, the worker was asymptomatic requiring no treatment for asthma. He was reassessed by the workers' compensation board to determine if he had permanent disability.

Introduction

Work-exacerbated asthma (WEA) and occupational asthma (OA) are clinical entities included in the broader term work-related asthma (WRA), which is adult asthma that worsens in the workplace (see Chapter 1). These respiratory conditions are the most prevalent work-related lung diseases in developing and industrialized countries (1) although they are often underdiagnosed. The population fraction of risk attributable to occupation has been estimated in a joint statement issued by the European and

TABLE 9.1 Optimal Assessment and Management Strategies Targeted for the Workplace and the Worker

	The Workplace		The Worker
Assessment	Existing or new agent with the potential of causing *sensitizer-induced OA* (structure-activity analysis)? Consider assessment of air (median, peak values), surface, biological monitoring, job-exposure matrix, using immunoassay procedures.	Identify agents with the potential of causing *irritant-induced OA or irritation*, alone or with other contaminants (pollutants).	Surveillance programs initiated by occupational or primary care physicians in workplaces with identified risks or after confirmation of index case(s): early referral to specialized centers (≤1 yr after onset of symptoms) to diminish risk of permanent sequelae.
	HMW agents: Use of more characterized recombinant occupational allergens for assessment of antibodies.	Obtain detailed SDS. Workplace site visit with hygienist.	Periodic ongoing surveillance in workplaces at risk, particularly for workers with biologic markers (Ig-mediated sensitization to HMW agent, other mucosal symptoms—nose, eye, skin).
	LMW agents: Improved analytical methods, direct-reading instruments, etc.		Tests (immunological, inflammatory, functional) carried out in hierarchical order to confirm the diagnosis of sensitizer-induced OA.
	Obtain detailed material SDS and verify they are accurate.		If worker is still at work, ongoing follow-up.
	Consider workplace visit with hygienist.		For irritant-induced asthma, obtain detailed clinical and occupational history as well as lung function tests.
			If diagnosis of OA is confirmed, reassess worker 2 years after diagnosis, at a time asthma is stable and worker is no longer exposed or, at the least, minimally exposed, for permanent impairment/disability.
Management	*General:*	**Reduction or cessation of exposure is essential.**	
	Improved monitoring strategies Propose TLVs for more numerous specific agents.		
	Specific to a workplace: **Reduction or cessation of exposure is essential.**	If inhalation accident or development of chronic airway obstruction and/or hyperresponsiveness without or with minimal evidence of other personal causes, refer to a medicolegal agency.	During investigation, treat asthma according to guidelines.
	Propose substitution of agent, change in process, improved hygiene, etc.		Propose cessation of exposure only when diagnostic evidence is sufficient and there is minimal risk for the worker.
			Propose referral to a medicolegal agency, this needing delicate decision-making and open discussion with the worker to avoid prejudice.
			Once the diagnosis of OA is confirmed, propose cessation of exposure (if possible) or, at the least, reduction of exposure.
			Treat residual asthma (ICS may accelerate improvement).
			Retraining/return to school/work reintegration programs with satisfactory financial compensation and psychosocial interventions.

Abbreviations: HMW, high-molecular-weight; ICS, inhaled corticosteroid; LMW, low-molecular-weight; OA, occupational asthma; SDS, safety data sheet; TLVs, threshold limit values.

American Thoracic societies to be 16% (95% CI 10%–22%), based on nine case-control and cohort studies of incident asthma (2).

The purpose of this chapter is to review the management of workers with WRA, using an informative case similar to the one used to illustrate the various steps in the assessment of WRA (as reviewed in Chapter 5). Irritant-induced asthma and reactive airways dysfunction syndrome (RADS) will not be considered here as the subject is covered in Chapter 19. A summary of various aspects related to the assessment and management of the workplace and of the worker is proposed in Table 9.1.

Several evidence-based guidelines on the management of WRA have been published or updated in the recent years (3–6).

The most relevant aspects of the management of workers suffering from this condition will be covered in this chapter in the form of questions. The management of WRA includes prevention, assessment, treatment, and compensation. This chapter focuses mainly on OA treatment, where other topics are covered in other chapters.

When suspecting OA, how should the asthma be treated, should the worker continue to work, and when should they file a claim for compensation (see case history at the beginning of this chapter, items 6-10)?

As reviewed in Chapter 5, the diagnosis of asthma should not rely only on history, as this is too often the case, but on objective evidence of either reversible airways obstruction or increased bronchial responsiveness. Once the diagnosis of asthma is confirmed, the physician has to determine if increased symptoms at work are due to asthma and if the worker has WEA or OA.

During the investigation, symptoms should initially be treated with an inhaled long-acting beta-2 agonist (LABA) combined to low-dose inhaled corticosteroids (ICSs) taken on demand (7). Ideally, during the investigation, regular treatment with ICS, LABA, and other controller medications should be avoided since such treatment might impair the ability to properly assess the relation of symptoms with work. However, if symptoms are too frequent or present at night, regular treatment of LABA–ICS and increased doses of ICS should be considered according to guidelines (7). The dose of ICS should be kept at a minimum dosage and the dose should not be modified during monitoring (7).

In order to reduce the socioeconomic burden related to a wrong diagnosis, it is highly recommended to avoid taking a subject off work before confirming WRA. However, if asthma symptoms are too severe and uncontrolled, work withdrawal may be necessary; this should be kept at a minimum to avoid loss of income and stress for the worker. Once asthma is controlled on a minimum dose of medication, the worker should be asked to return to work with continued monitoring while keeping the dose of controlled medication constant and not reduced. Indeed, too often, when taken off work, the patient is treated aggressively for asthma with rapid control and then returned to work while controller medication is reduced or even stopped—this per se may be enough to induce a flare-up of asthma, which may be misdiagnosed as due to work. Monitoring of PEF and nonspecific bronchial responsiveness (NSBR) assessed by the provocative concentration or dose of methacholine causing a 20% fall (PC20-M or PD-M) in the forced expiratory volume in 1 second (FEV_1), and if possible assessment of airway inflammation, may allow confirming OA. Specific inhalation challenges (SICs) may be required to confirm or exclude the diagnosis, as reviewed in Chapter 8. Although the investigation of WRA may be performed by any physician, referring the worker to a specialized center may facilitate the investigation and is usually recommended (8).

Deciding when it is appropriate to file a claim to either a workers' compensation board or the worker's insurances may be delicate and needs open discussion with the worker. Indeed, in some instances, it may be better to file a claim only when there are sufficient data either confirming the diagnosis of OA or making it likely as some employers may refuse to collaborate and may lay off a worker simply on presentation of a claim. Although in most countries, the worker is in theory protected by law against such dismissal, it should be kept in mind that this may occur and put the worker in a precarious psychosocial situation. Ideally, the worker should be kept at work until they are assessed by a compensation board and a final decision is made.

CASE HISTORY

With formoterol, the worker was able to continue to work, although he remained symptomatic and was awakened occasionally at night and was symptom free when he was off work for more than a day. He was referred to a specialized center in OA, where he had serial measurements of PC20-M and monitoring of PEF while he was still at work. He had significant and recurrent falls in PEF at night and during the day while working with improvement over weekends and during 2 weeks off for his holidays. His PC20-M improved from 2 mg/mL at the end of a working week, confirming the diagnosis of asthma, to 9.0 mg/mL at the end of his holidays. With these findings combined with positive skin tests to wheat to which he was regularly exposed, the diagnosis of OA to wheat was confirmed. A claim was filed to the workers' compensation board, which, upon reviewing the investigation, accepted the diagnosis of OA to flour.

Once the diagnosis of OA is confirmed, what is the best way to improve the outcome (see case history at the beginning of this chapter, items 10-12)?

Reducing exposure versus no exposure— Does it make a difference in OA?

The optimal intervention to address OA is cessation of exposure to the causative agent (4, 5, 9). Justification for this approach is suggested by a rigorous systematic Cochrane review of the literature and meta-analysis in which the outcome of OA was compared in workers with complete removal vs partial reduction of exposure (6). In this review, removal from exposure included either complete removal from the exposed environment or substitution of another agent to replace the causal agent (for example, substituting nonlatex medical gloves for powdered latex gloves). Reduction of exposure involved relocating the affected worker to another work area with less exposure; or educating workers to avoid exposures; or using personal protective equipment (PPE) such as respirators. Henneberger and coworkers (6) were unable to identify any randomized prospective controlled trials, so the review and meta-analysis was based on 26 nonrandomized controlled before-and-after studies with 1695 participants. Overall, it was felt that the quality of evidence for the outcomes assessed was very low and thus the findings of the review and meta-analysis were very uncertain. Still, findings from 18 studies comparing removal to continued exposure indicated that removal improves asthma symptoms when evaluated either as absence or improvement of symptoms. Findings from seven studies indicated that reducing exposure compared to continued exposure reduces asthma symptoms but does not improve FEV_1. Findings from 10 studies indicated that complete removal improves asthma symptoms and FEV_1 more than reduced exposure in those with OA due to LMW agents. It is of note that in the three studies evaluating for absence of symptoms as an outcome for those with OA due to HMW agents, the risk ratio favoring complete removal was 10.8, but it did not achieve statistical significance. Data for nonspecific airway hyperreactivity was not available for the comparisons of reduced vs continued exposure and complete vs reduced exposure. Findings from two studies indicated increased risk of complete removal leading to unemployment more often than reducing exposure. In four studies, complete removal was associated with a 20% to 50% decrease in income.

Thus, the current weight of evidence based solely on clinical outcomes favors complete removal from exposure over reduction in exposure. Whenever possible, the best approach to complete removal from exposure is substitution of another workplace agent for the sensitizing agent that caused OA. An excellent example is substitution in medical centers for medical gloves other than nonpowdered latex gloves (10). This approach allows the patient to continue their employment, and also protects others in the workplace from OA caused by the sensitizing agent. If removal of the worker from the workplace is the only way to achieve removal from exposure, the potential clinical benefits should be weighed against the potential adverse impact of unemployment and loss of income. The outcome of this assessment will vary depending on a variety of socioeconomic factors, including the patient's financial status, prospects for alternate employment, and the availability of a social safety net able to assist the patient in the event of job loss.

If reduction in exposure is pursued despite the risk for worse clinical outcomes, the best approach is to use a comprehensive set of interventions known as the hierarchy of controls. This hierarchy describes different types of interventions according to their likeliness of effectiveness. The most effective type of intervention has already been described, eliminating or substituting a less hazardous agent for the causative one. The next most effective type of intervention is engineering controls such as improved ventilation, including increased ventilation, directional and local exhaust ventilation, and filtration of air prior to its return. Engineering controls do not require worker adherence to be effective. In contrast, administrative or work practice controls are in general less effective than engineering controls because they depend on high levels of adherence. For example, they might include alterations to processes to aerosolize less dust. Using PPE such as respirators is generally viewed as the least effective intervention in the hierarchy of controls because so many things can go wrong. In the case of respirators, they must be worn whenever needed and each time they are worn they must fit and function properly. Respirators are best used as a last line of defense, not as the only line of defense.

In terms of timing of exposure removal, available data suggest that it should happen as quickly as possible before OA deteriorates into severe disease. OA has worse outcomes with longer duration between onset of symptoms and removal from exposure; and when asthma is more severe at the time of diagnosis (11). In a study involving long-term follow-up (average 11 years) of 78 subjects with OA caused by toluene diisocyanate (TDI), multivariate analysis showed that the PD20 methacholine at baseline was a significant predictor of follow-up PD20 with more severe airway hyperreactivity at baseline predicting more severe subsequent airway hyperresponsiveness (12). Another study evaluated 133 workers with OA due to either HMW or LMW agents after a mean interval of 8.7 years. Multivariate analysis showed that higher baseline PD20 methacholine and longer time interval since diagnosis were significantly associated with a higher follow-up PD20 (that is, less airway hyperreactivity) (13). Thus, studies evaluating prognostic factors suggest that early intervention prior to developing more severe asthma might lead to better outcomes.

Although OA does not commonly lead to mortality, fatal cases have happened when prolonged exposures occurred, likely leading to development of severe disease (14).

Medical management

Removal from exposure to the causative agent is the single most important measure in the management of OA, as it leads to the best health outcome, as discussed in the previous section. Other important actions are prescribing effective therapies according to asthma severity, along with instituting preventive strategies, such as appropriate avoidance of environmental triggers.

As in other forms of asthma, optimal management of patients with WRA requires an adequate pharmacological treatment, aiming to achieve asthma control and prevent exacerbations and decline in lung function (8). A stepwise treatment approach is used as indicated in international asthma guidelines, including high-intensity treatment if necessary (7). ICS used after cessation of exposure may offer further clinical and functional improvement after cessation of exposure (15). However, there is currently insufficient evidence that treatment with ICS and LABA is able to prevent the long-term deterioration of asthma in subjects who remain exposed to the agent causing OA (4).

About 16% of patients with OA have been found to have severe uncontrolled asthma (16) and consequently they need appropriate treatment (i.e. GINA step 5) (7). This may include prescription of oral corticosteroids and/or biologic agents. Omalizumab (anti-IgE monoclonal antibody) has been found to be effective in workers with severe OA who continue to be exposed to the causal agent (17). Omalizumab has shown clinical efficacy in OA caused by HMW agents, such as cereal flour in baker's asthma (18) as well as in OA caused by LMW agents, including isocyanates and acrylates (19). This treatment can enable some patients to remain in their jobs.

Allergen immunotherapy, either subcutaneous or sublingual, has been scarcely used in occupational rhinitis and asthma, and only with a few allergen extracts, such as cereal flour, latex, and laboratory animals (17). This treatment may allow some allergic workers to continue their work activity, but the long-term clinical outcome remains unknown. The main limitations of this treatment are the lack of standardized extracts, modest clinical improvement, and potential adverse side effects (17). Nevertheless, personalization of the diagnosis, immunologic assessment by allergenic components, and targeted therapies allow the individualization of treatment in workers with sensitizer-induced OA, which fits very well with the concept of precision medicine (20, 21).

Rehabilitation/work reintegration

Following the diagnosis of OA and once the decision is made for the worker to stop the exposure completely, vocational rehabilitation should be offered to the worker to reduce the psychosocial burden of the disease (22). There is a need for active communication between the treating physician, the affected worker, the employer, and the compensation board/insurance company to ensure the best chances for the worker to return to full employment in safe conditions. Factors to be considered that may affect patient preference and physician recommendations include aspects of the job, the skills of the worker, possible areas of relocation at work, options for retraining, planned age of retirement, extent of support from workers' compensation and other support systems, and additional socioeconomic factors (20).

In addition, if the worker has persistent asthma, they may need protection from environmental exposure to irritants, smoke, fumes, dust, and cold air. Follow-up of the worker in their new environment with appropriate adjustment in exposure or medication is necessary. Education and retraining are very important aspects in the management of WRA, for work rehabilitation and integration. New tools and technologies such as educational web-based programs (23), smartphone and tablet apps (24), as well as social media (25) can help to improve the management of OA, with the support of physicians, medicolegal institutions, and specialized centers.

CASE HISTORY

Upon review and acceptance of the diagnosis of OA by the workers' compensation board, the baker was referred to the workers' reintegration program. As the company was a small family business with no possibilities to find him a proper job where he would not be exposed to flour, he was given the opportunity to retrain in a new trade. He completed a truck driving course and was able to find a job with adequate income.

Compensating the worker for disability-impairment

Once OA has developed, there is good evidence that the specific sensitization to the offending agent is long lasting even following cessation of exposure and normalization of NSBR (26). Therefore, workers with OA should be considered as being permanently disabled as they cannot be re-exposed to their offending sensitizer and this may be associated with loss of income. As most subjects with OA have persistence of increased NSBR, with or without symptoms requiring medication, there is a need to assess if there is permanent impairment and disability after cessation of exposure. Most subjects reach a plateau of improved FEV_1 by 1 year and a plateau of improved NSBR by 2 years while other individuals do not. A scheme for compensation (27) has been proposed as discussed in Chapter 11A.

CASE HISTORY

When reassessed 2 years after cessation of working in the bakery, the worker was asymptomatic, requiring no asthma medication. He had a normal spirometry and PC20-methacholine >32 mg/mL, thus normal. He had reached maximal medical improvement (MMI), showed no objective findings for permanent pulmonary impairment, and received no further disability compensation.

Surveillance, prevention

Any case of OA should be considered a sentinel event. This topic is covered in Chapter 10 but should be considered as part of the management of OA.

Once work-exacerbated asthma is confirmed, what is the best way to improve outcome?

WEA has been defined as "preexisting or concurrent asthma that is worsened by workplace conditions" (28). Just as general environmental triggers such as smoke, perfume, and cold air can trigger exacerbation of non-WRA, a range of workplace triggers can exacerbate asthma, including asthma not originally caused by a workplace exposure. Examples include cleaning agents (29), passive exposure to tobacco smoke (30), and exposure to dust, smoke, chemicals, and senstizers across a range of industries (31). A review found a median prevalence in population studies of WEA among those with asthma of 21.5% (28). WEA has been reported as having features of asthma severity worse than OA (32) and the impact of WEA on work productivity and earning capacity has been reported as similar to OA (33). In another indication of potential severity, 72% of those filing for asthma-related workers' compensation claims in Ontario over a 5-year period fulfilled criteria for WEA (31).

Since WEA is common and is associated with substantial morbidity, appropriate management is important. Unfortunately, as noted in an authoritative statement in 2008, "Very few studies to date have evaluated different treatment or preventive strategies in WEA patients…" (3). However, a study was cited showing that Scottish bar workers with asthma had lower levels of exhaled nitric oxide and improved quality of life after implementation of smoke-free legislation, suggesting the importance of avoiding workplace triggers (30).

Because of limitations in published studies, the approach to managing WEA is based on expert opinion (3, 28, 34). Management should be optimized as recommended for any person with asthma and exacerbations (GINA 2020). As is the case for usual asthma management, reducing exposures that trigger exacerbations (including workplace exposures) is important. The hierarchy of controls that is used to eliminate or reduce exposures triggering WEA is the same as that previously described for exposures causing OA. An important goal is to enable patients with WEA to keep their jobs. Unfortunately, in cases where optimizing asthma management and limiting triggering work exposures to the degree possible fails to control WEA, job change to a workplace with fewer triggers may be necessary.

Conclusion and research needs

The management of WRA requires the ability of the treating physician to assess whether a worker can reasonably continue to work or should be removed from exposure, depending on clinical and social criteria. Once the diagnosis is confirmed, the treating physician should also follow the worker to ensure adequate medical treatment, refer for permanent disability assessment, and ensure the worker does not experience flare-ups of asthma when returning to work with a change of working condition.

Research should focus on:

- If a worker with suspected WRA is investigated, what is the effect of various medication on the pattern of PEF and NSBR?
- What represents the best outcome: reducing or avoiding exposure at work?
- What are the efficacy, sociopsychological impact, and costs of readaptation programs?
- At what interval after diagnosis (for various agents causing OA) should impairment/disability be assessed?

Disclaimer: The findings and conclusions in this report are those of the authors and do not necessarily represent the official position of the National Institute for Occupational Safety and Health.

References

1. Jeebhay MF, Quirce S. Occupational asthma in the developing and industrialised world: a review. Int J Tuberc Lung Dis. 2007;11:122–33.

2. Blanc PD, Annesi-Maesano I, Balmes JR, et al. The occupational burden of nonmalignant respiratory diseases. An Official American Thoracic Society and European Respiratory Society Statement. Am J Respir Crit Care Med. 2019;199:1312–34.

3. Tarlo SM, Balmes J, Balkissoon R, et al. Diagnosis and management of work-related asthma: American College Of Chest Physicians Consensus Statement. Chest. 2008;134:1S–41S.

4. Baur X, Sigsgaard T, Aasen TB, et al. Guidelines for the management of work-related asthma. Eur Respir J. 2012;39:529–45.

5. Fishwick D, Barber CM, Bradshaw LM, et al. Standards of care for occupational asthma: an update. Thorax. 2012;67:278–80.

6. Henneberger PK, Patel JR, de Groene GJ, et al. Workplace interventions for treatment of occupational asthma. Cochrane Database Syst Rev. 2019 Oct 8;10:Cd006308.

7. Ginasthma.org. Global strategy for asthma management and prevention. Updated 2020. https://ginasthmaorg/wp-content/uploads/2020/04/GINA-2020-full-report_-final-_wmspdf. 2020.

8. Tarlo SM, Lemiere C. Occupational asthma. N Engl J Med. 2014;370:640–9.

9. Tarlo SM, Balmes J, Balkisssoon R, et al. ACCP consensus statement: diagnosis and management of work-related asthma. Chest. 2008;134:1S–41S.

10. Kelly KJ, Wang ML, Klancnik M, et al. Prevention of IgE sensitization to latex in health care workers after reduction of antigen exposures. J Occup Environ Med. 2011;53:934–40.

11. Ameille J, Descatha A. Outcome of occupational asthma. Curr Opin Allergy Clin Immunol. 2005;5:125–8.

12. Padoan M, Pozzato V, Simon M, et al. Long-term follow-up of toluene diisocyanate-induced asthma. Eur Respir J. 2003;21:637–40.

13. Maghni K, Lemière C, Ghezzo H, et al. Airway inflammation after cessation of exposure to agents causing occupational asthma. Am J Respir Crit Care Med. 2004;169:367–72.

14. Ortega HG, Kreiss K, Schill DP, et al. Fatal asthma from powdering shark cartilage and review of fatal occupational asthma literature. Am J Ind Med. 2002;42:50–4.

15. Malo JL, Cartier A, Côté J, et al. Influence of inhaled steroids on the recovery of occupational asthma after cessation of exposure: an 18-month double-blind cross-over study. Am J Crit Care Respir Med. 1996;153:953–60.

16. Vandenplas O, Godet J, Hurdubaea L, et al. Severe occupational asthma: insights from a multicenter European cohort. J Allergy Clin Immunol Pract. 2019;7:2309–18.

17. Moscato G, Pala G, Sastre J. Specific immunotherapy and biological treatments for occupational allergy. Curr Opin Allergy Clin Immunol. 2014;14:576–81.

18. Olivieri M, Biscardo CA, Turri S, et al. Omalizumab in persistent severe bakers' asthma. Allergy. 2008;63:790–1.

19. Lavaud F, Bonniaud P, Dalphin JC, et al. Usefulness of omalizumab in ten patients with severe occupational asthma. Allergy. 2013;68:813–5.

20. Tarlo SM, Maestrelli P. Precision medicine in the area of work-related asthma. Curr Opin Allergy Clin Immunol. 2018;18:277–9.

21. Quirce S, Sastre J. Occupational asthma: clinical phenotypes, biomarkers, and management. Curr Opin Pulm Med. 2019;25:59–63.

22. Lipszyc JC, Silverman F, Holness DL, et al. Comparison of psychological, quality of life, work-limitation, and socioeconomic status between patients with occupational asthma and work-exacerbated asthma. J Occup Environ Med. 2017;59:697–702.

23. Lipszyc JC, Gotzev S, Scarborough J, et al. Evaluation of the efficacy of a web-based work-related asthma educational tool. J Asthma. 2016;53:1071–5.

24. Marcano Belisario JS, Huckvale K, Greenfield G, et al. Smartphone and tablet self management apps for asthma. Cochrane Database Syst Rev. 2013;27(11):cd010013.

25. Harber P, Leroy G. Social media use for occupational lung disease. Curr Opin Allergy Clin Immunol. 2017;17:72–7.

26. Lemière C. Persistence of bronchial reactivity to occupational agents after removal from exposure and identification of associated factors. Ann Allergy Asthma Immunol. 2003;90(Suppl):52–5.

27. American Medical Association. Guides to the evaluation of permanent impairment. In: Rondinelli RD, ed. The Pulmonary System. Chicago, IL. 2008:77–99.

28. Henneberger PK, Redlich CA, Callahan DB, et al. An Official American Thoracic Society statement: work-exacerbated asthma. Am J Respir Crit Care Med. 2011;184:368–78.

29. Siracusa A, De Blay F, Folletti I, et al. Asthma and exposure to cleaning products—a European Academy of Allergy and Clinical Immunology task force consensus statement. Allergy. 2013:1532–45.

30. Menzies D, Nair A, Williamson PA, et al. Respiratory symptoms, pulmonary function, and markers of inflammation among bar workers before and after a legislative ban on smoking in public places. JAMA. 2006;296:1742–8.

31. Lim T, Liss GM, Vernich L, et al. Work-exacerbated asthma in a workers' compensation population. Occup Med (Lond). 2014;64:206–10.

32. Lemière C, Boulet LP, Chabouillez S, et al. Work-exacerbated asthma and occupational asthma: do they really differ? J Allergy Clin Immunol. 2013;131:704–10.

33. Vandenplas O, Henneberger PK. Socioeconomic outcomes in work-exacerbated asthma. Curr Opin Allergy Clin Immunol. 2007;7:236–41.

34. Tarlo SM. Update on work-exacerbated asthma. Int J Occup Med Environ Health. 2016;29:369–74.

10

PREVENTION

Susan M. Tarlo,[1] Rolf Merget,[2] Eva Suarthana,[3] Julie McKibben,[4] and Jean-Luc Malo[5]
*[1]University Health Network and St Michael's Hospital, Toronto, Department of
Medicine, University of Toronto, Toronto, Ontario, Canada
[2]Institute for Prevention and Occupational Medicine of the German Social Accident
Insurance (IPA), Institute of the Ruhr University, Bochum, Germany.
[3]Département de médecine sociale et préventive, École de santé publique, Université de Montréal, Montréal, Québec, Canada
[4]Global Medical, Procter & Gamble Company, Cincinnati, Ohio, USA
[5]Hôpital du Sacré-Cœur de Montréal and Université de Montréal, Montréal, Québec, Canada*

Contents

WORKPLACE SCENARIO

You are a community health professional and have your main practice in workplaces. A nurse in one of the industries you are responsible for informs you of two situations:

1. There is a new industry under her responsibility that will hire 250 employees, in which glues containing acrylates will be used. What will you suggest to reduce risks of occupational asthma (OA)? (For answer, read section on primary prevention.)

2. In another industry that produces carpets and underlays, a small group of workers reported nasal and respiratory complaints that were potentially work-related. Because of their symptoms, a health survey is planned among all 50 workers. The expectation is that the total set of control measures will significantly reduce exposure for the workers who will also benefit from a permanent health surveillance program. The intention is also to reintegrate workers with OA in the workplace into areas in which exposure to the offending agent will be avoided or reduced. How will you tackle this request? (For answer, read section on secondary and tertiary prevention.)

Introduction and definitions

OA should be considered as a preventable condition (1). Efforts of prevention are justified on the basis of many societal (frequency and costs of the disease) and scientific (epidemiological and clinical evidence, amenable risk factors, efficient methods of prevention) convincing arguments (1). Prevention encompasses three aspects as follows.

Primary prevention consists of controlling hazards before disease has occurred (2). Prevention should start with the introduction of new chemicals and evaluation of their toxicity, including a theoretical approach (3). Then, agents have to be labelled or can only be used under certain conditions. Exposure standards defined by a level below which workers are unlikely to develop adverse effects should be evaluated as part of the hygiene approach (4). This has only been examined for a few agents causing OA such as flours (5), enzymes (6), and diiisocyanates (7). Combining exposure elimination or reduction to a medical approach is ideal. Exposure-reducing strategies have the greatest impact on the burden of disease (2, 8).

Secondary prevention involves medical surveillance with early detection of workers with sensitization or OA, preferably at a time when the condition is reversible.

Tertiary prevention involves medical management to minimize impairment with complete or partial removal and includes workers' compensation programs.

Prevention of sensitizer-induced OA

Primary prevention

Structure-activity relationships and respiratory sensitization potential

Structure-activity relationship (SAR) models have been developed for preproduct hazard identification as an alternative to more cumbersome and costly animal experiments, but also ethical considerations play a role. SAR can be mechanistic (qualitative) or statistical (quantitative), the latter being termed QSARs. For example, in the context of respiratory sensitization to low-molecular-weight (LMW) substances the formation of covalent bonds between the chemical and amino acid residues present within the structure of human protein molecules is assumed to be a key mechanism for sensitization. The molecular structures of LMW organic compounds of respiratory sensitizers are more likely to contain heteroatom (notably nitrogen or oxygen) containing functional groups than nonsensitizers, and a high sensitizing potential is assumed when two or more groups containing such heteroatoms are present in the same molecules (9). Also, electrophilic reaction chemistry is considered as a key mechanism for binding to electron dense amine groups in the side chains of amino acids, with the generation of hapten-protein conjugates, but further mechanisms have been reported (3, 10). Also in vitro tests of conjugation to protein molecules have been suggested as part of a tiered approach for prediction of a sensitizing potential (11).

QSARs link a chemical structure with sensitization mathematically (also called *in silico models*). It is of importance to accurately define sensitizers and nonsensitizers in these models, and it is obvious that irritant mechanisms constitute a major confounder. Misclassification can be expected to be relevant due to the low number of reported asthma cases for a large number of putative sensitizers. Over the years several QSARs have been proposed and refined (12). Some have been validated with external datasets. A negative predictive value (NPV) of 1.00 of various QSAR models has been described with much lower positive predictive values (PPV) that vary widely between the different models (13) but a more recent study calculated high PPV (0.96) and NPV (0.89) by combining the best performing SARs in a tiered approach (14).

A promising open access QSAR toolbox has been developed by the Organization for Economic Cooperation and Development (OECD) (www.qsartoolbox.org). The toolbox is a free software application that supports chemical hazard assessment by providing information and tools which can be used to find structurally and mechanistically defined analogues and chemical categories as sources for read-across (which means predicting endpoint information for one substance by using data for the same endpoint from other substances). Until now there has been no widely accepted QSAR model and the actual frequency of use of the QSAR models is unknown.

Exposure control options in the workplace

Control of exposure can be achieved by different control measures, and a hierarchy of measures has been defined (Table 10.1). The preferred method of exposure reduction for OA is substitution of the asthmagen agent. However, substitution is often not possible or practicable. The second best approach is exposure reduction. There are many options to reduce exposure; the strength of the source of the pollutant can be reduced or the formulation in which an agent is used can be modified: enzymes can be used in liquid form, gels, or encapsulated or granulated instead of using powdered forms. Changes can be made to the process, or general hygiene (good housekeeping) can be implemented. Often a combination of measures is required to reduce the exposure. Other options are isolation of the source (enclosure or segregation), ventilation (general or local), avoidance of exposure, and, last but not least, use of personal protective equipment (PPE). Often, optimal exposure reduction strategies consist of a combination of measures. One of the rare exceptions is latex, where considerable exposure reduction can be achieved by using nonpowdered instead of powdered gloves in healthcare environments.

TABLE 10.1 Hierarchy of Control Options for Airborne Contaminants in the Work Environment in Order of Priority (Top to Bottom) and Preference (Left to Right)

Control Measure	Agent	Process/Appliance	Working Environment	Work Practice
1. Elimination	Total substitution	Different process	Layout change	Automation, robotization, remote control
2. Reduction	Partial substitution change of form	Adjustment preventive maintenance specialized appliance	Good housekeeping	Correct work procedures, training, instruction, motivation, supervision
3. Isolation		Enclosure segregation	Glove box, safety cabinet segregation, high-exposure departments	Ensuring enclosure
4. Ventilation		Local exhaust ventilation, push-pull ventilation	Dilution ventilation, air douches, air curtains	Portable jets, low-volume high-velocity tools
5. Exposure avoidance			Booths for operators	Shorter shifts, fewer people, work schedules
6. Personal protection				Respiratory protection, gloves, clothing

Introduction of new agents and supervision of existing agents in the workplace

When a product is considered for use in a workplace, a review process should be set and examined by an expert committee in occupational health and safety in regards to possible health risks for workers (15). This review process should be based on consultation of relevant documents made available to workers by public laws of various countries, one being the REACH (Registration, Evaluation, Authorization and Restriction of Chemicals) regulation in force in Europe since 2007 (16). There are two important documents that should be examined: labels and safety data sheets (SDSs). "SDS and labels are for many workers the only available source of information on the products they use" (17). Warning design of labels should consider several aspects, related to the "receiver": noticeability (preeminence), wording, size, layout and placement, pictorial symbols, color/contrast, auditory warnings, and personal factors (age, cultural background, etc.), all those influencing the efficiency of safety communications (18). This information should not only provide explicit information but also influence behavior and individual perception of hazard, a topic of great interest for behavioral psychologists (19).

Safety data sheet

"A SDS is a technical document providing detailed information regarding ingredients, concentrations, and toxic properties of chemicals in the workplace; health effects; hazard evaluation for product handling, storage, and use; measures to protect workers; and emergency procedures. It serves as a supplement to label information, and copies must be readily accessible to employees" (15). The threshold for having to give information on the content of sensitizing products varies: 1.0% in the United States, 0.1% to 1.0% in Europe and Canada. Workers consulting physicians for possible OA are generally asked to bring SDSs of all products they are exposed to at work (Chapter 5). Although useful information might be found, it has been argued that SDSs may also not contain important health information (20), especially for cleaning products (21). Bernstein lists four "major limitations" of SDSs: omission of vital information regarding the generic chemical names, omission of listing of potential respiratory and skin sensitizing agents, failure to update regulation on permissible exposure levels, and no information regarding specific occupational lung or cutaneous disease (21). Several chemicals used as cleaning agents may not be identified as asthmagenic, the focus being put on irritating properties (22).

Respiratory protective equipment

Exposure reduction is the primary aim for preventing OA. Methods of control of agents causing OA, of sensitization, and of OA include elimination (i.e. powdered gloves in the case of latex), enclosure (i.e. in the case of enzymes in the detergent industry), improved ventilation and modified work practices (respiratory protective equipment [RPE], environmental monitoring, and medical surveillance at work) (1). In this, reduction at the source or elimination of the product, through engineering and work practice controls, is the priority target. This approach has been most successful in the case of latex through the use of nonpowdered gloves and enzymes in the detergent industry by encapsulation (see section "Effectiveness of Preventive Measures"). RPE should be regarded as alternatives in the primary and secondary prevention of OA. The use of RPE has been incorporated into more global preventive programs and it is difficult to know if wearing RPE per se reduces sensitization and OA. In addition, the evidence supporting the use of RPE to reduce exposure is limited to small case series, as discussed (23, 24).

The use of RPE in tertiary prevention might be considered in specific workplaces and for targeted tasks in the effort of trying to maintain a worker with OA in their workplace. Wearing a mask, especially positive pressure air supply mask in the case of vapors (diisocyanates), can result in reduction of exposure. It is still uncertain if workers with OA with reduced exposure have a worse medical outcome than those completely removed (25). For socioeconomic reasons, the option of keeping a worker with OA at work with reduced exposure can sometimes be considered (25).

A respirator is defined as "a personal protective device that is worn on the face, covers at least the nose and mouth, and is used to reduce the wearer's risk of inhaling hazardous airborne particles" (26). There are two main types of RPE: air-purifying respirators that remove contaminants from the air (half- and full-face masks, with cartridges or canisters) and air-supplying respirators that allow for fresh air supply, including positive pressure masks or personal powered respirators. The term "N95" describes a mask with a filter "that removes at least 95% of airborne particles during 'worst case' testing" (26). The choice of a particular RPE depends on the physical properties of the agent suspected to cause OA. These devices should be well fitted to the face, regularly checked for efficiency, and cleaned.

There are several pitfalls that limit the use of RPE, the first, and probably the most important, being interest and compliance. From data of the US Farm and Ranch Survey, Casey and Mazurek reported on 11,000 farmers exposed to organic dust and pesticides (27). Only 36% of farmers (or their spouse) had declared wearing a respirator or a dust mask in the past year. Farmers in grain production, with a history of asthma, and, more so, work-related asthma (WRA), were more likely to wear a RPE, particularly when they were exposed to pesticides (27). In an online survey of more than 1000 institutional organizations using laboratory animals for research (of which 198 replied) only 25% reported that RPE was required, although 80% offered it to employees (28). Ilgaz and coworkers examined the efficacy of air-fed respirators with charcoal and particle filters in 20 workers affected with OA due to metalworking fluid. This improved the area between the curves (ABC) score of peak expiratory flow (PEF) recording (Chapter 8) but not significantly, and work-related decline in PEF was unsatisfactory in 12 of the 20 workers. The authors therefore concluded that RPE has a limited role in protecting workers with OA (29). Another limitation of personal RPE is its lack of adequate protection for some types of work. Air-fed visors used for diisocyanate paint spraying need to be lifted for several reasons by workers, which results in undue exposure (30). Many workers do not tolerate wearing masks or having a positive pressure full face respirator because these devices are cumbersome and can impact on their work performance. In addition, due to airflow resistance, they can be difficult to tolerate by workers with airway obstruction. Workers can wear RPE for a limited portion of their work shift, with RPE offering only partial protection in such instances. In workplaces where there are risks of accidental leaks that may cause irritant-induced asthma and reactive airways dysfunction syndrome (RADS) (Chapter 19), workers should have an RPE on hand and rapidly be advised to wear it if there is a spill. Compliance with wearing gloves is also limited in the case of exposure to diisocyanates that are also absorbed through the skin (Chapter 14) and can cause sensitization and OA. In a study based on interviews, Ceballos and coworkers found that workers were not generally aware of the risk of dermal exposure to diisocyanates and concluded that there is a need for providing information in the use of protective gloves (31).

Exposure standards

The risk of sensitization and disease is a function of exposure and individual susceptibility. Genes may play an inciting or a protective role in the development of sensitized-induced OA (Chapter 3). This being said, the exposure and, more so, the intensity of exposure are considered to play a more important role than host markers such as genes and atopy, in the case of HMW agents, although the proportion for which each factor (i.e. exposure vs host markers) plays a role is a common object of legal apportionment. Many studies have shown an association, in a dose-response fashion in many instances, between the intensity of exposure and the frequency of sensitization to HMW and, more generally, sensitizer-induced OA as defined in epidemiological studies (Chapter 3). As a result, "These observations have changed the perspective for risk assessment and development of exposure standards for allergens considerably" (6). Furthermore, studies have shown that reducing exposure results in a diminution of sensitization and OA, as reviewed below for several occupational agents (enzymes, latex, diisocyanates, platinum salts, flours, and laboratory animals).

In the same way as permissible exposure limit (PEL) standards have been developed in the case of inorganic dusts (asbestos and silica dusts) to reduce the risk of pneumoconiosis and cancers (PEL of 0.1 fiber/cc^3 for the 8-hr time-weighted average [TWA] and an excursion limit of 1 fiber/cc^3 over a 30-min period for asbestos), the same approach was proposed for the prevention of OA, particularly in bakers (Chapter 12). Quantitative exposure data on both total inhalable dust and airborne allergens in UK (32) and Dutch (33) bakeries were thoroughly examined by researchers. The interpretation of these data was greatly enhanced by the availability of personal sampling devices, that keep being improved, more recently coupled with sophisticated immunoassays (34) (Chapter 6). The pioneered works by professor Dick Heederik from Utrecht, The Netherlands, have shown dose-response relationships between wheat flour allergen exposure and wheat sensitization, the association being steeper and stronger in atopic subjects (33). The authors of the aforementioned important publication concluded: "The existence of exposure-sensitization gradients suggests that work-related sensitization risk will be negligible when exposure levels will be reduced to average exposure concentration of 0.2 mg/m^3 wheat allergen or approximately 0.5 mg/m^3 inhalable dust during a work shift." This study also paved the way for establishing exposure standards for occupational allergens in European countries. Based on several studies, many from the same Netherlands-based group, the exposure limit for alpha-amylase was proposed at 0.9 ng/m^3 as detailed (6). These findings do not mean that the risk is nonexistent at levels below the proposed limits, with a potential identification of a "no-observed effect level," but, rather, acceptable if these limits are observed.

The situation is more complex for LMW agents, particularly diisocyanates, because of both respiratory and skin absorption, the possibility of biological monitoring by urinary sampling (35), and the effect of not only cumulative but also peak exposures in the risk of OA as shown for toluene diisocyanate (TDI) (7).

Secondary prevention

The objective of secondary medical prevention (medical surveillance) is to detect OA at an early stage in order to minimize the long-term effects.

Identification of high-risk workers

In designing a medical surveillance program for OA, the greatest effectiveness is ideally obtained from selecting workplaces with greatest exposure to known sensitizers, and workers that are most at risk. Epidemiological studies have revealed that there are personal risk factors for some causes of OA, such as atopy for HMW agents and smoking for some LMW agents such as platinum salts. Some socioeconomic factors have also been identified in the delay for submitting a claim for OA to a medicolegal agency (36). Being older and having children and a higher salary increase this delay. It might therefore be relevant to put an emphasis on these factors in a surveillance program. However, none of these factors offers a sufficiently high predictive value to be used in selecting workers at the time of placement in an area of exposure (1, 37). Also, the use of these individual risk factors poses some ethical questions in the sense that several of these risk factors such as atopy and smoking are present in a large proportion of the general public, which would lead to exclusion of a large part of the population from certain jobs. It would be more suitable to intervene early on at the career-counseling level in schools, to avoid having an asthmatic youth choose a career in baking or other higher risk job, without at least being advised of the risks that he or she would take (38).

Medical surveillance

The purpose of medical surveillance is early detection of an illness so that its progression can be slowed down or stopped by appropriate intervention. Secondary prevention of OA involves medical monitoring aimed at identifying the illness even before the onset of clinical symptoms (at the stage of early immunologic sensitization) or, at the very least, at an early stage of the illness. Systematic reviews have confirmed the beneficial effects of early removal of sensitized workers from the workplace in comparison with those who remain exposed (24, 25, 39–41). Medical monitoring must be carried out in parallel with primary prevention methods such as exposure reduction at the source. As noted above, even compliance to exposure standards does not entirely eliminate the individual risks of immune-allergic hypersensitivity.

Scientific evidence supporting the implementation of surveillance programs remains in large part indirect due to the inherent nature of intervention that does not allow for randomized trials. One report from Finland indicated that among workers included in medical surveillance programs who developed OA, the surveillance program only identified 18%, and the remainder were detected at doctor's appointments that were not related to the surveillance program, with a similar delay from the onset of symptoms (42). However, it is unknown whether the surveillance programs may have increased awareness by the workers that their symptoms may have been work-related, perhaps leading to earlier assessment. To date, the main justification for OA surveillance programs has been based on the fact that with early diagnosis, early removal from exposure to the causal agent, and less severe asthma at diagnosis, the worker with OA has a more favorable prognosis (25).

Educational programs

Taskforce documents have recommended improving worker education in order to reduce risks (38, 39). Such programs have been largely developed for the self-management of asthma in promoting action plans (43) and have been introduced for the prevention of OA in surveillance and programs (Chapter 5) such as laboratory animal workers (44). In one intervention in supermarket bakeries in South Africa, it is stated: "Furthermore, posters on specific dust reduction elements were also provided and mounted on bakery walls to reinforce the information provided in the training manual" (45). Ghajar-Khorsavi and coworkers have developed a web-based, work-related educational tool for asthma (46). This instrument was shown to be efficient in increasing and maintaining knowledge in WRA after 1 year (47).

Medical surveillance methodology
Testing

OA diagnosis is a procedure that first requires asthma confirmation and then subsequent evidence of work-relatedness. A sequential scheme for diagnosing OA is presented in Figure 10.1. The first step of the process includes an assessment of clinical and occupational history, of nonspecific bronchial hyperresponsiveness (NSBH), and of IgE-mediated sensitization to the suspected workplace agent if relevant (agent acting through an IgE-mediated mechanism) and available. The causality of exposure for the development of OA should then be confirmed by various means: serial PEF recordings, NSBH, induced sputum, or exhaled nitric oxide (FeNO) test off work vs at work and/or SIC. The protocol and tests used are contingent on available resources in the country and region.

Questionnaires

The administration of a brief respiratory questionnaire to at-risk workers as the first step in a surveillance program has been recommended by investigators (48) and the European Respiratory Society Task Force (49). Such a "screening" questionnaire should be administered every 6–12 months in order to allow for the necessary latency period for being affected by IgE-mediated sensitization. The questionnaire should also detect rhinitis symptoms that may precede or accompany OA (50) and may represent a risk factor for the subsequent onset of OA (51).

The diagnostic sensitivity and specificity of questionnaires are often unknown, but even if they are generally lacking in specificity, the important aspect is that they are most often sensitive, a characteristic required at the first step of surveillance.

The reproducibility of questionnaires administered in epidemiological studies and in a surveillance monitoring setting has been examined among UK bakers (52). In a health surveillance survey carried out by a supermarket company that operated 324 stores, only one-third of subjects with respiratory symptoms at work reported these in company-organized surveillance questionnaires versus an independent cross-sectional monitoring program undertaken in a randomly selected sample of 20 stores of the same company (52). The proclivity of workers to report work-related symptoms is dependent on their fear that their claims could affect their jobs. It is suspected that "workers in larger companies, where the possibilities of relocation with the same employer are higher may be more willing to admit the work-related asthma symptoms" (1). A short not yet fully validated self-administered questionnaire has been successfully used in surveillance of nearly 3000 workers exposed to isocyanate (48, 53). A validated short self-administered questionnaire has been used in a country-wide surveillance to identify bakery workers at risk of sensitization to wheat allergens in the Netherlands (54).

Spirometry and measurement of bronchial hyperresponsiveness

Spirometry does not contribute more over and above questionnaire alone (55, 56). As for the measurement of NSBH, it shows very high sensitivity and negative predictive value if it is carried out when workers are still working or were recently exposed (57).

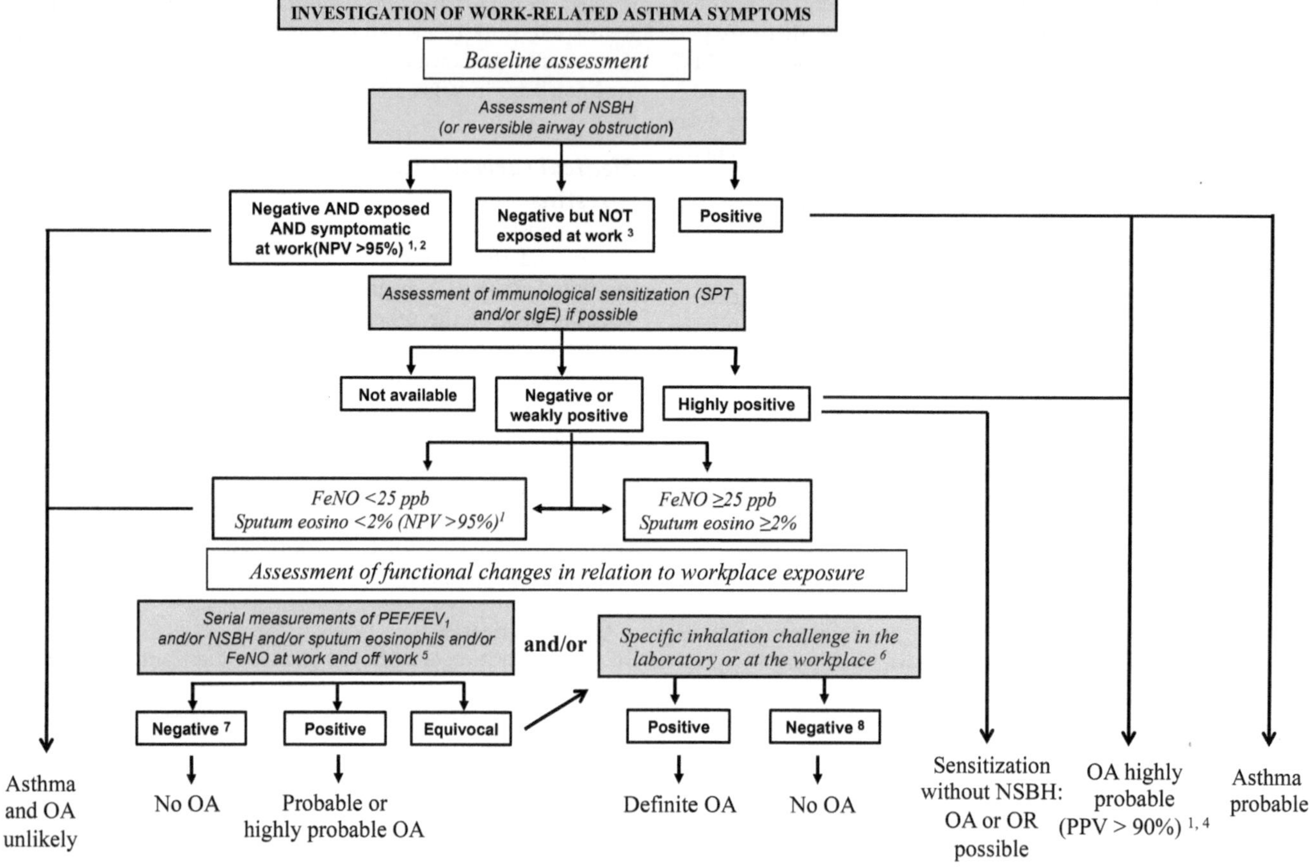

FIGURE 10.1 Proposed stepwise algorithm for diagnosing occupational asthma. (Slightly modified from Cullinan, P, Vandenplas O, Bernstein D. Assessment and management of occupational asthma. *J Allergy Clin Immunol Pract.* 2020;8(10):3264–75. By permission.) *Abbreviations:* eosino, eosinophils; FEV1, forced expiratory flow in 1 second; NPV, negative predictive value; NSBH, nonspecific bronchial hyperresponsiveness; OR, occupational rhinitis; PEF, peak expiratory flow; PPV, positive predictive value; sIgE, specific immunoglobulin E; SPT: skin-prick test.

[1] High negative predictive values (NPV) and positive predictive values (PPV) are applicable only for selected populations of subjects with a high pretest probability of OA (i.e. tertiary centers).

[2] Consider further investigation at the workplace if the clinical history is highly suggestive of OA since the absence of NSBH has been documented even after an asthmatic reaction induced by occupational agents.

[3] Consider either return to the workplace where the worker was symptomatic or specific inhalation challenge in the laboratory. If this is not possible for different reasons, a decision can be made on results of NSBH, immunological testing, and clinical judgment.

[4] In subjects with NSBH when immunological tests have been validated against SIC, increasing the cut-off value for a positive sIgE test ≥ 2.22 kU$_A$/L for wheat flour, ≥ 9.64 kU$_A$/L for rye flour, and ≥ 4.41 kU$_A$/L for latex provides a PPV for a positive SIC result above 95%.

[5] Especially useful when: the subject is exposed to multiple asthmagens at work; no agent known as causing OA has been identified at work; facility for SIC is not easily available; the conditions of exposure at work cannot be reproduced in the laboratory.

[6] Especially useful when: SIC can be performed efficiently and safely; the subject is no longer exposed at work; the highest level of diagnostic confidence is required; there is need to identify a particular agent; PEF records are inconclusive.

[7] Consider a SIC in the laboratory if the clinical history is highly suggestive of OA.

[8] Consider a workplace inhalation challenge or serial PEF recording at work if the clinical history is highly suggestive of OA.

Immunological tests

The identification of IgE-mediated sensitization to an occupational agent is a useful test in certain environments. In workers exposed to platinum salt, trimellitic anhydride, and enzymes, the skin-prick test (SPT) and/or specific IgE assessment provide a high predictive value for the development of OA (see Chapters 3, 7, and 18).

Predictive models

Clinical prediction models have been developed to estimate an individual's probability of the presence or occurrence of an outcome (e.g. OA, specific sensitization to workplace agent) to assist clinical decision-making (58). These models propose identifying workers at risk followed by more costly diagnostic investigation only carried out in individuals targeted by the model. The main objective of these models is to optimize risk estimation at a reasonable cost or in the absence of sparsely available and/or invasive diagnostic test. SIC as the reference test of OA is only available in a few specialized centers worldwide (see Chapter 8). These problems inspired a group of researchers to develop and validate models consisting of information from clinical interview and objective tests other than SIC (i.e. non-SIC based models) for diagnosing OA. This group first successfully developed the model in Canadian workers exposed to HMW agents (56) and validated them in European populations recently (58). The authors showed that the combined use of specific sensitization and assessment of bronchial responsiveness resulted in the highest diagnostic accuracy compared to adding only one of the tests to the clinical interview model. These models enable specialists with access to specific sensitization and NSBH tests to identify individuals at high risk of OA from HMW agents and refer them for more specialized investigations or initiate the treatment by removing them from exposure.

Effectiveness of preventive measures
Overview
Measuring the effectiveness of preventive measures for OA remains difficult due to the challenge that success is largely influenced by the amount of exposure reduction achieved, which is not available, and a lack of data showing the impact of prevention program components needed for exposure reduction. When available, air monitoring levels against a benchmark safe level below which exposures are least likely to result in health effects is one way to evaluate worker exposure. Unfortunately, many causative agents of OA do not have a threshold level below which no health effects are seen, so low numbers of occupational allergy and asthma are possible despite meeting and exceeding air monitoring safe levels further complicating effectiveness analysis. Removal of high-risk workers and implementing medical surveillance are known measures to reduce exposure. There are sparse data showing the effect of removing workers. The detergent, baking, and healthcare industries have been able to successfully implement comprehensive workplace hygiene programs that have contributed to a decline in worker exposures, thus reducing the burden of OA (Table 10.2)

Example of enzymes
After a large numbers of OA cases from enzymes was seen in the late 1960s, the detergent industry trade associations published guidelines that detail how to control enzyme exposures (primary prevention) and monitor employees for potential health effects including sensitization, allergy, and asthma (secondary prevention) (59, 60). After decades of following these comprehensive guidelines with deep penetration across a large number of workplaces, adherence to these guidelines results in near elimination of occupational allergy and asthma (OAA). However, there are examples of nonadherence which led to outbreaks of enzyme allergy and asthma (61, 62).

Primary preventive measures were implemented at the beginning of the 1970s in the detergent industry to reduce sensitization to enzymes: encapsulation to reduce dustiness, air monitoring of ambient concentrations of enzymes, improved equipment design and maintenance, standard spill control procedures, and training on the hazards of enzymes. A significant reduction in the incidence of OA was reported following these preventive strategies (63, 64). Larsen and colleagues showed a clear dose-response relationship for development of sensitization confirming that primary prevention via exposure control is achievable and effective at limiting OAA (65).

Medical surveillance programs are used to identify individuals with immunologic evidence of exposure to enzymes. IgE-mediated sensitization is the first step in the development of OAA. When the annual sensitization incidence rate is kept below 3%, the incidence of OAA is very low (62, 66). Full investigation of each sensitization to identify root causes of exposure and define action steps for remediation are critical to continuous improvement in exposure control.

For more details, see Chapter 18.

Latex
The effect of preventive measures on allergy and OA incidence due to latex is probably the one that has been the best documented. A number of studies have shown that replacing powdered latex gloves with latex gloves having a low allergen and powder content or synthetic elastomer gloves for nonsterile medical procedures, combined or not with medical surveillance, was associated with a very significant reduction of latex sensitization and OA incidence due to latex (67–70). For more details, see Chapter 18.

Diisocyanates
In 1983, the Canadian province of Ontario introduced an OA prevention program for isocyanates combining an information campaign for employers and workers, exposure standards of less than 5 ppb, and medical surveillance monitoring of workers (71, 72). A retrospective analysis of workers' compensation data showed that this prevention strategy had been followed by a reduction in accepted OA claims for isocyanates from 1990 onward, whereas accepted claims for other causes of OA had remained the same (72). Moreover, for workers compensated for OA, the time lapse between the start of symptoms and the diagnosis was shorter, and the asthma was less severe than for other causes of OA (73). Later similar studies in Ontario showed an ongoing reduction (74).

Similarly, a Quebec monitoring program in nearly 3000 workers exposed to diisocyanates, mainly body shop workers, showed earlier diagnosis of OA at a less severe stage as assessed by bronchial responsiveness. Two years after diagnosis, these workers had a better prognosis in terms of clinical remission of asthma and responsiveness (53). Moreover, the median cost for permanent impairment two years after diagnosis was reduced by nearly half. For more details, see Chapter 14.

Platinum salts
There is no study which examined the effectiveness of primary preventive measures in platinum salt asthma, with the exception of one study showing that allergy was completely avoided after substitution of chloroplatinates by tetraamine platinum dichloride (75).

Secondary prevention by medical surveillance programs has a long tradition in precious metals refineries. It has been shown in prospective cohort study in a catalyst production that immediate removal from exposure after SPT conversion from negative to positive resulted in an excellent prognosis (76). The importance of immediate removal from the workplace—preferably immediately after SPT conversion to positive—is also highlighted by a more recent retrospective longitudinal study of 96 German workers with sensitization to platinum salts. Workers included in this "real-life study" had a much worse prognosis but had not been removed from exposure until they reported asthma symptoms, and there was no association of outcomes with the duration of symptomatic exposure duration (77). For more details see Chapter 16.

TABLE 10.2 Secondary Prevention Studies (Coupled or Not with Primary Prevention) in Asthma in the Workplace

Type	Number of Subjects	Country/Province	Methods	Principal Results	References
Enzymes					
Longitudinal study for 7 yrs (1968–1975) (all subjects)	1642	UK	Skin test, questionnaire, spirometry, and every 6 months systematic follow-up Environmental component (encapsulation)	Incidence of sensitization to enzyme alcalase: 18% Diminution in incidence after 18 months Atopic subjects at risk Diminution of incidence of sensitization coincides with diminution of exposure	*1. Juniper, 1977*
Flour (alpha-amylase)					
Longitudinal observational study for 9 yrs (1993–2002) Systematic follow-up during the past 5 yrs of all employees	˜3450/yr	UK	Skin test, questionnaire, environmental approach	Incidence of symptomatic sensitization more important in bread department (amylase) Diminution of incidence from $2085/10^6$ workers during the first 5 yrs to $330/10^6$ millions	*2. Smith, 2004*
Latex					
Observational study for 5 yrs (1994–1999) (cases reported on a voluntary basis)	8000	Ontario	Environmental approach, teaching, voluntary medical surveillance	Diminution of cases from 25 (1994) to only 1 case in 1999	*3. Tarlo, 2001*
Observational study for 5 yrs (1996–2001) (cases with self-report)	3×10^6	Germany	Environmental approach Diffusion of information to workers	Diminution of reported cases from 90 in 1996 to 18 in 2001	*4. Allmers, 2002*
Laboratory animals					
Longitudinal study for 4 yrs (1991–1995) (all subjects)	159	US	Environmental approach Diffusion of information Systematic follow-up component	Diminution of incidence of 10.3% (1992) to 0% in 1994 and 1995	*5. Fisher, 1998*
Platinum salts					
Prospective cohort for 5 yrs (cases, sensitized compared to controls (nonsensitized)	159	Germany	Medical surveillance by questionnaire, skin tests, and spirometry If skin sensitization, worker is transferred Reassessment and comparison with 1:3 sensitized/ nonsensitized subjects	14 cases of sensitization vs 42 controls Loss or diminution of sensitization for all cases Symptoms, spirometry, bronchial responsiveness nondifferent in cases and controls at follow-up	*6. Merget, 1998*
Isocyanates					
Observational study from 1967–1992 (chemical plant of TDI)	313 cases and 158 controls	US	Environmental and medical surveillance	Diminution of number of visits to the clinical from 20.5 to 1 per 100 employment yrs Incidence of OA to TDI reduced from 1.8% to 0.7% Initial fall in FEV_1 with correction later	*7. Ott, 2000*
Cases of WSIB applications for OA	Variable	Ontario	Environmental and medical surveillance started in Ontario in 1983 for isocyanates; medical assessment and spirometry baseline each yr	Increase in number of cases from 1983 (n=5) to 1988–1990 (n=50–60) with diminution (n=20) with stable number (n=˜40) 1987–1993 for other causal agents OA to isocyanates less important for 1987–1993 period than for 1980–1986 period	*8. Radon, 2006*

Prospective follow-up of body shop workers (1995–2000) in 400 garages	~3000 per year	UK	Medical surveillance, questionnaire, and spirometry	Identification of 40 cases per year Cases referred: 20 cases saw a specialist; 9 confirmed cases of OA	*9. Mackie, 2008*
Prospective follow-up of body shop workers (2000–2004) (cases and controls referred by standard method)	2897	Quebec	Medical and environmental surveillance	Confirmation of 20 cases Cases of OA less affected in the same period at diagnosis and follow-up (2 yrs) vs controls Lower costs for impairment	*10. Labrecque, 2011*

Abbreviations: FEV$_1$, forced expiratory volume in 1 second; OA, occupational asthma; TDI, toluene diisocyanate; WSIB, Workplace Safety and Insurance Board of Ontario.

References: 1. *Juniper CP, et al. Bacillus subtilis enzymes: a 7-year clinical, epidemiological and immunological study of an industrial allergen. J Soc Occup Med. 1977;27:3–12;* 2. *Smith TA. Preventing baker's asthma: an alternative strategy. Occup Med. 2004;54:21–7;* 3. *Tarlo SM, et al. Outcomes of a natural rubber latex control program in an Ontario teaching hospital. J Allergy Clin Immunol. 2001;108:628–33;* 4. *Allmers H, et al. Primary prevention of natural rubber latex allergy in the German health care system through education and intervention. J Allergy Clin Immunol. 2002;110:318–23;* 5. *Fisher R, et al. Prevention of laboratory animal allergy. J Occup Env Med. 1998;40:609–13;* 6. *Merget R, et al. Effectiveness of a medical surveillance program for the prevention of occupational asthma caused by platinum salts: a nested case-control study. J Allergy Clin Immunol. 2001;107:707–12;* 7. *Ott MG, et al. Respiratory health surveillance in a toluene di-isocyanate production unit, 1967–97: clinical observations and lung function analyses. Occup Environ Med. 2000;57:43–52;* 8. *Radon K, et al. Do respiratory symptoms predict job choices in teenagers? Eur Respir J. 2006;27:774–8;* 9. *Mackie J. Effective health surveillance for occupational asthma in motor vehicle repair. Occup Med(Lond). 2008;58:551–5;* 10. *Labrecque M, et al. Medical surveillance programme for diisocyanate exposure. Occup Environ Med. 2011;68:302–7.*

Flours

The topic of prevention of occupational allergies in bakers has been extensively covered in a recent authoritative article (78). Meijster and colleagues reported the effectiveness of three different strategies to reduce OAA in bakers using a dynamic population-based model (79). This is one of the earliest studies to quantify the effect of prevention. The strategies evaluated were (1) industry-wide hygiene measures to reduce exposures, (2) health surveillance to identify workers sensitized to wheat and fungal alpha-amylase followed by immediate 90% reduction in exposures, and (3) pre-employment screening for atopy with atopic individuals not being hired. Hygiene measures and health surveillance strategies both showed significant reductions in disabling asthma and lower respiratory symptoms over the 20-year simulation period. Atopy screening at hiring showed little effect. By comparison, a randomized intervention that used several types of environmental control measures conducted in South Africa showed up to 80% reduction in flour dust and cereal antigen exposure (45). Smith and colleagues (80) reported results of a medical surveillance program carried out among workers exposed to cereal flours and alpha-amylase in industrial mills and bakeries over a 10-year period aimed at reducing exposure. Follow-up showed a reduction in the annual incidence of sensitization associated with respiratory symptoms of 21 to 4 per 10,000 workers. For more details, see Chapter 12.

Laboratory animals

The available studies showing the effect of prevention measures on OAA from laboratory animals is limited. What evidence is available seems to show a reduction in incidence of laboratory animal allergy can be achieved when following well-designed workplace management practices. Measures reported to be effective include regular training of workers on the hazard, use of PPE, individual cage ventilation or cage filters, HEPA room ventilation, use of dust-free bedding and HEPA vacuums, and medical surveillance (81, 82). For more details, see Chapter 13.

Tertiary prevention

Avoidance of exposure: complete or partial?

Once the diagnosis of OA is made, the worker should stop exposure rapidly. The delay between the onset of symptoms at work and removal is generally too long, which likely explains the persistence of asthma in the majority of workers diagnosis with OA. Too often, asthmatic subjects are not questioned on their workplace and are prescribed powerful inhaled steroid preparations, which may mask the symptomatology and delay consultation. Although complete removal from exposure may represent the ideal situation, practical issues may make this impossible. Therefore, one can consider partial removal since there are discrepancies on whether or not complete removal leads to a more satisfactory clinical and functional outcome (25, 40, 83).

Anti-inflammatory medication

Only one clinical trial has examined the effect of anti-inflammatory medication in addition to the cessation of exposure (84). In a crossover study that included 32 subjects with OA and removed from exposure who took either active preparation (1000 μg of beclomethasone daily) administered for 12 months followed by placebo for 6 months or vice versa, the authors showed that initiation of treatment with the active preparation followed by placebo resulted in better outcome.

Public health perspective

Continuous surveillance of data relevant to OA is essential for development of preventive public health strategies. This includes the systematic collection of data on incidence and causes of disease. Surveillance data may be obtained using various sources: (i) schemes collecting data on sentinel cases, (ii) occupational disease registers, (iii) medicolegal statistics, (iv) incidence studies in high-risk workplaces, and (v) general population studies on incidence of asthma in relation to occupation. All these sources of information are useful for public health (Chapter 3). Harber and Leroy have proposed that computer and information systems can substantially improve the efficiency of data sharing among key stakeholders represented by workers, employers, insurers, practitioners, and public health organizations (85). Decision-making algorithms and internet applications, in addition to current approaches, can be useful for the diagnosis and prevention of occupational respiratory diseases (85).

WORKPLACE SCENARIO

Regarding the second part of the workplace scenario proposed at the beginning of this chapter, it is mentioned that a small group of workers in a carpet and underlay industry complained of nasal and respiratory symptoms. Two approaches should be carried out in parallel: First, obtain detailed information on the content of all products used to produce carpets. If there is a sensitizing agent, most likely a diisocyanate, contact an industrial hygienist in order to reduce the levels of exposure by appropriate ventilation, confine procedures in well-ventilated rooms, and arrange use of appropriate respirators (air supplied and not only cartridge masks). Second, plan a cross-sectional assessment of at-risk workers by defining first the sample of workers at risk of exposure (beginning with the groups with highest exposure). Organize meetings with the workers followed by individual interviews if needed to inform them regarding the symptoms and consequences of possible OA and the surveillance interventions that are suggested (questionnaires, spirometry, and bronchial hyperresponsiveness). Referral to specialists can be considered afterward if required. Finally, there should be provision for repeating the assessments periodically.

For the workers with OA, tertiary prevention will include the possibility of offering a job in which they will no longer be exposed to the causal agent (and initiating compensation claims on their behalf if appropriate). In some instances, it might be possible to offer another job in which exposure is avoided or reduced by workers wearing a positive pressure mask for a limited period of time. If the workers no longer exposed remain with clinical asthma and increased bronchial responsiveness, inhaled steroids are recommended and particularly beneficial if they are taken as soon as possible after diagnosis. A medical follow-up visit is recommended 2 years after ending exposure to assess the severity of residual asthma and the need for medication, spirometry, and bronchial responsiveness (permanent disability assessment for compensation).

Conclusion and research needs

- Primary prevention targeted toward the reduction in exposure is effective in reducing the incidence of OA.
- Secondary medical surveillance for OA among workers at risk appears to be effective, although to a lesser extent than reducing exposure. More studies should be planned.
- Tools to evaluate the effectiveness of exposure reduction in OA cases should be assessed (e.g. are noninvasive parameters like FeNO better predictors of insufficient measures than symptoms or lung function?).

References

1. Cullinan P, Tarlo S, Nemery B. The prevention of occupational asthma. Eur Respir J. 2003;22:853–60.
2. Heederik D, Henneberger PK, Redlich CA, et al. Primary prevention: exposure reduction, skin exposure and respiratory protection. Eur Respir Rev. 2012;21:112–24.
3. Seed MJ, Agius RM. Progress with structure-activity relationship modelling of occupational chemical respiratory sensitizers. Curr Opin Allergy Clin Immunol. 2017;17:64–71.
4. Heederik D. Are we closer to developing threshold limit values for allergens in the workplace? Curr Opin Allergy Clin Immunol. 2001;1:185–9.
5. Baatjies R, Meijster T, Heederik D, et al. Exposure-response relationships for inhalant wheat allergen exposure and asthma. Occup Environ Med. 2015;72:200–7.
6. Heederik DJJ. Towards evidence-informed occupational exposure limits for enzymes. Ann Work Expo Health. 2019;63(4):371–4.
7. Collins JJ, Anteau S, Conner PR, et al. Incidence of occupational asthma and exposure to toluene diisocyanate in the United States toluene diisocyanate production industry. J Occup Environ Med. 2017;59(12):S22–S7.
8. Cullinan P, Muñoz X, Suojalehto H, et al. Occupational lung diseases: from old and novel exposures to effective preventive strategies. Lancet Respir Med. 2017;5:445–55.
9. Agius RM, Nee J, McGovern B, et al. Structure activity hypothesis in occupational asthma caused by low molecular weight substances. Ann Occup Hyg. 1991;35:129–37.
10. Sullivan KM, Enoch SJ, Ezendam J, et al. An adverse outcome pathway for sensitization of the respiratory tract by low-molecular-weight chemicals: building evidence to support the utility of in vitro and in silico methods in a regulatory context. Appl In Vitro Toxicol. 2017;3:213–26.
11. Sarlo K, Clark ED. A tier approach for evaluating the respiratory allergenicity of low molecular weight chemicals. Fund Appl Toxicol. 1992;18:107–14.
12. Jarvis J, Seed MJ, Stocks SJ, et al. A refined QSAR model for prediction of chemical asthma hazard. Occup Med (Lond). 2015;65:659–66.
13. Seed MJ, Cullinan P, Agius RM. Methods for the prediction of low-molecular-weight occupational respiratory sensitizers. Curr Opin Allergy Iimmunol. 2008;8:103-9
14. Dik S, Ezendam J, Cunningham AR, et al. Evaluation of in silico models for the identification of respiratory sensitizers. Toxicol Sci. 2014;142(2):385–94.
15. Heederik D, Houba R, Liss GM, et al. Protecting the worker and modifying the work environment. In: Asthma in the Workplace, 4th ed. CRC Press; 2013: Chapter 11, 138–49.
16. European Union. European Chemicals Agency (ECHA). Understanding REACH. echaeuropaeu.
17. Suleiman AM, Svendsen KV. Are safety data sheets for cleaning products used in Norway a factor contributing to the risk of workers exposure to chemicals? Int J Occup Med Environ Health. 2014;27(5):840–53.
18. Wogalter MS, Conzola VC, Smith-Jackson TL. Research-based guidelines for warning design and evaluation. Appl Ergon. 2002;33(3):219–30.
19. Laughery KR. Safety communications: warnings. Appl Ergon. 2006;37(4):467–78.
20. Nicol AM, Hurrell AC, Wahyuni D, et al. Accuracy, comprehensibility, and use of material safety data sheets: a review. Am J Ind Med. 2008;51(11):861–76.
21. Bernstein JA. Material safety data sheets: are they reliable in identifying human hazards? J Allergy Clin Immunol. 2002;110:35–8.
22. Saito R, Virji MA, Henneberger PK, et al. Characterization of cleaning and disinfecting tasks and product use among hospital occupations. Am J Ind Med. 2015;58(1):101–11.
23. Lemière C, Bernstein DI. Occupational asthma: management, prognosis, and prevention. UpToDate. 2020.
24. Nicholson PJ, Cullinan P, Newman Taylor AJ, et al. Evidence based guidelines for the prevention, identification, and management of occupational asthma. Occup Environ Med. 2005;62:290–9.
25. Henneberger PK, Patel JR, de Groene GJ, et al. Workplace interventions for treatment of occupational asthma. Cochrane Database Syst Rev. 2019;8(10):Cd006308.
26. CDC. Respirator Trusted-Source Information. https://wwwcdcgov/niosh/npptl/topics/respirators/disp_part/respsource1quest1html. 2018.
27. Casey ML, Mazurek JM. Respirator use among US farm operators with asthma: results from the 2011 Farm and Ranch Safety Survey. J Agromedicine. 2017;22(2):78–88.
28. Stave GM, Darcey DJ. Prevention of laboratory animal allergy in the United States: a national survey. J Occup Environ Med. 2012;54:558–63.
29. Ilgaz A, Moore VC, Robertson AS, et al. Occupational asthma; the limited role of air-fed respiratory protective equipment. Occup Med (Lond). 2019;69:329–35.
30. Clayton M, Baxter N. Air-fed visors used for isocyanate paint spraying–potential exposure when the visor is lifted. Ann Occup Hyg. 2015;59(9):1179–89.
31. Ceballos D, Reeb-Whitaker C, Glazer P, et al. Understanding factors that influence protective glove use among automotive spray painters. J Occup Environ Hyg. 2014;11(5):306–13.

32. Cullinan P, Lowson D, Nieuwenshuijsen MJ, et al. Work related symptoms, sensitisation, and estimated exposure in workers not previously exposed to flour. Occup Environ Med. 1994;51:579–83.

33. Houba R, Heederik D, Doekes G. Wheat sensitization and work-related symptoms in the baking industry are preventable. Am J Respir Crit Care Med. 1998;158:1499–503.

34. Raulf M, Buters J, Chapman M, et al. Monitoring of occupational and environmental aeroallergens–EAACI Position Paper. Concerted action of the EAACI IG Occupational Allergy and Aerobiology & Air Pollution. Allergy. 2014;69(10):1280–99.

35. Cocker J. Biological monitoring for isocyanates. Ann Occup Hyg. 2011;55(2):127–31.

36. Miedinger D, Malo JL, Ghezzo H, et al. Factors influencing duration of exposure with symptoms and costs of occupational asthma. Eur Respir J. 2010;36:728–34.

37. Tarlo SM, Liss GM. Prevention of occupational asthma–practical implications for occupational physicians. Occup Med (Lond). 2005;55:588–94.

38. Moscato G, Pala G, Boillat MA, et al. EAACI position paper: prevention of work-related respiratory allergies among pre-apprentices or apprentices and young workers. Allergy. 2011;66:1164–73.

39. Tarlo SM, Balmes J, Balkisssoon R5, et al. ACCP consensus statement: diagnosis and management of work-related asthma. Chest. 2008;134:1S–41S.

40. de Groene GJ, Pal TM, Beach J, et al. Workplace asthma interventions for treatment of occupational asthma: a Cochrane systematic review. Occup Env Med. 2012;69:373–4.

41. Beach J, Rowe BH, Blitz S, et al. Diagnosis and management of work-related asthma. Evid Rep Technol Assess (Summ). 2005;129:1–8.

42. Suojalehto H, Karvala K, Haramo J, et al. Medical surveillance for occupational asthma-how are cases detected? Occup Med (Lond). 2017;67(2):159–62.

43. Beauchesne MF, Levert V, El Tawi M, et al. Action plans in asthma. Can Respir J. 2006;13:306–10.

44. Fisher R, Saunders WB, Murray SJ, et al. Prevention of laboratory animal allergy. J Occup Environ Med. 1998;40(7):609–13.

45. Baatjies R, Meijster T, Heederik D, et al. Effectiveness of interventions to reduce flour dust exposures in supermarket bakeries in South Africa. Occup Environ Med. 2014;71(12):811–8.

46. Ghajar-Khosravi S, Tarlo SM, Liss GM, et al. Development of a web-based, work-related asthma educational tool for patients with asthma. Can Respir J. 2013;20(6):417–23.

47. Lipszyc JC, Gotzev S, Scarborough J, et al. Evaluation of the efficacy of a web-based work-related asthma educational tool. J Asthma. 2016;53(10):1071–5.

48. Pralong JA, Moullec G, Suarthana E, et al. Screening for occupational asthma by using a self-administered questionnaire in a clinical setting. J Occup Environ Med. 2013;55:527–31.

49. Wilken D, Baur X, Barbinova L, et al. What are the benefits of medical screening and surveillance? Eur Respir Rev. 2012;21:105–11.

50. Vandenplas O, Van Brussel P, D'Alpaos V, et al. Rhinitis in subjects with work-exacerbated asthma. Respir Med. 2010;104:497–503.

51. Moscato G, Vandenplas O, Van Mijk GR, et al. Occupational rhinitis. Allergy. 2008;63:969–80.

52. Brant A, Nightingale S, Berriman J, et al. Supermarket baker's asthma: how accurate is routine health surveillance? Occup Environ Med. 2005;62:395–9.

53. Labrecque M, Malo JL, Alaoui KM, et al. Medical surveillance programme for diisocyanate exposure. Occup Environ Med. 2011;68:302–7.

54. Suarthana E, Vergouwe Y, Moons KG, et al. A diagnostic model for the detection of sensitization to wheat allergens was developed and validated in bakery workers. J Clin Epidemiol. 2010;63(9):1011–9.

55. Mackie J. Effective health surveillance for occupational asthma in motor vehicle repair. Occup Med(Lond). 2008;58:551–5.

56. Taghiakbari M, Pralong JA, Lemière C, et al. Novel clinical scores for occupational asthma due to exposure to high-molecular-weight agents. Occup Environ Med. 2019;76:495–501.

57. Pralong JA, Lemière C, Rochat T, et al. Predictive value of nonspecific bronchial responsiveness in occupational asthma. J Allergy Clin Immunol. 2016;137:412–6.

58. Suarthana E, Taghiakbari M, Saha-Chaudhuri P, et al. The validity of the Canadian clinical scores for occupational asthma in European populations. Allergy. 2020;75(8):2124–6.

59. American Cleaning Institute. Guidance for the Risk Assessment of Enzyme-Containing Consumer Products. Accessed June 12, 2020. http://www.cleaninginstitute.org

60. International Association for Soaps Detergents and Maintenance Products. Guidelines for the Safe Handling of Enzymes in Detergent Manufacture. Accessed June 12, 2020. http://www.aise-net.org

61. Basketter DA, Kruszewski FH, Mathieu S, et al. Managing the risk of occupational allergy in the enzyme detergent industry. J Occup Environ Hyg. 2015;12(7):431–7.

62. Sarlo K. Control of occupational asthma and allergy in the detergent industry. Ann Allergy Asthma Immunol. 2003;90(Suppl):32–4.

63. Juniper CP, Roberts DM. Enzyme asthma: fourteen years' clinical experience of a recently prescribed disease. J Soc Occup Med. 1984;34:127–32.

64. Cathcart M, Nicholson P, Roberts D, et al. Enzyme exposure, smoking and lung function in employees in the detergent industry over 20 years. Occup Med. 1997;47:473–8.

65. Larsen AI, Cederkvist L, Lykke AM, et al. Allergy development in adulthood: an occupational cohort study of the manufacturing of industrial enzymes. J Allergy Clin Immunol Pract. 2020;8(1):210–8.e5.

66. Schweigert MK, Mackenzie DP, Sarlo K. Occupational asthma and allergy associated with the use of enzymes in the detergent industry—a review of the epidemiology, toxicology and methods of prevention. Clin Exp Allergy. 2000;30:1511–8.

67. Tarlo SM, Easty A, Eubanks K, et al. Outcomes of a natural rubber latex control program in an Ontario teaching hospital. J Allergy Clin Immunol. 2001;108:628–33.

68. Quirce S, Polo F, Figueredo E, et al. Occupational asthma caused by soybean flour in bakers—differences with soybean-induced epidemic asthma. Clin Exp Allergy. 2000;30:839–46.

69. LaMontagne AD, Radi S, Elder DS, et al. Primary prevention of latex related sensitisation and occupational asthma: a systematic review. Occup Environ Med. 2006;63:359–64.

70. Vandenplas O, Larbanois A, Vanassche F, et al. Latex-induced occupational asthma: time trend in incidence and relationship with hospital glove policies. Allergy. 2009;64:415–20.

71. Tarlo SM, Liss GM. Diisocyanate-induced asthma: diagnosis, prognosis, and effects of medical surveillance measures. Appl Occup Environ Hyg. 2002;17:902–8.

72. Tarlo SM, Liss GM, Yeung KS. Changes in rates and severity of compensation claims for asthma due to diisocyanates: a possible effect of medical surveillance measures. Occup Environ Med. 2002;59:58–62.

73. Liss GM, Tarlo SM, Macfarlane Y, et al. Hospitalization among workers compensated for occupational asthma. Am J Respir Crit Care Med. 2000;162:112–8.

74. Ribeiro M, Tarlo SM, Czyrka A, et al. Diisocyanate and non-diisocyanate sensitizer-induced occupational asthma frequency during 2003 to 2007 in Ontario, Canada. J Occup Environ Med. 2014;56(9):1001–7.

75. Linnett PJ, Hughes EG. 20 Years of medical surveillance on exposure to allergenic and non-allergenic platinum compounds: the importance of chemical speciation. Occup Environ Med. 1999;56:191–6.

76. Merget R, Schultze-Werninghaus G, Muthorst T, et al. Asthma due to the complex salts of platinum— a cross-sectional survey of workers in a platinum refinery. Clin Allergy. 1988;18:569–80.

77. Merget R, Pham N, Schmidtke M, et al. Medical surveillance and long-term prognosis of occupational allergy due to platinum salts. Int Arch Occup Environ Health. 2017;90:73–81.

78. Jeebhay MF, Baatjies R. Prevention of baker's asthma. Curr Opin Allergy Clin Immunol. 2020;20:96–102.

79. Meijster T, Warren N, Heederik D, et al. What is the best strategy to reduce the burden of occupational asthma and allergy in bakers? Occup Environ Med. 2011;68:176–82.

80. Smith TA. Preventing baker's asthma: an alternative strategy. Occup Med. 2004;54:21–7.

81. Bush RK, Stave GM. Laboratory animal allergy: an update. ILAR J. 2003;44(1):28–51.

82. Feary JR, Schofield SJ, Canizales J, et al. Laboratory animal allergy is preventable in modern research facilities. Eur Respir J. 2019;53.

83. Vandenplas O, Dressel H, Wilken D, et al. Management of occupational asthma: cessation or reduction of exposure? A systematic review of available evidence. Eur Respir J. 2011;38:804–11.

84. Malo JL, Cartier A, Côté J, et al. Influence of inhaled steroids on the recovery of occupational asthma after cessation of exposure: an 18-month double-blind cross-over study. Am J Crit Care Respir Med. 1996;153:953–60.

85. Harber P, Leroy G. Informatics approaches for recognition, management, and prevention of occupational of respiratory disease. Clin Chest Med. 2020;41:605–21.

11A

IMPAIRMENT AND DISABILITY EVALUATIONS
I. Psychosocial, Economic, and Medicolegal Aspects

Kim L. Lavoie,[1] Katelynn E. Dodd,[2] Jacek M. Mazurek,[3] Philip Harber,[4] Sheiphali Gandhi,[5] Paul D. Blanc,[6] Kjell Toren,[7] and Jean-Luc Malo[8]

[1]Department of Psychology, University of Quebec at Montreal (UQAM), Montreal, Quebec, Canada
[2]Respiratory Health Division, National Institute for Occupational Safety and Health, CDC, Morgantown, West Virginia, USA
[3]Surveillance Branch, Respiratory Health Division, National Institute for Occupational Safety and Health, CDC, Morgantown, West Virginia, USA
[4]Mel and Enid Zuckerman College of Public Health, University of Arizona, Tucson, Arizona, USA
[5]School of Medicine, University of California, San Francisco, California, USA
[6]School of Medicine, University of California, San Francisco, California, USA
[7]School of Public Health and Community Medicine, Sahlgrenska Academy, University of Gothenburg, Gothenburg, Sweden
[8]Hôpital du Sacré-Cœur de Montréal and Université de Montréal, Montréal, Québec, Canada

Contents

General considerations

In assessing the general "impact" or "burden" of health disorders or conditions such as asthma or occupational asthma (OA), one has to consider body functions and structure, as well as contextual individual and societal perspectives. Initially, considerations were focused on functions and structure by requesting physicians to assess "impairment." Even then, tools to assess alterations of functions were only proposed for pulmonary conditions that caused a restrictive lung defect or alteration in gas exchange, this being relevant for occupational pulmonary diseases (pneumoconiosis) due to exposure to inorganic dust such as silica and asbestos. Although scales have long been proposed for assessing impairment in the case of occupational lung diseases due to exposure to inorganic dusts, these were not adapted for asthma, a condition that shows an obstructive pattern, with features of reversibility when treated, and NSBH (1), its course being marked by instability (2) and long-term deterioration of airway caliber. Therefore in light of these characteristics, specific scales have been developed to assess impairment for asthma (3, 4). Moreover,

CASE HISTORY

A 32-year-old man is referred for disability evaluation. He was diagnosed with adult-onset asthma. He is using an inhaled steroid (in a combination product also containing a long-acting beta$_2$-agonist [LABA]).

He has been out of work for the past 2 years. At the time of his asthma diagnosis, he was employed as an auto body spray painter exposed to isocyanates and epoxy. He started that job after a high-school apprentice program and had respiratory symptoms for several years before a doctor told him he had asthma. No one told him that his condition might be work related. He had to give up his job after a few years because he missed many days due to his asthma. He found a job in a supermarket, but going in and out of the cold room made him cough, so he quit.

His current lung function shows a mildly reduced but highly increased nonspecific bronchial hyperresponsiveness (NSBH). In addition to his breathlessness and cough, he also expresses feelings of panic, depression, and hopelessness about his condition, including his economic situation. The garage he was employed in is owned by his brother-in-law.

besides considering the assessment of impairment, generally proposed by specialist physicians, in workers with OA, compensating and insurance agencies also take into account various aspects related to disability (psychosocial status, work- and non-work-related activity, societal participation, financial considerations, etc.). Therefore, the aspects related to quality of life (QOL), the psychosocial impact, as well as direct and indirect costs are also relevant to disability and will be addressed in this chapter.

The World Health Organization (WHO) has proposed a document on disability and impairment that includes the following statement:

"Disabilities is an umbrella term, covering impairments, activity limitations, and participation restrictions. An impairment is a problem in body function or structure; an activity limitation is a difficulty encountered by an individual in executing a task or action; while a participation restriction is a problem experienced by an individual in involvement in life situations. Disability is thus not just a health problem. It is a complex phenomenon, reflecting the interaction between features of a person's body and features of the society in which he or she lives. Overcoming the difficulties faced by people with disabilities requires interventions to remove environmental and social barriers" (5).

Impairment and disability

Definitions of impairment, disability, and handicap: Relevance and applications to asthma

While clinicians frequently use the terms *impairment* and *disability* interchangeably, these are two distinct, albeit interrelated, concepts. Clinicians may mistakenly characterize the former as "objective" and the latter as "subjective," yet this dichotomization offers little useful insights. Impairment refers to a measured decrement in function. In contrast, disability reflects how much the

impairment measured (for example, lung function impairment in respiratory disease) impedes or precludes altogether the individual's ability to perform expected daily-life activities, including work tasks. Therefore, disability is highly contextualized within the individual's environment.

Of note, these terms may also be confused with the term *handicap*. Handicap refers to the degree to which a person with a disability adapts to their impairment. Patients with asthma may have a handicap if their asthma impairs their lung function, that impairment negatively impacts their ability to work, and' affects their activities of daily living, and to adapt, they avoid specific types of employment. This chapter will not address handicap further, focusing on impairment and disability as constructs more relevant to the clinician assessing and treating asthma.

Impairment refers to a decrement in function below an expected norm. In respiratory medicine, this is particularly salient as physiologic testing standardly quantifies impairment in such terms. Classically, physiologic measurement of lung function relies on resting spirometry. In many cases, however, more sophisticated testing is performed. This can include lung volume measurements, the diffusion capacity for carbon monoxide (DLCO), and the utilization of oxygen at rest and exercise. The results of such testing are compared to the expected normative expected values for the individual based upon age, height, sex, and ethnicity to determine their absolute level of impairment.

The theoretical model underpinning modern thinking about disability is that this is a dynamic process in which impairment, through its impact on the individual in the context of life activities, leads to disablement. Consequently, disability is relative because of the full range of activities specific to an individual to which the disablement interferes (6). This distinction is particularly pertinent to respiratory disease in general and asthma in particular, given that the factors promoting respiratory disability transcend the results of physiologic laboratory testing. Examples include: the frequency and severity of acute exacerbations, medication side effects, and the necessity of recurrent medical visits, all of which disrupt an individual's daily work and life activities (7). Disability incorporates a spectrum of human activities. Vocations are particularly relevant, but so too are activities of daily living, both social and discretionary. For this reason, disability due to occupational respiratory disease, especially when uncontrolled, has negative impacts upon QOL (8–10).

"Work disability" represents a subcategory of disability pertinent to the compromised capacity for employment. The relative nature of work disability in asthma is easy to highlight by example. A person who develops exercise-induced asthma may become disabled at a job that requires running up and down the stairs; an identical twin with the same physiological impairment might not be disabled in a sedentary job. A similar scenario could apply to a person with asthma exacerbated by temperature changes whose job as a butcher involves frequent cold air challenges in the meat locker. More saliently, a person specifically sensitized may be disabled in a job when they cannot avoid the offending agent but could work in a similar vocation using a different work process, as in the case scenario presented at the beginning of the chapter (11).

The structure or organization of employment further complicates work disability as it pertains to OA. Jobs with minimal scheduling flexibility may lead to asthma disability due to the inability to miss days of work during exacerbations or for medical appointments. In contrast, a flexible work schedule or telecommuting would result in reduced disability, although the vocations may be indistinguishable. Again, this discrepancy reflects the relative nature of disability as it resides within the context of the individual's work environment.

Just as various methods of physiologic assessment can gauge limitations, work disability can be quantified by a wide range of measures. This can include disease-related cessation of work, change in job or job duties, lost work hours, or decreased productivity on the job (12). It is clear from the nature of these outcomes that they typically derive from a subjective report by the person with the disease (or absences documented by an employer or insurer), not the assessment of a treating clinician, another sharp demarcation from the process of establishing limitation.

Maintaining clear and distinct definitions of *impairment* and *disability* is crucial to developing a consistent and stepwise approach to the clinical assessment of the global impact of the disease on the day-to-day life of the person with asthma. These definitions are also critical to the medical-legal interface of clinical care, workers' compensation, and other social insurance support for disabled patients.

Overview of asthma morbidity in relation to disability

Asthma is a chronic condition that is relatively common among adults, manifested over a range of clinical severity. Thus, asthma carries the potential for morbidity sufficient enough to cause disability that affects many aspects of daily life. Moreover, asthma incidence and prevalence span the range of years encompassing working age, making it a disease particularly relevant to the specific question of occupational disability. Also of importance, the interplay between impairment and disability in asthma, as well as in other respiratory diseases, can be driven by multiple factors beyond the basic demographic features of disease. Asthma has another important characteristic with a major impact on work disability: the critical feature that asthma can be initiated de novo by exposures on the job or may be made worse by the conditions of employment. In addition, work disability also must assess the role that occupational factors are likely to play in worsening the manifestations of asthma, potentially leading to an even more pronounced work disability than already present.

The Global Burden of Disease study group has analyzed disability, defined as disability adjusted life years (DALYs), and mortality over time among multiple chronic respiratory diseases, e.g. including asthma as well as chronic obstructive pulmonary disease (COPD), pneumoconiosis, and interstitial lung disease (13). This worldwide assessment shows that for asthma, there was an improvement in DALYs for the period 1990–2017 as compared to other chronic respiratory diseases, where worsening health was observed. In addition, asthma mortality decreased in all socioeconomic groups, especially among men. Asthma mortality represents the most severe form of asthma exacerbation (and permanent work cessation). Other data show that occupational exposure to asthmagens is a strong risk factor for asthma mortality (14, 15). Nonetheless, there is no direct evidence that declining asthma mortality reflects a reduced prevalence of OA.

Based on US National Health Interview Survey (NHIS) data from the 1990s, 3.3% of US adults aged 35 to 64 years and 4.2% of those aged 15 to 34 years reported an episode of asthma or an asthma attack in the previous year, accounting for approximately 6,650,000 persons with this condition (16). Follow-up US NHIS data from 2001–2009 showed that the prevalence of current asthma had increased among adults from 6.9% at the beginning of the decade to 7.7% by 2009, 5.5% among men and 9.7% among women (17). It is important to note that the greater asthma prevalence among women compared to men above age 18 (as opposed to younger age) is a well-established pattern. A limitation of these data is that they include all adults above age 18 into older postretirement age and therefore are not restricted solely to those of working age. Data from the US National Health and Nutrition Examination Survey (NHANES) from 2001–2004, however, are consistent with these estimates, with a prevalence of current asthma of 9.9% among those aged 20–29 years, dipping to 7.1% among those aged 30–39 years, and climbing to 10.6% in those aged 50–59 years before falling off again in older age (18).

In adults with asthma, the relative proportion reporting activity limitations is substantial and in particular is impacted by comorbidity. For example, more than 8% of US adults with asthma reported 14 or more activity limitation days out of the previous 30; this proportion climbed to more than half of those with both asthma and serious psychological distress, with such comorbidity reported by 7% of those with asthma (19). Analysis of the Canadian Community Health Survey of persons aged 15 years and above found that 14% of those with asthma reported disability in the past 2 weeks due to physical health and 15.5% reported long-term disability specifically in terms of work limitations; these proportions climbed to 25% and 27%, respectively, among those with combined asthma and a concomitant mental disorder (20). Although these estimates are based on North American data, the phenomenon of asthma-associated disability being common and the substantial magnification of risk by comorbidity is likely to be generalizable.

Prospective data from Finland show that those with asthma alone have a 63% increased risk of long-term work disability; those with asthma and one other chronic condition have a 124% increased risk and those with two or more comorbidities, a 349% increased risk (12). Lower lung function, especially a reduced FEV_1, was a risk factor for all-cause disability pension (hazard ratio 1.7, 95% CI 1.2–2.2), adjusted for comorbidities, smoking, and body mass index (BMI) (21). This observation is further supported in a Finnish 10-year follow-up of 529 middle-aged persons with asthma, where comorbidities, especially gastroesophageal reflux disease, were associated with impaired work ability (22). Another Finnish cross-sectional study observed that in older workers, increasing age of onset of asthma was an important predictor for work disability (23).

Beyond comorbidity, there also is evidence to support the critical role played by sociodemographic factors in predicting individuals' and communities' health and well-being. The sociodemographic factors that have been linked to increased chronic disease morbidity and mortality in general include: age, sex and gender, education, income and income distribution, immigration status, civil status, and, saliently, employment status and working conditions (24). These factors have been shown to be significant risk factors for both the development and progression of various chronic diseases, including non-WRA (25). Though the impact of these factors remains relatively understudied among patients with OA, preliminary evidence suggests that they also are important to consider within the context of OA and warrant further attention.

Disability in adult asthma, including OA and work-exacerbated asthma

Asthma-related respiratory work disability can carry large consequences for work-life participation. Such respiratory work disability can take many forms. At one end of the spectrum, complete cessation of employment caused by asthma represents the most extreme manifestation of work disability. Altered presenteeism, that is, staying at the same job and with the same duties but with a self-assessed reduction in productivity due to asthma, can be placed at the other. In between fall disability in the form of changing job or job duties due to asthma or experiencing full or partial sick absence days. Asthma-related work disability occurs both among persons with OA and among those having asthma where the onset is unrelated to occupational exposures. In support of the latter scenario, work disability defined as sickness absence or disability pension utilization was significantly more common among persons with asthma exacerbations due to different triggering exposures outside work (11).

In a large prospective study by the European Community Respiratory Health Survey (ECRHS) comprising a European random population sample, it was found that during 9 years of follow-up, 4.9% of the subjects with asthma reported change of work due to respiratory problems, compared to 1.1% in the random control sample (26). Further, it was found that exposure to biological dust and gases and fumes in the subsample of persons with asthma markedly increased the risk of changing work because of respiratory complaints, compared to randomly selected population controls. Exposure to mineral dust (stone, quartz, sand, etc.), in contrast, was not associated with any increased risk for respiratory related change of work (work disability). Atopy was not a modifying factor in that study. In a large Norwegian cross-sectional study, job change among women due to respiratory symptoms was more common among certain occupations such as chefs, hairdressers, and cleaners (27). Among men, job change due to respiratory symptoms was seen among gardeners, sheet metal workers, and welders. Further analyses of occupational exposures show that both inorganic and organic dust increased the risk for respiratory-related job change. Severe asthma is a disease often refractory to therapy, and it will also affect a substantial subset of those with asthma. Severe asthma is clearly associated with work disability defined as self-reported decreased work ability (28, 29). In a Finnish cross-sectional study of 2613 adults with asthma, current asthma symptoms were a risk factor for both unemployment (OR 2.3, 95% CI 1.3–4.2) and work disability (OR 4.4, 95% CI 2.3–8.2) (30). These findings support the conclusion that work-related exposures induce asthma exacerbations, thus causing persons to change job duties or take a different position altogether.

In terms of sickness absence, the number of workdays lost by workers with asthma has been found to be related both to severity of asthma (31), and also to current exposure to vapors, gas, dust, and fumes, where such exposures seem to double the risk for respiratory sickness absence among subjects with asthma or respiratory symptoms (32). There are other studies indicating that employed asthmatics have reduced productivity (impaired presenteeism) because of their disease (33, 34).

Exacerbation of preexisting asthma is a scenario that has particular relevance to respiratory work disability. There are multiple studies indicating that occupational exposure to vapors, gas, dust, and fumes increases the prevalence of symptoms among asthmatics, hence increasing the risk for respiratory disability, a relationship affirmed in an American Thoracic Society Task Force report on WEA (35). Three studies are of particular relevance to this question. In a Finnish general-population based case-control study, workplace exposure to gas, dust, and fume (i.e. nonspecific exposures) and work in abnormal temperatures both increased the occurrence of asthma symptoms (36). In the previously cited ECRHS study, unplanned care for asthma was linked to high exposure to dust and fumes (37). Finally, in a Swedish general

population study, exposure to gas, dust, and fumes and to cold work also were associated with exacerbations of asthma (38).

Among workers with OA (work-caused asthma, as opposed to asthma unrelated in its etiology to workplace factors), longitudinal studies have consistently shown that OA is associated with a high risk of work disability, defined either as complete work cessation or reduced income levels (39). The magnitude of the effect appears to differ among countries, with the lowest asthma related work-loss rate observed in a Finnish population study (40).

In summary, both cross-sectional and longitudinal studies clearly have shown that persons with asthma are at increased risk for work disability defined in multiple different ways. Moreover, workplace exposures, disease severity, and comorbidities appear to interact with one another in promoting work disability.

Quality of life

Quality of life (QOL) is a construct to express an individual's perception of personal function in several domains (e.g. emotional, social interaction). Health-related QOL, specifically, subsumes these domains as they more directly encompass aspects of health and well-being. As used in this section QOL predominantly refers to health-related QOL, focusing on the individual and is distinct from the disease process itself. The assessment of QOL is often operationalized using standardized questionnaires or questions about self-perceived health well-being. Some health-related QOL questionnaires are asthma specific, while others are more general, for example the Short-Form-36 and Short-Form-12 batteries.

Published data convincingly demonstrate that QOL is affected by WRA (see Table 11A.1 for examples). An early study in 1989 reported that 70% of cases reported impacts on their social and emotional lives (41). QOL effects of WRA are generally greater than those of non-WRA.

A study of members of a community-based health maintenance organization using a simple telephonic instrument in the United States demonstrated that WEA has more effect on QOL than comparable asthmatics without WEA (42). However, a small clinical series of latex-associated respiratory allergies found only minimal impact on QOL using a modified Juniper scale (42). This anomalous result may occur because most of the cases were healthcare professionals and may have greater job flexibility than many other workers.

Because data are largely cross-sectional, the time course is poorly understood. Nevertheless, since some of the data are from cross-sectional surveys conducted several years after diagnosis it is clear that effects are long-lasting.

Causal pathways and interventions

Recent recognition of nonclinical effects indicate the need for posttreatment interventions (i.e. "quaternary prevention") to complement primary, secondary (screening), and tertiary (e.g. medication) prevention.

Future research is needed to understand the causal pathways among factors associated with QOL. For example, lower educational attainment may make it more likely to be employed by small employers or may affect future job flexibility. Longitudinal studies following transitions among disease, exposure, and employment status are needed to guide optimal interventions. In addition to single patient-oriented intervention trials, societal interventions are needed. For example, employers' willingness to accommodate and maintain employment can be responsive to legal requirements, such as the US Americans with Disabilities

TABLE 11A.1 Studies of Quality of Life

First Author/ Country	Year	Type	Condition	Findings	Comments
Venables (UK) (1)	1989	Follow-up survey 79 workers Various agents	OA	High proportion reported handicap ranging from 40% to 73% depending on activity	Suggests that clinical status and "handicap" not fully correlated
Malo (Canada) (2)	1993	Cases (n=134) matched to clinically and physiologically comparable non-WRE (n=91) Various agents	OA	Small difference in QOL when adjusted for asthma severity	Early insightful study
Al-Otaibi (Canada) (3)	2005	Case series 10 workers Latex	OA	Effect was small	Only latex as agent and may be atypical
Lowery (US) (4)	2007	Short standard questionnaire for WEA (n=136) and non-WRA (n=462) in a large general group	WEA	WEA worse in all domains of QOL Largest effect in social and concerns scales	Representative population base Female gender and lower education had worse effect
Vandenplas (European countries) (5)	2008	Review of other studies	WRA	Relatively few studies of QOL noted in the review	
Knoeller (US) (6)	2013	Large population-based study (~40,000) 9% with WRA	WRA non-WRA	WRA affected PR for all 4 scales in comparison to non-WRA WRA by HCP diagnosis had "limited activity" PR (value of 2.16)	More specific diagnosis (by HCP) had stronger associations than "possible WRA" Clinical asthma control did not affect association of WRA and QOL
Lipszyc (Canada) (7)	2017	Clinic series (77 participants) overall and in each domain	OA WRA	OA and WEA had similar QOL effects	Overall had "mild range" effect
Feary (UK) (8)	2020	Clinic series (71 participants)	OA	56% report "worse" QOL	

Abbreviations: CS, clinical specialty center; HCP, healthcare professional; OA, occupational asthma; PR, prevalence ratio; QOL, quality of life; WEA: work-exacerbated asthma; WRA, work-related asthma.

References: 1. Venables KM, et al. *Respir Med.* 1989;83:437–40. 2. Malo JL, et al. *J Allergy Clin Immunol.* 1993;91:1121–7. 3. Al-Otaibi S, et al. *Occup Med.* 2005;55:88–92. 4. Lowery EP, et al. *Qual Life Res.* 2007;16:1605–13. 5. Vandenplas O. *Expert Rev Pharmacoeconomics Outcome Res.* 2008;8:395–400. 6. Knoeller GE, et al. *Qual Life Res.* 2013;22(4):771–80. 7. Lipszyc JC, et al. *J Occup Environ Med.* 2017;59:697–702. 8. Feary J, et al. *Occup Med (Lond).* 2020 Apr 20.

Act. Availability of appropriate workers' compensation and job retraining must be arranged at a scale broader than the individual patient level. Causal pathway analysis may facilitate understanding (43).

Despite the intuitive appeal, it is still unclear whether clinical severity is an intermediate step in a causal pathway from WRA to financial/QOL consequences or if clinical severity is an effect modifier. QOL was worse in OA patients individually matched to non-OA patients with equivalent physiologic parameters (44). Thus, the difference in QOL was not due to disease severity per se. The authors postulate the difference would be even greater in countries that do not offer similar readaptation programs (44). A large US population-based survey showed that the strength of association of WRA with QOL was not affected by degree of asthma control (45). This contrasts with a large Canadian population-based study suggesting that adverse effects of WRA on productivity were much greater in those with poor asthma control (46). In WEA, the breathlessness scale had much weaker associations than did social or concerns scales of the QOL scale used, also suggesting clinical symptom manifestations per se were not the primary driver of QOL consequences of WEA (42).

In summary, WRA adversely affects QOL. The magnitude of effect of WRA is greater than that of non-WRA, and the effects are long-lasting. The adverse consequences of WRA are not primarily mediated through clinical severity. Better understanding of causal pathways in the future will greatly facilitate implementing successful preventive interventions at the personal and societal levels.

Psychological aspects

Overview

Significant psychological impacts are associated with the suspicion, investigation, and confirmation of the diagnosis of OA, as well as with the fact of living with OA, often with impairment in functional health that can be permanent. Most workers affected by OA have manual or blue-collar jobs (e.g. carpenters, bakers, spray painters, etc.), which are generally associated with less formal education and greater socioeconomic disadvantage, which in turn has been associated with greater psychiatric morbidity including depression, compared to workers occupying more white-collar or professional jobs (47, 48). This indicates that workers affected by OA may suffer from several potentially important health (and asthma) risk disparities that are associated with compensation issues (fear of losing a job with financial impact, becoming impaired/disabled, etc.) and social and economic inequalities, potentially increasing the risk for greater psychosocial impairment than subjects with non-OA.

Psychological impact of asthma

Psychological stress has long been considered an important asthma trigger, with references to asthma being related to emotional factors and being referred as a "neurotic affection" (see Chapter 2) warranting psychological interventions. Asthmatic attacks at night, which reflect an unstable condition, have been associated with "nightmares." Conditions mimicking or accompanying asthma, such as hyperventilation and vocal cord dysfunction, are also attributed to emotional factors. According to the American Psychiatric Association, "psychological factors affecting other medical conditions (PFAOMC) is a disorder that is diagnosed when a general medical condition is adversely affected by psychological or behavioral factors; these factors may precipitate or exacerbate the medical condition, interfere with treatment, or contribute to morbidity and mortality" (49). Asthma is among these conditions. A vast number of studies have demonstrated an association, causal or not, between asthma and various psychological factors that include various mood (depression, anxiety) (50) and panic (51) disorders, all affecting asthma management (52). Bronchi are innervated by C-fibers. Asthma is characterized by airway inflammation and there is evidence that a part of it is of neurogenic origin. Indeed, neuronal fibers close to the bronchial epithelium penetrate the basal membrane and are in contact with epithelial cells via transient receptor potential (TRP) channels (53), with the release of neuropeptides including substance P (Chapter 19).

Psychological impact of OA

Several studies have assessed QOL in subjects with asthma and OA as reviewed in this chapter. Questionnaires on QOL cover various domains, including emotions. With the availability of several psychological questionnaires (viz., psychiatric symptom index [PSI], Primary Care Evaluation of Mental Disorders [Prime-MD], Beck Anxiety and Depression Inventory [BAI, BDI], Whitley Hypochondriasis Index [WHI]), it became possible to examine various psychological impacts of OA. Yacoub et al. (54) found that workers with possible (at the time of investigation) and confirmed OA have higher levels of anxiety and depression. The most common psychiatric disorder was anxiety disorder, with 14 (35%) subjects having a possible (n=5) or probable (n=9) anxiety disorder. Levels of dysthymia (a chronic form of depression) were also high, with 22.5% of subjects having a possible (n=7) or probable (n=2) dysthymia (54). Two studies by Miedinger et al. (55, 56) assessed rates of psychiatric disorders and levels of psychological distress among 60 patients with OA 2 years after cessation of exposure to their sensitizing agent. They found that rates of mood (depressive) disorders were as high as 32%, with major depressive disorder affecting 13% of workers and 50% of patients experiencing clinically significant levels of psychological distress (55). One study of individuals with WRA found that depression was not only more prevalent among those with WRA (relative to those with non-WRA), but also associated with more adverse asthma outcomes (57). In a prospective study of 219 patients presenting to a tertiary center OA clinic (26% with final diagnoses of OA, 25% with final diagnoses of WEA), more than one-third had one or more psychiatric disorder (mostly anxiety and depressive disorders). Further, 7% had scores on the WHI indicating hypochondriasis, which was associated with a nearly four-fold lower risk of meeting the diagnostic criteria for any medical or asthma-related diagnosis, suggesting that hypochondriasis (a condition associated with fears of having medical illness without objective evidence) may account for a significant proportion of undiagnosable cases among patients presenting for evaluation of OA (58). Long-term psychological outcome is still impaired as assessed in a group of nearly 200 workers and seen up to 10 years after being investigated, the group with WEA (n=62) and OA (n=64) having comparable BAI and BDI scores (59). Lavoie et al. showed that patients with a psychiatric disorder at the time of OA investigation were nearly three times less likely to be employed 12–18 months postevaluation, irrespective of final diagnosis (OA, WEA, or no asthma), compared to those without a psychiatric diagnosis. Those with a psychiatric disorder at baseline also had higher rates of emergency visits (35%) compared to those without (19%), also irrespective of final diagnosis, indicating a higher degree of somatization in these patients (60). In a retrospective analysis of 77/166 workers seen from 10 to 15 years after diagnosis in two tertiary care clinics, 50 with OA and 27 with WEA, subjects with WEA behaved slightly less well than those with OA (61). Among 112 participants investigated for OA (40 with OA, 37 with non-OA, and 35 with no asthma), the drop in FEV_1 at the time of SIC was lower in subjects with OA and depression compared to subjects with OA and no depression. Depression was also associated with increased blood neutrophils and decreased blood lymphocytes, but only among subjects without asthma. This suggests that depression is associated with attenuated autonomic responses, particularly in participants with OA, and with dysregulated immune responses in participants without asthma (but who present with asthma-like symptoms) (62).

Psychological stress and psychiatric morbidity among persons with OA

The fact that OA is a chronic, debilitating illness that is caused by agents present in an individual's workplace may place an additional psychological burden in several ways. First, given the fact that symptoms are typically worse in the associated work environment, a diagnosis of OA often requires that workers be removed from the workplace, which may ultimately threaten the workers' ability to earn a living. These fears appear to be well founded and will be underscored in a following section on "Sociodemographic aspects". OA may not only affect income and employment opportunities but also have a detrimental impact on the workers' ability to perform valued life activities (VLAs), which have been shown to be related to psychological well-being in patients with a number of chronic health conditions (8). In a US population-based longitudinal study of which 139 subjects with asthma were identified, the mean proportion of activities affected out of 25 rated varied from 20% to 30% (8). It is likely that OA would be associated with similar, if not higher, levels of disability related to VLAs. These findings highlight the potential personal and financial burden of OA, and how a confirmed diagnosis of OA (even in cases where compensation claims are accepted) may be a source of significant psychological distress. Workers need not have a confirmed diagnosis of OA to experience the psychological burden of this disease. Simply experiencing asthma-like symptoms suggestive of OA may provoke anxiety about the potential consequences of a diagnosis. This includes being removed from the only work environment and culture a worker has ever known. Worker fears about the negative consequences of disclosing WRA symptoms and/or submitting a claim to workers' compensation might be associated with increased nondisclosure of symptoms to colleagues, perception of lack of understanding from managers (63), as well as to failing to file claims. Workers may even remain in their causative work environment, continuing to be exposed, just to avoid the negative social and economic consequences of an OA diagnosis (64). This, coupled with potential fears about how a diagnosis of OA may affect the ability to perform VLAs, may result in many workers not coming forward, "hiding" their symptoms, and remaining exposed to the causative work environment, at the costs to their health and well-being (65).

Sociodemographic aspects

Overall morbidity

Asthma is one of the most prevalent lung diseases. In 2016, an estimated 339 million people had asthma and 417,918 asthma deaths occurred worldwide (66). In the United States, an estimated 19.2 million adults aged ≥18 years had asthma in 2018 corresponding with a prevalence of 7.7% (67, 68). WRA accounts for an estimated 16% of adult incident asthma (69).

Gender differences

Gender differences in airway behavior are complex, occur throughout the human life span, and are related to biological (i.e. sex/genetics, airway structure/function, immunological and hormonal determinants) and sociocultural/environmental (i.e. gender-related) determinants (70, 71). In a meta-analysis of population-based occupational health studies, women had a higher risk for shortness of breath and asthma, while men had a greater risk of chronic phlegm and lower lung function, which shows that the manifestations of a disease are related to sex/gender (72). Current asthma prevalence among US adults is higher among women (9.6%) than men (5.5%) (67). Women with asthma have more frequent and severe asthma symptoms, increased activity limitation due to asthma, poorer asthma-related QOL, and increased healthcare utilization than men (73–75).

Although women's labor market participation is lower than men, workers with WRA are predominantly women (54%–60%) (76). This difference can be explained, in part, by differential distribution of male and female workers in different jobs, various responsibilities within the same occupation, different exposures, and varying exposure levels (71, 77). For example, men are more likely to work in the construction, agricultural, trades, and manufacturing sectors and women are more likely to work as professional (particularly in health and education-related occupations), service and sales workers, and clerks (76, 77). Also, women and men differ in the exposures associated with their WRA. White et al. reported that, compared to men, women were more likely to report exposure to miscellaneous chemicals, cleaning materials, indoor air pollutants, and mold and were less likely to report pyrolysis products, plant materials, isocyanates, and metals and metalloids (76). In a New Zealand study of workers, Eng et al. found that men were more likely to report exposure to dust and chemical substances while women were more likely to report exposure to disinfectants, hair dyes, and textile dust (77).

Healthcare and asthma medication utilization

Asthma is associated with a substantial burden, including lower productivity at work and school, and increased healthcare use. Individuals with WRA have more frequent physician visits for asthma, more emergency department visits, and more hospitalizations for asthma exacerbations than those with all other asthma (73).

WRA is more severe and less controlled than non-WRA and requires more medication to control (78). Dodd et al. reported that adults with WRA were more likely to be taking certain asthma medications, including anticholinergics, leukotriene pathway inhibitors, and methylxanthines, and were more likely to be taking two or more asthma controller medications than those with non-WRA (79). Proper management of asthma depends on several factors, including affordable access to healthcare. However, Knoeller et al. found that adults with WRA were more likely to experience a financial barrier to asthma care than those with non-WRA (80).

Measuring the current economic burden of asthma provides important information on the impact of healthcare utilization for asthma on society. Nurmagambetov et al. found that the annual per-capita incremental medical cost of asthma was $3,266 (in 2015 US dollars), including $1,830 for prescription medication, $640 for office visits, $529 for hospitalizations, $176 for hospital-based outpatient visits, and $105 for emergency room visits (81).

Employment, unemployment, and work productivity

WRA can cause permanent impairment, and patients are often advised to avoid or reduce exposure to the offending agent. Workers may leave their current workplace, train for a new position, or take early retirement, potentially leading to adverse social and economic outcomes including poor QOL (see section "Quality of Life"), decreased productivity (46, 82), and loss of income and unemployment (83, 84).

Gruffydd-Jones et al. found, on average, 9.3% of work hours were missed per week due to asthma symptoms, ranging from 3.5% (United Kingdom) to 17.4% (Brazil) (82). Study participants also reported a 36% productivity loss at work (i.e. both time off and productivity while at work), which ranged from 21% (United Kingdom) to 59% (Brazil). Among workers with WRA, Wong et al. observed a significantly greater productivity loss with impaired presenteeism and total productivity loss compared to those with non-WRA (46). The authors hypothesized that workers with WRA may work while unwell because they have reached their maximum allowable sick days and are unable to take further time off from work, or workers may not take sick days because of illness disclosure and potential fear of stigma from coworkers.

Changing or leaving jobs due to workplace exposure frequently results in loss of income and unemployment. Unemployment rates after diagnosis of WRA reported from various studies ranged from 14% (Finland) to 69% (United States) (84–86) and unemployment rate among individuals ever diagnosed with WRA was greater than among those with non-WRA (86). This variability in rates can be explained, in part, by differences in access to medical care and time from WRA onset to diagnosis (early WRA diagnosis favors recovery) (85); duration of exposure; opportunities to change jobs, re-educate, or take early retirement; compensation practices; worker education level; and asthma management and medication use (40, 80). Psychiatric disorders (anxiety and mood disorders) in workers with WRA also increase their likelihood of being unemployed (see section "Financial Impacts").

TABLE 11A.2 Key Considerations for Assessing Financial and Other Costs

Cost Elements

Direct Costs

  Health services

  Salary replacement

  Salary replacement and other compensation costs

Indirect Costs

  Lost productivity

  Absenteeism

  Labor replacement costs

  Opportunity cost

Nontangible Consequences

  Individual perception of health and social status (e.g. QOL)

  Workplace climate

Perspectives/Unit of Analysis

  Individual worker/patient

  Borne by worker personally versus paid by others

  Insurance costs such as workers' compensation

  Employers

  Society

Financial Data Sources

  Questionnaires to WRA cases

  Workers' compensation payments for accepted cases

  General payments for asthma care in patients with likely WRA

  Extrapolation from national asthma expenditures

Abbreviations: QOL, quality of life; WRA, work-related asthma.

Financial impacts

The impact of WRA extends far beyond direct clinical findings. Effects include economic consequences for the worker, family, employer, and society more generally. The impact on employment has changed little since 1989, when an early case series found 33% unemployed at 6 years, and 43% of those still working reported income loss (41). QOL (see section "Quality of Life") and economic impacts are closely related; this section describes the economic burdens, and QOL is described subsequently.

Methods of assessment

Categories of economic consequences are summarized in Table 11A.2. Costs may be described from the perspective of individual patients, employers, insurers, or society. Direct costs include medical costs for treatment and direct compensation costs. Direct costs are more easily ascertained than the indirect costs of lost productivity, lost income, transactional costs, and costs borne by other family members. Few studies employ standardized measures of productivity, absenteeism, and presenteeism (46). Intangible costs such as impact upon QOL and the reputation and latent liability of employers are difficult to monetize.

Data derive from varied sources that are not directly comparable. Each category has strengths and limitations as shown in Table 11A.3. Published data may underestimate the true cost since workers compensation payouts are limited to the minority of WRA cases awarded benefits. An indirect approach estimated $1 billion annually for treatment in the United States by apportioning 16% of the total asthma cost to WRA (87).

Financial consequences

Both WEA and OA have more adverse nonclinical consequences than general asthma (GA). Methods differ among studies; illustrative studies are summarized in Table 11A.4. WRA is often clinically more adverse and typically has greater healthcare costs and impact upon the finances of patients. WEA and OA have comparable financial costs.

In an 11 European multicenter study of SIC-confirmed OA, the prevalence of clinically severe asthma was much greater than for non-WRA (88). A review of several published studies found that loss of income from work was reported from 44% to 74% of subjects, without substantial differences between WEA and OA (89), and workers also used healthcare resources before diagnosis (73). Lower education, older age, and employment in smaller firms increase the adverse economic consequences (Table 11A.4).

Clinical disease severity is not the sole determinant of socioeconomic consequences. Studies suggest that social circumstances have greater impact than disease severity (89). A multicenter European case series showed that the severity was conditioned by factors such as the educational level of the patient (89). Spirometry results were similar in those employed and not employed at follow-up in Finnish cases of SIC-confirmed OA (90). However, payout from compensation schemes can be severity related, possibly reflecting the criteria employed (91). A study dissected the interrelationships between WRA and clinical asthma control with productivity, absenteeism, and presenteeism (46). It found that the independent effect of WRA itself was largely limited to those with the worst clinical control and acted primarily through presenteeism.

Removal from exposure improves symptoms, but studies from Canada, Finland, Italy, United Kingdom, and France show that diagnosis and removal adversely affects income (Table 11A.4).

How can costs be reduced? In addition to primary (e.g. reducing exposures) and secondary prevention (e.g. screening for early detection), economic consequences can be reduced by addressing relevant social and personal factors. Providing individual patient oriented medical services may reduce costs by addressing psychological consequences (60, 92) or facilitating remaining in the workforce (60). Differences in workers' compensation coverage for OA and WEA may lead to disparate consequences for the individuals (73). A comprehensive review in 2008 showed that long-term unemployment was lowest in Finland and Québec, which have "effective retraining programs" (89). In Finland, of the OA patients who were not working, most were on sick leave or in retraining rather than being truly unemployed (90).

How to assess impairment and disability in the compensation process?

General aspects of compensation for OA

Workers' compensation and related systems provide financial support, medical care, and facilitation of return to work. There are wide disparities between countries regarding the policies governing compensation for WRA, including eligibility, ascertaining causality, and evaluating the level of disability.

OA can be diagnosed more accurately by referring workers to a medicolegal agency with experts or a board of experts, although that is not always feasible. For OA, the diagnosis optimally is based on:

TABLE 11A.3 Data Sources

Source Type	Explanation	Examples	Strengths	Limitations
Specialized diagnostic centers	Regional centers specialized in WRA, often performing SIC	(1–4)	Excellent clinical assessment with minimal diagnostic misclassification Opportunity for in-depth assessment and follow-up	Most in Europe and Canada. Few in United States May be nonrepresentative, particularly for OA
Workers' compensation boards	Administrative boards of specialized positions conducting numerous evaluations at the request of the boards	(5)	Do not emphasize SIC and therefore may contain more WEA	No data on the majority of WRA cases who do not file a claim
General non-WRA asthma patients in clinical large practices	Identifies WRA cases among general non-WRA patients	e.g. asthma patients in an HMO (6)	Permits direct comparison of non-WRA and WRA cases from the same setting Likely to be representative	Significant probability of diagnostic misclassification
Community population surveys	WRA operationally defined among participants in large community populations service	US behavioral risk factor surveillance system (7, 8)	Least biased and includes persons with underdiagnosed asthma and underdiagnosed work-relatedness	General-purpose questionnaires or limited telephone interviews have potential for misclassification
"Ecologic studies" with no data about the individual subjects	Apportions total non-WRA costs from large (governmental) data repositories	Application of the US medical panel survey (9)	Very large medical expenditure database; not subject to local variation	No data on quality control Assumes WRA is similar to non-WRA Wise upon what estimate of attributable fraction
Data-linkage studies and "big data"	Cross-links databases with health, cost, labor, and employment data	Future possibility only	Allows precise granular data from multiple domains	Requires stringent personal confidentiality controls and collaboration from disparate agencies
Machine learning from EHRs	Use natural language processing and machine learning approaches to identify cases in large corpora of EHRs and associated data	Underutilized in occupational respiratory research in comparison to other areas of medicine	Avoids clinicians to diagnose WRA; detects novel relationships	Requires stringent personal confidentiality controls
Social media	Analysis of web information posted by large numbers of individuals	Amazon Mechanical Turk (MTurk) or Twitter analyses (10, 11)	Rapid, low-cost way to obtain diverse input Avoids a priori assumptions	Social media users may be unrepresentative Limited control over data quality May be computationally complex

Abbreviations: EHR, electronic health record; HMO, health maintenance organization; SIC, specific inhalation challenge; WEA, work-exacerbated asthma; WRA, work-related asthma.

References: 1. *Lemiere C, et al. J Allergy Clin Immunol. 2007;120:1354–9. 2. Lemière C, et al. J Allergy Clin Immunol. 2013;131:704–10. 3. Kauppi P, et al. Clin Respir J. 2011;5:143–9. 4. Feary J, et al. Occup Med (Lond). 2020 Apr 20. 5. Miedinger D, et al. Eur Respir J. 2010;36:728–34. 6. Lowery EP, et al. Qual Life Res. 2007;16:1605–13. 7. Knoeller GE, et al. Qual Life Res. 2013;22(4):771–80. 8. White GE, et al. J Asthma. 2013;50(9):954–9. 9. Blanc PD, et al. Am J Respir Crit Care Med. 2019;199:1312–34. 10. Harber P, Leroy G. J Occup Environ Med. 2015;57(4):381–5. 11. Harber P, Leroy G. J Occup Environ Med. 2019;61(6):484–90.*

a. Exposure at work to an agent that acts through an apparent or presumed sensitizing mechanism or history of exposure to an agent generated at abnormally high concentration and causing irritant-induced asthma;

b. evidence of a sensitizing process for HMW allergens (skin reactivity; specific IgE assessment);

c. physiological documentation of variable airway obstruction for periods at work and away from work and NSBR;

d. presence of airway inflammation (exhaled nitric oxide [FeNO] or induced sputum);

e. confirmation that exposure to the suspected agent in a hospital laboratory or at the workplace reproduces an asthmatic reaction that generally triggers NSBR and airway inflammation.

TABLE 11A.4 Work-Related Asthma Financial Impact Illustrative Studies

First Author	Year	Type	Condition	Findings	Comments
Venables UK (1)	1989	6-yr clinic interviews CSC	OA	33% not employed; 43% of those employed	High proportion also noted social and emotional had income loss consequences
Malo Canada (2)	1993	Case-control	OA	All left work and were receiving compensation	Discussed in QOL Section "Quality of Life"
Cannon UK (3)	1995	Follow-up study CSC	OA, WEA, non-WRA	30% earn much less income	50% report difficulty finding employment
Ameille France (4)	1997	3-yr follow-up	OA	44% left original job; 25% unemployed	Employment status outcome worse for employees in small companies and lower education workers
Moscato Italy (5)	1999	Follow-up study CSC	OA-S	Annual income fell 28% in those who left workplace	Removal from exposure was good for clinical measures but financially adverse
Lemière Canada (6)	2007	Clinic series CSC	OA-S and WEA	WRA had more healthcare visits than non-WRA	Very detailed clinical evaluations "WEA" cases all had been referred for SIC
Vandenplas Europe (7)	2008	Summary of multiple studies	WRA, OA, WEA	OA: 44%–74% have income loss 14%–69% unemployed	Worse employment outcomes with lower education, older age, and small companies
Miedinger Canada (8)	2010	Workers' compensation board	OA-S (SIC)	73% reported lower income after diagnosis	Defines cost from workers' compensation board view
Kauppi Finland (9)	2011	6-month status CSC (SIC)	OA (SIC)	49% not working, but only 2% unemployed	No difference in spirometry in those working and not working
Lemière Canada (10)	2013	Clinic series CSC (SIC)	OA-S, WEA	WEA and OA: similar costs before diagnosis Both WEA and OA had much greater healthcare cost than non-WRA	Remaining at same workplace more common in WEA (44%) than OA (23%) Benefited from linkage of clinic series to government healthcare databases
White US (11)	2013	National population-based sample	WRA	42% of WRA unemployed compared to 28% with non-WRA WRA more likely to state unable to work than non-WRA	Based on US behavioral risk factor study Unusually high percentage of asthma as WRA or possible WRA (48%)
Lipszyc Canada (12)	2017	Clinic series	OA, WEA	Income loss reported by 33% of WEA and 60% of OA More OA than WEA workers left the workplace	Directly compared OA and WEA
Wong Canada (13)	2017	Questionnaire including specific standardized productivity scales	WRA	Productivity, particularly presenteeism, worse for WRA than non-WRA with similar level of clinical asthma control	Unique study for its use of well-standardized productivity scales, but may have significant disease misclassification
Vandenplas Europe (14)	2019	Multicenter case series CSC	OA-S	Severe asthma appears more frequently with WRA and non-WRA and is associated with worse nonclinical effects	Sociodemographic characteristics influence outcome
Syamlal US (15)	2020	US Medical Expenditure Panel	WRA	Estimated $1 billion annual US healthcare cost	Included all persons with asthma
Feary UK (16)	2020	Follow-up self-reported impact survey	OA-S	24% unemployed; 78% had career impact	<50% filed a claim Despite adverse effects, 86% "glad diagnosis" made

Abbreviations: CSC, clinical specialty center; OA, occupational asthma; OA-S, sensitizer-induced OA; QOL: quality of life; SIC, specific inhalation challenge; WRA, work-related asthma; WEA, work-exacerbated asthma.

References: 1. Venables KM, et al. Respir Med. 1989;83:437–40. 2. Malo JL, et al. J Allergy Clin Immunol. 1993;91:1121–7. 3. Cannon J, Cullinan P, Taylor A Newman. Consequences of occupational asthma. BMJ. 1995;311:602–3. 4. Ameille J, et al. Eur Respir J. 1997;10:55–8. 5. Moscato G, et al. Occupational asthma. Chest. 1999;115:249–56. 6. Lemiere C, et al. J Allergy Clin Immunol. 2007;120:1354–9. 7. Vandenplas O. Expert Rev Pharmacoeconomics Outcome Res. 2008;8:395–400. 8. Miedinger D, et al. Eur Respir J. 2010;36:728–34. 9. Kauppi P, et al. Clin Respir J. 2011;5:143–9. 10. Lemière C, et al. J Allergy Clin Immunol. 2013;131:704–10. 11. White GE, et al. J Asthma. 2013;50(9):954–61. 12. Lipszyc JC, et al. J Occup Environ Med. 2017;59:697–702. 13. Wong A, et al. Asthma. 2017;54(5):537–42. 14. Vandenplas O, et al. J Allergy Clin Immunol Pract. 2019;7:2309–18. 15. Syamlal G, et al. MMWR Morb Mortal Wkly Rep. 2020;69(26):809–14. 16. Feary J, et al. Occup Med (Lond). 2020;70:231–23.

As for asthma, confirmation of the diagnosis of OA is too often made by clinical history alone. In many countries, for sensitizer-induced OA, medicolegal agencies rely on history of exposure to an agent present in tables of scheduled diseases and agents. Clinical history is sensitive but poorly specific. Adequate confirmation of the diagnosis is essential for the worker and the employer. Advising wrongly a worker to leave work because of the sole evidence of exposure to a known sensitizing agent and the onset of respiratory symptoms may lead to serious socioeconomic outcome for the worker and have financial impact for the employer and the public or private insurance company. Confirmation of the diagnosis is generally made by a combination of testing applied in a step-by-step approach and/or specific inhalation testing, the latter considered as the reference standard and the former nearly reaching the validity of specific inhalation testing (93).

Purpose of compensation process

The purpose of compensation is to assess temporary and permanent impairment. The temporary impairment, allocated when diagnosis is confirmed, makes the worker eligible for rehabilitation in which she/he can be offered either remaining with the same employer with ideally cessation of exposure to the offending agent, or finding or retraining into a new job, with financial compensation. This represents a very important aspect of the compensation, which has impact on psychological and psychosocial outcome as well as costs. Offering just a "lump sum" is not as satisfactory as allocating full social services.

Permanent impairment is allocated when the worker is in a steady asthmatic condition and has reached maximal medical improvement. For OA due to snow-crab, this occurs after 2 years (94) but information is lacking for other agents, although presumed to be similar, and is unknown for irritant-induced asthma. A first attempt to propose criteria (need for medication to control asthma; airway caliber; NSBH) occurred for workers with OA due to snow-crab and endorsed by the American Thoracic Society (ATS) and American Medical Association (AMA) (Table 11A.5). Although clinical and physiological indices generally seem to reach a plateau of improvement, inflammation and airway remodeling are still present long after (95).

WEA is managed differently by medicolegal agencies. In most countries, compensation is awarded only for asthma that has been caused by the workplace environment (i.e. OA) but not for WEA with exception (96). Offering temporary impairment seems an acceptable decision.

Apportionment refers to the allocation of responsibility for the impairment or disability among several sources. The medicolegal agencies should attempt to determine how much of the current dysfunction might be attributed to the work exposure, considering personal conditions (atopy and exposure to HMW agents, smoking). Another aspect of apportionment splits responsibility among several employers who may all have contributed to the illness.

Accommodation is the process by which workplace changes may ameliorate the work disability caused by WRA and/or OA. Accommodation may be provided by employers on a voluntary basis but several countries have specific laws requiring it. Several types of accommodation are relevant to WRA. Providing a completely different job may obviate ongoing exposure to a sensitizing agent. This is, however, difficult if the worker has highly specialized skills. Exposure control measures to reduce levels of dusts, irritant gases, or heavy exertion may produce significant reduction in workplace-related symptoms and are feasible for individuals with WEA.

Disability in OA

Assessment of disability is a complex process that considers the global impact that physiological impairment may have on the patient's functioning. Translation of impairment into disability is affected by nonmedical variables, including job conditions, age,

TABLE 11A.5 Rating of Asthma-Related Impairment

Impairment Score	Airway Obstruction (FEV₁ Post-BD)	Airway Hyperresponsiveness		Medication Need
		% FEV₁ Change Post-BD	PC20 (mg/mL) or Equivalent	
0	Greater than lower limit of normal	<10	>8	No medication
1	>70% of predicted value or lower limit of normal	10–19	>0.5–8	Occasional BD
2	60–69	20–29	>0.125–0.5	Daily BD or low-dose ICS (<1000 µg beclomethasone)
3	50–59	≥30	≤0.125	High-dose ICS (>1000 µg beclomethasone) or occasional oral steroids
4	<50	—	—	High-dose inhaled steroids and daily oral steroids

Summary classes of impairment: class 0—total score = 0; class I—total score = 1–3; class II—total score = 4–6; class III—total score = 7–9; class IV—total score = 10–11.

Abbreviations: BD, inhaled bronchodilator; ICS, inhaled corticosteroid.

Source: Table from Blanc PD, Harber P, Lavoie KL, Vandenplas O. Psychosocial, economic and medicolegal aspects. In: Malo JL, Chan-Yeung M, Bernstein DI. *Asthma in the Workplace.* 4th ed. CRC Press; 2013:169. Table derived from American Thoracic Society. Guidelines for the evaluation of impairment/disability in patients with asthma. *Am Rev Respir Dis.* 1993;147:1056–61.

gender, socioeconomic status, and factors related to QOL and psychological distress. Assessment of disability is a more administrative process that is generally managed by medicolegal agencies after they have received information on impairment that is examined by specialist physicians.

Summary

The psychosocial, economic, and medicolegal aspects of impairment and disability in WRA are complex and challenging. The diagnosis should be accurate but it is as important to consider medicolegal, financial, psychological, and ethical issues that have been presented and discussed in this chapter.

Research needs

- The socioeconomic consequences of WRA and its associated disability should be examined in well-powered, longitudinal worldwide studies, including in developed and developing economies.
- More data are needed on QOL and its interrelationship to disability, including in VLAs.
- Larger case series should better inform understanding of psychological illnesses among persons with asthma, especially in relation to working life. Intervention studies are needed to assess tertiary prevention efforts impacting WRA for work disability, including psychological interventions.
- The validity of criteria used to assess impairment should be examined; attempts should be made to improve scales; for this, there should be collaborative efforts of medicolegal agencies worldwide.
- Medicolegal agencies should try to set and validate factors to be considered in the assessment of disability.

Disclaimer: The findings and conclusions in this report are those of the authors and do not necessarily represent the views of the National Institute for Occupational Safety and Health in the case of authors Katelynn E. Dodd and Jacek M. Mazurek.

References

1. Chan-Yeung M. Evaluation of impairment/disability in patients with occupational asthma. Am Rev Respir Dis. 1987;135:950–1.
2. Harber P. Assessing occupational disability from asthma. JOM. 1992:120–8.
3. American Thoracic Society. Guidelines for the evaluation of impairment/disability in patients with asthma. Am Rev Respir Dis. 1993;147:1056–61.
4. American Medical Association. The pulmonary system. In: Rondinelli, RD, ed. Guides to the Evaluation of Permanent Impairment American Medical Association. 2008:77–99.
5. World Health Organization. International classification of functioning, disability and health ICF. Geneva, Switzerland: World Health Organization; 2001.
6. Verbrugge LM, Jette AM. The disablement process. Soc Sci Med. 1982;38:1–14.
7. Eisner MD, Iribarren C, Blanc PD, et al. Development of disability in chronic obstructive pulmonary disease: beyond lung function. Thorax. 2011;66(2):108–14.
8. Katz PP, Gregorich S, Eisner M, et al. Disability in valued life activities among individuals with COPD and other respiratory conditions. J Cardiopulm Rehabil Prev. 2010;30(2):126–36.
9. Katz PP, Yelin EH, Eisner MD, et al. Performance of valued life activities reflected asthma-specific quality of life more than general physical function. J Clin Epidemiol. 2004;57(3):259–67.
10. Feary J, Cannon J, Fitzgerald B, et al. Follow-up survey of patients with occupational asthma. Occup Med (Lond). 2020;70:231–4.
11. Karvala K, Uitti J, Taponen S, et al. Asthma trigger perceptions are associated with work disability. Respir Med. 2018;139:19–26.
12. Hakola R, Kauppi P, Leino T, et al. Persistent asthma, comorbid conditions and the risk of work disability: a prospective cohort study. Allergy. 2011;66(12):1598–603.
13. Li X, Cao X, Guo M, et al. Trends and risk factors of mortality and disability adjusted life years for chronic respiratory diseases from 1990 to 2017: systematic analysis for the Global Burden of Disease Study 2017. BMJ. 2020 Feb 19;368:m234.
14. GBD 2015. Chronic Respiratory Disease Collaborators. Global, regional, and national deaths, prevalence, disability-adjusted life years, and years lived with disability for chronic obstructive pulmonary disease and asthma, 1990–2015: a systematic analysis for the Global Burden of Disease Study 2015. Lancet Respir Med. 2017;5(9):691–706.
15. Torén K, Hörte LG, Järvholm B. Occupation and smoking adjusted mortality due to asthma among Swedish men. Br J Ind Med. 1991;48:323–6.
16. Mannino DM, Homa DM, Akinbami L, et al. Surveillance for asthma—United States, 1980–1999. MMWR. 2002;51:SS1–SS13.
17. Zahran HS, Bailey C, P Garbe. Vital signs: asthma prevalence, disease characteristics, and self-management education—United States, 2001–2009. MMWR. 2011;50:547–52.
18. McHugh MK, Symanski E, Pompeii LA, et al. Prevalence of asthma among adult females and males in the United States: results from the National Health and Nutrition Examination Survey (NHANES), 2001–2004. J Asthma. 2009;46(8):759–66.
19. McKnight-Eily LR, Elam-Evans LD, Strine TW, et al. Activity limitation, chronic disease, and comorbid serious psychological distress in U.S. adults–BRFSS 2007. Int J Public Health. 2009 Jun;54(Suppl 1):111–9.
20. Goodwin RD, Pagura J, Cox B, et al. Asthma and mental disorders in Canada: impact on functional impairment and mental health service use. J Psychosom Res. 2010;68(2):165–73.
21. Lindström I, Pallasaho P, Remes J, et al. Does lung function predict the risk of disability pension? An 11-year register-based follow-up study. BMC Public Health. 2020;20(1):165.
22. Hirvonen E, Karlsson A, Kilpeläinen M, et al. Development of self-assessed work ability among middle-aged asthma patients-a 10 year follow-up study. J Asthma. 2020 May;13:1–9.
23. Taponen S, Uitti J, Karvala K, et al. Asthma diagnosed in late adulthood is linked to work disability and poor employment status. Respir Med. 2019;147:76–8.
24. R Wilkinson, Marmot M. Social Determinants of Health: The Solid Facts. 2nd ed. Copenhagen: World Health Organization; 2003.
25. Mikkonen J, Raphael D. Social Determinants of Health: The Canadian Facts. Toronto: York University School of Health Policy and Management; http://www.thecanadianfacts.org
26. Torén K, Zock JP, Kogevinas M, et al. An international prospective general population-based study of respiratory work disability. Thorax. 2009;64:339–44.
27. Fell AKM, Abrahamsen R, Henneberger PK, et al. Breath-taking jobs: a case-control study of respiratory work disability by occupation in Norway. Occup Environ Med. 2016;73(9):600–6.
28. Eisner MD, Yelin EH, Katz PP, et al. Risk factors for work disability in severe adult asthma. Am J Ind Med. 2006;119:884–91.
29. Hiles SA, Harvey ES, McDonald VM, et al. Working while unwell: workplace impairment in people with severe asthma. Clin Exp Allergy. 2018;48(6):650–62.
30. Taponen S, Lehtimäki L, Karvala K, et al. Correlates of employment status in individuals with asthma: a cross-sectional survey. J Occup Med Toxicol. 2017;12:19.
31. Gonzalez Barcala FJ, La Fuente-Cid RD, Alvarez-Gil R, et al. Factors associated with a higher prevalence of work disability among asthmatic patients. J Asthma. 2011;48(2):194–9.
32. Kim JL, Blanc PD, Villani S, et al. Predictors of respiratory sickness absence: an international population-based study. Am J Ind Med. 2013;56(5):541–9.
33. Balder B, Lindholm NB, Lowhagen O, et al. Predictors of self-assessed work ability among subjects with recent-onset asthma. Respir Med. 1998;92(5):729–34.
34. Blanc PD, Trupin L, Eisner M, et al. The work impact of asthma and rhinitis: findings from a population-based survey. J Clin Epidemiol. 2001;54:610–8.
35. Henneberger PK, Redlich CA, Callahan DB, et al. An Official American Thoracic Society statement: work-exacerbated asthma. Am J Respir Crit Care Med. 2011;184:368–78.

36. Saarinen K, Karjalainen A, Martikainen R, et al. Prevalence of work-aggravated symptoms in clinically established asthma. Eur Respir J. 2003;22:305–9.

37. Henneberger PK, Mirabelli MC, Kogevinas M, et al. The occupational contribution to severe exacerbation of asthma. Eur Respir J. 2010;36(4):743–50.

38. Kim JL, Henneberger PK, Lohman S, et al. Impact of occupational exposures on exacerbation of asthma: a population-based asthma cohort study. BMC Pulm Med. 2016;16(1):148.

39. Vandenplas O, Toren K, Blanc P. Health and socioeconomic impact of work-related asthma. Eur Respir J. 2003;22:689–97.

40. Piirila PL, Keskinen HM, Luukkonen R, et al. Work, unemployment and life satisfaction among patients with diisocyanate induced asthma–a prospective study. J Occup Health. 2005;47:112–8.

41. Venables KM, Davison AG, Newman Taylor AJ. Consequences of occupational asthma. Respir Med. 1989;83:437–40.

42. Lowery EP, Henneberger PK, Rosiello R, et al. Quality of life of adults with workplace exacerbation of asthma. Qual Life Res. 2007;16:1605–13.

43. Lederer DJ, Bell SC, Branson RD, et al. Control of confounding and reporting of results in causal inference studies. Guidance for authors from editors of respiratory, sleep, and critical care journals. Ann Am Thorac Soc. 2019;16(1):22–8.

44. Malo JL, Dewitte JD, Cartier A, et al. Quality of life of subjects with occupational asthma. J Allergy Clin Immunol. 1993;91:1121–7.

45. Knoeller GE, Mazurek JM, Moorman JE. Health-related quality of life among adults with work-related asthma in the United States. Qual Life Res. 2013;22(4):771–80.

46. Wong A, Tavakoli H, Sadatsafavi M, et al. Asthma control and productivity loss in those with work-related asthma: a population-based study. J Asthma. 2017;54(5):537–42.

47. Theorell T, Hammarström A, Aronsson G, et al. A systematic review including meta-analysis of work environment and depressive symptoms. BMC Public Health. 2015;15:738.

48. Tsuno K, Kawachi I, Inoue A, et al. Long working hours and depressive symptoms: moderating effects of gender, socioeconomic status, and job resources. Int Arch Occup Environ Health. 2019;92(5):661–72.

49. Levenson JL, Dimsdale J, Solomon S. Psychological factors affecting other medical conditions: clinical features, assessment, and diagnosis. UptoDate. 2020.

50. Del Giacco SR, Cappai A, Gambula L, et al. The asthma-anxiety connection. Respir Med. 2016;120:44–53.

51. Favreau H, Bacon SL, Labrecque M, et al. Prospective impact of panic disorder and panic-anxiety on asthma control, health service use, and quality of life in adult patients with asthma over a 4-year follow-up. Psychosom Med. 2014;76(2):147–55.

52. Lavoie KL, Bacon SL, Barone S, et al. What is worse for asthma control and quality of life: depressive disorders, anxiety disorders, or both? Chest. 2006;130:1039–47.

53. Kabata H, Artis D. Neuro-immune crosstalk and allergic inflammation. J Clin Invest. 2019;130:1475–82.

54. Yacoub MR, Lavoie K, Lacoste G, et al. Assessment of impairment/disability due to occupational asthma through a multidimensional approach. Eur Respir J. 2007;29:889–96.

55. Miedinger D, Lavoie KL, L'Archeveque J, et al. Identification of clinically significant psychological distress and psychiatric morbidity by examining quality of life in subjects with occupational asthma. Health Qual Life Outcomes. 2011;9:76.

56. Miedinger D, Lavoie KL, L'Archevêque J, et al. Quality-of-life, psychological, and cost outcomes 2 years after diagnosis of occupational asthma. J Occup Environ Med. 2011;53:231–8.

57. Mazurek JM, Knoeller GE, Moorman JE. Effect of current depression on the association of work-related asthma with adverse asthma outcomes: a cross-sectional study using the Behavioral Risk Factor Surveillance System. J Affect Disord. 2012;136:1135–42.

58. Lavoie KL, Joseph M, Favreau H, et al. Prevalence of psychiatric disorders among patients investigated for occupational asthma. An overlooked differential diagnosis? Am J Respir Crit Care Med. 2013;187:926–32.

59. Moullec G, Lavoie KL, Malo JL, et al. Long-term socioprofessional and psychological status in workers investigated for occupational asthma in Québec. J Occup Environ Med. 2013;55:1052–64.

60. Lipszyc JC, Silverman F, Holness DL, et al. Comparison of clinic models for patients with work-related asthma. Occup Med (Lond). 2017;67:477–83.

61. Lipszyc JC, Silverman F, Holness DL, et al. Comparison of psychological, quality of life, work-limitation, and socioeconomic status between patients with occupational asthma and work-exacerbated asthma. J Occup Environ Med. 2017;59:697–702.

62. Paine NJ, Joseph MF, Bacon SL, et al. Association between depression, lung function and inflammatory markers in patients with asthma and occupational asthma. J Occup Environ Med. 2019;61:453–60.

63. Bradshaw LM, Barber CM, Davies J, et al. Work-related asthma symptoms and attitudes to the workplace. Occup Med (Lond). 2007;57(1):30–5.

64. Jong M, Neis B, Cartier A, et al. Knowledge, attitudes and beliefs regarding crab asthma in four communities of Newfoundland and Labrador. Int J Circumpolar Health. 2004;63(Suppl 2):337–42.

65. Howse D, Jeebhay MF, Neiss B. The changing political economy of occupational health and safety in fisheries-lessons from Eastern Canada and South Africa. J Agrarian Change. 2012;12:344–63.

66. World Health Organization (WHO) Newsroom, Fact Sheets. Asthma. Accessed June 18, 2020. https://www.who.int/news-room/fact-sheets/detail/asthma

67. U.S. Department of Health & Human Services (DHHS) CDC, NCEH. 2018 National Health Interview Survey (NHIS) Data. Accessed June 18, 2020. https://www.cdc.gov/asthma/nhis/2018/data.htm

68. US Department of Health & Human Services (DHHS) CDC. National Center for Health Statistics. National Health Interview Survey. Tables of Summary Health Statistics (2013–2018 NHIS). Accessed June 18, 2020. https://ftp.cdc.gov/pub/Health_Statistics/NCHS/NHIS/SHS/2018_SHS_Table_A-2.pdf

69. Blanc PD, Annesi-Maesano I, Balmes JR, et al. The occupational burden of nonmalignant respiratory diseases. An official American Thoracic Society and European Respiratory Society statement. Am J Respir Crit Care Med. 2019;199:1312–34.

70. Becklake MR, Kauffman F. Gender differences in airway behaviour over the human life span. Thorax. 1999;54:1119–38.

71. Moscato G, Apfelbacher C, Brockow K, et al. Gender and occupational allergy (GOA): Report from the task force of the EAACI Environmental & Occupational Allergy Interest Group. Allergy. 2020 Apr 12.

72. Dimich-Ward H, Beking K, Dybuncio A, et al. Occupational exposure influences on gender differences in respiratory health. Lung. 2012;190:147–54.

73. Lemiere C, Forget A, Dufour MH, et al. Characteristics and medical resource use of asthmatic subjects with and without work-related asthma. J Allergy Clin Immunol. 2007;120:1354–9.

74. Lisspers K, Ställberg B, Janson C, et al. Sex-differences in quality of life and asthma control in Swedish asthma patients. J Asthma. 2013;50(10):1090–5.

75. McCallister JW, Holbrook JT, Wei CY, et al. Sex differences in asthma symptom profiles and control in the American Lung Association Asthma Clinical Research Centers. Respir Med. 2013;107(10):1491–500.

76. White GE, Seaman C, Filios MS, et al. Gender differences in work-related asthma: surveillance data from California, Massachusetts, Michigan, and New Jersey, 1993-2008. J Asthma. 2014;51(7):691–702.

77. Eng A, Mannetje A, McLean D, et al. Gender differences in occupational exposure patterns. Occup Environ Med. 2011;68(12):888–94.

78. Le Moual N, Carsin AE, Siroux V, et al. Occupational exposures and uncontrolled adult-onset asthma in the European Community Respiratory Health Survey II. Eur Respir J. 2014;43(2):374–86.

79. Dodd KE, Mazurek JM. Asthma medication use among adults with current asthma by work-related asthma status, asthma call-back survey, 29 states, 2012–2013. J Asthma. 2018;55:364–72.

80. Knoeller GE, Mazurek JM, Moorman JE. Work-related asthma, financial barriers to asthma care, and adverse asthma outcomes: asthma call-back survey, 37 states and District of Columbia, 2006 to 2008. Med Care. 2011;49:1097–104.

81. Nurmagambetov T, Kuwahara R, Garbe P. The economic burden of asthma in the United States, 2008–2013. Ann Am Thorac Soc. 2018;15(3):348–56.

82. Gruffydd-Jones K, Thomas M, Roman-Rodríguez M, et al. Asthma impacts on workplace productivity in employed patients who are symptomatic despite background therapy: a multinational survey. J Asthma Allergy. 2019;12:183–94.

83. Vandenplas O, Henneberger PK. Socioeconomic outcomes in work-exacerbated asthma. Curr Opin Allergy Clin Immunol. 2007;7:236–41.

84. Dimich-Ward H, Taliadouros V, Teschke K, et al. Quality of life and employment status of workers with Western red cedar asthma. J Occup Environ Med. 2007;49(9):1040–5.

85. Gannon PFG, Weir DC, Robertson AS, et al. Health, employment, and financial outcomes in workers with occupational asthma. Br J Ind Med. 1993;50:491–6.

86. White GE, Mazurek JM, Moorman JE. Work-related asthma and employment status—38 states and District of Columbia, 2006–2009. J Asthma. 2013;50(9):954–9.

87. Syamlal G, Bhattacharya A, Dodd KE. Medical expenditures attributed to asthma and chronic obstructive pulmonary disease among workers—United States, 2011–2015. MMWR Morb Mortal Wkly Rep. 2020;69(26):809–14.

88. Vandenplas O, Godet J, Hurdubaea L, et al. Severe occupational asthma: insights from a multicenter European cohort. J Allergy Clin Immunol Pract. 2019;7:2309–18.

89. Vandenplas O. Socioeconomic impact of work-related asthma. Expert Rev Pharmacoeconomics Outcome Res. 2008;8:395–400.

90. Kauppi P, Hannu T, Helaskoski E, et al. Short-term prognosis of occupational asthma in a Finnish population. Clin Respir J. 2011;5:143–9.

91. Miedinger D, Malo JL, Ghezzo H, et al. Factors influencing duration of exposure with symptoms and costs of occupational asthma. Eur Respir J. 2010;36:728–34.

92. Lavoie KL, Favreau H, Paine NJ, et al. Prospective impact of psychiatric disorders on employment status and health care use in patients investigated for occupational asthma. J Occup Environ Med. 2016;58:1196–201.

93. Taghiakbari M, Pralong JA, Lemière C, et al. Novel clinical scores for occupational asthma due to exposure to high-molecular-weight agents. Occup Environ Med. 2019;76:495–501.

94. Malo JL, Cartier A, Ghezzo H, et al. Patterns of improvement of spirometry, bronchial hyperresponsiveness, and specific IgE antibody levels after cessation of exposure in occupational asthma caused by snow-crab processing. Am Rev Respir Dis. 1988;138:807–12.

95. Sumi Y, Foley S, Daigle S, et al. Structural changes and airway remodelling in occupational asthma at a mean interval of 14 years after cessation of exposure. Clin Exp Allergy. 2007;37:1781–7.

96. Tarlo SM, Liss G, Corey P, et al. A workers' compensation claim population for occupational asthma. Chest. 1995;107:634–41.

11B

IMPAIRMENT AND DISABILITY EVALUATIONS

II. Various Legislations

Mohamed F. Jeebhay,[1] Philip Harber,[2] Xaver Baur,[3] Marcos Ribeiro,[4] Hae-Sim Park,[5] Ilenia Folletti,[6] R. Hoy,[7] and Jean-Luc Malo[8]

[1]*Occupational Medicine Division, School of Public Health and Family Medicine, Faculty of Health Sciences, University of Cape Town, Cape Town, South Africa*
[2]*Mel and Enid Zuckerman College of Public Health, University of Arizona, Tucson, Arizona, USA*
[3]*University of Hamburg, Hamburg, Germany*
[4]*Section of Pulmonology, Department of Medicine, Health Science Centre, State University of Londrina, Parana, Brazil*
[5]*Ajou Research Institute for Innovative Medicine, Suwon, South Korea*
[6]*Department of Medicine and Surgery, Section Occupational Medicine, University of Perugia, Terni Hospital, Terni, Italy*
[7]*School of Public Health and Preventive Medicine, Faculty of Medicine, Nursing and Health Sciences, Monash University, Melbourne, Australia*
[8]*Hôpital du Sacré-Cœur de Montréal and Université de Montréal, Montréal, Québec, Canada*

Contents

Introduction—An international perspective

Occupational lung diseases due to inhalation of inorganic dusts, mainly asbestos and silica dusts, have principally and still represent the main concern of medicolegal agencies worldwide. In particular, mesothelioma and lung cancer related to exposure to asbestos dust are certainly the most important medicolegal issues due to the fact that these conditions are very often not amendable to treatment. Moreover, mesothelioma is reaching its peak frequency approximately since 2010. It is generally accepted that conditions that cause airway obstruction are less of a concern, although nearly 17% of the population risk of asthma can be attributable to the workplace (1). Moreover, asthma in the workplace affects younger workers than those due to inorganic dusts and has an important socioeconomic impact (2).

Medicolegal compensation of work-related asthma (WRA) covers two major aspects: (*i*) diagnosis, compensation, and readaptation of the worker at the time of referral; and (*ii*) long-term compensation for impairment and disability after the diagnosis.

First, with regard to diagnosis, schedules or tables of specific diseases, occupations, and etiological agents causing occupational asthma (OA) have been established by several compensation agencies. In those countries relying upon schedules, if a claimant develops a disease within the scope of an approved schedule, there is a strong presumption that compensation will be allowed. Therefore, there might be a lesser need for confirming the diagnosis with objective tools in the case where a worker with asthma is exposed to an agent that is on a list. On the other hand, if a worker claims for a disease not on the list, the presumption against compensation for that disease may direct the worker to seek other sources of social assistance if there is no possibility of changing the decision by confirming the diagnosis with objective tools. To ensure an even-handed approach when compensation is based on restrictive lists of diseases, it is essential that these lists be upgraded at frequent intervals to accommodate the regular addition of new agents causing OA or, alternatively, to allow for accepting claims if objective tools are used to confirm the diagnosis. Inequalities in such systems could arise if, despite evolving medical evidence, legislative revision of the list does not occur due to sociopolitical factors or the absence of an additional open clause to deal with agents that do not appear on the accepted list but for which objective evidence exists in support of a particular case.

Since such lists were deemed to be overly restrictive and were generally not amended in a timely manner when new scientific evidence mandated a change, many agencies eventually abandoned the use of scheduling for occupational diseases. It seems reasonable to abandon referral to lists of at-risk occupations and causal agents (when workers have asthma and have been exposed to an agent present on a list, this does not necessarily mean that they suffer from OA), provided that diagnostic tools allow for establishing the relationship of exposure to an agent or in a workplace and onset of asthma. Currently, despite expensive and sophisticated diagnostic methods being available for most health conditions, OA too often remains undiagnosed and incorrectly or insufficiently investigated by clinical and functional means, with the risk of wrong diagnosis and delay in removal from exposure. Diagnosing OA solely on the basis of a medical interview is not to be recommended. Questionnaires are sensitive but not specific (3, 4). Medicolegal decisions are often made without objective medical evidence. This is often the case in countries where the medicolegal system puts more emphasis on the legal aspects and not enough on medical considerations.

Aggravation of pre- or coexisting asthma is not, as a rule, accepted by medicolegal agencies, unless the workplace-aggravating factor is clearly identified. For example, in the event of a contamination with fungi in a damp workplace, an atopic asthmatic worker may receive compensation for time lost at work due to exacerbation of asthma.

Second, compensation should cover two aspects: (*i*) relevant readaptation programs at the time of diagnosis to ensure especially that young workers are offered a new job with retraining if necessary and financial compensation; and (*ii*) compensation for permanent impairment/disability assessed approximately 2 years after cessation of exposure at work.

Medicolegal compensation for occupational asthma around the world

North America
United States
The United States has over 60 different systems. General classes are summarized below. The first two focus upon workplace causation, whereas the latter two are based upon functional impairment and disability:

1. Workers' compensation: Workers' compensation benefits are provided to workers by their employer. Each state in the United States has a different workers' compensation system, but they all provide salary replacement, medical care, and some form of vocational rehabilitation.
2. Tort: Tort cases require lawsuits. Tort cases may be filed by persons whose exposure did not occur in the course of their employment. Unlike workers' compensation, it is necessary to demonstrate negligence (e.g. an isocyanate product manufacturer did not provide adequate warnings).
3. Disability insurance: Disability insurance benefits depend upon the level of functional impairment, regardless of whether the asthma was determined to be caused by work. The largest provider is the federal Social Security Disability Insurance system, which requires that the applicant be unable to compete in the labor market.
4. Mandatory accommodation: The Americans with Disabilities Act requires reasonable efforts to reduce the occupational burden of a disability (5).

Benefits and criteria vary by jurisdiction. Some states have a single workers' compensation insurer, which is usually a quasi-public agency (e.g. Washington state). In other states (e.g. California), there are multiple insurers. Large employers typically contract to third-party administrators.

Each state has a workers' compensation board (WCB) responsible for implementing procedures. Physicians submit reports. All states consider reports from primary treating physicians, but some place restrictions upon the physicians who perform examinations to resolve conflicts of interest. Experience and knowledge of evaluating physicians is heterogeneous since there are no government-mandated national or regional centers.

Some states have implemented "guidelines," sometimes misinterpreted as de facto requirements, but these may be rebutted by appropriate information.

Many states' workers' compensation systems use standardized diagnostic and treatment "guidelines." Depending on the jurisdictions, they are advisory or almost mandatory. The widely used guidelines of the American College of Occupational and Environmental Medicine (ACOEM) go beyond treatment and include a practical table of default criteria for ability to continue work based upon functional severity and the exposure level relative to the Occupational Safety and Health Administration (OSHA) standard (the US occupational exposure limit, OEL) (6). Each workers' compensation system specifies how the extent of impairment will be classified. Many states use the American Medical Association (AMA) Guides (7).

There are several incompletely resolved compensation issues in the United States:

a. Disability without impairment: The US systems are based on the concept that functional impairment determines disability. However, in the case of sensitizer-induced OA, there may be no impairment unless the worker returns to the prior workplace.
b. Lack of a scheduled list of sensitizing or exacerbating agents: This fosters disagreement about whether a specific agent may do so and may discourage some physicians from diagnosing OA for less well-known agents. Furthermore, there is no common terminology for estimating the likelihood that one or more exposures have caused irritant-induced asthma.
c. Work exacerbation: In contrast to de novo development of OA after documented exposures to occupational agents, exacerbation of preexisting asthma is subject to variable assessment.
d. Assessing long-term consequences: Some state systems require the initial examining physician to specify the need for future treatment in addition to determining the current impairment. This requires the physician to speculate about the course of OA many years in the future. Other state systems, however, allow reopening or reassessing a case.

e. Treatment guidelines: In some states, treatment guidelines are advisory, whereas in others they are almost mandatory. Two widely used workers' compensation guidelines (6, 8) show differences with the AMA guidelines (7).

f. Work accommodation: The ability to modify working conditions is a major determinant of the impact of WRA upon the individual and their family, which mainly depends on the employer.

g. "Second injury" benefits: Second injury funds that are available in some states reimburse insurers or employers for part of the cost of disability/treatment when that is superimposed on a preexisting similar impairment (i.e. apportionable responsibility).

Canada

Compensation for OA in Canada is not under the responsibility of the country itself but, rather, of provinces. In all provinces, compensation programs have eliminated the adversarial approach and "neutral" professionals representing neither the worker nor the employer are assigned by the WCB.

All provinces of Canada have workers' compensation provisions and information related to four of these is listed in Table 11B.1. In Quebec, claims are examined by three chest physicians sitting on four committees appointed by the Minister of Labour. In a case of suspected OA, claimants are referred to one of the two accredited centers where claimants are further investigated, mostly by performing specific inhalation challenges (SICs). It is felt that by considering the working population (4 to 5 million), two centers are sufficient to maintain the quality of expertise without delays. In the event a claim is accepted, workers are referred for readaptation that may include studies in order to train into a new field (a program that may run for 1–2 years) and permanent financial compensation for loss of salary in the event of a lower salary for the new job. Workers are reassessed 2 years after diagnosis to set permanent impairment/disability. This is based on a scale that was developed in Quebec in the 1980s (9) and on the level of bronchial obstruction and responsiveness to methacholine as well as to the need for medication to control residual asthma. This scale is based on the same criteria that were subsequently proposed by the American Thoracic Society (ATS) (10) and the AMA (7). In other Canadian provinces, claims are generally examined by WCB authorities who can request further assessment by specialists. SICs can be requested but are generally not. Reactive airways dysfunction syndrome (RADS) and irritant-induced asthma can be compensated and permanent disability is allocated based on the ATS and AMA scales either when the disease is stable or 1 to 2 years after diagnosis (see above same paragraph).

South America

Compensation systems in South American countries vary, but in general, it would appear that either National Social Security agencies or Ministries of Labour and some self-insurers are responsible for administering workers' compensation (Table 11B.1). In general, all three major WRA phenotypes are covered. The claims are evaluated by medical personnel employed by diverse institutions. While a specific list of agents causing OA is used, there is a possibility of an open system. More specialized diagnostic modalities are not specifically required for the claim to be evaluated. AMA guidelines are used in Brazil to assess the degree of permanent disablement and in most countries, compensation is awarded as a lump sum based on the degree of disablement. However, while removal from exposure in affected workers is possible, it is associated with income loss. Using cases diagnosed in the municipality of São Paulo, state of São Paulo, Brazil, an incidence of 17 cases per million registered individuals was demonstrated.

The social consequences of confirming the diagnosis of WRA are important for both the worker and the employer. In Brazil, WRA has great importance for its political and social aspects, so that four ministries are involved in its control: labor, justice, health, and social security.

The diagnosis of WRA in Brazil implies notification through the Work Accident Communication, which is a document of the Ministry of Social Security and Social Assistance, even if it does not imply removal from work. The Work Accident Report can be issued by the company, the union, or any health professional involved in the investigation of the case. With this document, the affected worker will be submitted to a medical examination by the National Institute of Social Security to assess the causal link and disability, criteria used in judging the right to social security benefits.

Europe

The European list of occupational diseases (11, 12), which is not legally binding but represents occupational diseases recognized in most European countries, currently includes diseases called by the following chemical agents: isocyanates (104.3), chlorine (115.1), formaldehyde (124), ammonia (109.3), bronchopulmonary ailments caused by dust from the intact metals (303), allergic rhinitis caused by the inhalation of substances consistently recognized as causing allergies and inherent to the type of work (304.07); allergic asthmas caused by the inhalation of substances consistently recognized as causing allergies and inherent to the type of work (304.06); lung diseases caused by the inhalation of dust and fibers from cotton, flax, hemp, jute, sisal, and bagasse (304.02); respiratory ailments caused by the inhalation of dust from cobalt, tin, barium, and graphite (304.04); chronic obstructive bronchitis or emphysema in miners working in underground coal mines (307); and bronchopulmonary ailments caused by dusts or fumes from aluminum or compounds thereof (309) or caused by dust from basic slags (310) (13). Irritant-induced asthma (with a few exceptions such as due to ammonia, oxides of nitrogen, sulfuric acid, chlorine) and occupational chronic obstructive pulmonary disease (COPD) are not included.

Some European countries have specific lists for the presumptive agents which in some cases (Austria, Germany, Switzerland) include an open list of airway irritants causing OA. As an example the legally binding German list of 85 occupational diseases comprises two major OA subgroups (including COPD cases), i.e. obstructive airways diseases (including rhinitis) caused by allergenic substances (4301), bronchial obstructive airways diseases caused by chemical irritative or toxic substances (4302); https://www.baua.de/DE/Angebote/Publikationen/Praxis-kompakt/F3.html; https://www.baua.de/EN/Service/Legislative-texts-and-technical-rules/Occupational-diseases/Occupational-diseases_node.html. An annual report summarizes for each occupational disease figures of all claims, acknowledged and compensated cases; the latest report of 2017 mentions for the aforementioned two major OA subgroups 1678, and 1460 claims, respectively, of which 375 and 219 were acknowledged; https://www.baua.de/DE/Themen/Arbeitswelt-und-Arbeitsschutz-im-Wandel/Arbeitsweltberichterstattung/SuGA/SuGA_node.html.

TABLE 11B.1 Review of Compensation for Work-Related Asthma in Various Countries

Country	Workforce	Claim	Responsible Administration	Who Submits the Claim?	Is OA Compensated?	Is RADS Compensated?	Is Work-Aggravated Asthma Compensated?	Evaluation of Case (Physician, Committee of Physicians Patient Interview/Exam, Dossier Review)
North America								
United States	143[a]	Varies by state or other entity (e.g. OWCP for federal employees) Some have single insurer (e.g. Washington state), whereas most have multiple private insurers	Employers responsible for costs either directly (self-insurance) or purchasing mandatory workers' compensation insurance	Injured workers or their representative	Yes	Yes	Yes	Physician examination used; no centrally defined panel of physicians
Canada (provinces) Québec	4–5	Agency	Agency of the Québec government; funded by the employers' premiums	Worker and physician	Yes	Yes	Yes in limited number	Board of specialists
Alberta	~2.5	Agency	Semipublic insurance agency	Worker and physician	Yes	Yes	Yes in limited number	Specialists
Ontario	~7.1	Agency	Agency of the Ontario government; funded by employers' premiums	Worker and physician	Yes	Yes	Yes	Treating physicians and specialists (if needed)
British Columbia	~2.5	Agency	Semipublic insurance agency	Worker or physician	Yes	Yes	Yes	Case manager and physician if needed
South America								
Argentina	16 (2019)	Ministry of Labour Agency of Labour Risk	Mandatory insurance with labor risk Insurance companies	Employers and workers	Yes	Yes but no specific statement	Yes but no specific statement	Labor risk insurance companies, physician, and treating physician
Brazil	100 (2019)	National agency (National Social Insurance Trust Fund) and mutual associations like private insurers	National insurance agency	Any physician, employer, or employee	Yes	Yes	No	No
Europe								
Austria	8	Branch-oriented statutory accident insurance institutions	Statutory employers' insurers	Any physician (employer and employee)	Yes	Yes	Yes	Specialist (physician)

Belgium[b]	4.87	National agency	Public insurance agency with equal number of representatives from trade unions and employers; insurance premium paid by employers	Any physician	Yes	Yes (by a work injury insurance fund)	No	Board of specialists (claimants undergo medical evaluation at the WCB office)
Denmark	2.88	National agency	Employers and government	Any physician, the workers, and the trade union	Yes	Yes	No	Specialists
Finland	2.64	National agency	Employers/insurers	Worker and physician	Yes	Yes	No	Specialists
France	28.35	Regional agencies	Employers	Worker	Yes	Yes	Variable	Social security/ practitioners
Germany[c]	41.01	Branch-oriented statutory accident insurance institutions	Statutory employers' insurers	Any physician (employer and employee)	Yes	Yes	Yes	Specialist (physician)
Italy	24.3	National	National insurance	Physician (any)	Yes	Yes (although RADS is not a term specified in the list of occupational diseases)	No	Board of specialists Evaluation by Italian workers' compensation authority (INAIL) physician
Norway	2.5	National agency and private insurance (compulsory)	Government employers and private insurers	Patient	Yes	Yes	Often	Specialist
Spain	23	Government agency	Employers and government agency	Employees	Yes	Yes	No	Board of specialists
Netherlands	8.6	No specific system	Employers and employees	Not submitted	No official acceptance	No official acceptance	No official acceptance	Insurance physicians and in civil cases chest and occupational physicians

(*Continued*)

TABLE 11B.1 Review of Compensation for Work-Related Asthma in Various Countries (*Continued*)

Country	Workforce	Claim	Responsible Administration	Who Submits the Claim?	Is OA Compensated?	Is RADS Compensated?	Is Work-Aggravated Asthma Compensated?	Evaluation of Case (Physician, Committee of Physicians Patient Interview/Exam, Dossier Review)
UK	30.8	Government agency	General taxation		Yes		No	Career specialists for assessing occupational diseases
Africa								
Nigeria	62.5	National social insurance trust fund	Employers	Workers/ representatives	No specific statement	No specific statement	No specific statement	Claimant's physician/ committee of physicians
South Africa	23.1	National agency and mutual associations	Employers	Employers/ workers	Yes	Yes	Yes	Claimant's physician
Tanzania	27	Workers' compensation fund	Employers	Workers/ representatives/ employers	Yes	Yes	Yes	Medical practitioner/ medical advisory panel organized by WCF
Tunisia	4.2	National Fund of Health Insurance-CNAM (private sector) Central commission (public sector)	Employers	Workers	Yes	Yes	Yes	Committee of physicians
Mozambique	13.2	Insurance schemes for private companies (medicolegal claim)	Employers	Employers/ workers	No specific statement	No specific statement	No specific statement	
Australia and New Zealand								
Australia	11.5	National and state agencies and some self-insurers	Compensation agency and the employer	Worker	Yes	Yes	Yes	Usually a physician; in some cases a panel of physicians
New Zealand	1.9	Government via Accident Compensation Corporation (ACC)	ACC: state-owned enterprise providing compulsory injury insurance	Worker	Yes	Yes	Not usually. New sensitization only	Respiratory physician ± occupational physician then dossier review by ACC occupational physician

Country	Specific List of OA Agents	Open List of OA Agents	Is a Positive SIC a Precondition for Claim Acceptance?	Is Specific IgE or Positive SPT a Precondition for Claim Acceptance?	Is NSBH a Precondition for Claim Acceptance?	No. of OA Cases/Yr	Degree of Disablement Compensated and Time Frames	Removal of Worker from Exposure	Permanent Disability Awarded
Asia									
South Korea	20.1	National agency	Employer/government	Worker	Yes	Yes	Yes	Board of occupational physicians	
North America									
US	No	Yes	No	No	Not explicitly required	4132 from 4 states (California, Massachusetts, Michigan, New Jersey) Includes 2825 new-onset, 834 work-exacerbated National data not available but these 4 states represent 18% of workers. By extrapolation: 23,000 workers	Distinguishes temporary disability (until max. medical improvement achieved) from permanent disability No defined time frame Many states use AMA guides[c] as basis of assessing impairment	Yes, can be arranged generally with income loss	Yes
Canada (provinces)									
Quebec	No	Yes	Yes, in most cases	Can help in diagnosis	Generally present	~40–50 (2010–2018)	Yes (AMA, 2 yrs after diagnosis)	Yes	Yes
Alberta	No	Yes	SIC not generally requested	Can help in diagnosis	No	~25–50 (2000–2019)	Yes	Yes	Yes
Ontario	No	Yes	No	If feasible	Generally present	10–15	Yes, when stable	Yes	Yes
British Columbia	No	Yes	SIC helpful	Can help in diagnosis	No		Yes, when stable	Yes (not mandatory)	Yes
South America									
Argentina	Yes	Yes	No	No	No	NA	Yes	Yes	Yes

(*Continued*)

TABLE 11B.1 Review of Compensation for Work-Related Asthma in Various Countries (*Continued*)

Country	Specific List of OA Agents	Open List of OA Agents	Is a Positive SIC a Precondition for Claim Acceptance?	Is Specific IgE or Positive SPT a Precondition for Claim Acceptance?	Is NSBH a Precondition for Claim Acceptance?	No. of OA Cases/Yr	Degree of Disablement Compensated and Time Frames	Removal of Worker from Exposure	Permanent Disability Awarded
Brazil	Yes	Yes	No	No	Not specifically required, but can help in diagnosis	National data not available Data from major cities showed 394 cases from 1995–2000	No defined time frame Many states use AMA guides	Yes, can be arranged generally with income loss	Yes
Europe									
Austria	No	Yes	No, but helps in diagnosis	No, but strengthens claim	No, if positive challenge or obstructive pattern present	185	Mostly 20%–30%, rarely up to 80%, until disease is stable	Mostly	Yes
Belgium	Yes	Yes	No	No (if positive SIC)	No (if positive SIC)	Mean of 77 claims accepted (1992–2002)	Yes, based on AMA guides plus additional factors (reduced chances on the job market) no systematic reassessment	Yes	Yes
Denmark	Multiple means	Yes	No	No	No	50–70	Depending on the reduced chances on the job market	Yes	Yes
Finland	Yes	Yes	No	No	No	148 (2009)	10%–100%	Yes	Yes
France	Yes	Yes	No	No	No, but pulmonary functional tests compulsory	222 (2009)	0%–100%	Yes	Yes
Germany	No, except isocyanates	Yes	No, but helps in diagnosis	No, but strengthens claim	No, if positive SIC or obstructive pattern	400 (2018)	Mostly 20%–30% Rarely up to 80% until disease is stable	So far yes in the future in case of significant risk of worsening	Yes

Italy	Yes	Yes	No	No	No	202 (2006)	6%–100% (yearly for 15 yrs, not compulsory)	Yes	Yes
Norway	No	Yes	No	No	No	174 (2000)	15%–100%	Yes	Yes
Spain	Yes	No	No	No	Not an absolute precondition	258–294 (2000–2003)	No	Yes	No
Netherlands	No	No	NA			None	None		No
UK	Multiple	With individual proof and due to sensitization	No	No	No	170 (2009)	At least 14% required	No requirement	Yes
Africa									
Nigeria	No	No	No	No	No, but pulmonary function essential	NA	NA	Yes	Yes
South Africa	Yes	No	No	Can help in diagnosis	No, but pulmonary function tests essential	82 (2017)	15%–100% (1–2 yr after diagnosis)	Yes	Yes (>30% pension)
Tanzania	No. uses ILO list (2010)	Yes	No	May be used for diagnosis	No, but pulmonary function tests required	3 (2019)	>0%–100%	Yes	Yes
Tunisia	Yes	No	No	No	No, but pulmonary function tests essential	24.42 per million/year	5%–100%	Yes	Yes (>15% pension)
Mozambique	No	No	NA	Not defined	Not defined	No information	NA	Yes	NA
Australia and New Zealand									
Australia	No	Yes	No, would rarely be	No, but would assist claim, if performed	No, but would assist claim, if performed	~70	Varies between agencies; in Victoria requires impairment >10%	Yes	Yes in some cases

(Continued)

TABLE 11B.1 Review of Compensation for Work-Related Asthma in Various Countries (*Continued*)

Country	Specific List of OA Agents	Open List of OA Agents	Is a Positive SIC a Precondition for Claim Acceptance?	Is Specific IgE or Positive SPT a Precondition for Claim Acceptance?	Is NSBH a Precondition for Claim Acceptance?	No. of OA Cases/Yr	Degree of Disablement Compensated and Time Frames	Removal of Worker from Exposure	Permanent Disability Awarded
New Zealand	No, recognized sensitizing agents inherent in the work process	Yes	No, but supportive information	No, but supportive information	Must fulfill diagnosis of asthma, + obstructive pattern history and serial PEF	18/yr average (2009–2011)	Entitlements to treatment, social rehabilitation wage replacement if incapacitated vocational rehabilitation and a lump sum based on AMA guides, once stable with options to reassess at 5 yrs	Yes, vocational rehabilitation and income replacement while changing to safe job role	Yes, on medical assessment, the vocational rehabilitation unsuccessful; 80% wage replacement until 65 yrs
Asia									
South Korea	Yes	Yes	Yes	No	No	15/yr average (2009–2011)	Yes	Yes	Yes

[a] US Department of Labor. Bureau of Labor Statistics. Table A-1. Employment status of the civilian population by sex and age. Accessed March, 2012. http://www.bls.gov/news.release/empsit.t01.htm.

[b] Data from the Fonds des Maladies Professionnelles–Fonds voor de Beroepsziekten (O. Vandenplas, personal communication).

[c] Also includes a small number of objectively evaluated cases with work-aggravated asthma or occupational COPD. Additionally, 1095 COPD cases from the hard coal mining industry were acknowledged as occupational diseases.

Information on Canadian provinces obtained thanks to Dr. Susan Tarlo (Ontario), Dr. Jeremy Beach (Alberta), Dr. Christopher Carlsten (British Columbia), and Dr. Jean-Luc Malo (Quebec).

Information on South American countries obtained thanks to Dr. Marcos Ribeiro (Brazil).

Information on Europe obtained thanks to Dr. Xaver Baur and Ilenia Folletti.

Information from United States obtained from Dr. Philip Harber.

Information from African countries obtained thanks to Dr. Femi Adewole (Nigeria), Dr. Hussein Mwanga (Tanzania), Dr. Vania Chongo Faruk (Mozambique), Dr. Maoua Maher (Tunisia), and Dr. Mohamed Jeebhay (South Africa).

Information on Australia and New Zealand obtained thanks to Drs. Malcolm Sims and Anthony Johnson (Australia) and Margaret Macky (New Zealand).

Information on South Korea obtained thanks to Dr. Hae Sim Park.

Abbreviations: AMA, American Medical Association; IgE, immunoglobulin E; NA, not available; NSBH, nonspecific bronchial hyperresponsiveness; OA, occupational asthma; OWCP Office of Workers' Compensation Programs; PEF, peak expiratory flow; RADS, reactive airways dysfunction syndrome; SIC, specific inhalation challenge; SPT, skin-prick test; WCB, workers' compensation board; WCF, workers' compensation fund.

Insurance and compensation systems are rather heterogeneous all over Europe (14) with statutory employer insurance requirements in some countries such as Austria, Finland, Germany, and Switzerland. In most European countries, work-aggravated asthma is not acknowledged as an occupational disease or not differentiated from new-onset asthma and occupational COPD (such as in Germany) (Table 11B.1) (15). In the Netherlands, there is a uniform health insurance system not differentiating occupational diseases from others.

In countries following a predefined implementation schedule for occupational disease, a claimant who develops a listed disease has a strong likelihood of receiving a compensation award. However, claims for a disease not on restricted lists are more likely to be unsuccessful, which usually encourages the worker to seek other sources of social assistance. In the United Kingdom, Germany, and France, an implementation schedule is used, which can be broadened in its application. In Germany, this is possible if new scientific evidence identifies a novel occupational cause in a well-defined occupational exposure context.

Since 2007, REACH (Registration, Evaluation, Authorization, and Restriction of Chemical substances—European community regulation on chemicals and their safe use) has been in force. REACH is intended to improve the protection of human health and the environment through the better and earlier identification of the intrinsic properties of chemical substances. The REACH regulation places greater responsibility on industry to manage the risks from chemicals and to provide respective safety information. Manufacturers and importers are obliged to gather information on the properties of their chemical substances, which will allow their safe handling, and to register the information in a central database run by the European Chemicals Agency in Helsinki.

Africa

Workers' compensation systems vary in different African countries and are to a large extent inherited from their European colonial past (Table 11B.1). The dominant economic activity in most African countries is in the informal sector, although OA is more commonly reported by the formal sector. OA in most countries is underrecognized, poorly diagnosed and managed, and continues to remain underreported and therefore inadequately compensated (16–21). A Tunisian study estimated that between 25% and 41% of workers with OA lose their jobs (21).

The compensation system in South Africa, with the largest economy in Africa, is relatively better developed having a long history of evolution to its current dispensation (22). Compensation for OA, as for other occupational diseases, is covered by specific workers' compensation legislation for nonminers except for asthma in platinum salt refinery workers, which is covered by specific legislation that compensates miners with occupational lung diseases. This law has different administrative procedures and provides for inferior benefits compared to compensation for nonminers (23).

The presumptive list of occupational diseases for nonminers that will bring it in line with the less restrictive International Labour Organization (ILO) list of occupational diseases (revised 2010), is yet to materialize (24). This ILO list includes a generic phrase "asthma caused by recognized sensitizing agents or irritants inherent to the work process." Nevertheless there exist specific "circular instructions" guidelines for the three major phenotypes of WRA containing explicit diagnostic criteria to be used for compensation application purposes (19).

The no-fault compensation system funded through premiums paid by employers based on risk rating of a particular industry provides cover for all current and ex-workers (except domestic and informal sector workers), while at the same time also proscribes workers recourse to civil litigation. As a result, tort litigation in the nonmining industry has been almost entirely eliminated. The worker does not need to demonstrate employer negligence, although additional compensation is payable should this be shown. Workers are reassessed 2 years after diagnosis to set permanent impairment/disability after being removed from the identified exposure where possible. The degree of impairment is based on a modification of the Quebec (9) and ATS (10) guidelines. In instances where sensitization persists after removal from exposure, 15% permanent disablement is awarded if the worker has normal lung function and no need for medication (25). If there is >30% disablement, a pension is awarded. Other benefits include medical costs, loss of wages for a limited period, and a death benefit for dependents should the worker's death be due to an occupational disease.

Some of the major shortfalls of the compensation system relate to compensation being largely based on the degree of impairment rather than total disability, inadequate cover for loss of earnings, and lack of compulsory rehabilitation or vocational training programs. Furthermore, the no-fault principle shields employers from the full costs of the disease and shifts the burden to society. In addition, the administrative procedures of this centrally administered fund are inefficient, resulting in major delays (1.5–2 years) in claim resolution (26, 27). There are no government-sponsored or government-mandated national or regional centers with responsibility for evaluating workers with suspected occupational diseases. Provincial pilot projects were established for a few years, which demonstrated both diagnostic and administrative efficiency outcomes, but these were closed down due to other sociopolitical factors (28). These inadequacies have highlighted the need for reform of the compensation system to ensure greater equity, accountability, and responsiveness to the needs of workers disabled as a result of occupational diseases, including asthma. This becomes even more important given that less than 10% of workers reported in a recent study of being aware of the workers' compensation law and its benefits (29).

Australia and New Zealand

Compensation systems in Australia and New Zealand vary with national and state agencies responsible for administering workers' compensation (Table 11B.1). In Australia, there are 11 main workers' compensation systems. Each of the eight Australian states and territories has developed its own workers' compensation scheme and there are also three Commonwealth schemes. In New Zealand, the Accident Compensation Corporation (ACC) is the entity responsible for administering the country's no-fault accidental injury compensation scheme. It is a compulsory, statutory requirement that all businesses with employees in Australia and New Zealand have workers' compensation insurance. The cost of insurance is calculated by governments and is determined by the wages of employees, level of risk associated with the industry, and the employer's claims history. In general, all three major WRA phenotypes are covered in Australia, although WEA is not covered in New Zealand. Claimants are generally evaluated by an independent specialist physician (pulmonology or occupational medicine). No specific list of agents is used since an open system that recognizes any potential asthmagenic agent is used. The diagnosis of WRA is generally based on expert opinion supported by pulmonary function results. Specific inhalational challenges are not required and are rarely performed in Australia and New Zealand. Determination of the degree of impairment is based on AMA guidelines.

Most systems provide payments for medical expenses and compensation for the period of time the worker is unable to return to work due to the condition. Systems generally also provide access to reasonable retraining expenses if the worker is unable to return to her/his previous occupation. In New Zealand, 80% of weekly earnings are awarded until the individual is vocationally independent or the individual is 65 years old. Lump-sum payments may be available through either no-fault benefits, common law damages (where an employer has been negligent), or both. Lump-sum payments are usually linked to demonstration of a threshold requirement, such as 10% whole person impairment in accordance with AMA guidelines. For workers without permanent impairment, the focus of the system is to return the worker to work. Workers have an ongoing responsibility to make efforts to return to work, which is regularly reviewed by insurers and statutory bodies. The worker's treating doctor has an important role in assessing and advising on a worker's capacity to engage in her/his preinjury or alternative employment. Each system has a different dispute management proposal.

Asia

The current situation of compensation system in Korea is listed in Table 11B.1. After a specific bronchoprovocation test carried out by specialists, workers can ask for compensation from the governmental agency. A reviewing committee appointed by the government makes the decision. Both WEA and RADS as well as OA can be compensated. A list of major etiologic agents is provided. Workers who get compensation have to leave exposure. The responsible specialists follow compensated workers regularly and then submit a report on whether extension may be needed. Information on the medicolegal situation in other Asian countries was not available at the time of preparation of this chapter.

Summary

United States

The United States does not have a single consistent system for compensating or even defining OA. There are significant differences among the 50 states and other jurisdictions. None employ "scheduled lists of agents," and therefore, workers may seek benefits for all forms of WRA. Adjudication of claims considers reports from numerous physicians rather than any central designated medical board. Workers may obtain (limited) salary maintenance, health services, and (limited) vocational rehabilitation benefits. The heterogeneity among systems creates the potential for inconsistent criteria.

Canada

Compensation for work accident and diseases is under the responsibilities of provinces. WRA is an accepted compensable disease in all Canadian provinces. However, the extent of information requested for accepting the cases and the type of compensation offered vary from one province to the next. Permanent impairment/disability is assessed and compensated.

Europe

Although there exists a formally agreed list of occupational diseases (including allergic rhinitis and asthma) in Europe, only a few countries have comparable insurance systems and legal regulations related to occupational diseases. Regulations for hazardous occupational substances have been in force (REACH program); however, preventive measures still require concrete improvement and harmonization.

South America

Increasing industrialization and rapid economic development associated with globalization have highlighted the need for more comprehensive laws and national occupational health systems that are responsive to the needs of workers who are injured or diseased. This includes improved access to early diagnosis and optimal health care and compensation benefits for workers with WRA.

Africa

Aside from South Africa, workers' compensation systems in the rest of Africa are poorly developed due to a large proportion of economic activity conducted in the informal sector. This trend is changing with increasing industrialization and globalization. The compensation system in South Africa is comparable to industrialized countries that recognize all types of WRA and provide for (limited) loss of wages, treatment, and compensation for permanent impairment/disability. Continued reliance on a national system with poor administrative processes poses major challenges.

Australia and New Zealand

The workers' compensation system for WRA in general is very similar to the dispensation in North America. Vocational rehabilitation programs are implemented with greater vigor than in many other countries across the globe.

Recommendations and research needs

The heterogeneity of compensation systems within and between countries as regards OA might be addressed by implementing clear and consistent definitions of terms, developing consensus statements defining the types of asthma that should be compensable, ensuring an open list of asthmagenic agents with access to recognized databases that provided updated information on implicated agents, and developing consensus positions about the extent of work exacerbation of asthma that warrants compensation. Devolution of highly centralized national systems to more accessible regionally based systems and the development of several regional centers of excellence for assessing OA for compensation will serve as models to raise the overall standard of the process and also facilitate the use of technically demanding tests such as SIC and immunological testing where appropriate. The cadre of physicians and other health professionals who understand both clinical physiology and workplace prevention strategies should be expanded through improved training and national certification. Since OA mainly affects young workers, it would be relevant to offer medical surveillance to high-risk working populations and ensure efficient and rapid referral to diagnostic and medicolegal agencies. Further research on the long-term consequences of WRA and potential accommodation methods is needed to guide recommendations to employers on long-term placement and accommodation of affected workers.

Due to fragmentation legislation, there is a need for harmonization of laws and regulations that pertain to surveillance, diagnosis, insurance cover, compensation, and prevention of occupational diseases. Addressing WRA depends on effective government regulation and enforcement, education, and implementation of best practices. For successful interventions, national and local governments, employers, occupational health service providers, and workers need to work together. The barriers between the workers' compensation systems and prevention-oriented agencies should be reduced by creating mandatory data sharing between WCBs/agencies and governmental occupational safety and health enforcement agencies.

References

1. Toren K, Blanc P. Asthma caused by occupational exposures is common—a systematic analysis of estimates of the population-attributable fraction. BMC Pulm Med. 2009;9:7.
2. Blanc PD, Annesi-Maesano I, Balmes JR, et al. The occupational burden of nonmalignant respiratory diseases. An Official American Thoracic Society and European Respiratory Society statement. Am J Respir Crit Care Med. 2019;199:1312–34.
3. Malo JL, Ghezzo H, L'Archevêque J, et al. Is the clinical history a satisfactory means of diagnosing occupational asthma? Am Rev Respir Dis. 1991;143:528–32.
4. Vandenplas O, Ghezzo H, Munoz X, et al. What are the questionnaire items most useful in identifying subjects with occupational asthma? Eur Respir J. 2005;26:1056–63.
5. United States Code. Americans with Disabilities Act of 1990, as amended. Cited March 27, 2020. https://wwwadagov/pubs/adastatute08htm 2009.
6. Jolly AT, Klees JE, Pacheco KA, et al. Work-related asthma. J Occup Environ Med. 2015;57(10):e121–9.
7. American Medical Association. The pulmonary system. In: Rondinelli, RD, ed. Guides to the Evaluation of Permanent Impairment American Medical Association. 2008:77–99.
8. ODG MCG. Industry-leading medical treatment and return to work guidelines. Accessed December 4, 2020. https://wwwmcgcom/odg/about-odg/ Cited.
9. Malo JL. Compensation for occupational asthma in Quebec. Chest. 1990;98:236S–9S.
10. American Thoracic Society. Guidelines for the evaluation of impairment/disability in patients with asthma. Am Rev Respir Dis. 1993;147:1056–61.
11. Commission of the European Communities. Commission recommendation concerning the European schedule of occupational diseases (notified under document number C(2003) 3297) (Text with EEA relevance). https://eur-lex.europa.eu/legal-content/EN/TXT/?qid=1594022872504&uri=CELEX:3 2003H0670 or https://eur-lex.europa.eu/eli/reco/2003/670/oj
12. Aw TC, Ahmed S, Choudat D, et al. Information notices on occupational diseases: a guide to diagnosis. Luxembourg: Office for Official Publications of the European Communities; 2009. https://osha.europa.eu/en/legislation/guidelines/commission-recommendation-concerning-the-european-schedule-of-occupational-diseases
13. Commission of the European Communities. Commission recommendation of 19 September 2003 concerning the European schedule of occupational diseases. J EU 2003;238:28–34.
14. Barth PS, Hunt HA. Worker's compensation and work-related illnesses and disease. Cambridge, MA: MIT Press; 1982.
15. Baur X, Sigsgaard T, Aasen TB, et al. Guidelines for the management of work-related asthma. Eur Respir J. 2012;39:529–45.
16. Syabbalo N. Occupational asthma in a developing country. Chest. 1991;99:528.
17. Esterhuizen TM, Hnizdo E, Rees D. Occurrence and causes of occupational asthma in South Africa—results from SORDSA's Occupational Asthma Registry, 1997–1999. S Afr Med J. 2001 Jun;91:509–13.
18. Mbaye I, Ndiaye M, Soumah M, et al. Medico-legal conditions of recognition and compensation of occupational asthma in Senegal. Dakar Med. 2004;49:121–6.
19. Jeebhay MF, Quirce S. Occupational asthma in the developing and industrialised world: a review. Int J Tuberc Lung Dis. 2007;11:122–33.
20. Hoy R. Occupational asthma in developing countries requires further research. Int J Tuberc Lung Dis. 2015;19:372.
21. Maoua M, El Maalel O, Boughattas W, et al. Epidemiology of occupational asthma in Tunisia: results of a first national study. Occup Diseases and Env Med. 2016;4:27–36.
22. Bachmann OM. Compensating for occupational lung disease. S Afr Med J. 1990 Feb 17;77:202–7.
23. Ehrlich R. A century of miner's compensation in South Africa. Am J Ind Med. 2012;55:560–9.
24. International Labour Organisation. ILO List of Occupational Diseases (revised 2010). Programme on Safety and Health at Work and the Environment (SafeWork). Geneva: International Labour Office; 2010.
25. Republic of South Africa. Department of Labour. Circular instruction regarding compensation for occupational asthma No. 176, Government Gazette 2003. Curr Allergy Clin Immunol. 2004;17:43–4.
26. Jeebhay MF, Omar F, Kisting S, et al. Outcome of worker's compensation claims submitted by the workers clinic in Cape Town. Occup Health S Afr. 2002;8:4–7.
27. Ehrlich R. Persistent failure of the COIDA system to compensate occupational disease in South Africa. S Afr Med J. 2012;102:95–7.
28. Ehrlich R, Adams S, Manjra S, et al. Fate of outstanding COIDA occupational disease claims following closure of the Western Cape Provincial Medical Advisory Panel in 2008 – an audit. Occ Health Southern Africa. 2015;21:6–10.
29. Pilusa ML, Mogotlane MS. Worker knowledge of occupational legislation and related health and safety benefits. Curationis. 2018;41:e1–e6.

Part IV
Specific Agents Causing Immunological Occupational Asthma

12

OCCUPATIONAL ASTHMA IN THE BAKING INDUSTRY

Paul Cullinan,[1] Torben Sigsgaard,[2] Mohamed F. Jeebhay,[3] Monika Raulf,[4]
Editor Susan M. Tarlo[5]

[1]*Department of Occupational and Environmental Lung Disease, Imperial College (NHLI) and Royal Brompton Hospital, London, UK*
[2]*Department of Public Health, Section for Environment, Work & Health, Aarhus University, Aarhus C, Denmark*
[3]*Occupational Medicine Division and Centre for Environmental & Occupational Health Research (CEOHR), School of Public Health and Family Medicine, Faculty of Health Sciences, University of Cape Town, Cape Town, South Africa*
[4]*Department of Allergology/Immunology of the German Institute of Prevention and Occupational Medicine of the Social Accident Insurance; Institute of the Ruhr-University Bochum, (IPA), Bochum, Germany*
[5]*Department of Medicine, St Michael's Hospital, University Health Network, University of Toronto, Toronto, Ontario, Canada*

Contents

CASE HISTORY

On leaving school at the age of 18 years, a young man went to work in an in-store supermarket bakery where he mixed and prepared doughs on a daily basis. Previously in good health, 6 months after starting work he developed rhinitis that he and his doctor attributed to hay fever. After a further 6 months he found himself wheezy and short of breath on playing football; he put these down to being unfit. Over the next 12 months he found that his symptoms were better on days when he was not at work, and that they remitted altogether during a fortnight's holiday. Subsequent investigations indicated that he was sensitized to wheat flour (specific IgE 15kU/L) and that, on serial measurement, his peak flow was clearly related to periods at or away from work. On the basis of his symptoms (characteristic of an airborne protein allergy), his specific sensitization, and the functional changes in his peak flow, a probable diagnosis of baker's asthma was made. His symptoms remitted entirely when he was allocated to a different job in the store.

Introduction

For thousands of years, bread has played an important part in the diet, history, and even politics of many cultures, particularly those of Europe and the Middle East. Historically, bread was made by hand; mechanization was first introduced for the laborious process of milling cereal grains and later for the preparation of doughs and the means for mass production such as Otto Rohwedder's machine for slicing and wrapping loaves, introduced first in Missouri, United States, in 1928. Today, the production of bread and associated foodstuffs takes place in one of two broad settings. "Plant" bakeries are highly mechanized and can produce very large volumes of bread with relatively few employees and relatively limited exposures to dust. "Craft" bakeries tend to employ more traditional methods and are often small, family retail businesses but increasingly are outlets of large corporations, or are located in supermarkets (Figure 12.1). Bread sales are subject to the whims of fashion and health. In more affluent countries there has been a demand for a greater variety of breads including, for example, gluten-free products; in poorer parts of the world urbanization has been associated with an increase in demand for ready-made food, much of it comprising bread.

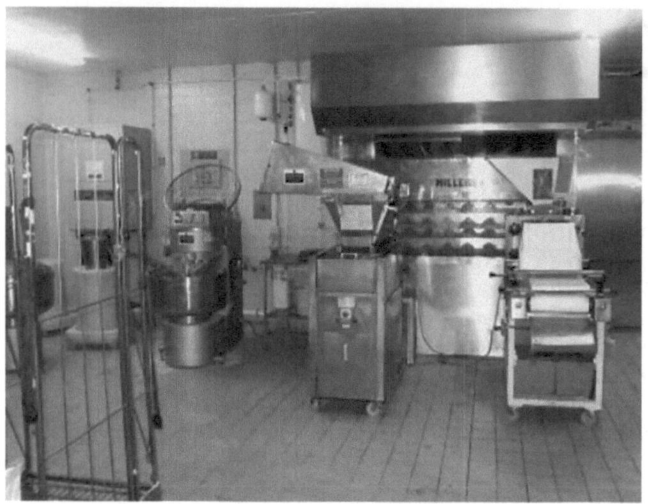

FIGURE 12.1 In-store (or "scratch") bakery situated within a large supermarket; two dough-mixing bowls are on the left.

Asthma in bakers and bakery workers is generally referred to as "baker's asthma." Although a useful shorthand, this terminology belies the observation that asthma caused by the same agents occurs in workers in related occupations such as flour milling, other food production, and in industries that produce and package enzymes and other ingredients for the baking sector. Asthma among bakers and millers is arguably the most familiar and, notoriously, the oldest (1) form of occupational asthma (OA). Until the beginning of the twentieth century, it was assumed that the disease was the result simply of the irritant effects of high dust exposures, but in 1929, de Besche (2) suggested for the first time that asthma in bakers is an allergic disease. Four years later, Baagöe (3) undertook the first systematic investigation of asthma and rhinitis in the baking industry. Since then there has been a substantial volume of clinical and epidemiological work aimed at unraveling the etiology and estimating the risks of allergic respiratory disease in bakery workers, and at devising methods to prevent them. The failure thus far to achieve effective primary prevention (4) is not through any deficiency in understanding the disease but the result of a lack of commercial and political will.

Allergens: nature and sources

Most studies indicate that wheat (*Triticum aestivum*) flour proteins are allergens for 60%–70% of symptomatic bakers (5), although other cereals like rye (*Secale cereale*), barley (*Hordeum vulgare*), oats (*Avena sativa*), and corn, and noncereal sources, enzymes, and insects may be involved because bakeries are complex environments (6). Wheat is in many parts of the world a major crop, and is immensely diverse, with over 25,000 different cultivars (7). Wheat flour is composed of starch (about 70%–75%), and four groups of proteins, namely glutenins, gliadins, globulins, and water/salt-soluble albumins. In addition, nonstarch polysaccharides (about 2%–3%), in particular arabinoxylans, and lipids (c. 2%) are minor but important constituents. Wheat, as a complex allergenic mixture, contains more vegetable proteins than the other two globally important cereals, corn and rice; more than 100 different protein spots can be detected as IgE-binding in wheat flour by means of high-resolution two-dimensional gel electrophoresis and immunoblotting (8, 9). Twenty-eight wheat

allergens are listed so far in the World Health Organization/ International Union of Immunological Societies (WHO/IUIS) Allergen Nomenclature database (www.allergen.org), from the wheat profilin (Tri a 12) up to Tri a 45 (10) (Table 12.1). These allergens are not only characterized with respect to baker's asthma; most are also ingested food allergens. Several wheat allergens isolated as native allergen or produced in recombinant form have been used in IgE assays in different systems (e.g. singleplex, multiplex, ELISA, immunoblotting) and with different groups of bakers; in many cases the IgE-reactivity of these allergens has only been identified in single studies and their clinical relevance is unclear. The highly diverse results may reflect differences in populations or in the different approaches used to identify IgE reactive proteins, making comparisons difficult (7, 11–13).

One study assessed a panel of 19 recombinant wheat flour allergens and two cross-reactive carbohydrate determinants (CCD) with singleplex technology for specific IgE quantification (CAP-FEIA system) in the sera of 101 bakers with OA from Germany, Spain, and the Netherlands, and of 29 pollen-sensitized control subjects without occupational exposure but with wheat-specific IgE (14).

The results indicate that different α-amylase inhibitors are important allergens for baker's asthma, but none of the single allergens reached the status of a major allergen. The geographical origin of the subjects had no significant influence on the sensitization patterns. Furthermore, the IgE-binding profile based on testing with the 19 recombinant wheat allergens and the two CCDs showed large interindividual variability. A combination of specific IgE testing to five components (Tri a 27, Tri a 28, tetrameric α-amylase inhibitor CM2 [Tri a 29.02], serine protease inhibitor-like allergen [Tri a 39], and 1-cys-peroxiredoxin [Tri a 32]), produced the highest diagnostic efficiency in receiver operating characteristic analyses, but this was still lower than the determination of specific IgE antibodies against the whole wheat flour extract.

Enzymes

During all steps of breadmaking, complex chemical, biochemical, and physical transformations occur, which affect and are affected by the various flour constituents. In addition, many substances are now used to influence the structural and physicochemical characteristics of the flour constituents in order to optimize their functionality (16). Enzymes are used to improve bread quality such as crumb softness and loaf microstructure, and to extend the shelf life of products (17). The most important enzymatic improvers are α-amylases, because they are effective in small quantities and have a very specific action on starch molecules. Amylases are members of the glycosyl hydrolases (EC.3.2.1.1) family 13 and are endo-acting enzymes responsible for hydrolyzing internal α-(1, 4)-glycosidic bonds and producing α-limit dextrins (18). Amylases can be prepared from either bacterial or fungal sources (e.g. *Bacillus, Pseudomonas, Aspergillus* species) and, depending on their origin, show only low cross-reactivity and have different temperature and/or pH optima. The choice for a particular application depends on the operating conditions in which the enzyme is required to perform. During baking processes, fungal α-amylase derived from *Aspergillus oryzae* is often used, added in small amounts (mg/kg flour) to baking flour, and denominated according to the WHO/IUIS as allergen Asp o 21 (53 kDa; formerly Asp o II) (19). It is classified as a respiratory sensitizer according to REACH, based on a document by the Dutch Expert Committee on Occupational Safety (DECOS, 2014),

TABLE 12.1 Relevant Airborne Wheat Allergens According to WHO/IUIS (Modified)

Allergen	Biochemical Name	Notes
Tri a 15	Wheat monomeric α-amylase inhibitor 0.28 (WMA-1-0.28)	Relevant in patients with baker's allergy, but not relevant for those with grass pollen allergy with wheat-specific IgE
Tri a 25	Thioredoxin	Not exclusive for baker's asthma
Tri a 27	Thiol reductase homologue	Relevant in patients with baker's allergy, but not relevant for those with grass pollen allergy with wheat-specific IgE
Tri a 28	Dimeric α-amylase inhibitor 0.19	Relevant in patients with baker's allergy, but not relevant for those with grass pollen allergy with wheat-specific IgE
Tri a 29 - Tri a 29.0101 - Tri a 29.0201	Tetrameric α-amylase inhibitor CM1 CM2	In contrast to Tri a 29.0201, Tri a 29.0101 is not exclusively recognized in patients with baker's allergy
Tri a 30	Tetrameric α-amylase inhibitor CM3	Relevant in patients with baker's allergy, but not relevant for those with grass pollen allergy with wheat-specific IgE
Tri a 31	Triosephosphate-isomerase (TPIS)	Not exclusively recognized by specific IgE from bakers
Tri a 32	1-cys-peroxiredoxin	Relevant in patients with baker's allergy, but not relevant for those with grass pollen allergy with wheat-specific IgE
Tri a 33	Serpin	Recognized by only 8% of patients with baker's asthma and 0% of grass-pollen allergic patients
Tri a 34	Glyceraldehyde-3-phosphate-dehydrogenase (GAPDH)	Recognized by only 5% of patients with baker's asthma and 0% of grass-pollen allergic patients
Tri a 35	Dehydrin	Recognized by only 2% of patients with baker's allergy and 0% of grass-pollen allergic patients
Tri a 39	Serine protease inhibitor-like protein (SPILA)	Recognized by 18% of patients with baker's allergy and 0% of grass-pollen allergic patients
Tri a 40*	WTAI-CM^2 17 protein (α-amylase inhibitor)	Recognized by 8% of IgE-positive bakers and 15% of IgE-positive grass-pollen allergic patients; addition of Tri a 40.0101 to the panel of recombinant allergen components had only minimal influence on diagnostic sensitivity and could not improve specificity

*http://*www.allergen.org (March 2020); remarks according to (14) and for Tri a 40* according to (15).

suggesting that the risks for the induction of sensitization and the elicitation of upper and lower respiratory symptoms in sensitized individuals may be increased with exposures in the low ng/m^3 range. In addition, enzymes derived from *Aspergillus niger* like glucoamylase and cellulase are also relevant in baker's asthma (20). Glucoamylase is an exohydrolase that removes glucose from the nonreducing end of the amylose. Between the α-amylases and the exohydrolases, glucoamylase and maltohydrolase (cleaving the disaccharide maltose from the nonreducing end of the amylose), there is a maximum sequence homology of 22%. Other baking industry enzymes such as hemicellulase or xylanase are used for the degradation of plant material and increase the solubility of cell wall arabinoxylans (21, 22). Beta-xylosidase (105 kDa) from *Aspergillus niger* is the main IgE-binding protein in a xylanase preparation and identified as Asp n 14 (23). The number of potential sensitizing "improver" enzymes used for commercial bread production has significantly increased in the last years (24) and more than 20 different single enzymes causing allergy in bakers have been reported, e.g. lipase, lysozyme, (25) phospholipase, and cellulase (26). Bakers and their employers are rarely aware of which enzymes are being used at any time and for most of them, with the important exception of fungal α-amylase, no IgE assay or skin-prick antigen is commercially available.

Other ingredients

Noncereal ingredients like buckwheat, soybean flour, nuts and seeds, eggs, and lupin flour also contribute—marginally—to the high prevalence of sensitization and respiratory allergy in bakers. Soybean (*Glycine max*) is not only a significant food allergen but soy flour is widely used as an additive in bread; inhalation of soybean flour has been associated with baker's asthma (7). The soybean allergens involved in baker's asthma are predominantly high-molecular-weight (HMW) proteins present both in soybean hull and flour. In contrast, relatively low-molecular-weight (LMW) proteins concentrated in the soybean hull Gly m 1 (7 kDa, the hydrophobic protein from soybean with two isoforms Gly m 1.0101 and Gly m 1.0102) and Gly m 2 (8 kDa, the defensin) are responsible for the asthma attacks during unloading of soybean at seaports in Spain (27). An additional ingredient used in bakeries is buckwheat (*Fagopyrum esculentum*), which is not taxonomically related to wheat (it belongs to the flowering plant family Polygonaceae) but is sometimes used as a wheat substitute. Cases of buckwheat allergy induced by occupational exposure in bakeries, but also in health food and crêpe production, have been described (28). Due to its high protein and low fat content, and the absence of gluten, the use of lupin flour in baked products has increased (29). In a study of van Kampen et al. (30) sera of 116 bakers with work-related allergic symptoms without known food allergies were assayed and specific IgE levels to wheat and rye flour, lupin, peanut, soy, and the recombinant birch allergen rBet v 1 were quantified. A third of the bakers were sensitized to lupin, 35% to peanut and 67% to wheat and/or rye flour. All lupin-positive bakers also had specific IgE to either wheat flour and/or peanut and lupin. Specific IgE significantly correlated with specific IgE to peanut, soy, wheat and rye flour; inhibition experiments indicated cross-reactivity between lupin and wheat in some cases. The apparently high sensitization rate could reflect significant lupin flour exposure in some bakeries although this was unquantified in this population. In general, the clinical significance of cross-reactivity with regard to baker's asthma remains to be clarified, especially when the use of lupin as a supplement or substitute has increased during baking processes.

Other noningredient allergens

The bakery environment is complex and there are several case reports of baker's asthma caused by molds (31) and insects, although these are of marginal importance to the burden of disease in bakers; nonetheless they should be kept in mind in the clinical setting if no sensitization to common bakery allergens is found (6). Storage mites (particularly those from the Glycyphagidae and the Acaridae families [Lepidoglyphus, Tyrophagus and Acarus genus, among others]) have been reported as bakery allergens (32) and in a cross-sectional study of Norwegian bakers with occupational rhinitis, different groups of storage mites were reported to be the most frequent cause of sensitization (33). These reports should be interpreted with care since the sensitization rates among bakers and the general population were similar and it is doubtful whether storage mite should be regarded as specific baker's allergen (34). The majority of insects (e.g. *Ephestia kuhniella*, *Tenebrio molitor*) in commercial cereal flour are "hidden," i.e. immature insects that are found within individual wheat kernels. The higher sensitization rates against mites and insects described in earlier studies may reflect the fact that wheat flours were less pure and more contaminated in the past, before the widespread use of pesticides in cereal cultivation (35).

Measurement of dust exposure and airborne allergens

Allergen exposure assessment should be based on (active) measurement of airborne concentrations, and in occupational studies, low-flow personal airborne sampling in the breathing zone is the recommended procedure (36). Personal sampling directly measures workers' exposures; stationary "area" sampling usually gives lower dust concentrations than the personal approach reflecting the general area situation. In some of the early measurement series, exposure to wheat in bakeries was assessed by traditional total dust measurements using gravimetric methods. This indirect approach is not useful in quantifying potent allergens that sensitize workers at exposures in the ng/m^3 range (37). Direct measurements of wheat protein allergens and the quantification of airborne enzyme concentrations with immunochemical methods are probably more valid (38). Nevertheless, in a dusty workplace such as a bakery, cereal flour allergen concentrations show a high correlation with inhalable dust content (39).

While several immunoassays are available and allow the quantification of specific allergen levels in personal dust samples, standardization is difficult. Differences between laboratories in methods for dust sampling, extraction, and wheat allergen measurements may induce large differences in reported allergen levels. In the European MOCALEX project, numerous immunoassays for the assessment of allergen concentrations in bakeries were established, validated, and optimized with regard to individual analytical parameters and processing steps. Based on this work, a polyclonal rabbit IgG inhibition EIA can be recommended as the most convenient assay for routine measurements of full-shift airborne wheat samples from a medium- to high-exposure bakery environment, while for analysis of samples with expected low amounts of wheat allergen, the highly sensitive wheat sandwich EIA is to be preferred (40). Additionally, in the same project, comparison of extraction methods using more than 400 filters with airborne flour dust collected in bakeries and flour mills in four

European countries using three different assays for the determination of wheat allergen concentrations, was undertaken. Based on these data it is recommended that the addition of Tween-20 is essential for optimal elution of wheat allergens from flour dust samples, especially at lower levels. Further but less strict recommendations are the use of conventional polystyrene tubes, simple shaking methods, and centrifugation after extraction—and that wheat dust extracts in phosphate-buffered saline (PBS)-Tween can be stored frozen for at least 4 months without addition of a stabilizing protein (41). The methods for quantifying fungal α-amylase airborne exposure assessment were also explored. The results indicated that for reliable personal exposure assessment of fungal α-amylase, repeated full-shift (about 8 hr) or half-shift (4 hr) measurements, with optimal elution conditions of PBS with 0.05% Tween-20 and quantification through the use of highly sensitive EIAs, are recommended (42).

Epidemiology

Prevalence and incidence

It is well documented that exposure to flour dust increases the risk of allergic sensitization, rhinitis, and asthma in various settings including highly mechanized plants, craft, and "in-store" supermarket bakeries.

Sensitization to wheat flour and fungal amylase has been evaluated in a large number of cross-sectional studies, either by skin-prick tests (SPTs) or by measuring allergen-specific IgE antibodies in sera. The prevalence of sensitization thus documented varies from 5% to 28% for wheat flour and from 2% to 16% for α-amylase (43, 44). The prevalence of sensitization to other bakery allergens, such as baker's yeast (*Saccharomyces cerevisiae*) and for other enzymes, such as xylanase, is considerably lower, and in most cases below 1%–2%. Recent studies suggest that sensitization to other fungal allergens (6.8%, n=117) such as *Aspergillus* species in bakers with work-related symptoms may also be important (45).

Longitudinal studies have demonstrated incidence rates for wheat flour sensitization between 2.2%–4.2% per person-year and for α-amylase of 2.5% per person-year. A more detailed comparison of studies is not possible since these tests have been performed using different methods, extracts, and cut-off points. Moreover, sparse data are available on background levels of sensitization; some occupationally unexposed individuals have specific IgE to "occupational" bakery allergens possibly due to nonoccupational exposures, while others have an increased propensity to develop general IgE-mediated sensitization (atopy) or cosensitization or cross-reactivity to other allergens, such as pollens.

A number of cross-sectional studies have shown that the prevalence of rhinitis is two- to four-fold higher than asthma-like symptoms (46). The prevalence of occupational rhinitis ranges between 18%–29%, while incidence rates are between 4.1%–13.1% per person-year (43, 44). Again, a detailed comparison of these studies is difficult as they incorporate variable (or missing) information on participation rates, methodology, and important risk modifiers such as atopy, gender, and smoking (46).

National registries, where they are kept, suggest that in many countries asthma in bakery workers is one of the most frequently occurring forms of OA. Data from the UK SWORD surveillance scheme (47) suggest that the annual incidence of asthma in bakery workers is between 29 and 41 cases per 100,000, putting this employment sector among the highest risk groups for developing OA. Disease registries in most other countries are consistent with the British data (48–51), although there are some notable exceptions (52). There is some evidence that in some countries the incidence may be falling (53), but this does not seem to be a general experience and it is seldom possible to reach firm conclusions about time trends from voluntary reporting schemes. Apart from registry-based estimates, incidence information for baker's asthma is available from studies across the industry. The prevalence of OA ranges between 4% and 13%, and incident rates are between 3–44 cases per 1000 person-years (44, 54).

Other work-related asthma (WRA) phenotypes such as work-exacerbated asthma (WEA) have been reported in bakers in African (prevalence=2.6%–3%) and European (10.4%) settings (55–57).

Studies of bakery apprentices

Several studies of apprentice bakers have been undertaken on the premise that cohorts of previously unexposed subjects will reveal the natural history of sensitization and disease. The first was a German cohort study in 880 apprentices with a 5-year follow-up of annual SPT. The study showed cumulative incidence data for sensitization of 12% in the second year, 19% in the third, 27% in the fourth, and 30% in the fifth year (58). Symptom incidence rates "compatible with allergic rhinitis or asthma" also increased from 0.2% to 7% in the third year but dropped to 4.8% after 5 years. A limitation of this study was the high loss to follow-up, particularly in the later years, which may have biased the estimates of prevalence and cumulative incidence.

This early study was followed by a number of apprentice studies in the baking and pastry industries in the past 25 years. These reported incidence rates for symptoms compatible with OA of around 10.0 per 100 person-years, as well as suggesting atopy and female gender as risk factors. For rhinitis, a higher incidence rate between 13.1 and 22.1 per 100 person-years was observed, while identifying sensitization to wheat flour at baseline and atopy as important risk factors. A more recent study of apprentices suggested, however, that atopy was not a risk factor for the earlier onset of OA (54).

As suggested by Herxheimer's early study (58), the incidence of new symptoms peaks early during the apprenticeship. In Figure 12.2, for example, the highest rate of new nasal and asthma symptoms occurs at about 4 months of follow-up. One interesting issue is the occurrence of asthma-like symptoms in relation to the presence of bronchial hyperresponsiveness (BHR) at the beginning of the vocational training. BHR appears to be associated with incident respiratory symptoms (59, 60) and a rise in inflammatory markers such as exhaled nitric oxide (FeNO) and sputum eosinophilia (61, 62).

Some studies have challenged assumptions derived from earlier work. In a cohort of Polish apprentices, there appeared to be no evidence of an "allergic march" since there was no difference between the time to onset of rhinitis and asthma (63). In a Danish study (60), the rise in incident asthma-like symptoms in an apprentice cohort was not paralleled by an increase in sensitization of the same magnitude, despite a very comprehensive battery of occupational allergens used. This again indicates that not only is allergic asthma a feature but nonallergic inflammation also has a role in the immunological reactions triggered by the initial exposure to bakery dust.

Determinants and exposure-response studies

Earlier studies were able to show exposure-sensitization relationships using general flour dust exposure data or worker perceptions on levels of "dustiness." Subsequent studies included specific quantitative exposure data on both inhalable dust and airborne allergens. In a population of newly exposed British bakery and mill workers, new work-related symptoms were closely related to flour aeroallergen exposure intensity (64). Positive SPT responses to mixed flour and to α-amylase were also more frequent with increasing exposure intensity, although this was confounded by atopic status. Similarly, in Dutch bakers, a strong and positive association was found between wheat flour allergen exposure and specific sensitization, particularly in atopic workers. In sensitized bakers, those with an elevated allergen exposure more often reported work-related symptoms. In this setting, the existence of exposure-sensitization gradients suggested that the risk of flour sensitization would probably be negligible at exposure levels of 0.2 µg/m³ wheat allergen or approximately 0.5 mg/m³ inhalable dust (65). Similar exposure-response relationships were also reported with respect to α-amylase (66). A further Dutch study of β(1→3)glucan found significant exposures in the baking industry and an association with wheat allergen concentrations but not with symptoms (67).

A reanalysis of the original Dutch study on wheat allergen exposure and sensitization has shown no indication of an

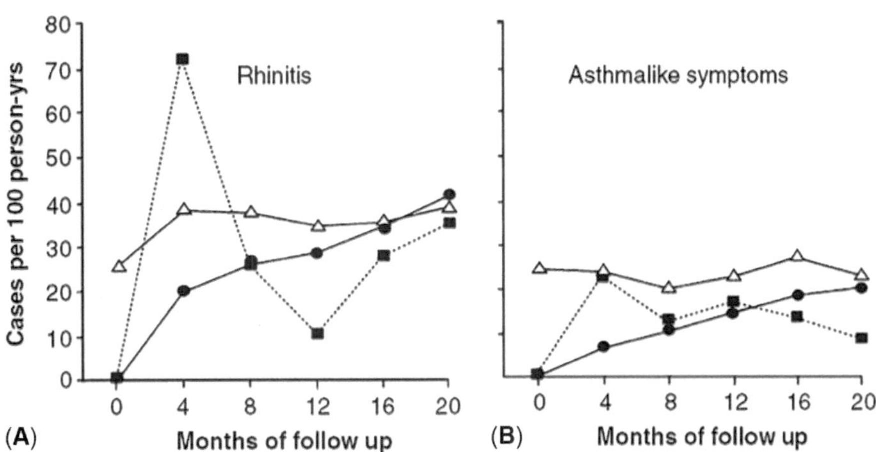

FIGURE 12.2 Incidence rates (■), cumulative incidence proportion (●), and prevalence (Δ) among bakery apprentices. (From Reference [60], by permission.)

exposure threshold, as has a more recent study in South African supermarket bakery workers (Figure 12.3). The risk of sensitization increases with increasing exposure intensity up to 10–15 µg/m³ wheat allergen concentration and flattens off at higher exposure levels. Interestingly, a similar analysis for symptomatic allergy, defined as sensitization in combination with either upper respiratory work-related symptoms (rhinitis) or asthma, results in a more sharply increasing exposure-response relationship, followed by a flattening, and then a reduction of the risk at higher exposure levels. Attenuation of risk at higher exposure levels is probably due to the healthy worker effect. Other factors such as wheat IgG4 showed no protective effect for sensitization, confirming the findings of previous studies; however, this needs to be established in longitudinal studies (68).

In a South African supermarket bakery intervention study, which demonstrated a greater than 50% reduction in flour dust exposures 1 year after a multifaceted intervention (69), a greater decline in the incidence of cereal flour sensitization (21% vs 6%) and mean FeNO in bakers with baseline FeNO at least 25 ppb (16.9 vs 7.7 ppb) was observed in the intervention compared to the control group (70). The study further demonstrated that belonging to the intervention group was a significant predictor of longitudinal

decline (≥10%) in FeNO over 1 year. This was particularly evident in bakers with work-related ocular-nasal symptoms at baseline (odds ratio 3.73, confidence interval 1.22–11.42). One of the limitations of this study was the short (1 year) follow-up, which could have possibly demonstrated further intervention effects had the period been extended.

Cohort studies have also shown that those who are sensitized to wheat or amylase have an elevated risk of developing work-related allergy (rhinitis, asthma) symptoms within a few years, indicating that work-related sensitization is an important risk factor for symptoms (71), although the initial incidence of respiratory symptoms seems to be independent of sensitization (60, 62). Some of these studies also suggest that the risk of sensitization attenuates after a few years and that fewer cases of sensitization occur after the first years of exposure. However, the length of follow-up of most studies does not allow firm conclusions on changes in risk over time.

Atopy is the most important risk modifier of work-related sensitization (Figure 12.4) (46). In most studies, atopy was defined as a positive SPT response to one or more common allergens (grasses, trees, house dust mites, etc.) and the risk of work-related sensitization estimated to be 5–20 times higher in atopic workers. A similar association was observed for incident asthma-like symptoms among apprentices (59, 60). Significantly, the inclusion of sensitization to grasses and pollens in its definition may have inflated the true importance of atopy, since there is some immunological cross-reactivity between these and wheat sensitization (see Table 12.1 in 'Allergens: nature and sources'). Other risk factors have also been investigated; only one study identified cigarette smoking as a risk factor for work-related sensitization (72). Rhinitis has been associated with an increased risk of developing OA due to cereal flour proteins. Two studies have suggested genetic risk factors; Toll-like receptor 4 (TLR4) and β2-adrenergic receptors (ADRB2) gene polymorphisms have been associated with work-related respiratory symptoms and wheat flour sensitization in bakery workers (46).

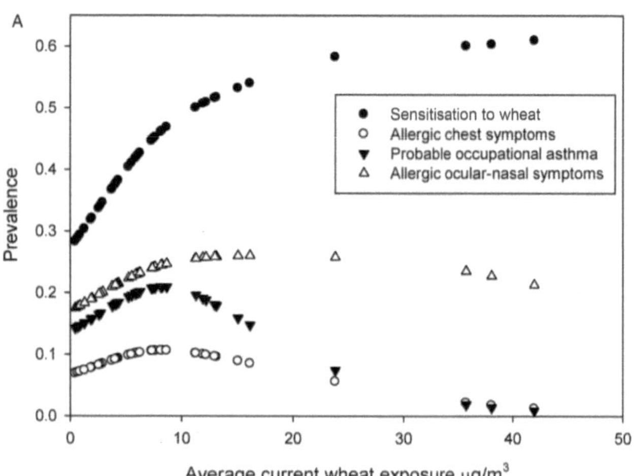

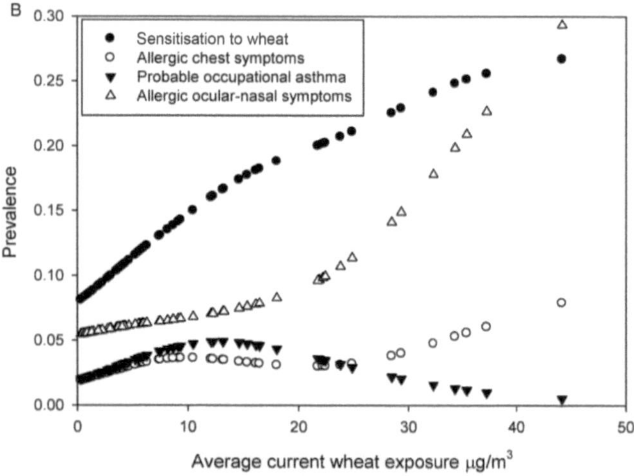

FIGURE 12.3 Relationship between various clinical endpoints and wheat allergen concentrations in **(A)** atopic (n=196) and **(B)** nonatopic (n=270) supermarket bakery workers (68). (By permission.)

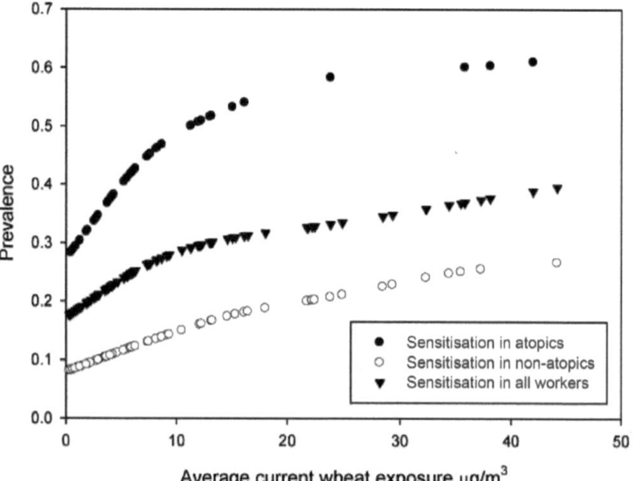

FIGURE 12.4 Relationship between wheat sensitisation and wheat allergen concentration among supermarket bakery workers (n=466), stratified by atopic status (68). (By permission.)

Diagnosis

The diagnosis of baker's asthma is frequently straightforward. Following an asymptomatic, "latent" period measured usually in months but sometimes of several years, patients develop the classic symptoms of an allergy to an airborne protein: rhinitis and chest tightness, wheeze, and breathlessness. The absence of rhinitis (which usually develops before the onset of asthma) in a baker with wheeze should prompt a consideration of other explanations for asthma. In most cases there is a clear relationship between periods at work and the development or worsening of symptoms. Symptoms may resolve within a few hours of leaving work, but can persist for 24 hours or more; in these circumstances, symptomatic improvement may not be appreciated over a day or two away from work but only during a more prolonged break. As with all types of OA, the diagnosis may be more challenging when there is a prior history of "constitutional" asthma.

Specific sensitization to bakery allergens can be identified either by SPT or in serum by detection of specific IgE antibodies. Where possible it is advisable that both techniques be used since there is some variability in the antigens prepared by different commercial producers of test materials (73) although with high-quality skin test extracts, there tends to be close agreement with in vitro assays. For example, in the study cited above, for a positive challenge with wheat flour the positive predictive value (PPV) of specific IgE determination was identical to that of SPT (74%), while in the case of rye flour SPT (91%) had a higher PPV than specific IgE (82%). Interestingly, the degree of sensitization is associated with a positive bronchial challenge, suggesting that some challenge tests with flour can be avoided in subjects with high-grade sensitization (74). While it has been suggested that intradermal testing with flour has a higher sensitivity than SPT, there are no studies that have made a direct comparison.

Most bakers with OA are sensitized to flour or other cereal allergens. Little information is available about the clinical relevance of other bakery allergens (see "Allergens: nature and sources") with the exception of baking enzymes. Most important among these is α-amylase but an increasing number and variety of other enzymes are used to "improve" bread and other baked goods. These are generally unidentified, which can cause problems in the consideration of bakers with clear work-related symptoms but no evidence of sensitization to either flour or α-amylase. One solution is to request a specialist laboratory to set up an IgE assay to the "improver mix" of enzymes. A less satisfactory alternative is to recognize that sensitization to nonamylase enzymes in the absence of sensitization to α-amylase appears to be very rare (24).

Both cross-sectional and longitudinal studies of bakers indicate that work-related nasal and bronchial symptoms occur with a higher frequency than sensitization. For example, in a longitudinal study of 186 Canadian pastry apprentices, 30 reported incident work-related symptoms of rhinoconjunctivitis, but only three of these developed a positive SPT to flour (75). Similar findings were described in a 20-month study of 87 bakery apprentices in Denmark, among whom the cumulative incidence of asthma-like symptoms was 21% but that of occupational sensitization rate just 6% (60). It is not entirely clear why bakers report work-related symptoms without evidence of sensitization to established bakery allergens; irritant mechanisms have been proposed, but, as above, in some cases there may be allergy to unidentified workplace antigens. A limited number of studies that included specific bronchial challenge tests suggest that symptomatic subjects without sensitization to known bakery allergens have a low risk of a positive response to challenge with flour, although some such cases have been reported (74). On the contrary, in subjects with established sensitization the likelihood of a positive challenge is high (76).

Bakers who are sensitized to flour may have additional sensitization to grass pollens although it is not clear that this is any more frequent than sensitization to other common aeroallergens. Cosensitization can be differentiated from cross-reactivity to plant pollen by radioallergosorbent test (RAST) inhibition (77); when flour was coupled to the solid phase, no inhibition by grass pollen could be shown in bakers, whereas this was clearly not the case in nonbakers with hay fever. Nonbakers with a high degree of sensitization to grass and birch pollen may show an allergic asthmatic reaction after inhalation of flour due to cross-reactivity (78). Bakers with OA are rarely sensitized to wheat pollen (79) and are very rarely intolerant to ingested bread, probably because heat, and perhaps gastric juices, denature wheat allergens.

Serial measurements of peak expiratory flow (PEF), or serial spirometry with portable electronic spirometers, ideally made at two to three hourly intervals from waking to sleep during a 4-week period that includes spells at and away from work, can identify WRA, with deterioration during periods at work and improvement during absence from work. These methods do not, however, identify the cause of any WRA and specific inhalation testing with relevant allergens may be indicated if the diagnosis cannot be made with sufficient confidence by noninvasive tests. Challenges with flour are usually undertaken by simulating the workplace using a dust-tipping method (80); alternatively, flour may be inhaled after being dispersed by dust dispersers (81) or Spinhaler devices (82). In all cases it is probably sensible to use flour or other ingredients from the patient's workplace. Powdered enzymes may be delivered similarly but are sometimes nebulized in an aqueous solution (80).

Management

The successful management of baker's asthma centers around the avoidance of further exposure to the cause of their disease. This can be achieved by a reduction in dust exposures at work, by the use of respiratory protection, or by a change of work (exposure cessation). In practice, because once sensitized, individuals react to very low concentrations of inhaled allergen, a reduction in dust exposure is impractical under the usual circumstances of bakery work. The use of respiratory protection is similarly impractical as a long-term solution but can allow an individual to continue in employment and provide time to consider and obtain alternative employment. In many cases—particularly in small "craft" bakeries—an alternative site of work in the bakery, where exposure to flour can be avoided, cannot be found and exposure is adequately avoided only by leaving work. In large bakeries, relocation at work is a more feasible solution, but even here, because of the dustiness of bakeries, avoidance of exposure sufficient to prevent the provocation of asthmatic symptoms may be difficult. In the rare cases of sensitization to bakery enzymes alone, work in a bakery where these are not used may be feasible.

Baking is a craft and many bakers enjoy and are proud of their work. For these reasons, and because of the adverse financial consequences of leaving work, some bakery workers with OA choose to remain in employment, despite being made aware that their asthma is likely to become increasingly severe and may become irreversible. In these cases, they should be advised to keep exposures to a minimum by careful work practices and the judicious use of respiratory protective equipment; their asthma and rhinitis should be treated sufficiently with inhaled corticosteroids and, where helpful, antihistamines; and they should be kept under regular medical review. A single case history suggests that treatment with omalizumab may allow patients to continue to work in baking in spite of severe asthma that is poorly controlled with standard asthma medication including oral steroids (83).

The evidence base for the effective management of bakery workers with occupational rhinitis alone (in the absence of asthma) is weak. Unsurprisingly, continuing allergen exposure in those with rhinitis causes continuing nasal symptoms, which may be difficult to manage effectively with medication and which can make the wearing of protective face masks very uncomfortable. Conversely, the avoidance of further exposure often leads to the resolution of (or at least improvement in) rhinitis. On these grounds, it would not be unreasonable to manage cases of lone rhinitis as one would asthma. However, rightly or wrongly, rhinitis is generally considered a less "serious" disease than asthma, and while there is reasonable evidence that occupational rhinitis, in general terms, increases the risk of subsequent OA, it is also clear that many bakery employees with rhinitis do not later develop asthma; it is currently not possible to distinguish these groups. In reality, the majority of cases of uncomplicated baker's rhinitis will continue to be exposed at work; management through exposure reduction and enhanced medical surveillance seems reasonable in such cases.

Prevention

Setting exposure standards

In the late 1990s, epidemiological studies incorporating detailed exposure assessment that allowed exposure-response modeling, suggested risks at (flour) dust exposures far lower than those previously considered. As a result, several countries felt able to set more stringent exposure standards. In the United States, the American Conference of Governmental Industrial Hygienists (ACGIH) adopted a threshold limit value for inhalable flour dust of 0.5 mg/m³ averaged over an 8-hour work shift (84). In Sweden, a standard for inhalable dust was set to 3 mg/m³ over 8 hours (85). In 2008, the Scientific Committee on Occupational Exposure Limits (SCOEL) EU declined to set a limit value but concluded that exposures at or below 1 mg/m³ of inhalable flour dust would protect the majority of exposed workers from the onset of disease although recognized that these concentrations may trigger symptoms in already sensitized workers (86). Values are based on no-observable adverse effect levels (NOAEL) obtained from the literature with or without adjustments for technical feasibility. Such levels can readily be met by most modern plant and in-store bakeries, with the possible exception of some activities that involve large quantities of flour dust during specific tasks (87). Notably, this approach has not yet been used to set exposure limits for α-amylase.

A different approach has been followed in the Netherlands (88). The Dutch Expert Committee on Occupational Safety (DECOS) expert-group concluded that a NOAEL could not be defined, since no exposure threshold is observable in Dutch and South African epidemiological studies. They therefore calculated the excess risk at a range of exposure levels, assuming a baseline sensitization rate to wheat allergens in the general population of 2%, concluding that an (acceptable) excess risk of 1% occurs at exposure levels of 0.2 mg/m³ (89). Using the same approach for α-amylase a safe level of 0.9 ng/m³ was proposed for all workers, irrespective of atopic status (90).

It has been demonstrated that interventions focusing on risk education and safe work practices have a limited effect on allergen exposures (91). In contrast, enzyme sensitization numbers were reduced after reducing bread improver exposures to below 1 mg/m³ (92). Experiences from the United Kingdom and Germany indicate that surveillance may be effective (93, 94). However, these entail multiple interventions and suffer from selection bias. A recent study showed that a general group-effect of a multifaceted intervention was hard to find, but was discernible in a symptomatic group (nose and eye symptoms) 1 year after the intervention (70).

Reduction of dust and allergen exposures

Real-time monitoring shows that tasks such as emptying and then compressing bags containing flour, dough improvers, or dusting dough are among the dustiest bakery tasks. Maintenance and spillage-cleaning with brooms or the use of pressurized air also lead to high exposures. Silo- and bin-cleaning tasks resulted in the highest dust exposure according to one study (87). A Canadian study of the potential determinants of dust exposures showed that the use of horizontal mixers is associated with higher dust exposures than the use of vertical mixers (geometric mean exposure 13.0 mg/m³ vs 3.8 mg/m³; $p < 0.001$) (95); and that the use of divider oil to prevent dough adhesion was associated with considerably lower exposures than dusting with flour (geometric mean exposure 0.43 mg/m³ vs 12.0 mg/m³; $p<0.001$) (95). Dough brakes, or "sheeters," used for kneading, lead to exposures that are several orders of magnitude higher than with the use of other, automated forming methods (87, 95). Using flour of a coarser particle size is an effective way of decreasing airborne dust levels, and in one study was an effective intervention (96). The use of reversible sheeters, in which dough is kneaded in a back-and-forth manner, leads to increased exposures, probably because rapid changes in the direction of the machine's belt-like surface can result in emissions of dust particles. The use of premixed flour/enzyme products has been associated with higher exposure to fungal α-amylase (39).

Automation can lead to lower exposure (97), although maintenance seems crucial (95). Flour-dusting can be performed using flow tables. Exposure to enzymes could be reduced by the use of encapsulated, micropelletized, or liquid/paste enzyme formulations. Compliance with good housekeeping, optimal work practices, and the identification of an appointed safety representative appear to result in lower dust exposures (98). Unfortunately, there is little evidence of any concerted effort to reduce dust exposures in bakeries; data from the United Kingdom collected between 1995 and 2003, for example, indicate no significant temporal reduction in flour dust exposures (99).

Other preventive approaches

A program in the Netherlands attempted to change the current focus on risk education to a "covenant" of bakeries, flour mills, and ingredient producers (100). In a before–after comparison, there was evidence in some sectors of an increase in the use of local exhaust ventilation and liquid improver formulations. These were not, however, accompanied by important reductions in flour or α-amylase exposures; indeed among general bakers, a strong *increasing* trend in exposure to α-amylase was observed. In a smaller study of UK bakery workers (101), those employees who reported that they had been "warned" of the risks of dust exposure were less likely to report work-related respiratory symptoms and less likely to have a specific sensitization, although it is unclear if these associations were unconfounded.

Using simulation techniques based on cross-sectional data to examine the effectiveness of several strategies to reduce the burden of baker's asthma (91), the most successful approach was one of rigorous health surveillance identifying sensitized or symptomatic workers and decreasing their individual exposures by 90% shortly after diagnosis, resulting in an estimated decrease of almost 60% in disease burden after 20 years.

In a later study, the same group compared interviews with self-reported questionnaires and found that a questionnaire would be the most efficient way to prescreen workers for a medical examination (102). It is worth noting here that symptom-based questionnaires delivered by employers or their occupational health representatives are (at least in the United Kingdom) insensitive in the routine surveillance of bakery employees (103, 104). In contrast, questionnaire-based prediction models delivered by external, disinterested agencies have a far higher diagnostic accuracy (103, 105), although it is perhaps difficult to see how they could be used for periodic examination of bakers at risk.

Summary and research needs

Respiratory allergies in bakers are probably as old as baking itself, and by and large we understand the important issues in unusual detail. The baking environment is, in allergenic terms, complex and in some respects increasingly so as the assortment of cereals and other flours is broadened to satisfy consumers with an unending taste for variety, and as the complexity of enzymatic "improvers" grows to increase productivity. There should therefore be research efforts to keep on characterizing new sensitizing agents. This information should be transferred rapidly to clinicians but it is helpful to keep in mind that the vast majority of cases of baker's asthma are attributable to either flour or α-amylase hypersensitivity, and that the clinical picture is almost invariably one of a classic airborne protein allergy with prominent rhinitis. Unhappily, attempts at primary prevention have proved largely unsuccessful although it seems clear that they must incorporate dust control (there being no option of either "eliminating" or substituting flour) through technological change, careful work practices and education, all means for which innovative strategies should be proposed and tested. The profits in breadmaking are, however, marginal and it has proved difficult to persuade employers to invest, or bakers, who tend to view their work as a "craft"—as an "art" even—to change their ways. Research investments should therefore be obtained from other sources.

References

1. Ramazzini B. Diseases of Bakers and Millers. Disease of workers—De Morbis Artificium. New York, NY: Hafner Publishing Company, Inc.; 1713:225–35.
2. De Besche A. Serologische Untersuchungen über 'allergische Krankheiten' beim Menchen. Acta Pathol Microbiol Scand. 1929;6:115–44.
3. Baagöe KH. Mehlidiosynkrasie als Ursache vasomotorischer rhinitis und asthma. Acta Medica Scandinavica. 1933;80(4–6):310–22.
4. Verma DK, Purdham JT, Roels HA. Translating evidence about occupational conditions into strategies for prevention. Occup Environ Med.2002;59(3):205–13; quiz 14.
5. Quirce S, Diaz-Perales A. Diagnosis and management of grain-induced asthma. Allergy Asthma Immunol Res. 2013;5(6):348–56.
6. Brisman J. Baker's asthma. Occup Environ Med.2002;59(7):498–502; quiz, 426.
7. Tatham AS, Shewry PR. Allergens to wheat and related cereals. Clin Exp Allergy. 2008;38(11):1712–26.
8. Posch A, Weiss W, Wheeler C, et al. Sequence analysis of wheat grain allergens separated by two-dimensional electrophoresis with immobilized pH gradients. Electrophoresis. 1995;16(7):1115–9.
9. Sander I, Flagge A, Merget R, et al. Identification of wheat flour allergens by means of 2-dimensional immunoblotting. J Allergy Clin Immunol. 2001;107(5):907–13.
10. Raulf M. Allergen component analysis as a tool in the diagnosis and management of occupational allergy. Mol Immunol. 2018;100:21–7.
11. Gómez-Casado C, Garrido-Arandia M, Pereira C, et al. Component-resolved diagnosis of wheat flour allergy in baker's asthma. J Allergy Clin Immunol. 2014;134(2):480–3.
12. Olivieri M, Biscardo CA, Palazzo P, et al. Wheat IgE profiling and wheat IgE levels in bakers with allergic occupational phenotypes. Occup Environ Med.2013;70(9):617–22.
13. Sander I, Rozynek P, Rihs HP, et al. Multiple wheat flour allergens and cross-reactive carbohydrate determinants bind IgE in baker's asthma. Allergy. 2011;66(9):1208–15.
14. Sander I, Rihs HP, Doekes G, et al. Component-resolved diagnosis of baker's allergy based on specific IgE to recombinant wheat flour proteins. J Allergy Clin Immunol. 2015;135(6):1529–37.
15. Sander I, Rihs HP, Brüning T, Raulf M. A further wheat allergen for baker's asthma: Tri a 40. J Allergy Clin Immunol. 2016;137(4):1286.
16. Goesaert H, Brijs K, Veraverbeke WS, et al. Wheat flour constituents: how they impact bread quality, and how to impact their functionality. Trends Food Sci Tech. 2005;16(1):12–30.
17. Park SH, Na Y, Kim J, et al. Properties and applications of starch modifying enzymes for use in the baking industry. Food Sci Biotechnol. 2018;27(2):299–312.
18. Trabelsi S, Ben Mabrouk S, Kriaa M, et al. The optimized production, purification, characterization, and application in the bread making industry of three acid-stable alpha-amylases isoforms from a new isolated Bacillus subtilis strain US586. J Food Biochem. 2019;43(5):e12826.
19. Baur X, Chen Z, Sander I. Isolation and denomination of an important allergen in baking additives: alpha-amylase from Aspergillus oryzae (Asp o II). Clin Exp Allergy. 1994;24(5):465–70.
20. Simonis B, Hölzel C, Stark U. Glucoamylase: a current allergen in the baking industry. Allergo J Int. 2014;23(8):269–73.
21. Baur X, Sander I, Posch A, Raulf-Heimsoth M. Baker's asthma due to the enzyme xylanase – a new occupational allergen. Clin Exp Allergy. 1998;28(12):1591–3.
22. Merget R, Sander I, Raulf-Heimsoth M, Baur X. Baker's asthma due to xylanase and cellulase without sensitization to alpha-amylase and only weak sensitization to flour. Int Arch Allergy Immunol. 2001;124(4):502–5.
23. Sander I, Raulf-Heimsoth M, Siethoff C, et al. Allergy to Aspergillus-derived enzymes in the baking industry: identification of beta-xylosidase from Aspergillus niger as a new allergen (Asp n 14). J Allergy Clin Immunol. 1998;102(2):256–64.
24. Jones M, Welch J, Turvey J, et al. Prevalence of sensitization to 'improver' enzymes in UK supermarket bakers. Allergy. 2016;71(7):997–1000.
25. Santaolalla M, De Barrio M, De Frutos C, et al. Double sensitization to enzymes in a baker. Allergy. 2002;57(10):957.
26. Elms J, Fishwick D, Walker J, et al. Prevalence of sensitisation to cellulase and xylanase in bakery workers. Occup Environ Med.2003;60(10):802–4.
27. Quirce S, Polo F, Figueredo E, et al. Occupational asthma caused by soybean flour in bakers–differences with soybean-induced epidemic asthma. Clin Exp Allergy. 2000;30(6):839–46.
28. Wieslander G. Review on buckwheat allergy. Allergy. 1996;51(10):661–5.
29. de Jong NW, van Maaren MS, Vlieg-Boersta BJ, et al. Sensitization to lupine flour: is it clinically relevant? Clin Exp Allergy. 2010;40(10):1571–7.
30. van Kampen V, Sander I, Quirce S, et al. IgE sensitization to lupine in bakers—cross-reactivity or co-sensitization to wheat flour? Int Arch Allergy Immunol. 2015;166(1):63–70.
31. Weiner A. Occupational bronchial asthma in a baker due to aspergillus; a case report. Ann Allergy. 1960;18:1004–7.
32. Tee RD, Gordon DJ, van Hage-Hamsten M, et al. Comparison of allergic responses to dust mites in U.K. bakery workers and Swedish farmers. Clin Exp Allergy. 1992;22(2):233–9.
33. Storaas T, Steinsvåg SK, Florvaag E, et al. Occupational rhinitis: diagnostic criteria, relation to lower airway symptoms and IgE sensitization in bakery workers. Acta Otolaryngol. 2005;125(11):1211–7.
34. Droste J, Myny K, Van Sprundel M, et al. Allergic sensitization, symptoms, and lung function among bakery workers as compared with a nonexposed work population. J Occup Environ Med. 2003;45(6):648–55.

35. Panzani R, Armentia A, Lobo R, et al. Tolerance mechanisms in response to antigens responsible for baker's asthma in different exposed people. J Asthma. 2008;45(4):333–8.

36. Raulf M, Buters J, Chapman M, et al. Monitoring of occupational and environmental aeroallergens–EAACI Position Paper. Concerted action of the EAACI IG Occupational Allergy and Aerobiology & Air Pollution. Allergy. 2014;69(10):1280–99.

37. Heederik D, Doekes G, Nieuwenhuijsen MJ. Exposure assessment of high molecular weight sensitisers: contribution to occupational epidemiology and disease prevention. Occup Environ Med. 1999;56(11):735–41.

38. Houba R, Van Run P, Heederik D, Doekes G. Wheat antigen exposure assessment for epidemiological studies in bakeries using personal dust sampling and inhibition ELISA. Clin Exp Allergy. 1996;26(2):154–63.

39. Baatjies R, Meijster T, Lopata A, et al. Exposure to flour dust in South African supermarket bakeries: modeling of baseline measurements of an intervention study. Ann Occup Hyg. 2010;54(3):309–18.

40. Bogdanovic J, Wouters IM, Sander I, et al. Airborne exposure to wheat allergens: measurement by human immunoglobulin G4 and rabbit immunoglobulin G immunoassays. Clin Exp Allergy. 2006;36(9):1168–75.

41. Bogdanovic J, Wouters IM, Sander I, et al. Airborne exposure to wheat allergens: optimised elution for airborne dust samples. J Environ Monit. 2006;8(10):1043–8.

42. Sander I, Zahradnik E, Bogdanovic J, et al. Optimized methods for fungal alpha-amylase airborne exposure assessment in bakeries and mills. Clin Exp Allergy. 2007;37(8):1229–38.

43. Jeebhay M, Baatjies R. Baker's allergy and asthma: a review of the literature. Curr Opin Allergy Clin Immunol. 2013;26:232–43.

44. Jeebhay MF, Baatjies R. Prevention of baker's asthma. Curr Opin Allergy Clin Immunol. 2020;20(2):96–102.

45. Wiszniewska M, Tymoszuk D, Nowakowska-Świrta E, et al. Mould sensitisation among bakers and farmers with work-related respiratory symptoms. Ind Health. 2013;51(3):275–84.

46. Jeebhay MF, Moscato G, Bang BE, et al. Food processing and occupational respiratory allergy—An EAACI position paper. Allergy. 2019;74(10):1852–71.

47. Meredith SK, McDonald JC. Work-related respiratory disease in the United Kingdom, 1989–1992: report on the SWORD project. Occup Med (Oxford, England). 1994;44(4):183–9.

48. Orriols R, Isidro I, Abu-Shams K, et al. Reported occupational respiratory diseases in three Spanish regions. Am J Ind Med. 2010;53(9):922–30.

49. Karjalainen A, Kurppa K, Virtanen S, et al. Incidence of occupational asthma by occupation and industry in Finland. Am J Ind Med. 2000;37(5):451–8.

50. Esterhuizen TM, Hnizdo E, Rees D. Occurrence and causes of occupational asthma in South Africa–results from SORDSA's Occupational Asthma Registry, 1997–1999. S Afr Med J. 2001;91(6):509–13.

51. Ameille J, Pauli G, Calastreng-Crinquand A, et al. Reported incidence of occupational asthma in France, 1996–99: the ONAP programme. Occup Environ Med. 2003;60(2):136–41.

52. Oh SS, Kim KS. Occupational asthma in Korea. J Korean Med Sci. 2010;25(Suppl):S20–5.

53. Paris C, Ngatchou-Wandji J, Luc A, et al. Work-related asthma in France: recent trends for the period 2001–2009. Occup Environ Med. 2012;69(6):391–7.

54. Rémen T, Acouetey DS, Paris C, et al. Early incidence of occupational asthma is not accelerated by atopy in the bakery/pastry and hairdressing sectors. Int J Tuberc Lung Dis. 2013;17(7):973–81.

55. Wiszniewska M, Walusiak-Skorupa J. Diagnosis and frequency of work-exacerbated asthma among bakers. Ann Allergy Asthma Immunol. 2013;111(5):370–5.

56. Baatjies R, Lopata AL, Sander I, et al. Determinants of asthma phenotypes in supermarket bakery workers. Eur Respir J. 2009;34(4):825–33.

57. Ade S, Adjobimey M, Agodokpessi G, et al. Asthma symptoms in bakeries at Parakou, Benin. Pulm Med. 2020;2020:3767382.

58. Herxheimer H. The skin sensitivity to flour of baker's apprentices. A final report of a long term investigation. Acta Allergol. 1973;28(1):42–9.

59. Demange V, Wild P, Zmirou-Navier D, et al. Associations of airway inflammation and responsiveness markers in non asthmatic subjects at start of apprenticeship. BMC Pulm Med. 2010;10:37.

60. Skjold T, Dahl R, Juhl B, Sigsgaard T. The incidence of respiratory symptoms and sensitisation in baker apprentices. Eur Respir J. 2008;32(2):452–9.

61. Demange V, Zmirou-Navier D, Bohadana A, Wild P. Do airway inflammation and airway responsiveness markers at the start of apprenticeship predict their evolution during initial training? A longitudinal study among apprentice bakers, pastry makers and hairdressers. BMC Pulm Med. 2018;18(1):113.

62. Tossa P, Paris C, Zmirou-Navier D, et al. Increase in exhaled nitric oxide is associated with bronchial hyperresponsiveness among apprentices. Am J Respir Crit Care Med. 2010;182(6):738–44.

63. Walusiak J, Hanke W, Górski P, Pałczyński C. Respiratory allergy in apprentice bakers: do occupational allergies follow the allergic march? Allergy. 2004;59(4):442–50.

64. Cullinan P, Lowson D, Nieuwenhuijsen MJ, et al. Work related symptoms, sensitisation, and estimated exposure in workers not previously exposed to flour. Occup Environ Med. 1994;51(9):579–83.

65. Houba R, Heederik D, Doekes G. Wheat sensitization and work-related symptoms in the baking industry are preventable. An epidemiologic study. Am J Respir Crit Care Med. 1998;158(5 Pt 1):1499–503.

66. Houba R, Heederik DJ, Doekes G, van Run PE. Exposure-sensitization relationship for alpha-amylase allergens in the baking industry. Am J Respir Crit Care Med. 1996;154(1):130–6.

67. Stuurman B, Meijster T, Heederik D, Doekes G. Inhalable beta(1->3)glucans as a non-allergenic exposure factor in Dutch bakeries. Occup Environ Med. 2008;65(1):68–70.

68. Baatjies R, Meijster T, Heederik D, Jeebhay MF. Exposure-response relationships for inhalant wheat allergen exposure and asthma. Occup Environ Med. 2015;72(3):200–7.

69. Baatjies R, Meijster T, Heederik D, et al. Effectiveness of interventions to reduce flour dust exposures in supermarket bakeries in South Africa. Occup Environ Med. 2014;71(12):811–8.

70. Al Badri FM, Baatjies R, Jeebhay MF. Assessing the health impact of interventions for baker's allergy and asthma in supermarket bakeries: a group randomised trial. Int Arch Occup Environ Health. 2020;93(5):589–99.

71. Cullinan P, Cook A, Nieuwenhuijsen MJ, et al. Allergen and dust exposure as determinants of work-related symptoms and sensitization in a cohort of flour-exposed workers; a case-control analysis. Ann Occup Hyg. 2001;45(2):97–103.

72. Musk AW, Venables KM, Crook B, et al. Respiratory symptoms, lung function, and sensitisation to flour in a British bakery. Br J Ind Med. 1989;46(9):636–42.

73. van Kampen V, Merget R, Rabstein S, et al. Comparison of wheat and rye flour solutions for skin prick testing: a multi-centre study (Stad 1). Clin Exp Allergy. 2009;39(12):1896–902.

74. van Kampen V, Rabstein S, Sander I, et al. Prediction of challenge test results by flour-specific IgE and skin prick test in symptomatic bakers. Allergy. 2008;63(7):897–902.

75. Gautrin D, Ghezzo H, Infante-Rivard C, Malo JL. Incidence and host determinants of work-related rhinoconjunctivitis in apprentice pastry-makers. Allergy. 2002;57(10):913–8.

76. Quirce S, Fernández-Nieto M, Escudero C, et al. Bronchial responsiveness to bakery-derived allergens is strongly dependent on specific skin sensitivity. Allergy. 2006;61(10):1202–8.

77. Sander I, Raulf-Heimsoth M, Düser M, et al. Differentiation between cosensitization and cross-reactivity in wheat flour and grass pollen-sensitized subjects. Int Arch Allergy Immunol. 1997;112(4):378–85.

78. Merget R, Sander I, van Kampen V, et al. Allergic asthma after flour inhalation in subjects without occupational exposure to flours: an experimental pilot study. Int Arch Occup Environ Health. 2011;84(7):753–60.

79. Armentia A, Díaz-Perales A, Castrodeza J, et al. Why can patients with baker's asthma tolerate wheat flour ingestion? Is wheat pollen allergy relevant? Allergol Immunopathol (Madr). 2009;37(4):203–4.

80. Suojalehto H, Suuronen K, Cullinan P. Specific challenge testing for occupational asthma: revised handbook. Eur Respir J. 2019;54(2).

81. Cloutier Y, Lagier F, Lemieux R, et al. New methodology for specific inhalation challenges with occupational agents in powder form. Eur Respir J. 1989;2(8):769–77.

82. Merget R, Heger M, Globisch A, et al. Quantitative bronchial challenge tests with wheat flour dust administered by Spinhaler: comparison with aqueous wheat flour extract inhalation. J Allergy Clin Immunol. 1997;100(2):199–207.

83. Pérez Pimiento A, Bueso Fernández A, García Loria J, et al. Effect of omalizumab treatment in a baker with occupational asthma. J Investig Allergol Clin Immunol. 2008;18(6):490–1.

84. ACGIH. American Conference of Governmental Industrial Hygienists. Documentation on Flour Dust. Cincinnati, OH: ACGIH; 1999.

85. Arbetarskyddsstyrelsen Hygieniska gränsvärden och ätgärder mot luftföroreningar. 2000; Stockholm, Sweden.

86. SCOEL. Recommendation from the Scientific Committee on Occupational Exposure Limits for Flour Dust. 2008. ec.europa.eu/social/BlobServlet?doc Id=3869&langId=en.

87. Nieuwenhuijsen MJ, Sandiford CP, Lowson D, et al. Peak exposure concentrations of dust and flour aeroallergen in flour mills and bakeries. Ann Occup Hyg. 1995;39(2):193–201.

88. DECOS. Wheat and Other Cereal Flour Dusts: An Approach for Evaluating Health Effects from Occupational Exposure. 2020; www.gr.nl. Gezondheidsraad, Den Haag, The Netherlands.

89. Health Council of the Netherlands. Wheat and other cereal flour dusts, publication no. 2017/10. The Hague; 2017.

90. Heederik DJJ. Towards evidence-informed occupational exposure limits for enzymes. Ann Work Expo Health. 2019;63(4):371–4.

91. Meijster T, Warren N, Heederik D, Tielemans E. What is the best strategy to reduce the burden of occupational asthma and allergy in bakers? Occup Environ Med. 2011;68(3):176–82.

92. Smith TA. Preventing baker's asthma: an alternative strategy. Occup Med (Lond). 2004;54(1):21–7.

93. Smith TA, Patton J. Health surveillance in milling, baking and other food manufacturing operations–five years' experience. Occup Med (Lond). 1999;49(3):147–53.

94. Hölzel C, Kühn R, Stark U, Grieshaber R. Risk-based surveillance program baker's asthma [in German]. Arbeitsmed Sozialmed Umweltmed. 2009(44):533–8.

95. Burstyn I, Teschke K, Kennedy SM. Exposure levels and determinants of inhalable dust exposure in bakeries. Ann Occup Hyg. 1997;41(6):609–24.

96. Mason HJ, Fraser S, Thorpe A, et al. Reducing dust and allergen exposure in bakeries. AIMS Allergy Immunol. 2017(1):194–206.

97. Jauhiainen A, Louhelainen K, Linnainmaa M. Occupational hygiene around the world: exposure to dust and α-amylase in bakeries. Appl Occup Environ Hyg. 1993;8(8):721–5.

98. Elms J, Robinson E, Rahman S, Garrod A. Exposure to flour dust in UK bakeries: current use of control measures. Ann Occup Hyg. 2005;49(1):85–91.

99. van Tongeren M, Galea KS, Ticker J, et al. Temporal trends of flour dust exposure in the United Kingdom, 1985–2003. J Environ Monit. 2009;11(8):1492–7.

100. Meijster T, Tielemans E, Heederik D. Effect of an intervention aimed at reducing the risk of allergic respiratory disease in bakers: change in flour dust and fungal alpha-amylase levels. Occup Environ Med. 2009;66(8):543–9.

101. Fishwick D, Harris-Roberts J, Robinson E, et al. Impact of worker education on respiratory symptoms and sensitization in bakeries. Occup Med (Lond). 2011;61(5):321–7.

102. Jonaid BS, Rooyackers J, Stigter E, et al. Predicting occupational asthma and rhinitis in bakery workers referred for clinical evaluation. Occup Environ Med. 2017;74(8):564–72.

103. Brant A, Nightingale S, Berriman J, et al. Supermarket baker's asthma: how accurate is routine health surveillance? Occup Environ Med. 2005;62(6):395–9.

104. Gordon SB, Curran AD, Murphy J, et al. Screening questionnaires for bakers' asthma–are they worth the effort? Occup Med (Lond). 1997;47(6):361–6.

105. Meijer E, Suarthana E, Rooijackers J, et al. Application of a prediction model for work-related sensitisation in bakery workers. Eur Respir J. 2010;36(4):735–42.

13

ASTHMA AND ALLERGY TO ANIMALS, FISH, AND SHELLFISH

Mohamed F. Jeebhay,[1] Karin Pacheco,[2] Andreas L. Lopata,[3] and Jean-Luc Malo[4]
[1]*Occupational Medicine Division and Centre for Environmental & Occupational Health Research (CEOHR), School of Public Health and Family Medicine, Faculty of Health Sciences, University of Cape Town, Cape Town, South Africa*
[2]*Division of Environmental & Occupational Health Sciences, Department of Medicine, National Jewish Health, and Division of Environmental & Occupational Health, University of Colorado School of Public Health, Colorado, USA*
[3]*James Cook University, Australian Institute of Tropical Health and Medicine, Queensland, Australia*
[4]*Hôpital du Sacré-Cœur de Montréal and Université de Montréal, Montréal, Québec, Canada*

Contents

Introduction

Allergens derived from animals, insects, fish, and shellfish are an important source of sensitization and symptoms at work. The highest animal exposures occur in farming, ranching, feed, and processing operations, but the important development of biological research in the past century has exposed workers to allergens derived from laboratory animals, an important cause of occupational asthma (OA).

Laboratory animals

Exposure

Laboratory animals, particularly rodents, are an important component of research. The use of laboratory animals is so ubiquitous and important, that animal use practices are regulated and monitored by a separate body, Association for Assessment and Accreditation of Laboratory Animal Care (AAALAC, www. aaalac.org) International. The vast majority of all animals used in research are mice and rats. Exposure to laboratory animals occurs in two primary settings: the animal care facility and the research laboratory. Air sampling and epidemiological research have identified certain job tasks where the exposure to animal allergens is particularly high, such as direct handling of animals (injections, shaving), cage cleaning, and changing filters of room ventilation systems. Exposure is less in feeding animals or, even less so, in working with unconscious animals.

Specific modifications of animal cages have significantly reduced animal allergen exposures, from a situation of open cages to the ventilated top cage (1, 2). Changes in cage bedding from sawdust and wood chips to noncontact absorbent pads also reduce exposure. The respirable fraction of inhaled animal particles is increased with direct animal handling (3). Male rodents produce more allergens than females. In animal facilities, many nonmouse handlers may have levels of mouse allergen exposure similar to mouse handlers.

Veterinarians work with a wide range of furred and feathered animals. All of these job categories have been associated with animal allergy (Table 13.1).

Causative agents

Table 13.1 lists the most commonly used laboratory and farm animals. It summarizes available knowledge on the source and nature of the allergen response for sensitization, allergy, and asthma, as well as their biological and immunological characteristics.

Clinical presentation

Similar to other high-molecular-weight (HMW) antigens, laboratory animal allergens trigger IgE-mediated disease characterized by rhinorrhea and sneezing, eye itching and watering, skin itching and hives, and/or cough, chest tightness, shortness of breath, and/or wheeze characteristic of asthma. Many sensitized workers first present with rhinitis and conjunctivitis, which may precede the onset of asthma (4). In a systematic review, it was found that rhinitis is more associated with OA than predictive of OA due to HMW agents (5). Most laboratory animal (LA) allergic disease develops within the first 2–3 years of exposure (6) although sensitization and asthma may occur up to 10 years from first exposure, particularly in nonatopic workers. Once sensitized, workers may develop life-threatening anaphylaxis to a rodent bite (7) and, on occasion, a systemic allergic response to an animal bite may be the first indication of a laboratory animal allergy (LAA) (8). Work exposures also include a number of irritants, including straw and wood chip bedding, animal dander, along with water and commercial detergents in cage wash, that, with repeated exposures, can cause a chronic irritant dermatitis.

Epidemiology

Exposure to animals is frequent at work. In a study of nearly 5000 Australian workers, 11% admitted being exposed to various animals including 3% as farming/animal workers (9). The prevalence of LAA symptoms is high (mainly oculonasal), nearly 20% in a study of researchers (10). For LAA defined as both animal-related symptoms and evidence of laboratory animal sensitization, the prevalence falls to 10% to 20% of exposed workers (11). Possible explanations include that sensitization to laboratory animals causes more symptoms than sensitization to common allergens (12), that exposures to animal allergens in the research workplace may be more intense than common allergen exposure, and that laboratory animal exposure encompasses a number of respiratory irritants such as animal bedding, cleaning agents, and animal waste. A study of 13,957 US workers over 48 years identified the highest adjusted prevalence ratio of asthma of 14.9 in the occupational group with animal and feather exposures (13).

A prospective cohort study of 417 apprentices in animal-health technology evaluated them from 8 to 44 months of follow-up by skin testing, questionnaire, and spirometry. Incident skin sensitization to at least one animal-derived allergen was 23%, which was much higher than in apprentices exposed to flour and latex. The incidence of probable OA was 2.7/100 person-years (28/1043 person-years) (6). The incidence of specific sensitization after 8 years of exposure (job-related to training) was 1.8/100 person-years in 242 participants (14). The 12-year incidence of LAA symptoms in a cohort of 495 LA workers with 2080 person-years of exposure was 2.26 (1.61–2.91) per 100 person-years (15).

Risk factors and modifiers

Atopy is the most important personal modifier for the development of laboratory animal sensitization. In one study of pharmaceutical workers exposed to rats (16), atopy was a significant risk factor for chest symptoms (OR=5.2 (1.9±16.9)) and for rat skin test positivity (OR=6.1, 95% CI:2.1±17.8). LAA also associates with allergy symptoms and positive skin tests to cat and dog (17). Cigarette smoking, on the other hand, does not increase risk for laboratory animal sensitization as reviewed by Siracusa et al. (18). Genetic susceptibility studies implicate HLA-DR7 with sensitization to rats (OR, 1.82; 95% CI:1.12–2.97), respiratory symptoms at work (OR, 2.96; 95% CI:1.64–5.37), and, most strongly, sensitization with symptoms (OR, 3.81; 95% CI:1.90–7.65), whereas HLA-DR3 was protective against sensitization (OR, 0.55; 95% CI:0.31–0.97) (19). Functional variants in genetic factors responsive to allergen and endotoxin also affect risk for symptoms and sensitization, including the TLR4 minor variant (20) that associates with atopy, and the endotoxin responsive CD14/-1619 G alleles with significantly lower lung function (21) in atopic workers, compared to those with the alternate genotype.

Prevention

As discussed in Chapter 10, prevention of LAA should be first aimed at reducing exposure to the occupational allergens, the intensity of exposure being the main determinant of both the occurrence (22) of symptoms of LAA and, more generally, the worsening of OA if exposure persists. Assessment (Chapter 5) and management (Chapter 9) of exposed workers should include health surveillance programs in which information and regular meetings are offered.

TABLE 13.1 Laboratory-Animal- and Farm-Animal-Derived Agents Causing Occupational Asthma

Animal	Source	Allergen(s)	Nature	Structural Information—Molecular Weight	Biological Role/ Human Immune Response	Properties
Rat *Rattus norvegicus*	Urine (also glandular) *4. Newman Taylor, 1977*	Rat nl.02 (alpha-2-globulin) *3. Santiago, 1998*	Lipocalin *1. Bayard, 1996*	LMW 17 kDa	Pheromones/IgE	Mature rats *2. Gordon, 1996* secrete more serum proteins in urine
	Fur/hair/saliva *5. Baker, 2001*		Albumin	HMW ≥22 kDa (fur), LMW <22 kDa (saliva)		
	Urine	Rat n 1.01	Lipocalin	21 kDa	Pheromone	
	Serum *6. Wood, 2001*		Albumin similar to mouse albumin	MW 68kDa		Allergenic in 24% of rat-sensitized workers
Mouse *Mus musculus*	Urine *4, Newman Taylor, 1977*	Mus ml (MUA)	Lipocalin (sequence homology with Schistosome antigen) *3. Santiago, 1998* Equ cl, Feld4	LMW 19 kDa	Pheromones	Urine of male contains ˜4 times more Mus ml than female
	Hair	Mus m2, Agl, Ag3 *7. Longbottom, 1987*	Glyco-Protein	LMW 16 kDa		Not found in urine
	Serum *6. Wood, 2001*		Similar to rat albumin	MW 68 kDa		Allergenic in 30% of mouse-sensitized workers
Guinea pig *Cavia porcellus*	Fur, dander, saliva, and urine (other allergens less potent)	Cav p1 Cav p2	Lipocalin *8. Fahlbusch, 2003*	MW: 20 kDa	IgE specific to guinea pig serum and albumin	Lipocalins share 60% homology with Bos d2 (cow)
Rabbit *Oryctola Gus cuniculus*	Fur, saliva, urine, and dander/pelt *9. Price, 1988*		Lipocalin	MW>250-4.4 kDa; MW<34 kDa, ≥18 kDa, and <21 kDa		
Ferret *Mustela Putorius furo*	Hair, urine, and pelt *11. Codina, 2001*		Albumin *10. Nugent, 2003*	MW: 66 kDa 103, 81, 28.8 14.8 kDa 17 and 34 kDa	IgE-mediated response	Allergens studied mostly in male ferret urine; X-reactivity to cat
Monkey (cotton-t-optamarin) *Saguinus oedipus*	Dander and urine *12. Petry, 1985*				IgE-mediated response	
Cow *Bos domesticus*	Hair, dander, urine	Bos d2: major allergen (and isoforms) *14. Rautiaine, 2001*	Lipocalin *13. Mäntyjärvi, 1996*	MW: 20 and 22 kDa (dander) and 20 kDa in urine also 14, 30, 55, 67–97 kDa *15. Heutelbech, 2000; 16. Santiago, 1997; 17. Ylonen, 1992*	Bos d2: weak immunogen 40; IgE and IgG responses + SIC	Monoclonal antibody to the 20 kDa allergen without X-reactivity to cat, dog, horse
Goat *Caprahircus* (Bovidae family)	Hair and dander *18. Ferrer, 2006*	Not identified	Not identified	LMW: 9–30 kDa	Specific IgE to goat and cow allergens; + SIC	Moderate to high X-reactivity to cow epithelium
Pig-(gut) *Sus*	Vapor from pig-gut soaking *19. Donnay, 2006*		Albumin gamma globulin	MW: 26 kDa	Specific IgE to goat and cow allergens; + SIC	Moderate X-reactivity to cat

(*Continued*)

TABLE 13.1 Laboratory-Animal- and Farm-Animal-Derived Agents Causing Occupational Asthma (*Continued*)

Animal	Source	Allergen(s)	Nature	Structural Information—Molecular Weight	Biological Role/Human Immune Response	Properties
Pig *Sus*	Hair, urine 20. *Brennan, 1985*	Not identified	Not identified	Not identified	+ SPT and specific IgE+ PEF	
Deer *Capreolus*	Hair dander 21. *Nahm, 1996*	Not identified	Lipocalin	MW: 110, 72, 59 45, 21 kDa	IgE-mediated	Possible X-reactivity with related species
Roe deer *Capreolus capreolus*	Hair, dander 22. *Carballada, 2006*	Not identified	Lipocalin	MW 16–20 kDa, 37 and 75 kDa	+ SPT specific IgE + conjunctival test	X-reactivity with cow allergens
Chicken *Gallus gallus*	Poultry- related antigens; mites, feathers, feed, droppings 23. *Bar-Sela, 1984*	Not identified	Not identified	Not identified	+ SPT to poultry antigens + specific IgE reaction; + SIC	
	Feathers 24. *Perfetti, 1997*	Not identified	Not identified	Not identified	+ SPT to feathers + FEV$_1$ at work	
Mink *Mustelidae*	Urine not pelt 25. *Gomez, 1996*	Not identified	Not identified	Not identified	+ SPT to urine, neg specific IgE, + SIC	

Abbreviations: FEV$_1$, forced expiratory volume in 1 second; HMW, high-molecular-weight; kDa, kilo Dalton; LMW, low-molecular-weight; MW, molecular weight; PEF, peak expiratory flow; SIC, specific inhalation challenge; SPT, skin-prick test.

Slightly modified from Pacheco K, Fautrin D, Lopata AL, Jeebhay MF. Asthma and allergy to animals. (From Malo JL, Chan-Yeung M, Bernstein DI, eds. Asthma in the Workplace. 4th ed. Boca Raton: CRC Press; 2013.)

References: 1. Bayard C, et al. Biochem Biophys Acta. 1996;1290:129–34; 2. Gordon S, et al. Clin Exp Allergy. 1996;26:533–41; 3. Santiago ML, et al. Int Arch Allergy Immunol. 1998;117:94–104; 4. Newman Taylor A, et al. Lancet. 1977:847–9; 5. Baker J, et al. Clin Exper Allergy. 2001;31:303–12; 6. Wood RA. ILAR J. 2001;42:12–6; 7. Longbottom JL, et al. Int Archs Allergy Appl Immunol. 1987;82:450–2; 8. Fahlbusch B, et al. Allergy. 2003;58:629–34; 9. Price JA, et al. Allergy. 1988;43:39–48; 10. Nugent NS, et al. J Allergy Clin Immunol. 2003;111:Suppl 2;S324; 11. Codina R, et al. J Allergy Clin Immunol. 2001;107:927; 12. Petry RW, et al. J Allergy Clin Immunol. 1985;75:268–71; 13. Mäntyjärvi R, et al. J Allergy Clin Immunol. 1996;97:1297–303; 14. Rautiaine J, et al. J Chromatogr B Biomed Sci Appl. 2001;763:91–8; 15. Heutelbeck AR, et al. Int Arch Occup Environ Health. 2009;82:1123–31; 16. Santiago AL, et al. Allergol Immunopathol (Madr). 1997;25:259–65; 17. Ylonen J, et al. Int Arch Allergy Immunol. 1992;99:112–7; 18. Ferrer A, et al. Ann Allergy Asthma Immunol. 2006;96:579–85; 19. Donnay C, et al. Allergy. 2006;61:143–4; 20. Brennan NJ. Irish Med J. 1985;78:321–2; 21. Nahm DH, et al. Ann Allergy Asthma Immunol. 1996;76:423–6; 22. Carballada F, et al. Ann Allergy Asthma Immunol. 2006;97:707–10; 23. Bar-Sela S, et al. J Allergy Clin Immunol. 1984;73:271–5; 24. Perfetti L, et al. Allergy. 1997;52:594–5; 25. Gomez I, et al. Allergy. 1996;51:364–5.*

Control of exposure

Various administrative (training, medical surveillance, etc.), engineering (robotic equipment, separately ventilated cages, negative pressure environments, downdraft tables, etc.), hygiene practice (restrictive access to animal rooms, clothing, etc.), and personal protective measures are used by institutions where laboratory animals are handled as detailed in a US national survey, in which, however, participation of centers was low (23). Measures designed to lower exposure to animal allergens succeeded in reducing the incidence of reported symptoms (24). A decline in the incidence of LAA to zero was observed in the last 2 years of a comprehensive program including education, engineering controls, administrative controls, use of personal protective equipment (PPE), and medical surveillance over a 5-year period (25).

Increasing local ventilation remains the most effective way of controlling exposure. The use of individually ventilated cage systems has been shown to reduce external airborne rat and mouse allergen concentrations, especially when operated at negative pressure to the environment. A study carried out in 750 laboratory animal workers has shown that individually ventilated cages not only reduce allergenic burden but also result in improving rates of sensitization (2). Control of exposure is a more effective and ethical way to reduce the incidence of sensitization and OA than focusing on host susceptibility characteristics such as atopy or sensitization to pets that represent unsatisfactory predictors (6).

Although this was proposed for other occupational agents (see Chapter 10), there are no occupational exposure standards for laboratory animal allergens. Exposure limits should be set "as low as reasonably practicable."

Medical surveillance

Health surveillance is recommended using a combination of questionnaires, assessment of IgE sensitization, and, if possible, nonspecific bronchial responsiveness (NSBR), especially in the first years after starting exposure (6).

Globally, it would be tempting to deduce that the use of various prevention means reviewed above has resulted in reducing the frequency of OA due to laboratory animals, as for OA due to many other occupational agents, as based on the interpretation of medicolegal registries or voluntary health surveillance programs (see Chapter 3) (26). At the least, reducing exposure by using individually ventilated cages has resulted in improving the frequency of sensitization to laboratory animals (2).

TABLE 13.2 Insects and Mites Causing Occupational Sensitization, Allergy, and Asthma

Animal	Industry/ Occupation	Disorders/ Symptoms	Allergens/Source	Structural Information (MW (dDa))	References
Coleoptera (**beetle**)					
Green weevil (*Sitophilus gr.*)	Grain mill, bakery	Rhinitis, asthma	Whole body (unknown)	5–199	*1. Lopata, 2005*
Bean weevil (*Bruchus lentis*)					*2. Stejskal, 2008*
Mealworm (*Tenebrio molitor*)					*3. Siracusa, 2003*
Ground bug (*Metopoplax ditomoides*)					*4. Bernstein, 2009*
Warehouse beetle (*Trogoderma variabile*)					*5. Armentia, 2006*
Orthoptera (**grasshopper**)					
Grasshopper (*Locusta migratoria*) (*Schistocerca gregaria*) (*Melanoplus sanguinipes*)	Research lab	Asthma, rhinitis, urticaria	Whole body, wings (unknown)	52–107	*1. Lopata, 2005*
Cricket (*Acheta domesticus*) (*Gryllus bimaculatus*)					*6. Tee, 1988*
					7. Burge, 1980
					8. Bartra, 2008
					9. Bagenstose, 1980
Lepidoptera (**butterfly**)					
Bottle stalk borer (*Chilo partellus*)	Research lab	Rhinitis, urticarial anaphylaxis	Whole body (unknown)		
Pine processionary moth larvae (*Thaumetopoea pityocampa*)	Forest workers, silk processors, aquarists				
Silkmoth larvae of the bee moth (*Galleria mellonella*)					
Diptera (**fly**)	Animal farm, research lab	Asthma, rhinitis, urticaria	Whole body (unknown), wings	40–67	*6. Tee, 1988*
Housefly (*Musca domestica*)	Geneticists, hydroelectric aquarists				*7. Burge, 1980*
Fruit fly (*Drosophila melanogaster*)					*8. Bartra, 2008*
Plant sheep blowfly (*Lucilia caprina*)					*9. Bagenstrose, 1980*
Caddis fly (*Hydropsyche recurvata*)					*10. Lopata, 2000*
Larvae of the red midge (*Chironomus thummi*)					*11. Tracy, 2011*
					12. Vega, 1999
					13. Vega, 2004
					14. Baldo, 1989
Hymenoptera (**bee**)					
Bumble bee (*Bombus terrestris*)	Beekeeper, woodworker	Anaphylaxis, local urticaria	Venom, body dust, whole body	Phospholipase A(PLA2) acid, phosphatase, hyaluronidase allergen C mellitin	*15. Kraut, 1994*
Honey bee (*Apis mellifera*)					*16. Miedinger, 2010*
Wasp (*Vespula squamosa*)					*17. Tas, 2007*
Woodworm (*Scleroderma dom.*)					*18. Focke, 2003*
					19. Lembo, 2008
Blattodea (*cockroach*)					
German cockroach (*Blatella germanica*)	Research lab, grain mill	Asthma, rhinitis, urticaria	Bla, gl, Blag2, Bla g5	Protease Tropomyosin 14–78	*20. Kochuyt, 1993*
American cockroach (*Periplaneta am.*)	Animal handler				*21. Perez-Pimiento, 2007*
Oriental cockroach (*Blatta orientalis*)					*22. Potter, 2005*
					23. de Groot, 2006
					24. Roll, 2005
Acari (**mites**)					
Storage mite					
Lepidoglyphus destructor, Tyrophagus, Putrescentiae, Blomia tropicalis, Choroglyplus, Arcuatus acaras	Grain mill, animal farm, silo	Asthma	Lep d2 Tyr p2		
House dust mite					
Dermatophagoides pteronyssinus	Grain mill, animal farm, office	Asthma	Group 1 allergens Group 3 allergens	Proteases Tropomyosin	*25. Jeebhay, 2007*
Dermatophagoides farinae					*26. Koistinen, 2006*
					27. Iversen, 1990
					28. van Hage-Hamsten, 1988
					29. Cuthbert, 1995
					30. Terho, 1985

(Continued)

TABLE 13.2 Insects and Mites Causing Occupational Sensitization, Allergy, and Asthma (*Continued*)

Animal	Industry/ Occupation	Disorders/ Symptoms	Allergens/Source	Structural Information (MW (dDa))	References
Spider mite					
Red spider mite (*Tetranychus urticae*)	Apple farm	Asthma, rhinitis,			*26. Koistinen, 2006*
European red mite *(Panonychus ulmi)*	Greenhouse	urticaria			*27. Iversen, 1990*
Two-spotted mite *(Tetranychus urticae)*	worker				*31. de Jong, 2004*
Citrus red mite *(Panonychus citri)*					*32. Vieluf, 1993*
					33. Reunala, 1983
					34. Jeebhay, 2007
					35. Kim, 1999
					36. Burches, 1996
Various insects and mites used in pest control	Greenhouse worker	Asthma			*37. Lindström, 2018*

Source: Slightly modified from Pacheco K, Fautrin D, Lopata AL, Jeebhay MF. Asthma and allergy to animals. In: Malo JL, Chan-Yeung M, Bernstein DI, eds. *Asthma in the Workplace.* 4th ed. Boca Raton: CRC Press; 2013.

Abbreviations: FEV ₁, forced expiratory volume in 1 second; HMW, high molecular weight; kDa, kilo Dalton; LMW, low-molecular-weight; MW, molecular weight; PEF, peak expiratory flow; SIC, specific inhalation challenge; SPT, skin-prick test.

References: 1. Lopata AL, et al. Allergy. 2005;60:200–5; 2. Stejskal V, Hubert J. Ann Agric Environ Med. 2008;15:29–3; 3. Siracusa A, et al. Clin Exper Allergy. 2003;33:507–10; 4. Bernstein JA, et al. J Allergy Clin Immunol. 2009;123:1413–6; 5. Armentia A, et al. Allergy. 2006;61:1112–6; 6.Tee RD, et al. J Allergy Clin Immunol. 1988;81:517–25; 7.Burge PS, et al. Clin Allergy. 1980;10:355–63; 8. Bartra J, et al. J Invest Allergol Clin Immunol. 2008;18:141–2; 9.Bagenstose AH, et al. J Allergy Clin Immunol. 1980;65:71–4; 10. Lopata AL, et al. J Allergy Clin Immunol. 2000:16–9; 11. Tracy JM, Lewis EJ. Curr Opin Allergy Clin Immunol. 2011;11:332–6; 12. Vega JM, et al. Clin Exp Allergy. 1999;29:1418–23; 13. Vega J, et al. Contact Dermatitis. 2004;50:60–4; 14. Baldo BA, et al. Clin Allergy. 1989;19:411–7; 15. Kraut A, et al. Occup Environ Med. 1994;51:408–13; 16. Miedinger D, et al. Occup Environ Med. 2010 Jul;67(7):503 2010;67:503; 17. Tas E, et al. Der Hautarzt; Zeitschrift fur Dermatologie, Venerologie, und verwandte Gebiet. 2007;58:156–60; 18. Focke M, et al. Allergy. 2003;58:448–51; 19. Lembo S, et al. Contact Dermatitis. 2008;58:58–9; 20. Kochuyt AM, et al. Clin Exp Allergy. 1993;23:190–5; 21.Perez-Pimiento A, et al. Occup Med. 2007;57:602–4; 22. Potter PC. Curr Opin Allergy Clin Immunol. 2005;18:68–71; 23. de Groot H. Curr Opin Allergy Clin Immunol. 2006;6:294–7; 24. Roll A, et al. J Inv All Clin Immunol. 2005;15:305–7; 25. Jeebhay MF, et al. Int Arch Allergy Immunol. 2007;144(2):143–9; 26. Koistinen T, et al. Int Arch Occup Environ Health. 2006;79:602–6; 27. Iversen M, et al. Clin Exp Allergy. 1990;20:211–9; 28. van Hage-Hamsten M, et al. Allergy. 1988;43:545–51; 29. Cuthbert OD, et al. Clin Exp Allergy. 1995;25:382–3; 30. Terho EO, et al. Allergy. 1985;40:23–6; 31. de Jong NW, et al. Ann Allergy Asthma Immunol. 2004;93:281–7; 32. Vieluf D, et al. Allergy. 1993;48:212–4.; 33. Reunala T, et al. Clin Allergy. 1983;13:383–8; 34. Jeebhay MF, et al. Int Arch Allergy Immunol. 2007;144:143–9; 35. Kim YK, et al. J Allergy Clin Immunol. 1999;104:1285–92; 36. Burches E, et al. Clin Exp Allergy. 1996;26:1262–7; 37. Lindström I, et al. J Allergy Clin Immunol Pract. 2018;6:692–4.

Farm animals

Whereas exposure to laboratory animals is by far the principal cause of OA in workers exposed to animals and is the one more extensively examined, other animals and animal-derived antigens have been incriminated (Table 13.2) (https://reptox.cnesst.gouv.qc.ca/en/occupational-asthma/Pages/occupational-asthma.aspx). Most of the publications are case reports except for a few publications that are cross-sectional studies or case series that are commented below. Cow dander is still the third most frequent cause of OA in Finland (Hille Suojalehto, personal communication). Hinze et al. described 45 subjects with confirmed OA in whom IgE sensitization to cow dander was demonstrated (27). The major allergen was Bos d2 and the level of this allergen correlated with sensitization. OA has been documented in 16 poultry workers by Bar-Sela et al. (28), the majority with evidence of atopy and IgE-mediated sensitization to poultry antigens. Egg protein as a cause of OA has been extensively studied (29). In a cross-sectional study of 188 workers, Blair Smith et al. found 14 (7%) with OA. The cause was liquid or dried aerosol of egg protein. Bird keepers (n=200) were evaluated in zoos (30). The most common agents were canary, parrot, and pigeon feathers. El-Ansary and coworkers described seven Sudanese subjects with occupational symptoms, including one with OA, to bat guano (31). All had IgE-mediated reactivity to bat droppings of three species. The prevalence of OA was 14%. Among animals identified as causing OA (see quoted website in Section "Farm animals"), there are monkeys, deer, mink, goat dander and cheese, pig and pig gut, penguin, sea anemone, bat guano, and frog. Many animal-derived allergens can also cause OA, including lactoserum, raw beef, bovine serum albumin, casein, nacre, sericin, and royal jelly.

Insects

Exposure

A wide range of jobs and workplaces include exposure to various allergenic arthropods (Table 13.2): entomologists and laboratory workers exposed to locusts, crickets, and flies; grain mill workers and dock loaders sensitized to storage mites and grain weevils; food workers sensitized to the food colorant, carmine (cochineal extract), as well as to beetles, weevils and cockroaches. Electrical power plant and sewer workers may come in contact with caddis flies, while loggers and lumber mill workers may become sensitized to the tussock moth. While fish and bait handlers are at risk from exposure to larvae from the mealworm beetle, superworm, bee moth, blowfly, and chironomids, workers in pet food and pet retail may become sensitized to superworms and fleas. Outdoor work activities bring workers in contact with a large array of insects such as storage and spider mites. Workers in the honey industry are exposed to honeybee body dust and venom. There has been a newfound interest in insects for human consumption as food or edible insect species used whole or as ingredients in processed food products such as snacks, resulting in increased demand for their farming and processing.

Causative agents

Matrix

Arthropods produce large amounts of respirable allergens found in dust particulates or aerosols, including feces: dried exuviae, scales, hairs, fragmented dead remains, and metabolic products, such as feces, venoms, and silks. Storage mites feed on a variety of substances and this varied diet allows them to expand into a wider variety of ecological niches.

Allergen source and identified allergens

There have been many attempts to identify and characterize allergens from insects (Table 13.2). The feces and the peritrophic membrane seem to be important allergen sources in Orthoptera and in mites. Studies on locusts identified allergens in feces (32). Epidemiological studies of workers exposed to housefly and blow fly have also generally utilized extracts from whole adult flies (33). Additional allergens have been identified in the wings of locusts, also implicated in housefly sensitivity as well as in butterfly and silk moth wings. Similar wing proteins are found in locusts, beetles, flies, and moths suggesting allergic cross-reactivity.

Honeybee dust is a major source of allergen for those employed in the honeybee production with venom from bees, wasps, hornets, and ants. Several major allergens have been characterized in mite and cockroach species using the molecular techniques. Because many allergens originate from fecal products, these proteins are often digestive enzymes such as the mites group 1 and group 3 allergens and the cockroach allergen Bla g 2 (Aspartic protease). Other allergens are regulatory proteins. Studies of cross-reactivity have established immunological relationships between cockroaches, house dust mites, and crustaceans, and suggest tropomyosin may be an important cross-sensitizing allergen (34). Comparisons between storage and house dust mites demonstrate limited allergenic cross-reactivity (35). Molecular cloning demonstrates that the Group 2 allergens from storage mites show only 40% sequence identity with the Group 2 allergens from dust mites.

Clinical presentation, risk factors, and modifiers

The most common manifestations of OA due to arthropods include rhinitis, conjunctivitis, urticaria, and/or asthma. Many exposed subjects who develop symptoms also demonstrate IgE antibodies to the responsible allergens. In many cases, the route of exposure is to airborne arthropod allergens. Insect sting allergies can also be associated with work-related anaphylaxis. The diagnosis of occupational anaphylaxis can be made with more certainty if the reaction is accompanied by elevated serum tryptase levels documented within 2 hours of the incident, but the insect can also be identified by skin testing. Skin testing should be performed at least 6 weeks after the reaction, or may be falsely negative as specific IgE may have been consumed in the reaction. However, once identified, immunotherapy for insect sting allergies is highly effective in reducing occupational risk. Although a history of atopy is associated with increased risk of symptoms, it has poor predictive value for specific allergic sensitization. Tropomyosin, a fibrous structural protein that polymerizes with actin and regulates skeletal muscle function, is considered a pan allergen important in allergic cross-reactivity between crustaceans (crab, shrimp, and lobsters), mollusks (snail and squid), insects (including mites, mosquitos, cockroach, and silverfish), and some parasites (such as anisakis and ascaris) (36).

Case reports and series

Most documentation of OA due to insects has been published as case reports (https://reptox.cnesst.gouv.qc.ca/en/occupational-asthma/Pages/occupational-asthma.aspx) (Table 13.2). Some case series or proper epidemiological studies with more numerous subjects have been published. As a general consideration, rearing insects for agricultural purposes is associated with higher posthire onset of asthma (37).

Locusts, grasshoppers, and cockroaches

Burge and coworkers studied 118 workers in a research center breeding locusts, 26% reporting respiratory symptoms and 32% showing immediate skin reactivity to extracts of two locusts and a moth. Atopy was a risk factor and higher specific IgG was associated with exposure and disease (38). Of 16 workers in a research laboratory, four had presumed OA and half, skin reactivity (39). Cockroach is also a frequent cause of sensitization (approximately 20% of more than a thousand workers in food storage in Africa) (40) and in more than a hundred seamen (41).

Fly species, larvae, and worms

Fruit fly (*Drosophila*) is a common cause of sensitization, with one-third of 22 workers being symptomatic and sensitized in a study (42), the same proportion in the case of sheep blowfly (33). More than 50% of 17 workers in an hydroelectric power plant reported work-related symptoms and showed immediate skin reactivity to Caddis fly extracts (43). Aquatic fly (*chironomid*) exposure was associated with increased specific IgE levels in 20% of more than 600 fish breeders (44). Larvae of insects and worms used for fish bait can cause symptoms in nearly one-third of anglers and workers in fish farms (45). Sensitization to *Anisakis* worm was present in 8% of fish-processing workers (46). Gum derived from silkworm has been incriminated as causing OA in one-third of silk workers (47).

Mites and storage pests

A large variety of storage mites has been described as causing sensitization and OA in greenhouse, farm, grain, apple, flower, and grape workers (see https://reptox.cnesst.gouv.qc.ca/en/occupational-asthma/Pages/occupational-asthma.aspx).

Venom systemic reactions/anaphylaxis

Outdoor workers can be affected by insect stings and experience systemic reactions as listed in Table 13.2.

Seafood: Fish and shellfish

Exposure

Fishing and the seafood-processing industry

Fishery capture and aquaculture production produced 171 million tons in 2016 and provided direct employment and revenue for 60 million people worldwide, mostly (99%) from developing countries, and especially from Asia (48). The proportion of those employed in capture fisheries has decreased from 83% (1990) to 68% (2016), while those employed in aquaculture increased from 17% to 32% over this period.

The International Labour Organisation (ILO) estimates that approximately 50% of the fishing population work aboard fishing trawlers, 30% in aquaculture production (marine and freshwater), and 20% work inland as capture fishers or land-based activities such as processing (49). A characteristic feature of employment in the industry is the seasonal nature of work due to seasonal weather variations and the migratory nature of marine species. In many countries, labor in the fishing industry is divided along gender lines with men mainly (85%) involved in harvesting and some processing of seafood at sea, whereas women are mainly employed in processing activities ashore and some inland capture (48, 50).

A large proportion (88%) of seafood harvests are used for direct human consumption while the remainder for nonfood sources such as fishmeal and fish oil. In 2016, it is estimated that 53% of seafood harvested was eaten fresh in most developing countries. This proportion is declining toward trends in industrialized countries, as marine seafood stocks decrease and aquaculture and processing activities take hold. The processed aquatic products are mainly filleted frozen products, as well as dried, salted, canned products, surimi products, and fishmeal. Most of these processing activities involve exposure to seafood allergens in various forms that can cause allergic disease and asthma.

Working populations with seafood contact

Workers are involved in either manual or automated processing of crabs, prawns, mussels, fish, and fishmeal in factories. Processing plants, in particular, vary in technology, with some smaller workplaces relying entirely on manual seafood handling whereas larger companies use modern highly automated processes. There is also great variation in processing procedures and preservation techniques for the different seafood types that include filleting, freezing, drying, cooking, smoking, and high-pressure techniques (50). Aside from seafood processors, other occupations associated with exposure to seafood include harvesting activities (fishermen, aquaculture, oyster shuckers, fishmongers, truck drivers, maintenance), food preparation activities (restaurant chefs and waiters), laboratory and pharmaceutical technicians and researchers, pet food production, and value adding (shell grinders and jewelry polishers) (51–53).

Food-processing techniques

Aerosols and particulates produced in the seafood-processing industry are not inert but are biologically active proteins. In addition to the natural allergens, there is increasing evidence that food-processing techniques such as heating, freezing, and high pressures have the ability to change the nature, dose, and allergenicity of food (54). During processing, the seafood is concentrated into major allergen source compartments from muscle, visceral contents, and skin slime/mucin (51). The allergenic potential of these proteins is dependent on the seafood type with crustacean proteins being more allergenic than fish proteins (51). In addition, byproducts such as protease enzymes from the gut, chitin from shellfish, and endotoxin from Gram-negative bacteria also promote airway inflammation when present in high concentrations. Furthermore, storage conditions may affect allergenicity by influencing the relative distribution of various IgE-reactive proteins (54). Fish kept on ice for several days showed additional allergens and displayed much higher IgE-binding capacity than fresh fish. These changes may be attributed to the natural development of components such as formaldehyde in fish tissue, possibly affecting the allergenicity of some proteins (54). Other studies suggest that exposure to raw seafood may be less sensitizing to individuals than cooked seafood during processing activities (52, 53, 55).

Preservatives such as sulfites are also commonly used in prawn processing (53).

Work processes generating seafood

Common work processes that generate bioaerosols include butchering or grinding; degilling, "cracking," and boiling of crabs; cleaning and brushing of crabs; "tailing" of lobster; "blowing" of prawn meat through shells; washing or scrubbing of shellfish; degutting, heading, and cooking/boiling of fish; mincing of seafood; and cleaning of the processing line or storage tanks with high-pressured water hoses (50, 51, 56) (Figure 13.1). Processes

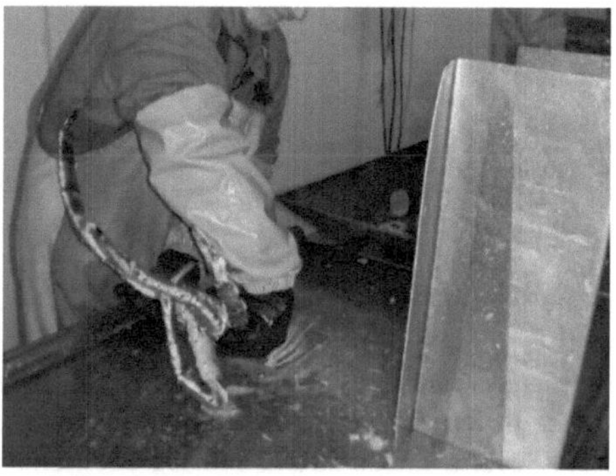

a. Degilling of crab

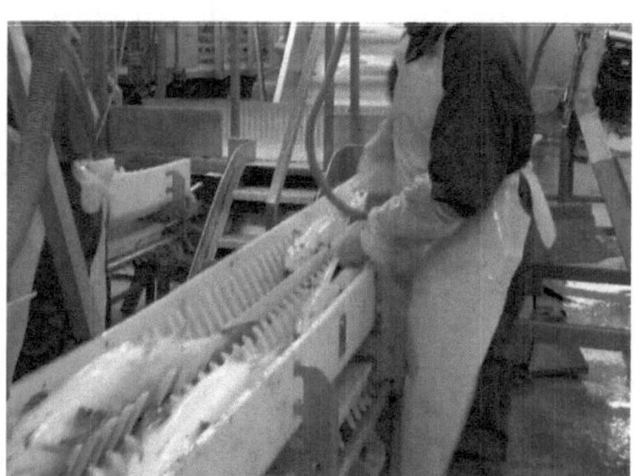

b. Degutting of salmon

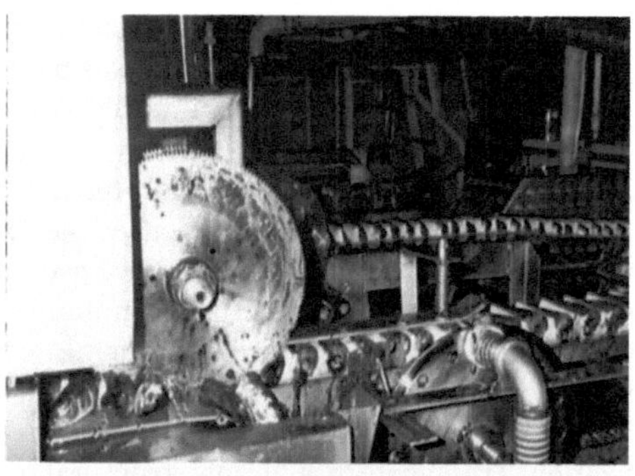

c. Degutting of pilchard

FIGURE 13.1 Work processes generating seafood bioaerosols. (Acknowledgment to Berit Bang and Mohamed Jeebhay picture archives.)

that generate dry aerosol particulates such as prawn blowing operations that use compressed air and fishmeal loading/bagging appear to generate higher levels of particulate than wet processes (prawn blowing with water jets) (50, 57). These aerosolized wet or dry particulates can subsequently be inhaled by workers and cause allergic respiratory disease.

Environmental exposure studies in seafood-processing plants from various countries have over the years demonstrated a wide range of aerosol concentrations, ranging from the lower limits of assay detection (LOD) to as high as 11 mg/m³ for total inhalable particulates, 6 mg/m³ for protein, and 75,000 ng/m³ for allergen levels (Table 13.3) (51, 52, 55).

A recent study of trends in OA and allergen levels in the United Kingdom from 2003–2017, reported allergen levels between 1–101,000 ng/m³ for shellfish (crab, prawn, scampi) tropomyosin and between LOD to 816 ng/m³ for salmon parvalbumin

(2017–2019) suggesting these levels had not declined over time (57). A Norwegian study showed differences in airborne tropomyosin concentrations in different parts of a plant where raw and cooked crab was processed (58). Some of the highest concentrations of particulates and allergens are detected during dusty fishmeal operations, and with crab processing aboard vessels at sea since processing occurs in confined spaces with poor ventilation. Particle concentrations are higher in factories with older processing machines and poor ventilation, with particles often in the respirable range (59, 60). In crab-processing environments at least 30% of airborne particulates are <5 μm in size and almost 100% are <1 μm in size in herring fish-filleting environments (51, 60). This suggests that most of these particles can reach the small airways. In addition, endotoxin levels can be relatively low in shrimp-processing plants, while much higher levels (103.7–136 EU/m³) were observed

TABLE 13.3 Exposure Assessment of Seafood-Handling Workers on Land and Aboard Vessels

Seafood Category	Particle Fraction Measured	Particulate Conc. (mg/m³) Range	Protein Conc. (mg/m³) Range	Allergen (ng/m³) Range	Endotoxin (EU/m³)
Crustaceans					
Crab (snow, Tanner,	Total inhalable	0.001–0.680	0.001–6.400	1–5061	32.6 (inhalable)
common, king)	Total inhalable	ND	0.011–0.048	0.1–76, raw (TM)	15.6 (respirable)
Crab (king)	Total inhalable	ND	0.003–0.027	1.3–5.1, cooked (TM)	LOD 24,000
Crab (edible)			0.003–0.047	0.4–72.2, raw (TM)	<1
			0.002–0.098	14.4–95.9, cooked (TM)	7–340
					7–20
Crab (snow)[a]	Total inhalable	ND	ND	79–21,093	ND
Prawn	Total inhalable	0.100–3.300	ND	ND	ND
Shrimp	Total inhalable	ND	ND	1500–6260	5.8–29.9 (inhalable)
Rock lobster	Thoracic	LOD, 0.661	LOD, 0.002	ND	ND
Scampi	Total inhalable	ND	ND	47–1042	ND
Finfish					
Whiff megrim/hake	Total inhalable	ND	ND	2–25	ND
	Respirable	0.040–3.570	ND	100–1000	ND
Salmon					
	Total inhalable	ND	ND	LOD, 1600	0.9–36.0
SalmonPollock	Total inhalable Total inhalable Total inhalable	NDND0.004	0.008–0.013NDND	0.20–358 (PA)20–186 (PA)ND	0.3–29.01.6–7.1 ND
Cod	Total inhalable	ND	ND	3800–5100	8.6–23.9
Pilchard	Thoracic	LOD, 2.954	LOD, 0.006	10–898	49
Herring	Total inhalable	ND	ND	300–1900	103.7
Herring	Total inhalable	ND	ND	63–9800	3–92
Fishmeal (anchovy)	Thoracic	LOD, 11.293	LOD, 0.004	69–75,748	136
Shark cartilage[b]	Respirable	0.920–5.140	ND	ND	ND
	Total inhalable	26.400–44.700	ND	ND	ND

[a] Processing aboard vessels; [b]Non-food-handling environment.

Abbreviations: ND, not done; LOD, limit of detection; TM, Tropomyosin; PA, Parvalbumin.

From References: **1.** Lopata AL, Jeebhay MF. *Curr Allergy Asthma Rep.* 2013;13(3):288–97. **2.** Shiryaeva O, et al. *Am J Ind Med.* 2014;57(3):276–85. **3.** Thomassen MR, et al. *Ann Occup Hyg.* 2016;60(7):781–94. **4.** Dahlman-Höglund A, et al. *Am J Ind Med.* 2012;55:624–30. **5.** Dahlman-Höglund A, et al. *Ann Occup Hyg.* 2013;57(8):1020–9.

in fish-gutting and fishmeal operations, and crab-processing plants (24,000 EU/m^3) (55, 58).

Causative agents

The seafood matrix

The three most important groups (phyla) of seafood organisms that are consumed and processed include the invertebrate Arthropods and Mollusca, and Pisces. All are associated with occupational allergy and asthma in high-risk populations (Table 13.4).

Exposures generated from processing seafood are complex. For example, aerosols generated in crab-processing plants demonstrate exoskeleton containing chitin, meat primarily muscle protein, gills, and kanimiso/internal organs. Fish juice produced in fish-filleting and canning plants contains various biogenic amines, degradation compounds associated with postmortem changes, digestive enzymes, skin slime/mucin, collagen, and fish muscle proteins. Furthermore, various nonseafood contaminants and additives have also been detected in the seafood matrix and may trigger allergic and respiratory symptoms. These include parasites (*Anisakis simplex*), protochordates (*Hoya* or sea squirt), red soft-coral, algae (dinoflagellates – *Hematodinium*), bacteria (Vibrio), and viruses (hepatitis A), marine or bacterial toxins (saxitoxins, scombroid toxin, histamine, and endotoxin), gases produced by anaerobic decomposition of fish (hydrogen sulfide), polyphosphates, nitrosamines, and residues of drugs used in aquaculture (e.g. antibiotics or hormones). Chemical additives (sulfites), spices (mustard, paprika, flour additives, and garlic), and hidden ingredients (casein) in canned or processed fish products add to the bioaerosol mix (51).

Allergen sources

Molecular characterization studies show that aerosolized seafood allergens are primarily HMW proteins and many are muscle components (Table 13.4) (61). Seafood allergens causing respiratory disease through inhalation in workers are often, but not always, the same as those causing seafood allergies through ingestion (62). In order to make this differentiation, the recent EAACI position paper highlighted this distinct form of inhalant food allergy, proposing the term *Class 3 food allergy* for such an entity (53). Immunological studies of serum obtained from crab/prawn processing workers with OA identified tropomyosin, a 34–39 kDa muscle protein, as the major allergen (57, 63, 64). Tropomyosin is also the major allergen in patients with ingestion-related food allergy (61). A minor inhalant shellfish allergen is the enzyme arginine kinase (40 kDa) identified in crab legs (65). Airborne snow crab tropomyosin and arginine kinase allergens are elevated in certain processing stations such as butchering and cooking activities compared to cleaning, packing, and storage activities (62). Studies suggest that cooked crab may be more allergenic than the raw form and is associated with higher tropomyosin levels (52, 53, 55, 58).

TABLE 13.4 Seafood and Associated Agents Causing Occupational Allergy and Asthma in Workers

Phylum	Class	Family Species (Common Name)	Allergen Name (Source)	Molecular Weight (kDa)
Arthropoda	Crustacea	Crab	Chi o 1 (tropomyosin - meat)	33
		Scampi, lobster, shrimp, shrimpmeal	Chi o 2 (arginine kinase - meat)	40
			Unidentified (meat, crab water)	4.4, 18.5, 25
		Prawn	Nep n DF9, Nep n 1 (tropomyosin - meat waste water)	30.2, 9780 35–3997
			Unidentified (dried whole body)	—
			Unidentified (raw, shrimp water)	
			Unidentified (cysts)	
			—	
Mollusca	Gastropoda	Abalone	—	—
	Bivalvia	Scallop	Unidentified (meat, viscera)	19–42
		Clam, oyster, mussel	—	—
	Cephalopoda	Octopus, squid	Unidentified (meat)	32, 43
		Cuttlefish	—	—
Pisces **(sub-phylum Chordata)**	Osteichthyes (bony fish)	Pilchard, anchovy	Sar sa 1, Sal s1 (parvalbumin - whole body, meat)	12, 36, 48, 60 (monomers/oligomers)
		Turbot Nile perch,[a] salmon, plaice, tuna, hake, cod, herring, trout, swordfish, (yellowfin) sole, pomfret, fishmeal (flour)	Glyceraldehyde-phosphate-dehydrogenase (whole body)	36 38, 58,61, 42, 29
			Unidentified (meat)	—
			Phosphoglucomutase, muscle actin, apolipoprotein Al (meat)	
			—	
	Chondrichthyes (cartilaginous fish)	Shark (cartilage)[a]	—	—
Other agents		Hoya (sea squirt), *Anisakis*, red soft coral, Daphnia, marine sponge, algae	—	—

[a]*Anaphylactic reaction.*

From References:　**1.** Jeebhay MF, et al. *Allergy.* 2019; Apr 6. doi:10.1111/all.13807. **2.** Lopata AL, et al. *Curr Allergy Asthma Rep.* 2013;13(3):288–97.

The muscle derived protein, parvalbumin, is one of the major airborne allergens responsible for asthma in fish-processing workers, as demonstrated for pilchard, herring, salmon, and other species (60, 66). Few other fish allergens have been demonstrated in the occupational setting and include glyceraldehyde-3-phosphate dehydrogenase, enolase, and aldolase (53). However, these enzymes are heat-sensitive, probably increasing the risk of sensitization while handling raw rather than cooked fish (52, 53, 55).

Some seafood allergens such as tropomyosin and arginine kinase are highly cross-reactive among shellfish species due to very similar IgE antibody binding protein regions (67). Workers allergic to one type of seafood may therefore develop allergic symptoms to other crustaceans (shrimp, lobster) as well as mollusca (oyster, squid, clam), insects (cockroach), parasites (*Anisakis*), and dust mites (61). Similarly, the major allergen parvalbumin demonstrated a high degree of cross-reactivity between different fish species (61). However, there appears to be no demonstrated cross-reactivity between shellfish and bony fish species.

Clinical presentation

Inhalation and skin contact are the main routes of exposure in workplace settings. In individuals exposed to seafood aerosols, both allergic and irritant reactions have been observed (52). Allergy is generally an IgE-mediated response to a seafood allergen present in the seafood matrix. There is also evidence from in vitro models that seafood digestive enzymes such as trypsin (from salmon, pilchard, and king crab) can activate protease-activated receptor-2 on epithelial cells and cause airway inflammation through IL-8 expression (53, 68).

Occupational seafood allergy can manifest with both upper and lower respiratory symptoms, as well as urticaria and protein contact dermatitis. Rhinitis and, less frequently, urticaria, are often associated with and may precede the development of chest symptoms. Systemic anaphylactic reactions have also been reported but are rare (51). Specific sensitization may be demonstrated by SPT or seafood-specific IgE (sIgE). In crab-processing workers, the PPVs of a positive crab extracts SPT or sIgE for OA confirmed by specific inhalation challenge (SIC) was 76% and 89%, respectively (69). A negative SPT does not exclude OA, whereas a positive test supports the diagnosis. The work-relatedness of asthma may be demonstrated by peak flow monitoring at and away from work or increased bronchial hyperresponsiveness (BHR) on return to work after a period away from work. In SIC for HMW proteins an early asthmatic reaction is more commonly observed, although dual reactions are possible. However, in crab-processing workers, isolated late asthmatic reactions are more frequent (70). The prognosis of OA is variable and depends on: (*i*) duration of exposure, particularly after symptom onset; (*ii*) FEV$_1$ and PC20 at the time of diagnosis; and (*iii*) type of agent involved. In crab-processing workers, those with shorter duration of exposure after symptom onset, and/or higher FEV$_1$ and PC20 at the time of diagnosis had a better prognosis (71). The same study also demonstrated that a plateau of improvement in spirometry was reached after a mean of 1 year after cessation of exposure, and after 2 years for NSBH (72). Although there was a concomitant decrease in sIgE to crab, no plateau was reached even at 5 years. Many workers continue to have abnormal lung function or asthmatic symptoms despite removal from exposure.

Irritant-induced asthma or reactive airways dysfunction syndrome (RADS) in seafood industries can be induced by exposure to high concentrations of irritants including sulfite preservatives and ammonia used as refrigerants. Asthma, triggered by exposure to sulfites in prawn- and lobster-processing workers, can simulate sensitizer-induced asthma (53, 73, 74), although the exact mechanism is unknown.

Epidemiology, risk factors, and modifiers
Epidemiology
Seafood allergy was first reported in 1937 by Arent de Besche in a fisherman who developed allergic symptoms and asthma when handling codfish (75). Since this sentinel event, many seafood species, from all three major seafood groupings, have been reported to cause occupational allergy and asthma (Table 13.4) (51–53).

Rhinitis
Various epidemiological studies show that ocular-nasal symptoms and allergic rhinitis are commonly encountered in seafood exposed workers. These are the first indicators of underlying allergic disease and commonly coexist with OA (51–53). Rhino-conjunctivitis (ORh) may precede or coincide with OA onset. The prevalence of seafood-associated ORh is between 5% and 24%, but it may well be an underestimate (53, 76).

Asthma
Epidemiological studies indicate that the prevalence of OA in seafood workers is between 2% and 36% (51–53). These differences in prevalence are partly due to varying definitions of OA. Furthermore, the allergenic potential of specific seafood proteins, as well as work processes (steam, organic dust, air blowing, water jets) causing high levels of airborne exposure, play a role. OA is more commonly associated with shellfish (4%–36%) than with bony fish (2%–8%). A recent study of OA in the UK seafood-processing industry for the period 1992–2017 demonstrated an excess incidence—the estimated annual OA incidence rate in seafood processors was 70 (95% CI:48.9, 91.1) per 100,000 workers compared with 2.9 (95% CI:2.8, 3.1) in all other industries (57). About 7% of workers with ingestion-related seafood allergy are estimated to also have asthma symptoms associated with inhalational seafood exposure (77). Conversely, there are isolated reports of workers (fishmonger handling shrimp and lobster, fish smoking factory worker handling trout, anchovy, salmon and sardines) with OA who subsequently developed ingestion-related allergic symptoms to the same seafood species (52, 53).

Risk factors and modifiers for occupational allergy and asthma associated with seafood
The etiology and development of allergic disease are due to an interaction between genetic, environmental, and host factors giving rise to different allergic disease phenotypes.

Environmental factors
Exposure-response relationships
There is increasing evidence that the risks of sensitization and OA are increased with higher exposures to seafood aerosols (51–53). Studies of prawn processors showed that a substantial proportion of workers experienced relief of allergic symptoms, including asthma, when compressed-air jets were replaced with cold-water jets for prawn meat extrusion and the wet weight of material filtered in air decreased from 1.8–3.3 mg/m^3 to 0.1–0.3 mg/m^3 (78). Similarly, the introduction of exhaust ventilation over gutting machines in a salmon-processing facility reduced respirable aerosol levels from a mean of 3.14 mg/m^3 to <0.01 mg/m^3 (79). As a result, no new cases of OA occurred over 24 months, compared to

a point prevalence of 8% over the prior 18-month period. Studies in crab processors have shown that cumulative exposure to snow crab allergens is positively associated with OA and allergy in a dose-response manner (80). Among pilchard and anchovy fish processors, the odds for WRA symptoms were three times greater (OR=3.53, CI=1.56–7.96) for workers exposed to fish antigen levels >90 ng/m^3 compared to those exposed to <30 ng/m^3 (81). A re-analysis of the exposure-response relationships using nonparametric methods showed evidence of clear dose–response relationships, more so with cumulative than current allergen exposures, for multiple outcomes including sensitization, work-related allergic ocular-nasal or chest symptoms, and probable OA (82). These relationships were modified by atopy and to a lesser extent smoking status, both associated with increased risks.

Workplace organization factors mediating exposure to seafood

Many environmental and organizational factors mediate hazardous exposures and worker vulnerability in the seafood industry. These include global ecological degradation and shifts in seafood production. Factors that are local and specific to the local context, include rural locations, migrant and seasonal workforce, divisions of labor along gender and ethnic lines, as well as shortcomings in occupational health and safety laws and interventions (83, 84). All these factors can lead to underdiagnosis, underreporting, and undercompensation of workers resulting in a poor quality of life for workers and their families.

Host factors

The following factors may increase the risk of OA in exposed workers. Atopy is the most important host factor associated with allergic sensitization and asthma to seafood allergens from crabs, prawns, cuttlefish, and pilchard (51–53). The presence of rhinitis has been associated with an increased risk of developing OA to a number of proteins including seafood (51–53). Smoking has been associated with an increased risk of sensitization to prawns, crab, and fish (pilchard, anchovy, and salmon) (51–53) and also augments the risk for OA in salmon- and crab-processing workers. This may be due to disruption of the natural epithelial barrier facilitating allergen entry or smoke acting as an adjuvant and enhancing allergenicity of inhaled allergens.

Prevention
Legislation, policies, and exposure standards
Currently, workplace exposure standards do not exist for seafood allergen exposures. However, these can only be developed and enforced once sampling methods and standardized assays for quantifying these allergens become widely available (53, 84, 85).

Workplace interventions and control measures
Exposure control measures by eliminating/reducing exposure (machine enclosure or local exhaust ventilation systems, repair of old machinery) or worker relocation are crucial to reducing the risk of occupational allergy and asthma. Identifying departments and activities with high aerosol exposure such as fishmeal bagging, gutting machines, cleaning and brushing crabs, compressed-air jets for prawn blowing, and using high-pressure water hoses for cleaning, should lead to the introduction of improved local exhaust ventilation systems and change in work processes to reduce aerosol exposures (84, 85).

Medical surveillance of workers
Regular medical surveillance and early diagnosis of workers in high-risk seafood industries such as crab and prawn processing are important strategies (51–53, 84, 85). Monitoring incident rates of disease can be used to inform the adequacy of exposure controls (57). Abbreviated questionnaires may allow early detection of allergic symptoms, which could prompt SPTs or sIgE if available. Surveillance may also identify allergy to previously unknown allergens that is newly introduced into the work environment before the product is released for broader public consumption. However, medical surveillance does not prevent the onset of disease, and cannot address workers who do not report symptoms for fear of losing their jobs. Exposure controls as mentioned above are the only means to prevent disease and keep workers in their jobs.

Increased worker awareness and training
Workers with seafood allergies and those working in high-exposure environments need to be educated on the health risks associated with handling seafood and its by-products and can use novel newly developed technologies as has been used in aquaculture (85, 86).

Immunotherapy modalities
While immunotherapy remains a theoretical possibility, it is still in the experimental stage, and has not yet been evaluated in workers with occupational allergy and asthma due to seafood (53, 87).

Conclusions and research needs

Animal, seafood, and insect allergy and asthma remain important occupational hazards in a wide range of jobs that include research, animal husbandry and care, harvesting, transportation, and processing animals for consumption and other human use. Laboratory animal allergy and asthma are probably the most well studied of this group of disorders, affecting members of academic, pharmaceutical, and veterinary industries. Allergy and asthma to seafood and insects may affect similar occupational groups as well as many workers in developing countries and other vulnerable populations (migrant, rural, and seasonal workers) with limited access to occupational interventions or other means of exposure protection. The research and intervention needs enumerated in this section must therefore apply to all worker populations at risk.

Some research needs are common to all these occupations, and include (53, 84):

- The relative contribution of respiratory versus cutaneous sensitization to specific allergens in relation to different phenotypic manifestations
- Characterization of different phenotypes of occupational inhalant food allergy and asthma through sentinel group surveillance/exposure cohorts in longitudinal studies from developing countries
- Development of commonly accepted high-quality sampling methods, analytical assays, and quantification techniques for allergens and other components in complex mixtures
- Detailed exposure-response studies using standardized allergen immunoassays to establish the utility of exposure threshold limits for inhalant allergens

- Appreciation of host modifiers that affect the dose–response relationships, and characterizing their effects in populations with varying degrees of susceptibility
- The adjuvant effects associated with the presence of associated agents in the food matrix such as pro-inflammatory agents (e.g. toxins, preservatives, enzymes)
- The relevance of the food matrix physical state (e.g. raw versus cooked seafood) in influencing the risk of inhalant seafood allergy and asthma
- Impact of increased farming and production of insect-derived food proteins on allergic sensitization among exposed workers
- The immunological mechanisms through which patients with food-induced OA and/or occupational rhinitis tolerate the ingestion of the same food
- Identifying and characterizing major inhalant allergens (e.g. seafood) and their clinical relevance in causing inhalant allergy and asthma
- Evaluating the effectiveness of intervention packages (exposure control/best practice/medical surveillance) for common high-risk sensitizers

References

1. Gordon S, Preece R. Prevention of laboratory animal allergy. Occup Med (Lond). 2003;53:371–7.
2. Feary JR, Schofield SJ, Canizales J, et al. Laboratory animal allergy is preventable in modern research facilities. Eur Respir J. 2019;53.
3. Pacheco KA, McCammon C, Thorne PS, et al. Characterization of endotoxin and mouse allergen exposures in mouse facilities and research laboratories. Ann Occup Hyg. 2006;50:563–72.
4. Elliott L, Heederik D, Marshall S, et al. Progression of self-reported symptoms in laboratory animal allergy. J Allergy Clin Immunol. 2005;116:127–32.
5. Balogun RA, Siracusa A, Shusterman S. Occupational rhinitis and occupational asthma: association or progression? Am J Ind Med. 2018;61:293–307.
6. Gautrin D, Infante-Rivard C, Ghezzo H, et al. Incidence and host determinants of probable occupational asthma in apprentices exposed to laboratory animals. Am J Respir Crit Care Med. 2001;163:899–904.
7. Hesford JD, Platts-Mills TAE, Edlich RF. Anaphylaxis after laboratory rat bite: an occupational hazard. J Emerg Med. 1995;13:765–8.
8. Kampitak T, Betschel SD. Anaphylaxis in laboratory workers because of rodent handling: two case reports. J Occup Health. 2016;58(4):381–3.
9. El-Zaemey S, Carey RN, Darcey E, et al. Prevalence of occupational exposure to asthmagens derived from animals, fish and/or shellfish among Australian workers. Occup Environ Med. 2018;75:310–6.
10. BA Muzembo, Eitoku M, Inaoka Y, et al. Prevalence of occupational allergy in medical researchers exposed to laboratory animals. Ind Health. 2014;52(3):256–61.
11. Venables KM, Tee RD, Hawkins ER, et al. Laboratory animal allergy in a pharmaceutical company. Br J Ind Med. 1988;45:660–6.
12. Simoneti CS, Ferraz E, de Menezes MB, et al. Allergic sensitization to laboratory animals is more associated with asthma, rhinitis, and skin symptoms than sensitization to common allergens. Clin Exp Allergy. 2017;47:1436–44.
13. Laditka JN, Laditka SB, Arif AA, et al. Work-related asthma in the USA: nationally representative estimates with extended follow-up. Occup Environ Med. 2020;77:617–22.
14. Gautrin D, Ghezzo H, Infante-Rivard C, et al. Long-term outcomes in a prospective cohort of apprentices exposed to high-molecular-weight agents. Am J Respir Crit Care Med. 2008;177:871–9.
15. Elliott L, Heederik D, Marshall S, et al. Incidence of allergy and allergy symptoms among workers exposed to laboratory animals. Occup Environ Med. 2005;62:766–71.
16. Cullinan P, Cook A, Gordon S, et al. Allergen exposure, atopy and smoking as determinants of allergy to rats in a cohort of laboratory employees. Eur Respir J. 1999;13:1139–43.
17. Gautrin D, Infante-Rivard C, Dao TV, et al. Specific IgE-dependent sensitization, atopy and bronchial hyperresponsiveness in apprentices starting exposure to protein-derived agents. Am J Respir Crit Care Med. 1997;155:1841–7.
18. Siracusa A, Marabini A, Folletti I, et al. Smoking and occupational asthma. Clin Exp Allergy. 2006;36:577–84.
19. Jeal H, Draper A, Jones M, et al. HLA associations with occupational sensitization to rat lipocalin allergens: a model for other animal allergies? J Allergy Clin Immunol. 2003;111:795–9.
20. Pacheco K, Maier L, Siulveira L, et al. Association of TLR4 alleles with symptoms and sensitization to laboratory animals. J Allergy Clin Immunol. 2008;122:896–902.
21. Pacheco KA, Rose CR, Silveira LJ, et al. Gene-environment interactions influence airways function in laboratory animal workers. J Allergy Clin Immunol. 2010;126:232–40.
22. Nieuwenhuijsen MJ, Putcha V, Gordon S, et al. Exposure-response relations among laboratory animal workers exposed to rats. Occup Environ Med. 2003;60:104–8.
23. Stave GM, Darcey DJ. Prevention of laboratory animal allergy in the United States: a national survey. J Occup Environ Med. 2012;54:558–63.
24. Botham PA, Lamb CT, Teasdale EL, et al. Allergy to laboratory animals: a follow up study of its incidence and of the influence of atopy and pre-existing sensitisation on its development. Occup Env Med. 1995;52:129–33.
25. Fisher R, Saunders WB, Murray SJ, et al. Prevention of laboratory animal allergy. J Occup Environ Med. 1998;40(7):609–13.
26. Walters GI, Kirkham A, McGrath EE, et al. Twenty years of SHIELD: decreasing incidence of occupational asthma in the West Midlands, UK? Occup Environ Med. 2015;72:304–10.
27. Hinze S, Bergmann KC, Lowenstein H, et al. Cow hair allergen (Bos d2) content in house dust: correlation with sensitization in farmers with cow hair asthma. Int Arch Allergy Immunol. 1997;112:231–7.
28. Bar-Sela S, Teichtahl H, Lutsky I. Occupational asthma in poultry workers. J Allergy Clin Immunol. 1984;73:271–5.
29. Blair Smith A, Bernstein DI, London MA, et al. Evaluation of occupational asthma from airborne egg protein exposure in multiple settings. Chest. 1990;98:398–404.
30. Swiderska-Kiełbik S, Krakowiak A, Wiszniewska M, et al. Occupational allergy to birds within the population of Polish bird keepers employed in zoo gardens. Int J Occup Med Environ Health. 2011;24:292–303.
31. El-Ansary EH, Gordon DJ, Tee RD, et al. Respiratory allergy to inhaled bat guano. Lancet. 1987;1:316–8.
32. Lopata AL, Fenemore B, Jeebhay MF, et al. Occupational allergy in laboratory workers caused by the African migratory grasshopper Locusta migratoria. Allergy. 2005;60:200–5.
33. Kaufman GL, Gandevia BH, Bellas TE, et al. Occupational allergy in an entomological research centre. I Clinical aspects of reactions to the sheep blowfly Lucilia cuprina. Br J Ind Med. 1989;46:473–8.
34. Purohit A, Shao J, Degree JM, et al. Role of tropomyosin as a cross-reacting allergen in sensitization to cockroach in patients from Martinique (French Caribbean island) with a respiratory allergy to mite and a food allergy to crab and shrimp. Eur Ann Allergy Clin Immunol. 2007;39:85–8.
35. de Jong NW, Groenewoud GC, van Ree R, et al. Immunoblot and radioallergosorbent test inhibition studies of allergenic cross-reactivity of the predatory mite Amblyseius cucumeris with the house dust mite Dermatophagoides pteronyssinus. Ann Allergy Asthma Immunol. 2004;93:281–7.
36. McKenna OE, Asam C, Araujo GR, et al. How relevant is panallergen sensitization in the development of allergies? Pediatr Allergy Immunol. 2016;27(6):560–8.
37. Suarthana E, Shen A, Henneberger PK, et al. Post-hire asthma among insect-rearing workers. J Occup Environ Med. 2012;54:310–7.
38. Burge PS, Edge G, O'Brien IM, et al. Occupational asthma in a research centre breeding locusts. Clin Allergy. 1980;10:355–63.
39. Soparkar GR, Patel PC, Cockcroft DW. Inhalant atopic sensitivity to grasshoppers in research laboratories. J Allergy Clin Immunol. 1993;92:61–5.
40. Lopata AL, Jeebhay MF, Groenewald M, et al. Sensitisation to three cockroach species in Southern Africa. J Allergy Clin Immunol. 2005;18:62–6.
41. Oldenburg M, Latza U, Baur X. Occupational health risks due to shipboard cockroaches. Int Arch Occup Environ Health. 2008;81:727–34.
42. Spieksma FTM, Vooren PH, Kramps JA, et al. Respiratory allergy to laboratory fruit flies (Drosophila melanogaster). J Allergy Clin Immunol. 1986;77:108–13.
43. Kraut A, Sloan J, Silviu-Dan F, et al. Occupational allergy after exposure to caddis flies at a hydroelectric power plant. Occup Environ Med. 1994;51:408–13.
44. Liebers V, Baur X. Chironomidae haemoglobin Chi t1-characterization of an important inhalant allergen. Clin Exp Allergy. 1994;24:100–8.
45. Siracusa A, Marcucci F, Spinozzi A, et al. Prevalence of occupational allergy due to live fish bait. Clin Exp Allergy. 2003;33:507–10.

46. Nieuwenhuizen N, Lopata AL, Jeebhay MF, et al. Exposure to the fish parasite Anisakis causes allergic airway hyperreactivity and dermatitis. J Allergy Clin Immunol. 2006;117:1098–105.

47. Uragoda CG, Wijekoon PMB. Asthma in silk workers. J Soc Occup Med. 1991;41:140–2.

48. Rome Italy: FAO. Food and Agriculture Organization. The state of world fisheries and aquaculture. 2018. Accessed June 28, 2020. http://wwwfaoorg/3/i9540en/i9540enpdf

49. International Labour Organisation. Safety and health in the fishing industry. Geneva. 1999.

50. Jeebhay MF, Robins TG, Lopata AL. World at work: fish processing workers. Occup Environ Med. 2004;61:471–4.

51. Jeebhay MF, Robins TG, Lehrer SB, et al. Occupational seafood allergy: a review. Occup Environ Med. 2001;58:553–62.

52. Jeebhay MF, Cartier A. Seafood workers and respiratory disease: an update. Curr Opin Allergy Clin Immunol. 2010;10(2):104–13.

53. Jeebhay MF, Moscato G, Bang BE, et al. Food processing and occupational respiratory allergy—A EAACI Position Paper. Allergy. 2019;74:1852–71.

54. Lopata AL. Allergenicity of food and impact of processing. In: Ahmed J, Ramaswamy HS, Kasapis S, Boye JI, eds. Novel food processing; effects on rheological and functional properties. USA: CRC Press LLC; 2010:459–78.

55. Lopata AL, Jeebhay MF. Airborne seafood allergens as a cause of occupational allergy and asthma. Curr Allergy Asthma Rep. 2013;13(3):288–97.

56. Shiryaeva O, Aasmoe L, Straume B, et al. Respiratory effects of bioaerosols: exposure-response study among salmon-processing workers. Am J Ind Med. 2014;57(3):276–85.

57. Mason HJ, Carder M, Money A, et al. Occupational asthma and its causation in the UK seafood processing industry. Ann Work Expo Health. 2020;64:817–25.

58. Thomassen MR, Kamath SD, Lopata AL, et al. Occupational exposure to bioaerosols in Norwegian crab processing plants. Ann Occup Hyg. 2016;60(7):781–94.

59. Dahlman-Höglund A, Renström A, Larsson PH, et al. Salmon allergen exposure, occupational asthma, and respiratory symptoms among salmon processing workers. Am J Ind Med. 2012;55:624–30.

60. Dahlman-Höglund A, Renström A, Acevedo F, et al. Exposure to parvalbumin allergen and aerosols among herring processing workers. Ann Occup Hyg. 2013;57(8):1020–9.

61. Ruethers T, Taki AC, Johnston EB, et al. Seafood allergy: a comprehensive review of fish and shellfish allergens. Mol Immunol. 2018;100:28–57.

62. Abdel Rahman AM, Gagné S, Helleur RJ. Simultaneous determination of two major snow crab aeroallergens in processing plants by use of isotopic dilution tandem mass spectrometry. Anal Bioanal Chem. 2012;403(3):821–31.

63. Gill BV, Rice TR, Cartier A, et al. Identification of crab proteins that elicit IgE reactivity in snow crab-processing workers. J Allergy Clin Immunol. 2009;124:1055–61.

64. Abdel Rahman AM, Lopata AL, O'Hehir RE, et al. Characterization and de novo sequencing of snow crab tropomyosin enzymatic peptides by both electrospray ionization and matrix-assisted laser desorption ionization QqToF tandem mass spectrometry. J Mass Spectrom. 2010;45(4):372–81.

65. Abdel Rahman AM, Kamath SD, Lopata AL, et al. Biomolecular characterization of allergenic proteins in snow crab (Chionoecetes opilio) and de novo sequencing of the second allergen arginine kinase using tandem mass spectrometry. J Proteomics. 2011;74(2):231–41.

66. Beale JE, Jeebhay MF, Lopata AL. Characterisation of purified parvalbumin from five fish species and nucleotide sequencing of this major allergen from Pacific pilchard, Sardinops sagax. Mol Immunol. 2009;46(15):2985–93.

67. Nugraha R, Kamath SD, Johnston E, et al. Conservation analysis of B-cell allergen epitopes to predict clinical cross-reactivity between shellfish and inhalant invertebrate allergens. Front Immunol. 2019;10:2676.

68. Larsen AK, Seternes OM, Larsen M, et al. Purified sardine and king crab trypsin display individual differences in PAR-2-, NF-KB-, and IL-8 signaling. Toxicol Environ Chem. 2011;93:1991–2011.

69. Cartier A, Malo JL, Ghezzo H, et al. IgE sensitization in snow crab-processing workers. J Allergy Clin Immunol. 1986;78:344–8.

70. Cartier A, Malo JL, Forest F, et al. Occupational asthma in snow crab-processing workers. J Allergy Clin Immunol. 1984;74:261–9.

71. Hudson P, Cartier A, Pineau L, et al. Follow-up of occupational asthma caused by crab and various agents. J Allergy Clin Immunol. 1985;76:682–7.

72. Malo JL, Cartier A, Ghezzo H, et al. Patterns of improvement of spirometry, bronchial hyperresponsiveness, and specific IgE antibody levels after cessation of exposure in occupational asthma caused by snow-crab processing. Am Rev Respir Dis. 1988;138:807–12.

73. Madsen J, Sherson D, Kjoller H, et al. Occupational asthma caused by sodium disulphite in Norwegian lobster fishing. Occup Environ Med. 2004;61:873–4.

74. Steiner M, Scaife A, Semple S, et al. Sodium metabisulphite induced airways disease in the fishing and fish-processing industry. Occup Med (Lond). 2008;58:545–50.

75. De Besche A. On asthma bronchiale in man provoked by cat, dog, and different other animals. Acta Med Scand. 1937;42:237–55.

76. Moscato G, Vandenplas O, Van Mijk RG, et al. Occupational rhinitis. Allergy. 2008;63:969–80.

77. Jeebhay MF, Robins TG, Miller ME, et al. Occupational allergy and asthma among salt water fish processing workers. Am J Ind Med. 2008;51:899–910.

78. Gaddie J, Legge JS, Friend JAR, et al. Pulmonary hypersensitivity in prawn workers. Lancet. 1980;2:1350–3.

79. Douglas JDM, McSharry C, Blaikie L, et al. Occupational asthma caused by automated salmon processing. Lancet. 1995;346:737–40.

80. Gautrin D, Cartier A, Howse D, et al. Occupational asthma and allergy in snow crab processing in Newfoundland and Labrador. Occup Environ Med. 2010;67:17–23.

81. Jeebhay MF. Occupational Allergy Associated with Saltwater Bony Fish Processing in South Africa. Doctor of Philosophy (Industrial Health). University of Michigan; 2003.

82. Jeebhay MF, Baatjies R, Lopata AL. Exposure-response relationships for allergy and asthma associated with seafood exposures. iFISH5—The Fifth International Fishing Industry Safety & Health Conference. St. Johns, Canada; June 2018 (abstract book). (abstract 6C.4).

83. Howse D, Jeebhay MF, Neiss B. The changing political economy of occupational health and safety in fisheries—lessons from Eastern Canada and South Africa. J Agrarian Change. 2012;12:344–63.

84. Bonlokke JH, Bang B, Aasmoe L, et al. Exposures and health effects of bioaerosols in seafood processing workers—a position statement. J Agromedicine. 2019;24(4):441–8.

85. Jeebhay MF, Lopata AL. Occupational allergy in the fish processing industry—towards preventive strategies. Curr Allergy Clin Immunol. 2006;19:34–7.

86. Marques F, Bettoni G, Adeoye A, et al. AquaSafe: aquaculture occupational safety and health in the palm of your hand. Brazilian Journal of Agricultural Research. 2020;26:59–66.

87. van der Ventel ML, Nieuwenhuizen NE, Kirstein F, et al. Differential responses to natural and recombinant allergens in a murine model of fish allergy. Mol Immunol. 2011;48:637–46.

14

POLYISOCYANATES AND THEIR PREPOLYMERS

Athena T. Jolly,[1] Piero Maestrelli,[2] Carrie A. Redlich,[3] Jean-Luc Malo,[4] and David I. Bernstein[5]
[1]Medical Consultant to Huntsman International LLC, Pennsylvania, USA
[2]University of Padova, Padova, Italy
[3]Pulmonary Section & Occupational and Environmental Medicine Program, Yale School of Medicine, New Haven, Connecticut, USA
[4]Hôpital du Sacré-Cœur de Montréal and Université de Montréal, Montréal, Québec, Canada
[5]Division of Immunology, Allergy and Rheumatology, University of Cincinnati College of Medicine, Cincinnati, Ohio, USA

Contents

Introduction

Polyisocyanates, a group of low-molecular-weight (LMW) cross-linking agents, are one of the most commonly identified causes of occupational asthma (OA). Polyisocyanates are generally synthesized by reaction of amines or their hydrochlorides with phosgene and are unique in their ability to catalyze the production of polyurethane, a product of great cultural and commercial importance.

The common feature of all polyisocyanates is the presence of more than two N=C=O groups which react with other compounds, most commonly polyols, to produce a wide array of polyurethane products, including foams, coatings, sealants, elastomers, and adhesives. Diisocyanate (DI) monomers (Figure 14.1), the forerunners of all polyisocyanates, were first discovered in the late 1840s by Wurtz (1). One prototype, toluene diisocyanate (TDI) was developed by I.G. Farben in Germany during World War II for the manufacture of polyurethane, while another, hexamethylene diisocyanate (HDI), was developed by H. Reinke to create a melt spinnable fiber that would circumvent DuPont's nylon patents (1). A number of related compounds have subsequently been developed and utilized commercially, with methylene diphenyl diisocyanate (MDI), naphthalene diisocyanate (NDI), and isophorone diisocyanate (IPDI) being the other major DI. The structure of the moiety attached to the N=C=O group (aliphatic or aromatic) and the number of N=C=O groups and polymers can alter the vapor pressure and reactivity. DI biurets, dimers, trimers, polymers, and prepolymers (Figure 14.2), which are less volatile than their related monomers, are being used. For example, TDI and HDI are volatile at room temperature, whereas MDI is a solid at room temperature, which is heated and dissolved in solvents to use. Newer polyisocyanates, mainly polymeric and prepolymeric formulations, which typically have lower vapor pressures than their parent DI are increasingly being used (Figure 14.2) (2). While DI or polyisocyanate more accurately describes the number of N=C=O groups, the terms *isocyanate* and *diisocyanate* are both commonly used to refer to this group of chemicals, and are used interchangeably in this chapter.

Uses and common exposures settings

DI, produced in a relatively small number of large production plants, are used to make various polyisocyanates for the production of polyurethane products. The use of polyisocyanates has

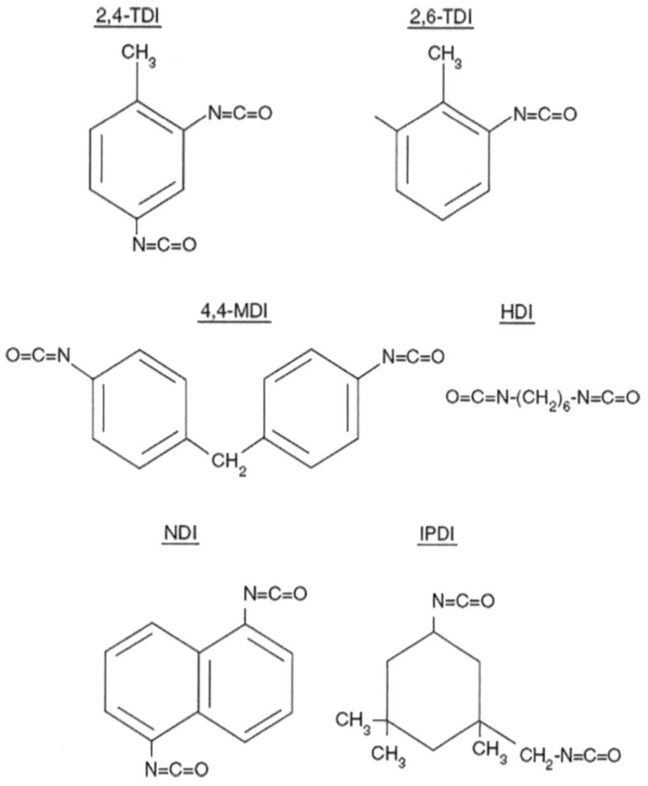

FIGURE 14.1 Diisocyanate chemicals.

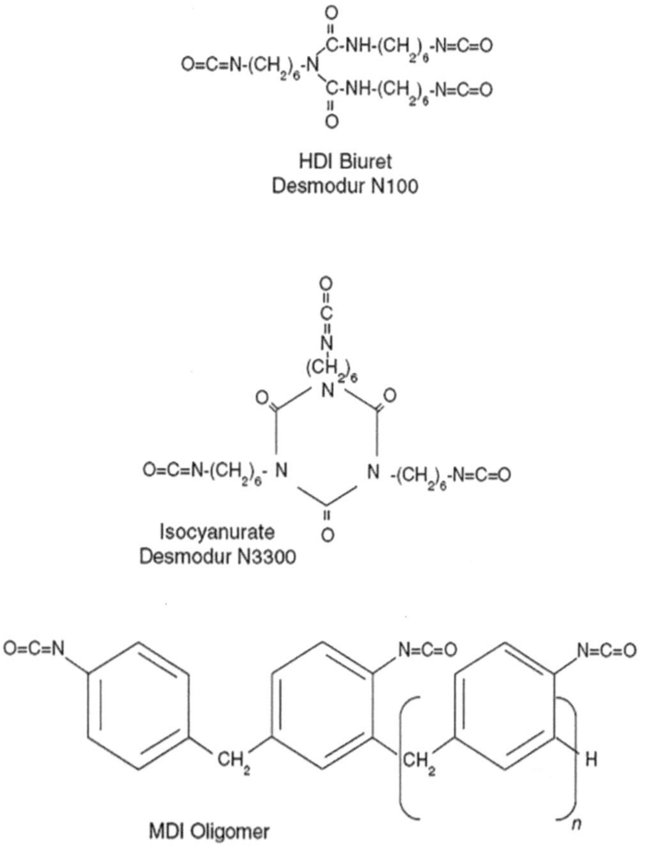

FIGURE 14.2 Common polyisocyanate compounds.

TABLE 14.1 Selected Industries and Uses with Potential Exposures to Diisocyanates

Industry	Polyurethane Products/Processes
Building and construction	Spray foam insulation, composite wood products, sealers, adhesives, paints, coatings, caulk, roofing materials
Automotive/transportation/ships/airplanes	Molded/composite parts, seats, acoustic panels, truck bed liners, protective coatings, engine parts
Clothing, footwear, and leisure	Manufacture of textiles, coated fabrics, human-made leather, shoe soles, sports equipment, inflatable rafts, food storage, and packaging products
Paint/coatings	Manufacturing, automotive and industrial paints, removal of paints and varnishes with heat
Foundry, casting, and machining	Molds for casting, resins, binders, machine parts, and protective coatings
Tunneling/mining	Spray or injected foams and coatings, rock, land consolidation, stabilization, prevent water incursion
Furniture, home furnishings	Wood composites, adhesives, foam mattresses, cushions, varnishes
Appliances and electronics	Thermal insulation refrigerators and freezers, tubing and wiring, encapsulate microelectronic components, cables and circuit boards
Medical care	Orthopedic casting, surgical implants, prostheses, catheter tubing, bedding

increased steadily as new applications and uses have been developed (Table 14.1). Polyurethanes are typically two-part systems, one containing the DI and the other part the polyols and other components, enabling a diverse array of polyurethane products and applications that use the same basic reactive $N=C=O$ building block. These other components can include solvents, blowing agents, amine and other catalysts, fire-retardants, surfactants, dyes, and fillers. When mixed together, the isocyanate reacts with the polyol (an exothermic reaction) to produce the cured polyurethane product. Aliphatic isocyanates such as HDI polymers are used primarily in external coatings and paints. Aromatic isocyanates, primarily MDI and TDI, are used to produce numerous products, flexible and rigid foams, adhesives, binders, sealants, and elastomer. Building and construction represent a large market for polyurethanes, including roofing, composite and engineered wood products, foam insulation, protective coatings, adhesives, and sealants. MDI and TDI are used extensively in the automobile industry for production of foam cushions, dashboards, other parts, and truck bed linings. The home furnishings, apparel, and footwear industries also increasingly depend on polyurethane products, such as foam mattresses, furniture, coated fabrics, synthetic leather, shoe soles, and sporting equipment. Various industrial processes use polyurethanes, including mold and core processes in foundries, machine parts, and adhesives. Polyurethane products are also used in the medical industry, including wound dressings, orthopedic casting, surgical implants, prostheses, and catheter tubing.

Aliphatic and cycloaliphatic DI, such as HDI and IPDI (Figure 14.1), and their related polymers are used in smaller quantities, primarily for light stable weather-resistant coatings such as auto body paints and outdoor coatings.

Worker exposures to DI can occur during primary production, in large secondary production facilities, in smaller end-user settings, such as spray coatings and foam applications, and during the thermal degradation of polyurethane products (2). The number of end users of polyurethane products greatly exceeds the number of workers involved in the production of DI, and these end users typically work in small companies. Two-part polyurethane systems are typically mixed, and then poured, sprayed, injected, or coated. Opportunities for respiratory and skin exposure are highly variable depending on the product, processes, engineering controls, co-exposures, and other factors. In addition, curing times, the time needed for the free N=C=O groups to fully react with the polyols can be highly variable, from seconds to many hours, with slow curing products having greater potential for exposure. Once fully cured, polyurethane products do not cause immune or toxic effects.

Environmental DI exposures can potentially occur with the application and use of polyurethane products in homes, schools, and healthcare facilities, such as certain glues, spray foam home insulation products, application of orthopedic casting, or manipulating polyurethane products such as cutting engineered woods. Whether some cured products such as foam mattresses may have free isocyanate groups remains open for debate (3) but even if present, such DI exposures are very low, way below workplace exposures.

DI should be distinguished from monoisocyanates such as methyl isocyanate, a potent volatile chemical used to produce pesticides, which can cause upper and lower respiratory tract irritant symptoms (Chapter 19), acute lung injury (pulmonary edema), and chronic health effects, including chronic obstructive pulmonary disease (COPD) and pulmonary fibrosis.

This chapter reviews important specific aspects of DI-induced OA, including clinical assessment, epidemiology, genetics, toxicity, airway inflammation, environmental sampling, surveillance of exposed workers, management, long-term outcomes, and future research directions.

Clinical manifestations and assessment

DI are potent sensitizers and, at high concentrations, can be irritants. Soon after the first commercial production of TDI, respiratory symptoms were recognized in exposed workers. Fuchs and Valade in 1951 described the development of asthma in seven of nine workers exposed to TDI (4). Exposure to DI can lead to a variety of health effects such as asthma, reactive airways dysfunction syndrome (RADS), irritant-induced asthma (Chapter 19), hypersensitivity pneumonitis (Chapter 24), rhinitis, and dermatitis. Immunologic OA is the most common of these conditions.

Workers with immunologic OA due to DI can be described using phenotyping characteristics (5, 6) and "clusters" of phenotypes according to an algorithm proposed in the severe asthma research program of the National Heart Lung and Blood Institute (7) (Chapters 5 and 9). Vandenplas et al. compared several characteristics in 544 and 635 subjects with confirmed OA, respectively, to HMW and LMW agents (17% represented by DI). Subjects with OA to LMW agents had a higher risk of severe exacerbations (RR:1.32, 95%CI:1.0–1.7), chest tightness, and late asthmatic reactions and a shorter latency period (6). Mason and coworkers identified three clusters of characteristics in 187 workers with OA

confirmed by specific inhalation challenge (SIC), mainly exposed to TDI (7). Of these, one cluster included almost half of subjects who were younger and showed a shorter duration of exposure and latency before onset of symptoms (8). Other specific features are interesting in the case of OA due to DI. The latency period between the onset of exposure and the onset of symptoms is generally comparable to what occurs after exposure to Western red cedar but shorter than for HMW agents (9). Immunologic OA due to DI can also develop after exposure to high levels (10) and can follow RADS (11). In some subjects, exquisite sensitivity to DI can occur, and exposure to low levels of the sensitizing agent, as low as 1 ppb for short intervals, can induce an attack of asthma. As for OA due to other LMW agents, the majority of affected subjects are nonatopic and nonsmokers (Chapter 3). By contrast, with HMW agents, rhinitis symptoms are less common (6) but it is uncertain if they more commonly precede chest symptoms (6, 12). Asthmatic responses following inhalational exposure are more frequently delayed than with HMW agents, but may also be atypical, which is not of the classical immediate, late, or dual types (Chapter 8). Moreover, tachyphylaxis may develop when workers are exposed on consecutive days (Chapter 8).

Epidemiology and risk factors

As detailed in Chapter 3, several different approaches have been used to assess the incidence and prevalence of DI-induced OA, workplace exposures and trends, with selected studies presented in Tables 14.2 and 14.3. Despite the extensive use of DI for over 70 years, there has been a relative paucity of epidemiologic studies investigating risks of exposure and dose-response relationships. Another important source of information has been surveillance data, which has been primarily on voluntary reporting, compensation data, or occupational disease registries.

Findings using these different approaches can be challenging to compare, given the many different DI formulations, measuring airborne and skin exposures, the variable diagnostic criteria and outcome measures, and the lack of consistent markers of sensitization, as exists with most HMW antigens. Epidemiological studies of DI-exposed workers evaluating asthma as the endpoint are particularly prone to the healthy worker effect (13, 14). Additionally, DI-induced OA commonly develops in the first 1 to 2 years of exposure (9, 14–16). Thus, longitudinal studies of inception cohorts (new employees or apprentices) are needed to accurately estimate incidence and prevalence of DI-induced OA in different exposure settings (Table 14.3).

These limitations should be considered in evaluating the incidence and prevalence of isocyanate asthma and trends over time. The annual incidence of TDI asthma, based on data primary TDI manufacturing plants, has been about 1% or lower. A longitudinal study of 197 US TDI-producing workers found an incidence of TDI-induced asthma of 0.9% (Collins, 2017, Table 14.3). However, in this study, 4 of 32 workers (12.5%) with less than 1 year of job tenure developed likely TDI asthma, suggesting a healthy worker effect and a possible higher incidence despite low TDI exposure (mean TDI levels of 0.65 ppb). The same study also suggested that acute unexpected exposure events, although challenging to measure, increased risk of DI-induced OA.

Most workers with exposure to isocyanates work in settings where polyurethane products are produced or applied in end-user settings, rather than primary production. The prevalence of isocyanate-induced OA reported in these settings has been variable, from less than 1% to over 30% in certain groups of exposed

TABLE 14.2 Selected Cross-Sectional Studies of Isocyanate Exposed Workers: Prevalence of Isocyanate Asthma/Symptoms

Study (First Author/Yr)	Agent	Process/Occupation	Study Group Number	Prevalence Isocyanate-Asthma (%)
1. Bruckner, 1968	TDI	R&D	26	19%
2. Tanser, 1973	MDI	PU rigid foam	57	7%
3. White, 1980	TDI	PU seat covers	57	30%
4. Baur, 1981	TDI	Plastics, varnish	195	28%
5. Tse, 1985	MDI	Foundry	76	13%
6. Seguin, 1987	PMDI	Paint shops	51	11.8%
7. Liss, 1988	MDI	Foundry	27	31%
8. Wang, 1988	TDI	Adhesive	38	0% to 85% symptoms
9. Huang, 1991	TDI	Varnish 3 factories	48	0% to 27%
10. Vandenplas, 1993	HDI	Spraying	9	45% (hypersensitivity pneumonitis)
11. Bernstein, 1993	MDI	Injection mold plant	243	4%; OR 36%
12. Kim, 1997	TDI	Spraying	81	10%
13. Woellner, 1997	MDI	Wood products	~130	14%
14. Ucgun, 1998	HDI	Spray painters	312	9.6%
15. Redlich 2001	HDI	Auto body shop	75	0 % (34% HDI-IgG)
16. Pronk, 2007	HDI	Spray painters	241	8.3% OA symptoms 20% OR symptoms
17. Cassidy, 2010	HDI	Workers in two producing plants	100	0%
18. Hathaway, 2014	Aliphatic diisocyanates	Workers in two producing plants	73	0%

Abbreviations: HDI, hexamethylene diisocyanate; IgG, immunoglobulin G; MDI, methylene diphenyl diisocyanate; OA, occupational asthma; OR, occupational rhinitis; PMDI, polymeric methylene diphenyl diisocyanate; PU, polyurethane; R&D, research and development; TDI, toluene diisocyanate.

References: **1.** Bruckner HC, Avery SB, Stetson DM, et al. *Arch Environ Health.* 1968;16:619–25. **2.** Tanser AR, Bourke MP, Blandford AG. *Thorax.* 1973;28:596–600. **3.** White WG, Morris MJ, Sugden E, et al. *Lancet.* 1980:756–60. **4.** Baur X, Fruhmann G. *Chest.* 1981;80:73S–6S. **5.** Tse KS, Johnson A, Chan H, et al. *Allergy.* 1985;40:314–20. **6.** Séguin P, Allard A, Cartier A, et al. *JOM.* 1987;29:340–4. **7.** Liss GM, Bernstein DI, Moller DR, et al. *J Allergy Clin Immunol.* 1988;82:55–61. **8.** Wang J-D, Huang P-H, Lin J-M, et al. *Am J Ind Med.* 1988;14:73–8. **9.** Huang J, Wang XP, Chen BM, et al. *Arch Environ Contam Toxicol.* 1991;21(4):607–11. **10.** Vandenplas O, Malo JL, Dugas M, et al. *Am Rev Respir Dis.* 1993;147:338–46. **11.** Bernstein DI, Korbee L, Stauder T, et al. *J Allergy Clin Immunol.* 1993;92:387–96. **12.** Kim H, Kim YD, Choi J. *Environ Res.* 1997;75(1):1–6. **13.** Woellner RC, Hall S, Greaves I, et al. *Am J Ind Med.* 1997;31:56–63. **14.** Ucgun I, Ozdemir N, Metintas M, et al. *Allergy.* 1998;53:1096–100. **15.** Redlich CA, Stowe MH, Wisnewski AV, et al. *Am J Ind Med.* 2001;39(6):587–97. **16.** Pronk A, Preller L, Raulf-Helmsoth M, et al. *Am J Respir Crit Care Med.* 2007;176:1090–7. **17.** Cassidy LD, Molenaar DM, Hathaway JA, et al. *J Occup Environ Med.* 2010;52:988–94. **18.** Hathaway JA, Molenaar DM, Cassidy LD, et al. *J Occup Environ Med.* 2014;56(1):52–7.

workers (Table 14.2). The wide range of prevalence figures can be related to variable work settings, processes, engineering controls, and use of personal protective equipment (PPE), as well as different diagnostic criteria and study designs. Higher prevalence figures are related in general to higher airborne exposures such as spray painting and heating and also to skin exposure. Findings, mainly descriptive, suggest that intermittent peak exposure events and skin exposure increase the risk of DI-induced OA (14, 16–18).

Surveillance data have shown that DI remains one of the most commonly reported causes of OA, although several recent surveillance reports have shown reduced number of cases (Table 14.3). This decline has been attributed primarily to reduced workplace exposures as well as effective surveillance.

Similar to other occupational agents, exposure, and more so, the intensity of exposure, remains the principal determinant (Chapter 3). Besides cumulative exposure, intermittent peak exposures likely play a role (14), especially exposure without respiratory protection to TWA-8 values, indicative of peak events (19). Works principally carried out by Redlich, her colleagues, and others have convincingly shown the importance of skin absorption for sensitization to polyisocyanates (17). Like for most LMW agents, atopy is not a risk factor (Chapter 3). Smoking does not seem to play a role as reviewed (20). Genetic aspects are discussed below.

Uptake, distribution, and excretion of polyisocyanates

The total retention rate of isocyanate during human respiratory exposure is estimated to be between 60% and 91% (21). It has been estimated by dosimetry that total respiratory uptake of HDI vapor, in the case of nasal breathing in humans, is 97% and that, by the 10th–15th airway generation, isocyanate is almost all deposited and absorbed (22). Animal radioisotopic tracing studies with ^{14}C-labeled vapors demonstrate that both MDI and TDI bind to the epithelial linings of the airway in animals and become broadly distributed throughout the circulatory system, primarily conjugated with albumin (23). In clinical studies, HDI has been shown to bind to keratin-18 in the bronchial epithelium and albumin in the fluid that lines the airway epithelium. By using polyclonal MDI specific IgG, Wisnewski et al. showed penetration of MDI in the lower airways and uptake by macrophages (24) while Hettick and coworkers showed the presence of MDI-conjugated protein (albumin) in bronchoalveolar lavage (BAL) (25). The majority of inhaled isocyanate is excreted in the urine within hours of exposure, which represents a useful biomarker of exposure (see below/above), although timing of the sampling is critical. The persistence of isocyanates in vivo, in the airways in humans, following occupational exposure remains uncertain. Such a retention

TABLE 14.3 Selected Longitudinal Studies of Isocyanate Exposed Workers

Study	Agent	Process/ Occupation	Study Group N (Follow-Up N Freq Unclear)	Outcomes Annual Incidence of WRA or Change FEV_1	Follow-Up (Years)	Diagnosis/ Testing
Primary Production						
1. Woodbury, 1956	TDI	TDI production	25	5.0%	1	MD
2. Peters, 1968; 3. Peters, 1970; 4. Peters, 1974	TDI	TDI production	38	Decline FEV_1	3	PFTs
5. Wegman, 1974; 6. Wegman, 1977; 7. Wegman, 1982	TDI	TDI production	112 to 37	Decline FEV_1	4	PFTs
8. Adams, 1975	TDI	TDI production	565	5.6%	11	MD
9. Porter, 1975	TDI	TDI production	300	0.9%	18	PFTs
10. Butcher, 1977 11. Diem, 1982	TDI	TDI production	277	3%	5.5	PFTs
12. Weill[a], 1979; 13. Weill, 1981	TDI	TDI production	277	1.0%	5	PFTs
14. Musk, 1982	TDI	TDI production	259 to 94	FEV_1 neg	10	PFTs
15. Omae, 1984	TDI	TDI production, research	106 (87 TDI production) 39 controls	FEV_1 neg 7.5% (8/106) acute asthmatic reaction, diagnosis unclear	2	
16. Jones, 1992	TDI	TDI production	386	0.7% FEV_1 neg	4	PFTs
17. Ott, 2000	TDI	TDI production	297	1.1%	29	PFTs
18. Bodner, 2001	TDI	TDI production	305	FEV_1 neg	26	PFTs
19. Cassidy, 2010	HDI	HDI production	100 + control	FEV_1 neg	> 10 yrs	PFTs
20. Collins, 2017	TDI	TDI production	197	0.9% (7 cases, 3 had acute exposure event) 9% (3/32 employed < 1 year) TDI odor, release common	5 yrs 32 < 1 yr	MD, PFTs, questionnaire
21. Clark, 1998 22. Clark, 2003	TDI	TDI foam 12 UK factories	780 f/up 251	8 left resp illness FEV_1 neg	5	PFTs
23. Petsonk[a], 2000	MDI	Wood products	214 144 f/up	10% to 14%	2	WRA symptoms, air levels ND
24. Grammer, 1988	HDI	Spray painters	150 126 f/up	0%–1% 21% HDI-IgG	1.5	Immunology SIC
25. Dragos, 2009	HDI	Apprentices in spray painting	298	4.4%	1.5	Questionnaire, methacholine testing, specific IgG
26. Gui, 2014[a]	TDI	Foam-producing workers	49	12.4% with "TDI-related health effects"	1	Symptoms
27. Ribeiro, 2014	Polyisocyanates	Workers' compensation registry	112 claims for OA	27% of claims	5 (Jan 2003–Dec 2007)	Symptoms, objective testing

(Continued)

TABLE 14.3 Selected Longitudinal Studies of Isocyanate Exposed Workers (*Continued*)

Study	Agent	Process/Occupation	Study Group N (Follow-Up N Freq Unclear)	Outcomes Annual Incidence IA or Change FEV$_1$	Follow-Up (Years)	Diagnosis/Testing
28. Jarolímek, 2017	Polyisocyanates	National Registry of Occupational Diseases; 247 companies from the automotive industry in Czechia		% of occupational diseases (including "allergic asthma") rose from 1.7% to 11.4%	13–14 yrs (2001–2014)	Medical diagnosis
29. Stocks, 2015	Polyisocyanates	UK vehicle repair industry	235 reports in SWORD	Significant decline (OR=0.9)	8–9 yrs (2006–2014)	Medical diagnosis
30. Lefkowitz, 2015	Polyisocyanates	Surveillance program in California, New Jersey, Massachusetts, and Michigan		368 cases of work-related asthma (329 with OA)	15 yrs (1993–2008)	Medical diagnosis

[a] Inception cohort.

Abbreviations: FEV$_1$, forced expiratory volume in 1 second; HDI, hexamethylene diisocyanate; OA, occupational asthma; MD, medical diagnosis; PFT, pulmonary function test; SIC, specific inhalation challenge; TDI, toluene diisocyanate; WRA, work-related asthma.

References: **1.** Woodbury JW. *Indust Med.* 1956;25:540–3. **2.** Peters JM, Murphy RL, Pagnotto LD, et al. *Arch Environ Health.* 1968;16(5):642–7. **3.** Peters JM. *Proc R Soc Med.* 1970;63:372–5. **4.** Peters JM. *Ann NY Acad Sci.* 1974;221:44–9. **5.** Wegman DH, Pagnotto LD, Fine LJ, et al. *J Occup Med.* 1974;16(4):258–60. **6.** Wegman DH, Peters J.M, Pagnotto L, et al. *Br J Ind Med.* 1977;34(3):196–200. **7.** Wegman DH, Musk AW, Main DM, et al. *Am J Ind Med.* 1982;3:209–15. **8.** Adams WG. *Br J Ind Med.* 1975;32(1):72–8. **9.** Porter CV, Higgins RL, Scheel LD. *Am Ind Hyg Assoc J.* 1975;36(3):159–68. **10.** Butcher BT, Jones RN, O'Neil CE, et al. *Am Rev Respir Dis.* 1977;116:411–21. **11.** Diem JE, Jones RN, Hendrick DJ, et al. *Am Rev Respir Dis.* 1982;126:420–8. **12.** Weill H. *J Allergy Clin Immunol.* 1979;64:662–4. **13.** Weill H. *Chest.* 1981;80(1 Suppl):54–7. **14.** Musk AW, Peters JM, DiBerardinis L, et al. *JOM.* 1982;24:746–50. **15.** Omae K. *Int Arch Occup Environ Health.* 1984;55(1):1–12. **16.** Jones RN, Rando RJ, Glindmeyer HW, et al. *Am Rev Respir Dis.* 1992;146:871–7. **17.** Ott MG, Klees JE, Poche SL. *Occup Environ Med.* 2000;57:43–52. **18.** Bodner KM, Burns CJ, Randolph NM, et al. *J Occup Environ Med.* 2001;43(10):890–7. **19.** Cassidy LD, Molenaar DM, Hathaway JA, et al. *J Occup Environ Med.* 2010;52:988–94. **20.** Collins JJ, Anteau S, Conner PR, et al. *J Occup Environ Med.* 2017;59 Suppl 12:S22–S7. **21.** Clark RL, Burgler J, McDermott M, et al. *Int Arch Occup Environ Health.* 1998;71:169–79. **22.** Clark RL, Bugler J, Paddle GM, et al. *Int Arch Occup Environ Health.* 2003;76:295–301. **23.** Petsonk EL, Wang ML, Lewis DM, et al. *Chest.* 2000;118:1183–93. **24.** Grammer LC, Eggum P, Silverstein M, et al. *J Allergy Clin Immunol.* 1988;82:627–33. **25.** Dragos M, Jones M, Malo JL, et al. *Occup Environ Med.* 2009;66:227–34. **26.** Gui W, Wisnewski AV, Neamtiu I, et al. *Am J Ind Med.* 2014;57:1207–15. **27.** Ribeiro M, Tarlo SM, Czyrka A, et al. *J Occup Environ Med.* 2014;56(9):1001–7. **28.** Jarolímek J, Urban P, Pavlínek P, et al. *Int J Occup Med Environ Health.* 2017;30(3):455–68. **29.** Stocks SJ, Jones K, Piney M, et al. *Occup Med.* 2015;65:713–8. **30.** Lefkowitz D, Pechter E, Fitzsimmons K, et al. *Am J Ind Med.* 2015;58:1138–49.

of isocyanates and, more generally, of antigens with the resulting ongoing immune activation and inflammation might explain the persistence of asthma even after cessation of exposure (Chapter 11A). HDI vapor binds to airway epithelial cells for >18 hours post-exposure, but it is unknown if this binding can persist (26). Also, HDI exposed subjects exhibit an acute (as assessed 2 hours after exposure) increase in the percentage of human peripheral blood mononuclear cells with a recovery after 24 hours (27). DI are also absorbed through the skin as outlined above in this section (17).

Genetics

Aspects related to the genetics of OA are presented and discussed in Chapter 4. Tables 14.4 and 14.5 focus on studies that examined human leukocyte antigen (HLA) and non-HLA genes in workers exposed to polyisocyanates. The following text that is related to OA due to polyisocyanates is also taken from Chapter 4.

Associations with HLA genes

Bignon et al. (Table 14.4) demonstrated that HLA DQB1*0503 and the allelic combination DQB1*0201/0301 were associated with susceptibility to DI asthma, whereas the DQB1*0501 allele and the DQA1*0101-DQB1*0501-DR1 haplotype appeared to be protective.

Mapp et al. (Table 14.4) confirmed the association with HLA-DQB1*0503 and reported that the DQA1*0104 allele was increased in DI-induced OA. The "protective" allele HLA-DQB1*0501 was confirmed in this cohort. In another study, confirmed OA was significantly associated with aspartic acid residue at position 57 of HLA-DQB1*0503 (Table 14.4). It is noteworthy that the HLA alleles associated with DI-induced OA reported in European workers were not replicated in Asian workers. DRB1*15-DPB1*05 and HLA DRB1*1501-DQB1*0602-DPB1*0501 were reportedly associated with TDI-asthma in Koreans (Table 14.4).

Genes associated with innate immunity, Th-2 immunity, oxidative stress, and epithelial cells

Single nucleotide polymorphisms (SNPs) associated with immune response genes (IL-4Rα, IL-13, and CD14) were evaluated in workers with confirmed OA. Increased frequencies of IL-4RA I50V allele and combinatorial genotypes of IL4RA (I50V), IL-13 (R110Q), and CD14 (C159T) were associated with OA due to DI in those workers exposed to HDI, suggesting an exposure-specific interaction (Table 14.5).

Since isocyanates are known to cause oxidative injury to respiratory epithelial cells, antioxidant defense genes have been examined in workers with OA due to DI. Given that

TABLE 14.4 HLA Genes Involved in Susceptibility to OA

Exposure	Sample Size (Case/Control)	Gene/Variant (OR, RR, or p)	Effect Size	References
Diisocyanates (TDI)	28/16	HLA-DQB1/*0503	RR 9.8	*1. Bignon, 1994*
		HLA-DQB1/*0201/ 0301	RR 9.5	
		HLA-DQB1/*0501	RR 0.1	
		HLA-DQA1/*0101 *0102	RR 0.04	
Diisocyanates (TDI)	30/126	HLA-DQB1/*0503	RR 2.9	*2. Balboni, 1996*
		HLA-DQB1/*0501	RR 0.04	
		HLA-DQB1/*0503	p=0.009	
		HLA-DQA1/*0501	p=0.01	
		HLA-DQA1/*0101	p=0.004	
		HLA-DQA1/*0104	p=0.005	
Diisocyanates (TDI)	84/127	HLA-DRB1/*1501 DQB1/*0602-DPB1/ *0501	OR 4.4 (1.5–13.1)	*3. Choi, 2009*
Diisocyanates (MDI, TDI, HDI)	73/67	HLA-E rs1573294,	OR 6.3 (2.4–17)	*4. Yucesoy, 2014*
		HLA-B rs1811197,	OR 7.7 (2.3–26)	
		HLA-DOA rs3128935	OR 20 (2.9–135)	
		HLA-DQA2 rs7773955	OR 8.4 (3–23)	

Abbreviations: HDI, hexamethylene diisocyanate; MDI, methylene diphenyl diisocyanate; TDI, toluene diisocyanate.

References: **1.** Bignon JS, et al. *Am J Respir Crit Care Med.* 1994;149:71–5. **2.** Balboni A, et al. *Eur Respir J.* 1996;9:207–10. **3.** Choi JH, et al. *Int Arch Allergy Immunol.* 2009;150:156–63. **4.** Yucesoy B, et al. *J Occup Environ Med.* 2014;56(4):382–7.

glutathione protects epithelial cells against toxicity from isocyanates (Table 14.5), Piirla et al. examined the polymorphisms of the glutathione S-transferase (GST) genes (GSTM1, GSTM3, GSTP1, and GSTT1) in workers with OA due to DI. GSTM1 null genotype was associated with an increased risk of OA. Mapp et al. (Table 14.5) reported a lower frequency of the GSTP1 Ile105Val Val/Val genotype in subjects with TDI-asthma and airway hyperreactivity (AHR). In another study, the N-acetyltransferase (NAT1) slow acetylator genotype was found to be associated with an increased risk of OA (OR, 2.5; 95% CI, 1.32–4.91). The risk of OA was higher among workers exposed to TDI (OR, 7.8; 95% CI, 1.18–51.6), suggesting an exposure-specific association (Table 14.5).

Genome-wide association studies (GWAS) offer a powerful approach to scan the entire genome for disease-associated SNPs. In a GWAS conducted in Korean workers with OA due to DI, significant associations were reported between catenin alpha 3 (CTNNA3) polymorphisms (rs10762058, rs7088181, rs4378283, and rs1786929) and TDI-asthma (Table 14.5). CTNNA3 proteins play an important role in cell-cell adhesion thereby having potential to impact the effects of TDI exposure on airway epithelial cells. A GWAS study performed in Caucasian workers with established OA due to DI did not confirm the findings (i.e. CTNNA3 SNPs) in the Korean study but did identify 11 OA-associated SNPs exceeding genome-wide significance (p <5 × 10⁻⁸) (Table 14.5). Next-generation sequencing (NGS) was performed in 91 OA cases of 14 loci containing OA-associated SNPs identified in the GWAS. NGS and bioinformatic analysis was used to detect and prioritize 21 OA-associated SNPs; 4 of these SNPs located on ATF, CDH17, TACR1, and FAM71A exhibited functional effects on gene regulation (Table 14.5).

Toxicity and oxidative effects

Isocyanate toxicity and sensitization were often studied independently, assuming that the two characteristics were unrelated. However, a number of studies have begun to suggest a possible link between the "toxic" properties of isocyanates and the development of allergy. The main areas that may interconnect toxicity and allergy are (*i*) glutathione, (*ii*) oxidative stress, and (*iii*) epithelial barrier disruption.

After access in the respiratory tract, isocyanate N=C=O groups can "conjugate" with host molecules (proteins) by means of nucleophilic addition or get "hydrolyzed" with water, which results in the production of amines (28). In 1997, Day et al. (29) showed that isocyanates react rapidly with the reduced form of glutathione (GSH), a thiol present in the lower airways and one of the major antioxidants of the fluid lining the airways, and that GSH–TDI conjugates could be found inside airway cells of exposed animals (30). Wisnewski et al. subsequently tested the hypothesis that GSH reacts with MDI to form quasi-stable conjugates, capable of mediating the formation of MDI-conjugated "self" protein antigens, which may participate in MDI-induced inflammation (31). These findings fit with in vivo toxicology studies in rats where decreased levels of GSH are observed inside the airway epithelium and increased levels of GSH in the fluid lining the airways upon acute exposure (Chapter 4). In animals, drugs that reduce systemic levels of GSH also increase toxicity of isocyanates (Chapter 4). Physiological levels of GSH prevent two processes, which are thought to be central to isocyanate sensitization, isocyanate conjugation to human proteins, and toxicity toward airway epithelial cells (32). However, human gamma-glutamyl transpeptidase-1 is able to cleave GSH-MDI

TABLE 14.5 Non-HLA Genes Involved in Susceptibility to OA

Exposure	Sample Size (Case/Control)	Gene/Variant (OR, p Value)	Effect Size	References
Diisocyanates (TDI, HDI, MDI)	109/73	GSTM1 null	OR 1.9 (1.0–3.5)	*1. Piirila, 2001*
Diisocyanates (TDI)	109/73	NAT1 slow Acetylator	OR 2.5 (1.3–4.9)	*2. Wikman, 2002*
Diisocyanates (TDI)	92/39	GSTP1 Val/Val	OR 0.2 (0.1–1.1)	*3. Mapp, 2002*
Diisocyanates (TDI, HDI, MDI)	62 OA, 75 exposed without OA	IL4RA, CD-14 and IL-13 Polymorphisms significantly associated with OA due to HDI, alone or in combination	p values ≤0.05	*4. Bernstein, 2006*
Diisocyanates (TDI)	132/114	CYP1A1 (wheeze) TNF-308 A (dry cough)	OR 12 (1.1–110) OR 2.2 (0.7–7)	*5. Broberg, 2008*
Diisocyanates (MDI)	141–158 exposed	GSTP1 isoleucine/ isoleucine (lower respiratory symptoms)	Not statistically significant	*6. Littorin, 2008*
Diisocyanates (TDI)	84/263 Genome-wide association study	CTNNA3/rs 10762058 CTNNA3/rs 7088181 CTNNA3/rs 4378283	OR 4.9 (2.3–10.5) OR4.9 (2.3–10.6) OR 4.4 (2.1–9.2)	*7. Kim, 2009*
Diisocyanates (TDI)	103/60	ADR/Arg16Gly A>G Leu134Leu G>A + Arg175 Arg C>A	OR 15.4 (1.81–131.1)	*8. Ye, 2010*
Diisocyanates (TDI)	70–128 exposed	GSTP1 105 modified toluene diamine (TDA) metabolites GSTP1 105 protective for OA	p <0.005 and p< 0.008 for TDA in plasma (allele-dosage effect)	*9. Broberg, 2010*
Diisocyanates (HDI)	368 exposed workers, 103 with diagnosis confirmed by SIC; 115 with symptoms but negative SIC	IL-4RA(150V)II+ CD14 (C159T) CT IL-4RA(150V)II+IL-13(R110Q) RR+ CD14 (C159T) CT	OR 3.08 (1.2–7.6) OR 3.86 (1.26–12.0)	*10. Bernstein, 2011*
Diisocyanates (TDI, HDI, MDI)	132/147 exposed a-symptomatic/132 exposed negative challenges	CTNNA3 alpha catenin rs7088181 CTNNA3 alpha catenin rs10762058	OR 9.05 (1.69–48.54) vs asymptomatic workers OR 6.82 (1.65–28.24) vs asymptomatic workers	*11. Bernstein, 2012* *12. Bernstein, 2013*
Diisocyanates (TDI, HDI, MDI)	95/116 ex-posed symptomatic negative challenges/142 exposed asymptomatic	SOD2 rs4880 GSTM1 (null) GSTP1 rs762803 EPHX1 rs2854450 + various genotype combinations	p = 0.004 p = 0.047 p = 0.021 p < 0.001	*13. Yucesoy, 2012*
Diisocyanates (MDI, TDI, Naphthalene diisocyanate)	24 exposed workers	GSTM1 null shows higher concentrations of diamine metabolites in urine GSTP1 modifies diamine levels in plasma and urine	Regression lines comparing diamine in plasma and urine	*14. Tinnerberg, 2014*
Diisocyanates (TDI, HDI MDI)	Genome-wide association study 74 workers with OA confirmed by SIC; 824 nonexposed healthy controls	ODZ3, HERC2, CDH17 + other single nucleotide polymorphisms	All significant OR	*15. Yucesoy, 2015*
Diisocyanates (TDI, HDI, MDI)	95/142 asymptomatic exposed	PTGS1 rs5788 TGFB1 rs1800469 TNF rs1800629 PTGS2 rs20417	OR = 0.38 (0.17–0.89) OR = 0.38 (0.18–0.74) OR = 2.08 (1.03–4.17) OR = 6.40 (1.06–38.75)	*16. Yucesoy, 2016*

| Diisocyanates (TDI, HDI, MDI) | 91 OA 238 unexposed controls nucleotide | 130 risk variants significantly (p ≤0.05) associated with OA; 5 regulatory polymorphisms, 3 with luciferase reporter activity | | *17. Bernstein, 2018* |
| Diisocyanates (TDI, HDI, MDI) | 108 patients with OA | GSTP1 slow activity associated with NSBH (at the follow-up but not at diagnosis) | OR=4.6 (1.6–13.3) | *18. Leppilahti, 2019* |

Abbreviations: HDI, hexamethylene diisocyanate; MDI, methylene diphenyl diisocyanate; OR: odd ratio; SIC, specific inhalation challenge; TDI, toluene diisocyanate.

References: **1.** Piirila P, et al. *Pharmacogenetics.* 2001;11:437–45. **2.** Wikman H, et al. *Pharmacogenetics.* 2002;12:227–33. **3.** Mapp CE, et al. *J Allergy Clin Immunol.* 2002;109:867–72. **4.** Bernstein DI, et al. *Ann Allergy Asthma Immunol.* 2006;97:800–6. **5.** Broberg K, et al. *Environ Health.* 2008;7:15. **6.** Littorin M, et al. *Int Arch Occup Environ Health.* 2008;81(4):429–41. **7.** Kim SH, et al. *Clin Exp Allergy.* 2009;39:203–12. **8.** Ye YM, et al. *Allergy Asthma Immunol Res.* 2010;2(4):260–6. **9.** Broberg KE, et al. *Pharmacogenet Genomics.* 2010;20:104–11. **10.** Bernstein DI, et al. *J Allergy Clin Immunol.* 2011;128:418–20. **11.** Bernstein DI, et al. *Toxicol Sci.* 2012;131:242–6. **12.** Bernstein DI, Kashon M, Lummus ZL, et al.. *Toxicol Sci.* 2013;131(1):242–6. **13.** Yucesoy B, et al. *Toxicol Sci.* 2012;129:166–73. **14.** Tinnerberg H, et al. *Int Arch Occup Environ Health.* 2014;87(4):365–72. **15.** Yucesoy B, et al. *Toxicol Sci.* 2015;146(1):192–201. **16.** Yucesoy B, et al. *J Immunotoxicol.* 2016;13:119–26. **17.** Bernstein DI, et al. *J Allergy Clin Immunol.* 2018;142(3):959–69. **18.** Leppilahti J, et al. *Front Med (Lausanne).* 2019;6:220.

and –HDI conjugates. Therefore, the potential reversibility of GSH-isocyanate conjugates suggests that GSH-mediated pathway not necessarily fulfill a conventional detoxification role for DI, since cleaved isocyanate may carbamoylate other molecules (32). Indeed, there are data supporting a pathogenetic role of GSH in response to DI exposure. GSH-TDI reaction products were capable of transferring TDI to albumin, recognized as a major carrier for TDI in vivo (33). In addition, GSH-MDI conjugates, delivered intranasally in mice, induce innate immune responses characterized by products of alternative macrophage activation, such as chitinase and IL-12/IL-23. Whether the interaction of GSH with DI in humans is weighted toward protective or toxic effects remains undetermined.

HDI induced increase of reactive oxygen species (ROS), through enzymatic inhibition of superoxide dismutase 1 in human dendritic cells. ROS promoted ERK phosphorylation and downstream transcriptional increase of several genes including heme oxygenase-1 (OH-1), involved in the protection against ROS (34). However, the expression of HO-1 and ferritin light chain (FTL) and the synthesis of other antioxidant proteins such as thioredoxin, glutathione peroxidase, peroxiredoxin, and catalase were found to be suppressed by TDI in a dose- and time-dependent manner in a human epithelial cell line (35). Human neutrophil apoptosis induced by DI was found to be mediated by mitochondrial production of ROS and elevation of proinflammatory cytokine response, such as IL-8, IL-6, IL-1 beta, IL-10, interferon-gamma (IFN-γ), and tumor necrosis factor (36). In a murine model, a role for toll-like receptor 4 deficiency has also been proposed for inducing apoptosis and related airway hyperresponsiveness and inflammation (37). These findings indicate the importance of oxidative stress in DI-induced toxicity, but their implication for DI-induced asthma has to be elucidated.

Disruption of epithelial cell-cell integrity is essential for the initiation and perpetuation of airway inflammatory response in asthma. Autophagy of human bronchial epithelial cells has been described in TDI-induced inflammation and airway remodeling (38). A compromised epithelial barrier caused by abnormal cytoplasmic retention of alpha-catenin and E-caderin redistribution has been reported in TDI-induced murine asthma (Chapter 4). Interaction of TDI with transient receptor potential (TRP) vanilloid 4 and TRP ankyrin 1 contribute to alpha-catenin and E-caderin dysfunction in the same mouse model of TDI asthma (39). Thymic stromal lymphopoietin (TSLP) is a likely IL-7 cytokine highly expressed in barrier epithelial cells, which can activate group 2 innate lymphoid cells (ILC2) and drive strong Th2 and Th17 response with release of IL-4, IL-5, IL-13, IL17 and TNF-alpha. Inhibition of TLSP by anti-TLSP antibodies attenuates airway inflammation induced by TDI in mice (Chapter 4).

Animal studies

The reader is referred to Chapter 4 in which animal studies, including those performed in regards to polyisocyanates, are reviewed.

Airway inflammation and immune responses

Isocyanate-induced asthma is associated with an inflammatory response, like other types of asthma. Initial sensitization may result from cutaneous exposure, leading to respiratory tract inflammation elicited by inhalation (17, 40), the resulting immune response being both innate and adaptive (41). Indeed, most animal models of isocyanate-induced asthma have been carried out by first sensitizing the animal through skin exposure with subsequent elicitation of the response by bronchial exposure, as reviewed (Chapter 4). Epithelial cells exposed to DI can stimulate lymphocyte proliferation. Increases in CD45+ T cells and eosinophils in the airways have been detected in BAL, endobronchial biopsy, and induced sputum (42, 43) of workers exposed to DI. The increased numbers of CD45+ T cells and eosinophils observed in isocyanate-induced asthma are similar to those observed in non-OA (44). However, some inflammatory changes in the airways differ from non-OA, particularly for the participation of neutrophils. Increased neutrophils and levels of IL-8, a cytokine that induces neutrophil chemotaxis, have been documented in airway secretions of DI-exposed individuals (43). Blockade of the nod-like receptor protein 3(NLRP3)/caspase inflammasome pathway, a pivotal mediator of chronic inflammatory diseases, improves neutrophilic airway inflammation caused by TDI in mice (45).

In a bronchial biopsy study of workers with DI-induced OA, Bentley et al. (46) observed increased CD25+ T cells and total activated eosinophils. Originally, these authors proposed that the CD25+ T cells represented activated effector T-cell types, since CD25 comprises part of the IL-2 receptor. However, it has been appreciated that CD25 is also highly expressed by regulatory T cells (Treg) with the capacity to modulate dendritic cell activity (47).

Two related studies have characterized human T-cell lines derived from endobronchial biopsies of workers with OA due to TDI (48, 49) suggesting that CD8+ T cells, that secrete IFN-γ, may predominate (49), whereas CD4+ T cells, that make Th₂-type cytokines, predominate in non-OA "atopic" asthma (48). However, in situ characterization of endobronchial biopsies has yielded somewhat conflicting results, since demonstrated Th2-type CD4+ T cells found in the airways of workers with OA, that may be indistinguishable from that reported in "nonoccupational" asthma (49). The presence of Th2-type cytokines/chemokines as well as of Th1- and Th17-associated cytokines has been shown in both animal models and in workers with OA due to DI (50–53) as well as a role for innate immunity (41). Cytokines like IL-33 and TSLP, derived from airway epithelial barrier, may activate group 2 innate lymphoid cells (ILC2). Indeed, increased levels of TSLP were detected in sputum supernatant of subjects exposed to high concentration of TDI and putative ILC2 cells were identified in bronchial biopsies of subjects with TDI-induced OA using immunohistochemistry (54, 55).

Analysis of bronchial biopsies has been used to demonstrate polyisocyanate binding to macromolecules in the airway epithelium, with keratin-18 being a predominant in vivo target (56, 57). The role of isocyanate–epithelial cell protein conjugates remains unclear, but they might act as antigens that drive airway inflammation following exposure, possibly in an "auto-immune"-like manner. Indeed, Choi et al. (58) demonstrated increased levels of antikeratin antibodies in subjects with OA due to DI. Activation of the transient receptor potential melastatin 8 (TRPM8) of epithelial cells by DI exposure led to increases in the mRNA of various interleukins (59).

The localized cellular inflammatory response in the lungs of individuals with respiratory disease may also be reflected in the peripheral circulation. In subjects with OA due to DI, increases in peripheral blood levels of CD8+ T cells have been reported following exposure in vivo (60), while in vitro, skewing of the T-cell repertoire in response to isocyanate antigen has been noted (61). In one report by Bernstein et al. (61), isocyanates induced a preferential usage of particular T-cell antigen receptor genes variable region (V)β_1 and Vβ_5, while a study by Wisnewski et al. (52) demonstrates a strong preferential induction of Vγ_9Vδ_2 T cells, a subset of which express an unusual CD8$\alpha\alpha$+ variant.

Direct innate immune effects of isocyanates on monocytes or macrophages could contribute to the underlying pathogenesis of OA due to DI. Support for this hypothesis was provided by in vitro studies conducted by Lummus (62), demonstrating a unique profile of cellular responses to isocyanate antigens, which included specific increases in monocyte chemotactic protein-1. Initial studies indicate that DI antigen-induced MCP-1 production in vitro may be the best diagnostic indicator of DI-induced asthma short of SIC (63). Subsequently, Wisnewski et al. reported that human mononuclear cells take up HDI–human serum albumin conjugates (27). These cells, cultured in vitro, also produce chemokines such as MCP-1 and pattern recognition receptors (i.e. chitinases).

In summary, the aforementioned studies suggest that pathogenesis of DI-induced OA is polymechanistic with several distinct asthma endotypes.

Diagnosis

Clinical presentation of polyisocyanate sensitizer-induced OA and sudden-onset irritant-induced OA differs, the former being progressive, elicited by inhalation of subirritant concentrations of polyisocyanates, and the latter acute, induced by acute exposure to high irritant concentrations. Diagnosis of sensitizer-induced OA is often difficult, especially when the asthma is of the delayed type occurring hours after exposure. The diagnostic assessment is similar to the approach used for other types of OA (Chapter 5).

A careful occupational and medical history is critical. Workers with OA due to DI may associate their asthma with a particular process and relate the onset after exposure to high levels of polyisocyanates during an accident or spill. Obtaining the relevant safety data sheets (SDSs) is important, being aware that content may not be complete. Assessment of the type of process (e.g. spraying, heating), quantity of DI used, industrial hygiene controls and PPE, as well as monitoring data, if available, can help assess the extent of exposure.

In addition to employment history, duration and timing of exposure, and knowledge of past and current hobbies, asthma symptoms during a work period with improvement on the weekends or holidays is suggestive but not conclusive of WRA (Chapter 5). Additional testing adds greater diagnostic certainty.

Differential diagnosis should include other upper and lower airways associated dysfunction syndromes. Urticaria, anaphylaxis, and eczema have occasionally been reported (64). Although polyisocyanates may be absorbed through the skin, contact dermatitis rarely accompanies OA. Hypersensitivity pneumonitis may be associated with OA (see Chapter 24) and upper airway involvement can coexist (see Chapter 22).

Confirmation of the diagnosis through assessment of spirometry, NSBH, serial PEF, workplace and laboratory specific inhalation tests, as well as immunological and inflammatory testing is described in detail in Chapters 8 and 7.

Laboratory testing

The few tests available from research laboratories include serological (isocyanate-specific antibody measurements) or cellular measurements of isocyanate-specific proliferative or cytokine responses. Radioimmunoassay testing (RAST) as well as enzyme-linked immunosorbent assay (ELISA), particularly a "sandwich" modification using monoclonal antibodies (65, 66), for detection of isocyanate serum-specific IgE adducts to various isocyanates (67) have been proposed. Although such assays even when optimized with respect to DI–human serum albumin (HSA) antigen-binding characteristics possess high specificity as reviewed (pooled specificity for all types of isocyanates = 0.94, 95% CI:0.88–0.97), test sensitivity is too low to use it to rule out OA due to DI, that is 0.27, 95% CI:0.19–0.39 (68). However, when specific IgE is present, particularly at higher levels (69), it is highly supportive of OA (70). Histamine release that has been detected after SIC may identify subjects who react in an IgE-dependent way (71). Serum levels of specific IgE may become undetectable after an undetermined period away from exposure (69, 72). ELISAs or western blots for isocyanate-specific IgG are often helpful in confirming prior immunological exposure to isocyanates and may be highly elevated in cases of isocyanate-induced HP (Chapter 24). Such antibodies can be found in nonsymptomatic exposed workers and appear more relevant to exposure than disease, which is a useful feature in the context of exposure biomonitoring (18).

In detecting polyisocyanate immunologic reactions, the role of the polyisocyanate protein conjugate used as the "antigen" is extremely important. Most clinical studies to date have used albumin as the carrier, a good choice based on current in vivo studies in animal and clinical studies. Hemoglobin is another possible protein but hemoglobin-TDI antigenicity was found to be approximately 30% that of HSA-TDI (73). Methods to prepare suitable antigenic preparations remain relatively unstandardized between laboratories and new methods for producing "polyisocyanate antigens" continue to evolve (Chapter 7). Conjugate preparation influences binding of specific antibodies but serologic detection of the exposure-induced polyclonal antibody response may not be significantly affected by these differences (74).

The lymphocyte proliferation test used for assessing potential in vitro sensitizing properties of various chemicals (Chapters 17 and 19) and to detect beryllium sensitization has shown some promise (75). The MCP-1 assay exhibited sensitivity and specificity of 79% and 91%, respectively, in identifying workers with confirmed OA due to DI (63). Cross-reactivity between different types of isocyanates remains hypothetical and could not be shown in an animal model (76).

Bronchoprovocation testing

Commonly known as SIC, it is reviewed in detail in Chapter 8. SIC elicits early (~30%), or, more commonly, dual (~35%) and late phase (~35%) asthmatic reactions in workers with a history of asthma induced by TDI (77). Inhalation challenge is considered the reference standard for confirming a diagnosis of OA in an individual worker (78, 79) and is a useful research tool. Ideally, a positive SIC should be reproduced by demonstrating a fluctuation in PEF when serially assessed at work and away from work although this may not be feasible if the worker has been away from work (80). Testing should only be performed in specialized centers and conducted by experienced personnel with all safety measures in place as recommended by international guidelines (78, 79).

There is limited availability of SIC testing around the world. Facilities are complex and expensive requiring well-ventilated exposure chambers for generation and monitoring of DI concentrations, and well-trained personnel. Adverse effects are infrequent though of concern, with 20% of subjects requiring inhaled bronchodilator, mainly after controlled exposure to LMW agents such as polyisocyanates (81). Challenges with DI are highly specific if the test is positive. False negative results may occur if the appropriate polyisocyanate or dose challenge is not utilized or if specific bronchial sensitivity to an agent has decreased after removal from exposure (Chapter 8). The pattern of bronchoconstrictive reactions to polyisocyanates is not necessarily linear from one day of exposure to the next consecutive day (Chapter 8).

Workplace challenge study through assessment of serial measurements of PEF at and away from work or exposure is an alternative method of documenting work-related changes in lung function (Chapter 8) (82). Generally, workers are instructed to record their PEF, activities, symptoms, and use of bronchodilators. The frequency and duration of the recordings and their effect on sensitivity and specificity has been studied and a minimum of four readings per day for 4 weeks, including periods at and away from exposure are recommended although more frequent readings and longer assessment periods may increase the value of the test. There are different interpretive methods for analysis of serial PEF data: visual analysis by experts of plotted values; examining percent diurnal variability; assessing differences in the mean values between days off work and on exposure days (see Chapter 8).

Concordance of timings of reactions during SIC and work challenge has provided further validation for confirming clinical relevance (80).

Based on published recommendations for assessing symptomatic workers for OA while still at work, Bernstein developed printed and audio guidance for the primary care physician utilizing serial PEF in evaluating workers during a 2-week period of work-related exposure and 2 weeks of nonexposure to polyisocyanates (83).

Industrial hygiene

Air sampling

Quantifying polyisocyanates is complex and depends on the reactivity of the N=C=O group. Sampling strategies (work area or personal) and methods, particularly for gases and vapors, have been described (Chapter 6). Impingers, made of glass or polyethylene, and reagent-impregnated filters in cassettes can collect and stabilize isocyanates (Chapter 6) (84). In the case of isocyanates, exposures frequently contain mixtures of different polymeric products. In addition, there are several different exposure metrics or units used to express isocyanate exposures, making it difficult to compare findings. Methods of sample analysis using liquid and gas chromatography coupled to mass spectrometry have been developed and can be used for biological monitoring in urine (85). A method for assessing dermal exposure consisting of thin medical-grade cotton gloves impregnated with a reagent, has been proposed (86).

Occupational exposure limits (OELs)

Current isocyanate occupational exposure limits (OELs) are predominantly for DI monomers, with few for polyisocyanates, even though exposure to polyisocyanastes is increasingly important (2). In the United States, the Occupational Safety and Health Administration (OSHA) has a ceiling permissible exposure limits for TDI and MDI monomers (20 ppb) but no other permissible exposure limits, and no time-weighted average standard for DI. The American Conference of Governmental Industrial Hygienists (ACGIH) recommended an 8-hr threshold limit value (TLV) time-weighted average (TWA) of 1 ppb and a short-term exposure limit (STEL) of 5 ppb in 2016 but no standard for polyisocyanates (87). A risk assessment yielded a prospective OEL of 0.4 ppb, below the current ACGIH TWA of 1 ppb (88). While dermal exposure may also be an important route of sensitization, especially with less volatile DI such as MDI, there are no regulatory standards for skin exposure. Importantly, once sensitized, workers can respond to very low exposure levels, below the TWA. Thus, airborne workplace DI levels below current OELs do not "rule out" the diagnosis of DI-induced OA.

Biomonitoring

Metabolites of MDI can be chemically hydrolyzed to form the free diamine 4,4′-methylenedianiline (MDA) that can be assessed in urine (89) by liquid chromatography/tandem mass spectrometry method (85) as a biomarker of MDI. Such monitoring is currently used in surveys of workers potentially exposed to DI, detectable levels being found in 2.6% of 196 spray-painters in Australia (90). Bello and coworkers found that 25% of urine samples obtained from 31 workers exposed to MDI showed elevated MDA levels (84).

Besides urinary markers of isocyanate exposure, serological markers of exposure and OA have been studied. Autotaxin-lysophosphatidic acid serum levels were significantly correlated with urinary markers (toluene diamine) of exposure to TDI in 118 exposed workers (91). Serum periostin (92) and folliculin (93) levels were higher and clusterin/progranulin levels lower (93) in subjects with OA due to TDI. Albumin-adducts of MDI as assessed in serum may be associated with OA (94), although this assessment was not discriminative for OA in another study (95). Albumin-adducts of HDI have been associated with exposure, suggesting that exposure-specific IgG, such as HDI-IgG or MDI-IgG, may be useful as a biomarker to monitor exposure (18).

Outcome and management

Although asthma symptoms can improve after removal from exposure, follow-up studies of workers with OA due to DI have shown that asthma symptoms and NSBH can persist in a large proportion of workers. Table 14.6 summarizes findings from several studies that have examined the outcome of OA due to isocyanates. These studies invariably showed a deleterious clinical and functional outcome. Moreover, the duration of exposure and the duration of symptomatic exposure are associated with a poorer prognosis. Reduction of exposure to HDI and medical surveillance have been associated with a diminution of cases of compensation for OA (96) and better outcome 2 years after removal from exposure (97). Reduction of exposure should focus on average and peak working area airborne concentrations (14) as well as dermal protection. Respiratory protective equipment (Chapter 10) can be considered for the purpose of reducing exposure and keeping subjects with OA at work if this is required to avoid deleterious socioeconomic outcome.

Although the clinical and functional phenotypes of OA due to HMW and LMW agents can differ (6), it is not clear if the outcome of OA differs for these two broad classes of agents. One study carried out in Ontario, Canada, suggested a better

TABLE 14.6 Selected Studies on Outcome of Occupational Asthma Due to Diisocyanates after Removal from or Diminution of Exposure

Authors/Yr Publication	Number of Subjects	Duration of Follow-Up (yrs)	Main Findings
1. Innocenti et al., 1981	37	Mean interval of 40 months	Disappearance of symptoms in 86% of workers Chronic bronchitis in 24% Annual decline in FEV_1 of 68 mL
2. Paggiaro et al., 1984	27 workers (12 left exposure, 15 still exposed)	~2 yrs after first assessment	67% of those who left exposure vs 93% of workers who stayed exposed with asthma symptoms Improved spirometry but persistence of NSBH in those who left exposure Lower FEV_1 in subjects who stayed exposed
3. Hudson et al., 1985	10/31 workers with OA due to diisocyanates	~2 yrs after first assessment	No improvement in NSBH Longer duration of exposure in workers with persistent symptoms
4. Moller et al., 1986	7 subjects with OA due to TDI	Mean of 4.5 yrs after first assessment	6 of the 7 still symptomatic after cessation of exposure and with NSBH
5. Lozewicz et al., 1987	50/56 workers with OA due to various isocyanates	> 4 yrs after first assessment	82% of subjects still symptomatic 50% with NSBH to histamine, 53% to cold air
6. Rosenberg et al., 1987	20 workers with OA due to various isocyanate compounds	Removed from exposure for an average of 19 months	50% of workers still symptomatic Asymptomatic subjects younger and with shorter exposure
7. Mapp et al., 1988	35 workers with OA due to TDI	30 workers seen after an average removal from exposure of ~10 months	Persistence of symptoms and NSBH Better recovery in younger subjects and those with a shorter duration of exposure
8. Banks et al., 1990	6 workers with OA due to TDI	Workers seen for 5 yrs Still exposed minimally	No clinical and no functional improvement
9. Pisati et al., 1993	60 workers with OA due to TDI	17 remained exposed, 43 stopped	Clinical and functional deterioration in workers who remained exposed 29% of workers completely recovered Longer duration of symptoms and exposure related to less favorable outcome
10. Marabini et al., 1994	40 workers with OA due to TDI	70% no longer exposed	No difference in outcome in subjects who left exposure or continued to be exposed
11. Tarlo et al., 1995	136 workers with OA due to various isocyanates and 89 workers with OA due to other agents (WCB decision based on objective tests in 43%)	89% removed from exposure Assessment at a mean of 1.9 yrs after initial assessment as part of a medical surveillance program	64% of the group exposed to isocyanates with asthma cleared or improved at follow-up Better clinical and functional outcome in the group with OA due to isocyanates

12. Piirila et al., 2000	91/245 workers with OA due to various isocyanates	"Clinically" assessed ~10 yrs after diagnosis	82% still symptomatic. More favorable outcome in subjects exposed to HDI and positive specific IgE
13. Talini et al., 2013	45 workers with OA due to TDI	Reassessed after a mean interval of ~11 yrs. 71% removed from exposure for a mean interval of ~6 yrs	Better clinical and functional outcome in workers no longer exposed. Shorter duration of exposure related to improved NSBH
14. Ruëgger et al., 2014	35 workers exposed to various isocyanates	Reassessed after a mean interval of ~12 yrs. 86% no longer exposed	Clinical improvement. Deterioration in spirometry. No change in NSBH. Outcome related to duration of exposure

Abbreviations: HDI, hexamethylene diisocyanate; NSBH, nonspecific bronchial hyperresponsiveness; OA, occupational asthma; TDI, toluene diisocyanate; WCB, workers' compensation board.

References: **1.** Innocenti A, et al. *Med Lavoro.* 1981;3:231–7. **2.** Paggiaro PL, et al. *Clin Allergy.* 1984;14:463–9. **3.** Hudson P, et al. *J Allergy Clin Immunol.* 1985;76:682–7.**4.** Moller DR, et al. *Chest.* 1986;90:494–9. **5.** Lozewicz S, et al. *Br J Dis Chest.* 1987;81:14–27. **6.** Rosenberg N, et al. *Clin Allergy.* 1987;17:55–61. **7.** Mapp CE, et al. *Am Rev Respir Dis.* 1988;137:1326–9. **8.** Banks DE, et al. *Chest.* 1990;97:121–5. **9.** Pisati G, et al. *Br J Ind Med.* 1993;50:60–4. **10.** Marabini A, et al. *Med del Lavoro.* 1994;85:134–41. **11.** Tarlo SM, et al. *Occup Environ Med.* 1997;54:756–61.**12.** Piirila PL, et al. *Am J Respir Crit Care Med.* 2000;162:516–22. **13.** Talini D, et al. *Int Arch Allergy Immunol.* 2013;161(2):189–94. **14.** Rüegger M, et al. *J Occup Med Toxicol.* 2014;9:21.

prognosis in workers exposed to isocyanates (98). However, the fact that these workers were followed in the context of a medical surveillance program may favor a better prognosis (98). Also, it is still uncertain if complete avoidance of exposure encompasses a better outcome than reduction, as discussed in a meta-analysis (99). Interestingly, subjects with increased specific IgE levels may behave more favorably (99). Adding inhaled steroids to reduction or avoidance of exposure may enhance improvement (100). Finally, whereas continuing exposure in subjects with OA results in an accelerated fall in FEV_1, the annual decline in FEV_1 after leaving exposure was found to be 27 mL/yr in 86 workers removed from exposure after diagnosis (22% with OA due to DI), which is comparable to healthy adults (101).

Exposure to isocyanates at concentrations below OELs is not associated with an accelerated fall in FEV_1 unless such exposure causes symptoms of asthma, hypersensitivity pneumonitis, or irritant-induced asthma (102).

Surveillance and prevention

Given the persistence of DI-induced OA despite efforts to reduce exposures, medical surveillance of isocyanate-exposed workers, along with efforts to minimize both skin and airborne exposure, is recommended. As presented (see section Epidemiology and risk factors) and in Chapter 10, there is evidence that medical surveillance has resulted in reducing the number of claims for OA due to isocyanates and the long-term clinical and functional consequences. Medical strategies for surveillance, discussed in Chapter 5, have been implemented in US TDI production workers (103). However, medical surveillance is rarely mandated and does not appear to be routinely performed on many DI-exposed workers.

Surveillance data can be helpful in the identification of high-risk exposures such as paint application on large objects, a work process that cannot reasonably be done in a paint shop, indirect exposure, exposure during cleanup, and dermal exposure (104). As with other occupational agents, the key to prevention is exposure reduction, with a focus on both respiratory and skin exposure. Use of gloves offering satisfactory protection by examining permeation features (105) using innovative glove sampling of isocyanates (86) is recommended.

Implementation of medical surveillance programs, along with efforts to reduce airborne and skin isocyanate exposures, should lead to reduced isocyanate-induced lung diseases.

Future directions in research

Elimination of DI is unlikely given the expanding use of polyurethane across numerous work sectors. Questions regarding disease pathogenesis, exposure risk factors, susceptibility, optimal diagnostic strategies, and prevention remain. Future studies to address outstanding issues are discussed below:

* *Exposure assessment and biomarkers*

Exposure risk factors, such as the route of exposure (respiratory, skin), peak exposures, chemical composition, and co-exposures, remain poorly defined, hindering preventive efforts. Better methods, including use of biomarkers, are needed to monitor workplace exposures to DI, especially skin exposure and infrequent exposure events. Such biomarkers can be used to better understand exposure risk factors and also monitor the effectiveness of industrial hygiene controls and PPE.

* *Define possible immunologic mechanisms*

It is unlikely that IgE-mediated immune mechanisms alone explain OA. However, genetic studies suggest that the immune response genes are associated with OA. Further investigation of alternative immune responses may yield new insights.

* *Genetic studies*

It is likely that multiple and diverse genes contribute to the pathogenesis of OA. Investigations on genetic variants should be carried out in the context of multicenter studies for increasing the power of the analysis with increased numbers of participants; furthermore, efforts should be made to replicate results in multiple worker populations of different genetic background. Next-generation DNA sequencing may facilitate identification of functional gene variants that may yield new insights into mechanisms of disease.

- *Diagnosis*

The recognition and diagnosis of isocyanate-induced OA remains challenging. Similar to other agents, effective approaches are needed to increase awareness of DI-induced OA among clinicians, workers, and industry. Incorporating clinical support systems into electronic medical records should increase recognition of possible WRA (106). However, there remains a need to optimize diagnostic tests (questionnaires, assessment of NSBH, PEF, and inflammation in induced sputum [Chapter 8]), especially tests that are readily available to practicing physicians.

- *Surveillance and prevention*

Better surveillance methods are needed and should focus on identifying exposure risks and early disease.

References

1. Urlich H. Chemistry and Technology of Isocyanates. West Sussex, England: John Wiley & Sons Ltd; 1996.
2. Bello D, Woskie SR, Streicher RP, et al. Polyisocyanates in occupational environments: a critical review of exposure limits and metrics. Am J Ind Med. 2004;46:480–91.
3. Krone CA, Klingner TD, Ely TJTA. Polyurethanes and childhood asthma. Med Sci Monit. 2003;9:HY39–HY43.
4. Fuchs S, Valade P. Étude clinique et expérimentale sur quelques cas d'intoxication par le Desmodur T (diisocyanate de toluylene 1-2-4 et 1-2-6). Arch Mal Profess. 1951;12:191–6.
5. Cullinan P, Vandenplas O, Bernstein D. Assessment and management of occupational asthma. J Allergy Clin Immunol Pract. 2020;8:3264–75.
6. Vandenplas O, Godet J, Hurdubaea L, et al. Are high- and low-molecular-weight sensitizing agents associated with different clinical phenotypes of occupational asthma? Allergy. 2019;74:261–72.
7. Mason P, Scarpa MC, Liviero F, et al. Distinct clinical phenotypes of occupational asthma due to diisocyanates. J Occup Environ Med. 2017;59:539–42.
8. Moore WC, Meyers DA, Wenzel SE, et al. Identification of asthma phenotypes using cluster analysis in the Severe Asthma Research Program. Am J Respir Crit Care Med. 2010;181(4):315–23.
9. Malo JL, Ghezzo H, D'Aquino C, et al. Natural history of occupational asthma: relevance of type of agent and other factors in the rate of development of symptoms in affected subjects. J Allergy Clin Immunol. 1992;90:937–44.
10. Butcher BT, Jones RN, O'Neil CE, et al. Longitudinal study of workers employed in the manufacture of toluene-diisocyanate. Am Rev Respir Dis. 1977;116:411–21.
11. Leroyer C, Perfetti L, Cartier A, et al. Can reactive airways dysfunction syndrome (RADS) transform into occupational asthma due to "sensitisation" to isocyanates? Thorax. 1998;53:152–3.
12. Balogun RA, Siracusa A, Shusterman S. Occupational rhinitis and occupational asthma: association or progression? Am J Ind Med. 2018;61:293–307.
13. Redlich CA, Stowe MH, Coren BA, et al. Diisocyanate-exposed auto body shop workers: a one-year follow-up. Am J Ind Med. 2002;42:511–8.
14. Collins JJ, Anteau S, Conner PR, et al. Incidence of occupational asthma and exposure to toluene diisocyanate in the United States toluene diisocyanate production industry. J Occup Environ Med. 2017;59(Suppl 12):S22–S27.
15. Ott MG, Klees JE, Poche SL. Respiratory health surveillance in a toluene diisocyanate production unit, 1967–97: clinical observations and lung function analyses. Occup Environ Med. 2000;57:43–52.
16. Petsonk EL, Wang ML, Lewis DM, et al. Asthma-like symptoms in wood product plant workers exposed to methylene diphenyl diisocyanate. Chest. 2000;118:1183–93.
17. Redlich CA. Skin exposure and asthma: is there a connection? Proc Am Thorac Soc. 2010;2:134–7.
18. Wisnewski AV, Stowe MH, Nerlinger A, et al. Biomonitoring hexamethylene diisocyanate (HDI) exposure based on serum levels of HDI-specific IgG. Ann Occup Hyg. 2012;56:901–10.
19. Plehiers PM, Chappelle AH, Spence MW. Practical learnings from an epidemiology study on TDI-related occupational asthma: part II-exposure without respiratory protection to TWA-8 values indicative of peak events is a good indicator of risk. Toxicol Ind Health. 2020:748233720947203.
20. Siracusa A, Marabini A, Folletti I, et al. Smoking and occupational asthma. Clin Exp Allergy. 2006;36:577–84.
21. Monso E, Cloutier Y, Lesage J, et al. What is the respiratory retention of inhaled hexamethylene di-isocyanate? Eur Respir J. 2000;16:729–30.
22. Schroeter JD, Kimbell JS, Asgharian B, et al. Inhalation dosimetry of hexamethylene diisocyanate vapor in the rat and human respiratory tracts. Inhal Toxicol. 2013;25(3):168–77.
23. Kennedy AL, Wilson TR, Stock MF, et al. Distribution and reactivity of inhaled ^{14}C-labeled toluene diisocyanate (TDI) in rats. Arch Toxicol. 1994;68:434–43.
24. Wisnewski AV, Liu J. Immunochemical detection of the occupational allergen, methylene diphenyl diisocyanate (MDI), in situ. J Immunol Methods. 2016;429:60–5.
25. Hettick JM, Law BF, Lin CC, et al. Mass spectrometry-based analysis of murine bronchoalveolar lavage fluid following respiratory exposure to 4,4'-methylene diphenyl diisocyanate aerosol. Xenobiotica. 2018;48(6):626–36.
26. Wisnewski AV, Lemus R, Karol MH, et al. Isocyanate-conjugated human lung epithelial cell proteins: a link between exposure and asthma? J Allergy Clin Immunol. 1999;104:341–7.
27. Wisnewski AV, Liu Q, Liu J, et al. Human innate immune responses to hexamethylene diisocyanate (HDI) and HDI-albumin conjugates. Clin Exp Allergy. 2008;38(6):957–67.
28. Wisnewski AV, Liu J, Redlich CA, et al. Polymerization of hexamethylene diisocyanate in solution and a 260.23 m/z [M+H](+) ion in exposed human cells. Anal Biochem. 2018;543:21–9.
29. Day BW, Jin R, Basalyga DM, et al. Formation, solvolysis, and transcarbamoylation reactions of bis(S-glutathionyl) adducts of 2, 4- and 2, 6-diisocyanatotoluene. Chem Res Toxicol. 1997;10:424–31.
30. Lange RW, Day BW, Lemus R, et al. Intracellular S-Glutathionyl adducts in murine lung and human bronchoepithelial cells after exposure to diisocyanatotoluene. Chem Res Toxicol. 1999;12:931–6.
31. Wisnewski AV, Liu J, Redlich CA. Connecting glutathione with immune responses to occupational methylene diphenyl diisocyanate exposure. Chemico-biological interactions. 2013;205(1):38–45.
32. Pauluhn J. Acute inhalation toxicity of polymeric diphenyl-methane 4, 4'-diisocyanate in rats: time course of changes in bronchoalveolar lavage. Arch Toxicol. 2000;74:257–69.
33. Wisnewski AV, Liu J, Colangelo CM. Glutathione reaction products with a chemical allergen, methylene-diphenyl diisocyanate, stimulate alternative macrophage activation and eosinophilic airway inflammation. Chem Res Toxicol. 2015;28:729–37.
34. Silva A, Nunes C, Martins J, et al. Respiratory sensitizer hexamethylene diisocyanate inhibits SOD 1 and induces ERK-dependent detoxifying and maturation pathways in dendritic-like cells. Free Radic Biol Med. 2014;72:238–46.
35. Kim SH, Choi GS, Ye YM, et al. Toluene diisocyanate (TDI) regulates haem oxygenase-1/ferritin expression: implications for toluene diisocyanate-induced asthma. Clin Exp Immunol. 2010;160:489–97.
36. Mishra PK, Khan S, Bhargava A, et al. Regulation of isocyanate-induced apoptosis, oxidative stress, and inflammation in cultured human neutrophils: isocyanate-induced neutrophils apoptosis. Cell Biol Toxicol. 2010;26(3):279–91.
37. Chen S, Deng Y, He Q, et al. Toll-like receptor 4 deficiency aggravates airway hyperresponsiveness and inflammation by impairing neutrophil apoptosis in a toluene diisocyanate-induced murine asthma model. Allergy Asthma Immunol Res. 2020;12(4):608–25.
38. Jiao B, Chen Y, Yang Y, et al. Toluene diisocyanate-induced inflammation and airway remodeling involves autophagy in human bronchial epithelial cells. Toxicol In Vitro. 2020;270:105040.
39. Yao L, Chen S, Tang H, et al. Transient receptor potential ion channels mediate adherens junctions dysfunction in a toluene diisocyanate-induced murine asthma model. Toxicol Sci. 2019;168(1):160–70.
40. Wisnewski AV, Xu L, Robinson E, et al. Immune sensitization to methylene diphenyl diisocyanate (MDI) resulting from skin exposure: albumin as a carrier protein connecting skin exposure to subsequent respiratory responses. J Occup Med Toxicol. 2011;6:6.
41. Shin YS, Kim MA, Pham LD, et al. Cells and mediators in diisocyanate-induced occupational asthma. Curr Opin Allergy Clin Immunol. 2013;13(2):125–31.
42. Maestrelli P, Calcagni PG, Saetta M, et al. Sputum eosinophilia after asthmatic responses induced by isocyanates in sensitized subjects. Clin Exp Allergy. 1994;24:29–34.
43. Lemière C, Pelissier S, Tremblay C, et al. Leukotrienes and isocyanate-induced asthma: a pilot study. Clin Exp Allergy. 2004;34:1684–9.

44. Robinson DS, Hamid Q, Ying S, et al. Predominant T_{H2}like bronchoalveolar t-lymphocyte population in atopic asthma. New Engl J Med. 1992;326:298–304.

45. Chen S, Yao L, Huang P, et al. Blockade of the NLRP3/Caspase-1 axis ameliorates airway neutrophilic inflammation in a toluene diisocyanate-induced murine asthma model. Toxicol Sci. 2019;170(2):462–75.

46. Bentley AM, Maestrelli P, Saetta M, et al. Activated T-lymphocytes and eosinophils in the bronchial mucosa in isocyanate-induced asthma. J Allergy Clin Immunol. 1992;89:821–8.

47. Shi HZ, Li S, Xie ZF, et al. Regulatory CD4+CD25+ T lymphocytes in peripheral blood from patients with atopic asthma. Clin Immunol. 2004;113(2):172–8.

48. Del Prete GF, De Carli M, D'Elios MM, et al. Allergen exposure induces the activation of allergen-specific Th2 cells in the airway mucosa of patients with allergic respiratory disorders. Eur J Immunol. 1993;23(7):1445–9.

49. Maestrelli P, DelPrete GF, DeCarli M, et al. CD8 T-cell clones producing interleukin-5 and interferon-gamma in bronchial mucosa of patients with asthma induced by toluene diisocyanate. Scand J Work Environ Health. 1994;20:376–81.

50. Park HS, Jung KS, Kim HY, et al. Neutrophil activation following TDI bronchial challenges to the airway secretion from subjects with TDI-induced asthma. Clin Exp Allergy. 1999;29:1395–401.

51. Maestrelli P, Occari P, Turato G, et al. Expression of interleukin (IL)-4 and IL-5 proteins in asthma induced by toluene diisocyanate (TDI). Clin Exp Allergy. 1997;27:1292–8.

52. Wisnewski AV, Herrick CA, Liu Q, et al. Human gamma/delta T-cell proliferation and IFN-gamma production induced by hexamethylene diisocyanate. J Allergy Clin Immunol. 2003;112:538–46.

53. Chen R, Zhang Q, Chen S, et al. IL-17F, rather than IL-17A, underlies airway inflammation in a steroid-insensitive toluene diisocyanate-induced asthma model. Eur Respir J. 2019;53(4).

54. Yu G, Zhang Y, Wang X, et al. Thymic stromal lymphopoietin (TSLP) and toluene-diisocyanate-induced airway inflammation: alleviation by TSLP neutralizing antibody. Toxicol Lett. 2019;317:59–67.

55. Blomme EE, Provoost S, Bazzan E, et al. Innate lymphoid cells in isocyanate-induced asthma: role of microRNA-155. Eur Respir J. 2020;56:1901289.

56. Kennedy AL, Stock MF, Alarie Y, et al. Uptake and distribution of 14C during and following inhalation exposure to radioactive toluene diisocyanate. Toxicol Appl Pharmacol. 1989;100(2):280–92.

57. Redlich CA, Karol MH, Graham C, et al. Airway isocyanate-adducts in asthma by exposure to hexamethylene diisocyanate. Scan J Work Environ Health. 1997;23:227–31.

58. Choi JH, Nahm DH, Kim SH, et al. Increased levels of IgG to cytokeratin 19 in sera of patients with toluene diisocyanate-induced asthma. Ann Allergy Asthma Immunol. 2004;93(3):293–8.

59. Kim JH, Jang YS, Jang SH, et al. Toluene diisocyanate exposure induces airway inflammation of bronchial epithelial cells via the activation of transient receptor potential melastatin 8. Exp Mol Med. 2017;49(3):e299.

60. Finotto S, Fabbri LM, Rado V, et al. Increase in numbers of CD8 positive lymphocytes and eosinophils in peripheral blood of subjects with late asthmatic reactions induced by toluene diisocyanate. Br J Ind Med. 1991;48:116–21.

61. Bernstein JA, Munson J, Lummus ZL, et al. T-cell receptor V beta gene segment expression in diisocyanate-induced occupational asthma. J Allergy Clin Immunol. 1997;99(2):245–50.

62. Lummus ZL, Alam R, Bernstein JA, et al. Diisocyanate antigen-enhanced production of monocyte chemoattractant protein-1, IL-8, and tumor necrosis factor by peripheral mononuclear cells of workers with occupational asthma. J Allergy Clin Immunol. 1998;102:265–74.

63. Bernstein DI, Cartier A, Cote J, et al. Diisocyanate antigen-stimulated monocyte chemoattractant protein-1 synthesis has greater test efficiency than specific antibodies for identification of diisocyanate asthma. Am J Respir Crit Care Med. 2002;166:445–50.

64. Bernstein DI, Korbee L, Stauder T, et al. The low prevalence of occupational asthma and antibody-dependent sensitization to diphenylmethane diisocyanate in a plant engineered for minimal exposure to diisocyanates. J Allergy Clin Immunol. 1993;92:387–96.

65. Lemons AR, Siegel PD, Mhike M, et al. A murine monoclonal antibody with broad specificity for occupationally relevant diisocyanates. J Occup Environ Hyg. 2014;11(2):101–10.

66. Wisnewski AV, Liu J. Molecular characterization and experimental utility of monoclonal antibodies with specificity for aliphatic di- and polyisocyanates. Monoclon Antib Immunodiagn Immunother. 2020;39(3):66–73.

67. Lemons AR, Bledsoe TA, Siegel PD, et al. Development of sandwich ELISAs for the detection of aromatic diisocyanate adducts. J Immunol Methods. 2013;397(1–2):66–70.

68. Lux H, Lenz K, Budnik LT, et al. Performance of specific immunoglobulin E tests for diagnosing occupational asthma: a systematic review and meta-analysis. Occup Environ Med. 2019;76(4):269–78.

69. Tee RD, Cullinan P, Welch J, et al. Specific IgE to isocyanates: a useful diagnostic role in occupational asthma. J Allergy Clin Immunol. 1998;101:709–15.

70. Budnik LT, Preisser AM, Permentier H, et al. Is specific IgE antibody analysis feasible for the diagnosis of methylenediphenyl diisocyanate-induced occupational asthma? Int Arch Occup Environ Health. 2013;86:417–30.

71. Blindow S, Preisser AM, Baur X, et al. Is the analysis of histamine and/or interleukin-4 release after isocyanate challenge useful in the identification of patients with IgE-mediated isocyanate asthma? J Immunol Methods. 2015;422:35–50.

72. Baur X, Chen Z, Flagge A, et al. EAST and CAP specificity for the evaluation of IgE and IgG antibodies to diisocyanate-HSA conjugates. Int Arch Allergy Immunol. 1996;110:332–8.

73. Mhike M, Hettick JM, Chipinda I, et al. Characterization and comparative analysis of 2,4-toluene diisocyanate and 1,6-hexamethylene diisocyanate haptenated human serum albumin and hemoglobin. J Immunol Methods. 2016;431:38–44.

74. Hagerman LM, Law BF, Bledsoe TA, et al. The influence of diisocyanate antigen preparation methodology on monoclonal and serum antibody recognition. J Occup Environ Hyg. 2016;13(11):829–39.

75. Avery SB, Stetson DM, Pan PM, et al. Immunological investigation of individuals with toluene diisocyanate asthma. Clin Exp Immunol. 1969;4:585–96.

76. Pollaris L, Devos F, De Vooght V, et al. Toluene diisocyanate and methylene diphenyl diisocyanate: asthmatic response and cross-reactivity in a mouse model. Arch Toxicol. 2016;90(7):1709–17.

77. Mapp CE, Boschetto P, Dal Vecchio L, et al. Occupational asthma due to isocyanates. Eur Respir J. 1988;1:273–9.

78. Vandenplas O, Suojalehto H, Aasen TB, et al. Specific inhalation challenge in the diagnosis of occupational asthma: consensus statement. Eur Respir J. 2014;43:1573–87.

79. Suojalehto H, Suuronen K, Cullinan P. Specific challenge testing for occupational asthma: revised handbook. Eur Respir J. 2019;54(2):pii:1901026.

80. Burge PS, Moore VC, Robertson AS, et al. Do laboratory challenge tests for occupational asthma represent what happens in the workplace? Eur Respir J. 2018;51.

81. Vandenplas O, D'Alpaos V, Evrard G, et al. Incidence of severe asthmatic reactions after challenge exposure to occupational agents. Chest. 2013;143:1261–8.

82. Moore V, Jaakkola M, Burge P. A systematic review of serial peak expiratory flow measurements in the diagnosis of occupational asthma. Ann Respir Med. 2010;1:31–40.

83. Bernstein DI. A Guide For The Primary Care Physician In Evaluating Diisocyanate Exposed Workers For Occupational Asthma International Isocyanate Institute. 2017. https://diiamericanchemistry.com/Primary-Care-Physician-Asthma.html.

84. Bello A, Xue Y, Gore R, et al. Assessment and control of exposures to polymeric methylene diphenyl diisocyanate (pMDI) in spray polyurethane foam applicators. Int J Hyg Environ Health. 2019;222(5):804–15.

85. Lépine M, Sleno L, Lesage J, et al. A validated liquid chromatography/tandem mass spectrometry method for 4,4'-methylenedianiline quantitation in human urine as a measure of 4,4'-methylene diphenyl diisocyanate exposure. Rapid Commun Mass Spectrom. 2019;33(6):600–6.

86. Harari H, Bello D, Woskie S, et al. Development of an interception glove sampler for skin exposures to aromatic isocyanates. Ann Occup Hyg. 2016;60(9):1092–103.

87. (ACGIH) American Conference of Governmental Industrial Hygienists. Documentation of the Threshold Limit Values and Biological Exposure Indices, 7th ed. 2016 supplement (ACGIH Publication #0100DocS16). 2016.

88. Daniels RD. Occupational asthma risk from exposures to toluene diisocyanate: a review and risk assessment. Am J Ind Med. 2018;61:282–92.

89. Pearson RL, Logan PW, Kore AM, et al. Isocyanate exposure assessment combining industrial hygiene methods with biomonitoring for end users of orthopedic casting products. Ann Occup Hyg. 2013;57:758–65.

90. Hu J, Cantrell P, Nand A. Comprehensive biological monitoring to assess isocyanates and solvents exposure in the NSW Australia motor vehicle repair industry. Ann Work Expo Health. 2017;61(8):1015–23.

91. Broström JM, Ye ZW, Axmon A, et al. Toluene diisocyanate: induction of the autotaxin-lysophosphatidic acid axis and its association with airways symptoms. Toxicol Appl Pharmacol. 2015;287(3):222–31.

92. Lee JH, Kim SH, Choi Y, et al. Serum periostin levels: a potential serologic marker for toluene diisocyanate-induced occupational asthma. Yonsei Med J. 2018;59(10):1214–21.

93. Pham DL, Trinh TH, Ban GY, et al. Epithelial folliculin is involved in airway inflammation in workers exposed to toluene diisocyanate. Exp Mol Med. 2017;49(11):e395.

94. Sabbioni G, Vanimireddy LR, Lummus ZL, et al. Comparison of biological effects with albumin adducts of 4,4'-methylenediphenyl diisocyanate in workers. Arch Toxicol. 2017;91(4):1809–14.

95. Luna LG, Green BJ, Zhang F, et al. Quantitation of 4,4'-methylene diphenyl diisocyanate human serum albumin adducts. Toxicol Rep. 2014;1:743–51.

96. Tarlo SM, Liss GM, Yeung KS. Changes in rates and severity of compensation claims for asthma due to diisocyanates: a possible effect of medical surveillance measures. Occup Environ Med. 2002;59:58–62.

97. Labrecque M, Malo JL, Alaoui KM, et al. Medical surveillance programme for diisocyanate exposure. Occup Environ Med. 2011;68:302–7.

98. Tarlo SM, Banks D, Liss G, et al. Outcome determinants for isocyanate induced occupational asthma among compensation claimants. Occup Environ Med. 1997;54:756–61.

99. Henneberger PK, Patel JR, de Groene GJ, et al. Workplace interventions for treatment of occupational asthma. Cochrane Database Syst Rev. 2019;10:Cd006308.

100. Malo JL, Cartier A, Côté J, et al. Influence of inhaled steroids on the recovery of occupational asthma after cessation of exposure: an 18-month double-blind cross-over study. Am J Crit Care Respir Med. 1996;153:953–60.

101. Anees W, Moore VC, Burge PS. FEV1 decline in occupational asthma. Thorax. 2006;61:751–5.

102. Ott MG, Diller WF, Jolly AT. Respiratory effects of toluene diisocyanate in the workplace: a discussion of exposure-response relationships. Crit Rev Toxicol. 2003;33:1–59.

103. Cassidy LD, Doney B, Wang ML, et al. Medical monitoring for occupational asthma among toluene diisocyanate production workers in the United States. J Occup Environ Med. 2017;59 Suppl 12:S13–S21.

104. Reeb-Whitaker C, Anderson NJ, Bonauto DK. Prevention guidance for isocyanate-induced asthma using occupational surveillance data. J Occup Environ Hyg. 2013;10(11):597–608.

105. Mäkelä EA, Henriks-Eckerman ML, Ylinen K, et al. Permeation tests of glove and clothing materials against sensitizing chemicals using diphenylmethane diisocyanate as an example. Ann Occup Hyg. 2014;58(7):921–30.

106. Harber P, Redlich CA, Hines S, et al. Recommendations for a clinical decision support system for work-related asthma in primary care settings. J Occup Environ Med. 2017;59:e231–e5.

15

WESTERN RED CEDAR AND OTHER WOOD DUSTS

Moira Chan-Yeung,[1] **Vivi Schlünssen,**[2] **David Fishwick,**[3] **and Jean-Luc Malo**[4]
[1]Department of Medicine, Faculty of Medicine, University of British Columbia, Vancouver, British Columbia, Canada
[2]Department of Public Health, Environment, Occupation and Health, Danish Ramazzini Centre, Aarhus University,
Aarhus C, and the National Reseach Center for the Working Environment, Copenhagen, Denmark
[3]University of Sheffield and Centre for Workplace Health, Health and Safety Executive (HSE) Science and Research Centre, Buxton, UK
[4]Hôpital du Sacré-Cœur de Montréal and Université de Montréal, Montréal, Québec, Canada

Contents

Introduction

Exposure to wood dust is a common occurrence in all countries because of its traditional use for fuel and for construction for human habitation. Respiratory illnesses associated with exposure to wood dust such as asthma, hypersensitivity pneumonitis (HP), organic dust toxic syndrome, chronic bronchitis, and mucous membrane irritation syndrome are found among woodworkers. For most kinds of wood dusts, the nature of the responsible chemical compound remains unknown; in others, the disease is caused by exposure to molds or bacteria growing on the wood chips, bark, or materials or chemicals used to bond the wood strips or boards together.

Most cases of occupational asthma (OA) caused by wood dusts were published as case reports, with the exception of OA due to Western red cedar (*Thuja plicata*), which has been studied extensively because it affects vast number of workers in the primary industries of the west coast of North America and carpenters using this wood in countries where red cedar is exported. For this reason, Western red cedar (WRC) asthma will be discussed in detail first.

In addition to respiratory illnesses, other health effects have been described. Contact dermatitis is a common complaint among woodworkers, and in many cases, it is not the wood dust itself that causes the dermatitis but contaminants.

Occupational asthma due to Western red cedar (*Thuja plicata*)

WRC is an important wood species in the Pacific Northwest region. In these areas, WRC accounts for approximately 20% of the total volume of sound wood. WRC has been used extensively for poles, shakes, shingles, and lumber for exterior construction because of its well-known high durability. WRC asthma affects sawmill workers, shingle and shake mill workers, workers in remanufacturing plants, carpenters, construction workers, and cabinetmakers.

Chemical composition of WRC

WRC is different from other species because of its unusually high contents of chemical extractives (1, 2). Cedar wood extractives may be separated by steam distillation into volatile

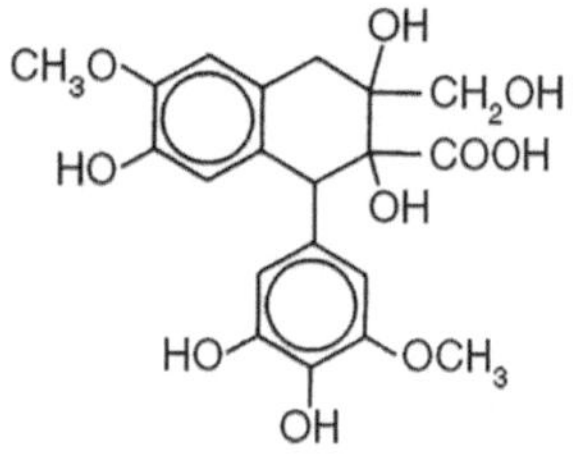

FIGURE 15.1 Structural formula of plicatic acid.

and nonvolatile fractions. The volatile fractions account for only 1%–1.5% of the heartwood (without bark), whereas the nonvolatile fractions account for 5%–15%. Of these, plicatic acid (PA) with a molecular weight of 440 Da, constituting about 90% by weight of the nonvolatile components, has been found to induce WRC asthma. The structural formula of PA is shown in Figure 15.1.

Inhalation challenge testing with PA induced similar types of asthmatic reaction as an aqueous extract of the WRC dust in patients with the disease with negative controls. The volatile fractions also contain some compounds that are natural fungicides responsible for the resistance of the wood against decay. Some compounds have beta-adrenergic receptor-blocking properties (3, 4). The significance of these compounds in the pathogenesis of WRC asthma has yet to be determined.

Clinical features

The clinical picture of patients with WRC asthma is characteristic. After a period of steady exposure, usually between 6 weeks and 3 years, but sometimes as long as 10 years, they develop cough, chest tightness, and wheeze. Some patients experience rhinorrhea several weeks before the onset of respiratory symptoms. In the majority of patients, respiratory symptoms occur initially after work and at night waking them with cough and wheeze. Later, cough, wheeze, and dyspnea occur during the day and the nocturnal symptoms become more distressing. Symptoms usually improve during weekends and holidays initially; with continuous exposure, they become persistent with no remission.

The characteristics of 232 patients proven to be suffering from WRC asthma by inhalation provocation test are shown in Table 15.1 (5). The features of note are that in this group of patients, the proportion of atopic subjects was 31.4%, same as those of the general population, and the high percentage of nonsmokers and ex-smokers, 94.8% (6).

Specific challenge tests can be performed either using fine red cedar dust or using a crude extract of WRC dust or PA. Exposure testing with fine WRC dust can be carried out using the "realistic" method (7) in Chapter 8 or by aerosolization of the crude WRC extract or PA (8). Three main types of asthmatic reaction—isolated immediate, isolated late, and biphasic or continuous asthmatic reaction—have been induced during specific challenge testing. Systemic or alveolar reaction has not been observed. The proportion of patients with late asthmatic reaction is high (89.2%), either as isolated late or part of biphasic or continuous reaction. Recurrent nocturnal asthma over several nights after one single inhalation challenge test has been documented (9).

Patients with a biphasic asthmatic reaction usually have a significantly lower lung function, a greater degree of nonspecific airway hyperresponsiveness (AHR) and a longer period between the onset of symptoms and diagnosis than patients with isolated immediate or late asthmatic reaction (10).

TABLE 15.1 Characteristics of 232 Patients with Documented Western Red Cedar Asthma

Age (yr) Mean ± SD	41.9 ± 11.8
Duration of exposure before onset of symptoms (yr)	4.1 ± 5.6
Smoking habit (%)	
Nonsmoker	66.8
Ex-smoker	28.0
Current smoker	5.2
Atopy (%)	
Positive skin test against one or more common allergens	31.4
Type of asthmatic reaction induced (%)	
Isolated immediate	10.8
Isolated late	42.3
Biphasic or continuous	46.9
Specific IgE antibodies against PA-HSA[a] (%)	20.1

Source: Summary of data in reference (5).

[a] Radioallergosorbent test (RAST) value greater than 2 was considered as a positive test.

Abbreviation: PA-HSA, plicatic acid-human serum albumin conjugate.

Diagnosis

The diagnosis of WRC asthma is based on the presence of a compatible history and objective evidence that exposure to WRC dust causes respiratory symptoms and lung function changes.

Prolonged recording of peak expiratory flow (PEF) every 2 hours during waking hours for 2 weeks at work and 1 week away from work had been found by Côté et al. (11) to be both sensitive and specific in the diagnosis of WRC asthma when compared with the results of specific challenge test with PA. The addition of measurements of AHR did not improve the sensitivity and specificity of PEF monitoring (12, 13).

Both crude WRC extract and PA or PA conjugated to human serum albumin (PA-HSA) failed to give specific reactions on skin testing. The recent finding that a blood-based gene expression biomarker panel may distinguish PA positive and PA negative subjects before inhalation challenge testing is exciting if proven in a much larger study, as it allows the diagnosis of WRC asthma without the time-consuming inhalation provocation test (14).

Outcome

The majority of the patients with WRC asthma did not fully recover years after they left exposure. A follow-up study of the 232 patients about 4 years after the diagnosis showed that of the 136 patients who left the industry, only 55 (40.4%) recovered completely, while the remaining 81 (59.6%) continued to have asthma (5). Early diagnosis and early removal from exposure was associated with complete recovery.

Patients who failed to recover after they left exposure continued to require medications for their asthma. Bronchoalveolar lavage (BAL) studies in these patients showed persistent airway inflammation with a higher total cell count, eosinophil and neutrophil counts, and an increase in protein and albumin in the lavage fluid compared with those who recovered (15). These findings were confirmed in a later study when an increase in circulating IFN-gamma, the canonical Th1 cytokine, in addition to sputum eosinophilia were found in those who failed to recover (16).

All patients who continued to work with WRC had respiratory symptoms and required medications even though most of them used personal protection. They had more severe airflow obstruction and a greater degree of AHR on follow-up examination (17).

The diagnosis of WRC asthma has considerable socioeconomic implications for the worker and their family. In follow-up studies, patients who became unemployed because of WRC asthma had their monthly income reduced substantially (18). They had significantly reduced quality-of-life scores compared to those who were relocated to jobs with no exposure WRC dust (19, 20).

Pathogenesis

The clinical feature of WRC asthma is one of allergic disease. The changes in the airway in WRC asthma are similar to those in allergic asthma. During late asthmatic reactions induced by PA, increase in eosinophils and albumin and sloughing of bronchial epithelial cells were found in BAL fluid (21). Multiple bronchial biopsies carried out in three patients 24 hours after inhalation challenge showed denudation of the bronchial epithelium, thickened basement membrane, and infiltration of eosinophils in the bronchial epithelium and submucosa—similar to patients with allergic asthma and AHR (22).

Using the radioallergosorbent test (RAST) method, specific IgE antibodies to PA-HSA were found in only 30% of WRC asthma patients (23), while skin tests were negative. The specific IgE antibodies to PA-HSA conjugate failed to passively sensitize human lung fragments (24). There are findings suggestive of the involvement of T lymphocytes in the pathogenesis: (1) increased numbers of T lymphocytes and activated T lymphocytes in the bronchial mucosa of patients; (2) proliferation of T lymphocytes in about 30% of patients when stimulated with PA-HSA conjugate (25); and (3) certain human leukocyte antigen (HLA) types are associated with predisposition to while others with protection from WRC asthma (26).

Prevalence and determinants

The prevalence of work-related asthma (WRA) is related to the degree of dust exposure; the higher the dust concentration, the higher the prevalence.

Brooks et al. (27) studied 74 cedar shake mill workers. OA was found among 24% of sawyers, 10.5% of packers, 5% of splitters, and in none of the deckmen. The average dust exposure concentrations of these workers were 6.8, 4.8, 3.6, and 0 mg/m^3, respectively. Vedal et al. (28) studied 652 cedar sawmill workers. Of the 334 workers with personal wood dust exposure, 301 were exposed to less than 1 mg/m^3, 20 to between 1 and 2 mg/m^3, and 13 to levels above 2 mg/m^3. The prevalence of WRA, defined by symptoms, was 6% and 5% in the low- and medium-exposure group and 15% in the high-exposure group.

After the initial survey in 1982, 26 workers with AHR and a history of WRA were invited to have a specific challenge test. Eleven workers developed a specific reaction to PA challenge. The prevalence rate of WRC asthma, defined as specific responsiveness to PA, was 1.7%. During the subsequent 6 years, six workers developed WRC asthma at the rate of one per year, giving an incidence of 0.3% per year even though the level of exposure in the sawmill was low with very few personal samples above 2.5 mg/m^3 (29).

Host susceptibility probably plays a role in WRC asthma since only a small proportion of exposed subjects develop the disease. Atopy and smoking are not important risk factors in WRC asthma (12). A study found that HLA antigens may play a role. Individuals with HLA class II antigens, DQB 0302 and DQB 0603, were found to be more susceptible to WRC asthma, while those with DQB 0501 were protected from the disease (25), similar to patients with diisocyanate-induced asthma when DQB 0503, HLA class II antigen, was found to confer susceptibility (30).

Permissible concentration of red cedar dust

There are very few epidemiologic studies to address the issue of permissible concentration. The workers' compensation board of British Columbia has arbitrarily lowered the permissible concentration of WRC dust from 5 mg/m^3 to 1 mg/m^3.

Asthma due to other wood dusts and other agents present in wood dust

Industries where wood is processed and used are often characterized by the simultaneous use of several wood species. This hampers the possibility for assessing the causal association between specific types of wood and the development of asthma among exposed workers. There is a vast number of publications on asthma due to various wood dusts exposure. An extensive list of wood dusts causing OA with information and key references can be found in a website table (see https://reptox.cnesst.gouv.qc.ca/en/occupational-asthma/Pages/occupational-asthma.aspx). In addition, an authoritative review on wood-specific sensitization that mainly includes asthmatic cases has been published (31). Most papers are case reports or clinical case series, where the diagnosis is generally made by the history combined with specific inhalation challenge (SIC) testing or peak expiratory flow (PEF) monitoring, often combined with skin-prick test (SPT) or specific IgE to the appropriate extracts of wood dust. Some of these studies in which two or more cases have been described are presented in Table 15.2.

Epidemiological studies

As reviewed by Jacobsen and colleagues, several epidemiological studies show an increased frequency of self-reported asthma (3%–14%) among workers exposed to wood dusts (32, 33). A meta-analysis on wood dust exposure and risk of asthma including 19 studies showed an overall poled RR of 1.5 (95% CI:1.3–1.9) (34). In a review among furniture and wood-processing workers and asthma including 55 articles it was concluded that working in the wood sector increased the risk of asthma (RR=1.5, 95% CI:1.25–1.87) (35), a figure corresponding to results obtained from a Finnish register-based population (36). In a random prospective cohort of 237 children recruited as nonasthmatic teenagers, and followed for 50 years, Tagiyeva and colleagues showed that exposure to wood dust was independently associated with adult-onset wheeze and airway obstruction (37).

Many cross-sectional studies, often including not exposed controls, have been carried out in sawmills, furniture, pellet, and parquet industries. In several studies, workers were exposed to pine dust. These studies are summarized in Table 15.3. Exposure to hard and soft wood dusts generally results in increased frequency of asthma or symptoms of asthma, work-related or not. In the SWORD surveillance study of OA, between 1991 and 2007, occupational sensitization to medium-density fiberboard (MDF) was reported in 21 cases (38).

Workers processing and handling wood may also concurrently be exposed and develop OA to agents such as molds, bacteria, natural volatile components of fresh wood, and chemicals in glue and biohazards, mostly endotoxins (see section "Sensitization to Specific Allergens"). Several agents, including molds, may, apart from asthma, cause HP (Chapter 24), alone or associated with OA, which, in epidemiological setting, can hardly be disentangled. Monoterpenes are volatile substances naturally occurring in pine

TABLE 15.2 Causes of OA Due to Various Wood Dusts

Agent	Occupation	Type of Report and Number of Subjects	Prevalence	Skin Test	Specific IgE	Other Immunologic Tests	Broncho-provocation Test	Other Evidence	References
Eastern white cedar (*Thuja occidentalis*)	Sawmill	ES (3)	4%–7%	ND	ND	ND	+	PC20	*1. Malo, 1994*
California redwood (*Sequoia sempervirens*)	Wood carvers	CS (2)	NA	—	ND	Negative precipitins	+		*2. Chan-Yeung, 1976*
Cedar of Lebanon (*Cedra libani*)	Joinery workers	CS (6)	NA	17% +	ND	100% negative precipitins	ND		*3. Greenberg, 1972*
Cocabolla (*Dalbergia retusa*)	Woodworkers	CS (3)	NA	100%	ND	ND	ND	Improvement on removal	*4. Eaton, 1973*
Iroko (*Chlorophora excelsa*)	Woodworkers	CS (9)	NA	4/9 with + negative intradermal test	ND	ND	+	PEF	*5. Ricciardi, 2003*
Oak (*Quercus robur*)	Construction	CS (3)	NA	ND	ND	ND	+		*6. Malo, 1995*
Abiruana (*Pouteria*)	Furniture factory	CS (2)	NA	+	ND	Negative	+		*7. Booth, 1976*
African maple (*Triplochiton scleroxylon*)	Construction, carpentry, sauna building	CS (2) CS (2)	NA NA	+ 100%+	+ 100%+	Passive transfer	+ +		*8. Hinojosa, 1984* *9. Reijula, 1994*
Tanganyika aningré	Woodworkers	CS (3)	NA	100% +	100% –	100% –	100%+ Precipitin		*10. Paggiaro, 1981*
Ramin (*Gonystylus bancanus*)	Woodworker	CS (2)	NA	+	+	ND	+		*11. Hinojosa, 1986*
Fernambouc (*Caesalpinia echinata*)	Bow making	ES (36)	33.3%	100% –	ND	ND	100% of 1+		*12. Hausen, 1990*
Cinnamon (*Cinnamomum zeylanicum*)	Store workers	ES (40)	22.5%	ND	ND	ND	100% of 1 +		*13. Uragoda, 1984*
Blackwood (*Acacia melanoxylon*)	Furniture	CS (3)	NA	ND	ND	ND	+	PEF	*14. Wood-Baker, 1997*
Unidentified agent in coniferous wood	Sawmills of Eastern Canada and US	CS (11)	NA	ND	ND	ND	+	PEF	*15. Malo, 1986*

Abbreviations: CS: case series; ES: epidemiological survey; NA: not assessed; ND: not done; PEF: peak expiratory flow. Includes studies with two or more subjects with OA. Slightly modified from https://reptox.cnesst.gouv.qc.ca/en/occupational-asthma/Pages/occupational-asthma.aspx.

References: **1**. Malo JL, et al. *Am J Respir Crit Care Med.* 1994;150:1697–701. **2**. Chan-Yeung M, Abboud R. *Am Rev Respir Dis.* 1976;114:1027–31. **3**. Greenberg M. *Clin Allergy.* 1972;2:219–24. **4**. Eaton KK. Respiratory allergy to exotic wood dust. *Clin Allergy.* 1973;3:307–10. **5**. Ricciardi L, et al. *Ann Allergy Asthma Immunol.* 2003;91:393–7. **6**. Malo JL, et al. *Chest.* 1995;108:856–8. **7**. Booth BH, et al. *J Allergy Clin Immunol.* 1976;57:352–7. **8**. Hinojosa M, et al. *J Allergy Clin Immunol.* 1984;74:782–6. **9**. Reijula K, et al. *Thorax.* 1994;49:622–3. **10**. Paggiaro PL, et al. *Clin Allergy.* 1981;11:605–10. **11**. Hinojosa M, et al. *Clin Allergy.* 1986;16:145–53. **12**. Hausen BM, Herrmann B. *Dtsch Med Wochenschr.* 1990;115:169–73. **13**. Uragoda CG. *Br J Ind Med.* 1984;41:224–7. **14**. Wood-Baker R. *Aus NZ J Med.* 1997;27:452–3. **15**. Malo JL, et al. *J Allergy Clin Immunol.* 1986;78:392–8.

and other coniferous trees, and liberated mainly during handling of fresh wood. Terpenes cause irritation of the mucous membranes and increased nonspecific bronchial hyperresponsiveness (NSBH) at high concentrations (39). Processing of wood composites may also expose workers to formaldehyde, a cause of irritant-induced and immunological OA (39).

TABLE 15.3 Exposure to Wood Dust and Risk of Asthma in Selected Cross-Sectional Studies

Type of Industry	Types of Wood	Number of Subjects	Smokers (%)	Asthma (%)	Dust Level (mg/m³)	Main Findings	References
Sawmill	Various jobs and woods	W: 168 C: 30	W: 33 C: 30	W: 8.3–13.4 C: 5.9	Inhalable dust GM: 0.6–11.5	Higher prevalence of asthma in joinery compared to saw and chip mill workers Association of symptoms and lung function	1. Mandryk, 1999
Sawmill	Pine	W: 772 C: 592	31%–57%	18% (OR: 1.6)	Qualitative (hygienists)	Asthma more common than in the control population Asthma more common in low- and high-exposure groups	2. Douwes, 2001
Sawmill	Mixture of soft and hard wood	W: 546 C: 565	23.6 23.2	Suggestive of OA W: 19.4 C: 4.4	GM: 3.86 (min: 0.9; max: 52.4)	High prevalence of OA Same prevalence of OA in low- and high-exposed workers	3. Rongo, 2002
Sawmill	Spruce, fir	W: 111	31%	"asthmatic syndrome" 50%	Mean: 1.7 (min: 0.2; max: 8.5)	Elevated fungi exceeding suggested limits Elevated fungi related to "bronchial syndrome" (cough and phlegm) Junior workers more affected by irritation Lung function not affected by bioaerosol nor dust levels	4. Rusca, 2008
Furniture	Various, mainly pine	Workers M: 1665 F: 368 Controls M: 262 F: 212	>20 cig/d 309 (19%) 57 (16%) 77 (31%) 40 (19%)	Physician-diagnosed M: 83 (4.9 %) F: 43 (12.2% M: 12 (6.1%) F: 12 (6.7%)	Inhalable dust GM: 0.95	Dose-response relationship between dust exposure and asthma symptoms Interaction for asthma between female gender and dust exposure Pine wood more harmful	5. Schlunssen, 2002
Furniture	Various, mainly pine		> 20 cig/d 37%	Symptoms n=244	Inhalable dust W: 0.96	Asthma related to dust level more pronounced among atopics Work-related asthma symptoms related to level of exposure in nonatopic workers	6. Schlunssen, 2004
Furniture	Rubber tree (*Hevea brasiliensis*) (+ cyano acrylate)	W: 73 C: 76	NA	Wheezing W: 15.5 C: 11.8	Inhalable dust min: 0.38 max: 2.93	Dose-dependent risk of wheezing and respiratory symptoms	7. Sripaiboonkij, 2009
Furniture	Particle- and fiber-board	W: 23 glue-paint: 35 C: 25	39 43 40	Improved symptoms in vacations 45 51 28	NA	Asthma and rhinitis more frequent in workers exposed to wood dust and glue/paint, the latter two groups having impaired ABC, OASYS-2 and methacholine scores	8. Paraskevaidou, 2019

(Continued)

TABLE 15.3 Exposure to Wood Dust and Risk of Asthma in Selected Cross-Sectional Studies (*Continued*)

Type of Industry	Types of Wood	Number of Subjects	Smokers (%)	Asthma (%)	Dust Level (mg/m³)	Main Findings	References
Furniture				wheezing	Inhalable dust	Increased frequency of respiratory symptoms and wheezing	9. *Asgedom, 2019*
	Particle-board (Eucalyptus)	W: 147 C: 73	0	45 2.7	GM: 4.66	Lung function not altered	
Small-scale cabinet maker industries				Wheeze	Respirable dust (mg/m³)	More symptoms in workers inverse correlation between lung function and exposure	10. *Holness, 1985*
	Hard and soft wood	W: 50 C: 50	70% 75%	W: 18 (36%) C: 10 (20%)	W: 0.29 C: 0.25		
Woodworking plant plant	Meranti, mainly	W: 982 (Males: 496; Females: 434)	50% 7%	Wheezing 1.6% 1.8%	GM: 1.13–3.21	Current exposure not related to respiratory symptoms nor functional results	11. *Borm, 2002*
Wood pellets plants	Spruce, pine, monoterpenes	W: 39	W: 10	Asthma medication W: 13 C: 5	GM: 1.7	More asthma medication Lower lung function	12. *Löfstedt, 2017*
Parquet manufacture				Work-relatedness wheezing	Duration of exposure: 17.4 yrs	More symptoms and lower function, related to duration of exposure	13. *Bislimovska, 2015*
	Hard wood	W: 37 C: 37	W: 0	W: 33 C: 0			
Carpentry				Work-related respiratory symptoms	NA	Work-related respiratory symptoms more frequent on exposure to wood dust than diisocyanates	14. *Campo, 2010*
	Various, diisocyanates	Apprentices (101)	46	50			

Abbreviations: C: controls; F: females; GM: geometric mean; M: males; NA: not assessed; OR: odds ratio; W: workers.

References: 1. Mandryk J, Alwis KU, Hocking AD. Am J Ind Med. 1999;35:481–90. 2. Douwes J, et al. Am J Ind Med. 2001;38:608–15. 3. Rongo LMB, et al. J Occup Environ Med. 2002;44:1153–60. 4. Rusca S, et al. Int Arch Occup Environ Health. 2008;81:415–21. 5. Schlunssen V, et al. J Occup Env Med. 2002;44:82–98. 6. Schlunssen V, et al. 2004;61:504–11. 7. Sripaiboonkij P, et al. Occup Environ Med. 2009;66:442–7. 8. Paraskevaidou K, et al. J Asthma. 2019;17:1–10. 9. Asgedom AA, et al. Int J Environ Res Public Health. 2019;16(12). 10. Holness DL, et al. JOM. 1985;27:501–6. 11. Borm PJ, et al. Occup Environ Med. 2002;59:338–44.12. Löfstedt H, et al. Ups J Med Sci. 2017;122:78–84.13. Bislimovska D, et al. Open Access Maced J Med Sci. 2015; 15;3:500–5.14. Campo P, et al. Ann Allergy Asthma Immunol. 2010;105:24–30.

Symptoms, asthma, and sensitization associated with wood dust exposure

Nasal symptoms and functional capacity

Nasal symptoms are commonly reported in woodworkers, in addition to the well-described association between exposure to certain woods and the development of nasopharyngeal carcinoma. Relatively historic work by Wilhelmsson (40) specifically addressed the issue of nasal hypersensitivity in woodworkers; noting that a high proportion, 16% of all workers, complained of such symptoms, although their presence did not relate to precipitating antibodies to mold and wood antigens.

Studies addressing these issues have described nasal symptoms in wood exposed workers that are associated with exposure to wood dust (41), duration of exposure (40), prolonged mucociliary clearance time (42), impaired olfactory function (42), eosinophil and cytokine levels in nasal lavage fluid (43) (the latter in small numbers of workers exposed to MDF), changes in lung function (44), and also various lifestyle issues such as smoking and perceived stress (45).

The relationship between nasal reactivity, as measured by histamine challenge, and the presence of symptoms remains less clear (46). The presence of work-related nasal symptoms (i.e. worse at work or better on days away from work) has also been shown to relate to levels of wood dust exposure (47, 48).

Various studies have importantly also assessed the potential causative role for coexisting microbiological exposures. One study measured not only wood dust exposure, but also a variety of other candidate exposures that may be linked to nasal symptoms. Personal exposures to fungi, bacteria, endotoxin, and (1–>3)-beta-D-glucan were measured at different woodworking sites, including logging sites, sawmills, wood-chipping sites, and joineries. The prevalence of common respiratory and nasal symptoms was significantly higher among woodworkers than controls, and certain dose-response relationships with work-related symptoms were identified.

Researchers have also focused on the important issues of altered nasal functional capacity. Notably, Schlünssen confirmed an increase in perceived nasal obstruction after exposure to wood dust using a self-rated visual analogue scale in a group of woodworkers (47). Regression analysis showed positive correlations between concentration of dust and change in mucosal swelling measured by acoustic rhinometry. Rhinomanometry has also been used to assess nasal function in MDF exposed workers (49), showing that nasal obstruction is more common in exposed workers, although not all studies identify differences in rhinomanometry between those with and without wood-related rhinitis (50).

General respiratory symptoms

Respiratory complaints are also commonly reported in woodworkers. Epidemiological and workplace-based studies may document, but not make definitive diagnoses of, for example, OA. A recent comprehensive review (35) of woodworkers identified that cough and chest tightness were the most frequently reported although a wide range of prevalence was seen between studies. Chronic bronchitis was also identified as variably prevalent in these workers (51). Wiggans et al. also considered a variety of studies that documented work-related symptoms specifically, more suggestive of occupational sensitization or OA (35).

The most commonly reported symptoms were wheeze and cough, although inconsistently defined between studies.

While OA might be regarded as the most important diagnosis to consider in woodworkers, there is an emerging, and also fairly long-standing, literature highlighting the risks of HP (see Chapter 24). Of course, multiple candidate causes are identified, and include *C. Corticale* incriminated in maple bark disease and wood-trimmers' disease, birch dust contaminated with *Pantoea agglomerans* and *Microbacterium barkerii* (52) and *Rhizopus microspores* (53) exposure in sawmill workers. HP is also described in precombustion biomass fuel process workers, who have the potential for wood and other bioaerosol exposures (54). Wood dust exposure might also cause interstitial lung disease apart from HP. In the United Kingdom, Hubbard and colleagues obtained lifetime occupational histories from 218 patients with cryptogenic fibrosing alveolitis and 569 matched controls, and found ORs of 1.7 (1.1–2.9) for wood dust and metal exposure (55). Similar results were obtained in a meta-analysis that included five studies that showed a pooled OR of 1.97 for wood dust (56).

Additional work has attempted to construct dose-response relationships between levels of wood dust exposure to dust and self-reported symptoms, with at first sight conflicting findings. While certain studies identify such relationships, for example with cough and bronchitis (51), in others the relationship is less clear. Such differences may be explained by methodological approaches, differing populations, and control methods used to reduce wood dust exposures.

Further studies have identified high levels of work-related cough and phlegm in hardwood workers (57) in comparison to nonexposed workers, and that symptom levels related to the duration of wood dust exposure. Different exposure scenarios have also been explored, with wood pellet workers (58) identified to complain of an excess of cough and nasal symptoms, and also an increased requirement for asthma medication use. Also, cellulose exposure itself as a cause of asthma, in the absence of sensitization to IgE to pine wood or xylanase (59) has been linked to asthma. Particleboard workers (60), who also had potential exposure to formaldehyde and endotoxin, also display excess of many respiratory and nasal symptoms, attributed primarily to eucalyptus, the raw material used in the board construction.

Sensitization to specific allergens

A relatively small number of workplace-based studies have specifically addressed the sensitization of workers to wood-based allergens, and when this has been done varying techniques for assessment and definitions of sensitization were used. Other occupational hazards may also constitute a risk of sensitization

in these workplaces, including acrylates, varnishes, epoxy resins, and monoterpenes, although aspects of these agents are not considered further here (see Chapter 18).

A comprehensive review has summarized sensitization to airborne wood allergens in woodworkers (31). Wilhelmsson identified that wood furniture workers had a 3% rate of sensitization to molds, and 2% to wood (40). Most workers so sensitized also had positive SPTs to other common allergens although the relationship with symptoms was less clear. Carosso furthered this work by assessing IgE in workers to extracts of woods from individual work environments (61). Positive skin-prick reactions were identified to a variety of woods including walnut, oak, mansonia, chestnut, framire and abies, with obeche, douglas, and white poplar being the most common. Positive reactions were seen most commonly in those workers with self-reported asthma.

Subsequently, Skorska identified high levels of sensitization, as judged by an intradermal method, to fungal species in workers using wood composites (62) to manufacture furniture. It was concluded that early allergic reactions to microorganisms associated with wood dust were common among workers in the furniture industry and that these responses may have clinical relevance.

Skovsted et al. reported their findings from a Danish study of furniture workers that identified no significant differences in the rates of positive IgE pine between differences in atopy (63). In the same year, Ricciardi interestingly reported the absence of iroko-specific IgE in a group of asthmatic patients with suspected OA who had all sustained a fall in PEF on SIC to iroko extract (64). Subsequent study of carpentry apprentices (also diisocyanate exposed) identified not only high levels of reported respiratory and nasal symptoms, but also that 9% of the population had positive SPTs (65).

Schlünssen has investigated the relationship between wood dust exposure levels, respiratory symptoms, and specific sensitization again in furniture workers (66). In a large number of Danish furniture factories and two reference factories, the point prevalence of pine and beech sensitization among current woodworkers was 1.7% and 3.1%, respectively. Interestingly, no differences in sensitization was found between woodworkers and references, although the prevalence of wood dust sensitization was associated with the current level of wood dust exposure. The study also assessed the levels of proteinogenic IgE epitopes, as defined by sIgE binding to pine or beech wood not being reduced by the glycogenic substance horseradish peroxidase (HRP) (67). There was a suggestion that IgE testing to woods may have more clinical significance if the IgE epitopes were proteinogenic.

In addition, a relatively large number of studies have associated a wide variety of wood species exposure and the development of human allergic endpoints. These are a hybrid group of case reports and results of clinical assessments in exposed workers. These are comprehensively recently reviewed (31). More than forty individual woods have been implicated, using evidence from a variety of studies, including case reports of respiratory problems and positive SICs associated with sawdust.

More recent case reports add to this body of literature, including the role of softwood (68) again utilizing proteinogenic epitope identification. An additional case attributed OA to samba (*Triplochiton Scleroxylon*) exposure in a maker of model airplanes supported by the presence of specific sensitization and a positive SIC (69).

Specific testing for sensitization is evidently not always useful in confirming a diagnosis of OA. Two of the three cases of OA due to MDF exposure, each confirmed by positive SICs to MDF dust, were tested for specific soft and hard wood mix IgE and found to be negative (38).

Other conditions associated with wood dust exposure: chronic bronchitis and airflow obstruction

Chronic bronchitis and airflow obstruction

While it is well known that exposure to a number of wood dusts can induce asthma, it is less well recognized that such exposure also gives rise to symptoms of chronic bronchitis and airflow obstruction. This issue has been addressed in recent general population-based studies, several cross-sectional and a few longitudinal studies.

Population-based studies

Results from the European Community Respiratory Health Survey (ECRHS) showed that metal and mineral dusts but not wood dusts were among the agents associated with incident symptoms of chronic bronchitis in the 20-year prospective cohort of nearly 9000 participants (70). A recent register-based study from Denmark could not confirm an association between cumulative organic dust exposure and incident COPD (71). Exposure-response relations between cumulative organic dust exposure and incident cases according to the patient national register COPD code (using the International Classification of Diseases, ICD-10) were examined in individuals born during 1950–1977 ever employed in the farming or wood industry (n=175,409). Cumulative exposures were assigned as based on industry-specific employment history (1964–2007), combined with time-dependent farming and wood industry-specific exposure matrices. Subanalysis including only wood dust exposed workers revealed the same result. Of note, the authors were not able to properly adjust for smoking. A meta-analysis did not consider wood dust as significantly associated with COPD (72). In the US National Health Interview Survey with 40,000 adult participants, exposure in the forestry and fishing sectors was associated with a population-attributable fraction of COPD of 0.02% only (73).

Cross-sectional and longitudinal studies

Many cross-sectional studies have been carried on in workers exposed to wood dusts. Some are listed and their principal results summarized in Table 15.4. Most conclude that there is an excess of symptoms of chronic bronchitis and reduced lung function. In some studies, these are significantly associated with the degree of exposure.

Acute and chronic changes in lung function

Cross-shift changes in spirometric values were detected in several studies, most often of small amplitude, 2.5% in the study by Holness et al. (74), 5.7% to 7.1% according to Mandryk et al. (44), but reaching asthmatic range (17.8%) in one survey (75). However, based on a publication from the Danish furniture industry cohort, cross-shift decline in lung function does not seem to be associated with a long-term decline in lung function (76).

The annual decline in lung function in exposed workers was also significantly greater than the control group in a longitudinal study with a follow-up of 4–13 years among 234 Western red cedar sawmill workers (77). Workers were stratified by average exposure levels. A significant exposure-response relationship

was found between cumulative dust exposure and decline in FVC. In workers exposed to cedar dust without asthma, airflow obstruction was associated with average levels of exposure as low as 0.3 mg/m³. Glindmeyer and colleagues studied lung function decline in workers over 5 years from 10 selected plants in the United States (78). The 1164 workers were followed with symptoms, spirometry, and personal dust sampling. In this study that did not include workers exposed to Western red cedar, annual FEV_1 decline was significant only in the milling (32 mL/yr) (obstructive pattern) and the sawmill-planing plywood (59 mL/yr) (restrictive pattern) facilities and associated to residual particulate matter and not wood solids (78).

In summary, as suggested in a meta-analysis that retained 14 studies including three in woodworkers (77–79), there might be some association between exposure to organic dust such as wood dust and lung function decline but results remain inconsistent (80).

Summary

In this chapter, OA and the various effects of wood dust exposure on the upper and lower airways have been reviewed. In rare instances, specific IgE antibodies have been demonstrated and the responsible allergenic fraction identified. One would postulate that a type I allergic reaction is likely to be responsible for the clinical manifestations in these subjects. However, the causal inference of IgE toward wood dust has been questioned, since a substantial amount of IgE epitopes recognized by the immune system are sugars of no clinical significance (68). Therefore, type I allergy is probably of minor importance for OA and occupational rhinitis caused by wood dusts. Chronic bronchitis with or without airflow obstruction unrelated to smoking (Chapter 25) and HP (Chapter 24) are also found among woodworkers. As more woods are being used for various purposes such as building houses and furniture making either in industry or at home as hobbies, physicians should be cognizant of their exposure as a cause of ill health.

Research needs

The important questions to be addressed by research should include the following:

- The pathogenic mechanisms of OA due to most wood species and specific responsible agents have yet to be clearly identified.
- Better exposure characterization for workers with mixed exposures where wood is a predominant and more minor exposure. What is the permissible exposure limit for various wood dusts?
- Optimization of diagnostic approaches including the utility of noninvasive markers of airway inflammation, induced sputum examination, exhaled nitric oxide (FeNO), exhaled breath condensate, and other exhaled breath fingerprinting.
- Efficient interventions at work to reduce wood dust exposure.
- Evidence-based approaches to cost-efficient health surveillance at work for wood dust exposed workers.

Future research, on individual workers and in workplaces and epidemiological studies, should consider all these areas, and how to develop better estimates of clinically relevant sensitization.

TABLE 15.4 Exposure to Wood Dust, Chronic Bronchitis, and/or COPD

Type of Industry	Types of Wood	Number of Subjects	Smokers (%)	Chronic Bronchitis and/or COPD (%)	Dust Level (mg/m^3)	Main Findings	References
Cross-sectional studies							
Sawmills	Various	W: 103 C: 58	67–76	CB symptoms W: 21–24 C: 9.6	Mean dust concentration: (highest): 10.4	Symptoms of CB similar in the high- and low-exposure groups but higher than in C	*1. Halpin, 1994*
Sawmill	Spruce Pine	W: 94 C: 165	43.6 27.9	Usual phlegm 26.6 13.3 Lower values of FEV1 and FEV_1/FVC	Respirable dust: 1.35	More airway obstruction in exposed workers	*2. Hessel, 1995*
Mills	Various	W: 72 C: 262	47.2 39.7	Chronic phlegm W: 16.7 C: 10 Airway obstruction higher in W	Respirable dust: 0.2–11.2	Negative effect of exposure on symptoms and airway caliber in exposed workers	*3. Liou, 1996*
Joinery/ sawmill/ chipping	Various	W: 168 C: 30	33.0 30.0	Lower FEV_1 CB symptoms W: 30–31 C: 12	Inhalable dust, GM: 0.6–11.5	More important symptoms and airway obstruction in exposed woodworkers	*4. Mandryk, 1999*
Sawmill				"Bronchial syndrome"		Elevated fungi exceeding suggested limits	*5. Rusca, 2008*
	Spruce Fir	W: 111	31%	56	Mean: 1.7 (min: 0.2; max: 8.5)	Elevated fungi related to "bronchial syndrome" (cough and phlegm) Junior workers more affected by irritation Lung function not affected by bioaerosol nor dust levels	
Sawmill	Western red cedar	W: 652	33.0	Phlegm 17	Mean: 0.46	More symptoms and lower functional values in higher exposure groups	*6. Vedal, 1986*
Woodworkers	Maple Pine	W: 1157	29.2	Airflow obstruction	Average: 0.2–4.5	Airflow obstruction associated with dust exposure	*7. Whitehead, 1981*
Woodworking plant	Meranti, mainly	W: 982 (Males: 496; Females: 434)	50% 7%	Bronchitis 3.9 4.4	GM: 1.13–3.21	Negative association between yrs of employment and airway caliber in men but not in women	*8. Borm, 2002*
Manufacture oriented strand board	Various, formaldehyde	W: 99 C: 165	W: 51.5 C: 27.9	Reduced $FEV_1/$ FVC ratio More symptoms	GM: 0.27	Symptoms of CB and more airway obstruction	*9. Herbert, 1994*
Furniture	Various, mainly pine	Workers M: 1665 F: 368 Controls M: 262 F: 212	> 20 cig/d 309 (19%) 57 (16%) 77 (31%) 40 (19%)	CB symptoms M: 138 (8.8%) F: 16 (4.6%) M: 16 (8.9%) F: 10 (5.6%)	Inhalable dust GM: 0.95	Chronic bronchitis associated with smoking but not by exposure to wood dust	*10. Schlunssen, 2002*

(Continued)

TABLE 15.4 Exposure to Wood Dust, Chronic Bronchitis, and/or COPD (*Continued*)

Type of Industry	Types of Wood	Number of Subjects	Smokers (%)	Chronic Bronchitis and/or COPD (%)	Dust Level (mg/m³)	Main Findings	References
Furniture	Pine Board fiber	Nonsmokers W: 145 C: 152		COPD FEV_1: 2.65 L FEV_1: 3.2 L CB symptoms W: 24.1 C: 10.5	Mean total dust: 3.82	Nonsmoking workers exposed to pine and and board dust have more symptoms and greater risk of airflow obstruction	*11. Shamssain, 1992*
Furniture	Particleboard (eucalyptus)	W: 147 C: 73	0	CB symptoms 31 5.5	Inhalable dust GM: 4.66	Increased frequency of respiratory symptoms and wheezing Lung function not altered	*12. Asgedom, 2019*
Furniture	Various	W: 90 C: 53	NA	COPD	Duration of exposure	Lower FEV_1 in exposed workers, related to duration of exposure	*13. Carosso, 1987*
Furniture	Various	W: 328 C: 328	W: 57 C: 64	COPD	Average dust concentration: 2.04	Lower FEV_1 in exposed workers. Higher FEV_1 values if exposure < 10 yrs and dust concentration ≥ 4	*14. Osman, 2009*
Furniture	Various, varnishes, lacquers, etc.	W: 48 C: 41	W: 58.3 C: 51.2	COPD	NA	Lower functional values in exposed workers, in smokers and nonsmokers	*15. Milanowski, 2002*
Small-scale cabinetmaker industries				Sputum	Respirable dust (mg/m³)	Inverse correlation between lung function and exposure	*16. Holness, 1985*
	Hard and soft wood	W: 50 C: 50	70% 75%	W: 30 (60%) C: 20 (40%)	W: 0.29 C: 0.25		
Longitudinal							
Furniture (6-yr follow-up)	Various	W: 1112 C: 235	W: 30 C: 37	CB symptoms + airflow obstruction (= COPD)	Inhalable dust: 3.3–3.8 × yr	Female but not male woodworkers have a dose-dependent association of exposure with onset COPD + accelerated decline in lung function	*17. Bolund, 2018*

Abbreviations: C, controls; CB, chronic bronchitis; COPD, chronic obstruction pulmonary disease; F, females; M, males; NA, not assessed; W, workers.

References: *1. Halpin DMG, et al. 1994;51:166–172. 2. Hessel PA, et al. Chest. 1995;108:642–6. 3. Liou SH, et al. Am J Ind Med. 1996;30:293–9. 4. Mandryk J, et al. Am J Ind Med. 1999;35:481–90. 5. Rusca S, et al. Int Arch Occup Environ Health. 2008;81:415–21. 6. Vedal S, et al. Arch Environ Health. 1986;41:179–83. 7. Whitehead LW, et al. Am Ind Hyg Ass J. 1981;42:178–86. 8. Borm PJ, et al. Occup Environ Med. 2002;59:338–44. 9. Herbert FA, et al. Arch Environ Health. 1994;49:465–70. 10. Schlunssen V, et al. J Occup Env Med. 2002;44:82–98. 11. Shamssain MH. Thorax. 1992;47:84–7. 12. Asgedom AA, et al. Int J Environ Res Public Health. 2019;16(12). 13. Carosso A, et al. Br J Ind Med. 1987;44:53–6. 14. Osman E, Pala K. Int J Occup Med Environ Health. 2009;22:43–50. 15. Milanowski J, et al. Ann Agric Environ Med. 2002;9:99–103. 16. Holness DL, et al. JOM. 1985;27:501–6. 17. Bolund ACS, et al. Ann Work Expo Health. 2018;62:1064–76.*

The risks of developing symptoms, and clinically relevant sensitization, can then be better predicted, and thus prevented, by considering risk factors that include personal characteristics, wood dust exposure profiles, and other physiological and immunological measures.

References

1. Gardner JA. *Chemistry and Utilization of Western Red Cedar.* Dept of Forestry Publication No. 1023, Ottawa Department of Forestry; 1963.

2. Barton GM, MacDonald BF. *The Chemistry of Utilization of Western Red Cedar.* Dept of Fisheries & Forestry Publication No. 1023, Ottawa Department of Forestry; 1971.

3. Belleau B, Burba J. Occupancy of adrenergic receptors and inhibition of catechol o-methyl transferase by toropolones. J Med Chem. 1963;6:755–9.

4. Shida T, Mimaki K, Sasaki N, et al. Western red cedar asthma: occurrance in Oume City, Tokyo and results of inhalation test using "Nezucone" aromatic substance of Western red cedar. Areugi - Jap J Allergology. 1971;20:915–21.

5. Chan-Yeung M, MacLean L, Paggiaro PL. Follow-up study of 232 patients with occupational asthma caused by Western red cedar (Thyja plicata). J Allergy Clin Immunol. 1987;79:792–6.

6. Chan-Yeung M, Lam S. Occupational asthma. Am Rev Respir Dis. 1986;133:686–703.

7. Vandenplas O, Malo JL. Inhalation challenges with agents causing occupational asthma. Eur Respir J. 1997;10:2612–29.

8. Chan-Yeung M, Barton GM, McLean L, et al. Bronchial reactions to Western red cedar. CMAJ. 1971;105:56–61.

9. Cockcroft DW, Cotton DJ, Mink JT. Nonspecific bronchial hyperreactivity after exposure to Western red cedar. Am Rev Respir Dis. 1979;119:505–10.

10. Paggiaro PL, Chan-Yeung M. Pattern of specific airway response in asthma due to Western red cedar (Thuja plicata): relationship with length of exposure and lung function measurements. Clin Allergy. 1987;17:333–9.

11. Côté J, Kennedy S, Chan-Yeung M. Sensitivity and specificity of PC 20 and peak expiratory flow rate in cedar asthma. J Allergy Clin Immunol. 1990;85:592–8.

12. Chan-Yeung M, Lam S, Koerner S. Clinical features and natural history of occupational asthma due to western red cedar (thuja plicata). Am J Med. 1982;72:411–5.

13. Cartier A, L'Archevêque J, Malo JL. Exposure to a sensitizing occupational agent can cause a long-lasting increase in bronchial responsiveness to histamine in the absence of significant changes in airway caliber. J Allergy Clin Immunol. 1986;78:1185–9.

14. Yang CX, Singh A, Kim YW, et al. Diagnosis of Western red cedar asthma using a blood-based gene expression biomarker panel. Am J Respir Crit Care Med. 2017;196:1615–7.

15. Chan-Yeung M, Leriche J, Maclean L, et al. Comparison of cellular and protein changes in bronchial lavage fluid of symptomatic and asymptomatic patients with red cedar asthma on follow-up examination. Clin Allergy. 1988;18:359–65.

16. Carlsten C, Dybuncio A, Pui MM, et al. Respiratory impairment and systemic inflammation in cedar asthmatics removed from exposure. PLOS ONE. 2013;e57166.

17. Côté J, Kennedy S, Chan-Yeung M. Outcome of patients with cedar asthma with continuous exposure. Am Rev Respir Dis. 1990;141:373–6.

18. Marabini A, Ward H, Kwan S, et al. Clinical and socioeconomical features of subjects with red cedar asthma—a follow up study. Chest. 1993;104:821–4.

19. Dimich-Ward H, Taliadouros V, Teschke K, et al. Quality of life and employment status of workers with Western red cedar asthma. J Occup Environ Med. 2007;49(9):1040–5.

20. He JQ, Chan-Yeung M, Carlsten C. Airway hyperresponsiveness and quality of life in Western red cedar asthmatics removed from exposure. PLOS ONE. 2012;7(12):e50774.

21. Lam S, LeRiche J, Phillips D, et al. Cellular and protein changes in bronchial lavage fluid after late asthmatic reaction in patients with red cedar asthma. J Allergy Clin Immunol. 1987;80:44–50.

22. Tse KS, Chan H, Chan-Yeung M. Specific IgE antibodies in workers with occupational asthma due to western red cedar. Clin Allergy. 1982;12:249–58.

23. Frew A, Chan H, Dryden P, et al. Immunologic studies of the mechanisms of occupational asthma caused by Western red cedar. J Allergy Clin Immunol. 1993;92:466–78.

24. Frew AJ, Chan H, Lam S, et al. Bronchial inflammation in occupational asthma due to Western red cedar. Am J Respir Crit Care Med. 1995;151:340–4.

25. Frew A, Chang JH, Chan H, et al. T-lymphocyte responses to plicatic acid-human serum albumin conjugate in occupational asthma caused by western red cedar. J Allergy Clin Immunol. 1998;101:841–7.

26. Horne C, Quintana PJE, Keown PA, et al. Distribution of HLA class II DQB1 alleles in patients with occupational asthma due to Western red cedar. Eur Respir J. 2000;15:911–4.

27. Brooks SM, Edwards JJ, Apol A, et al. An epidemiologic study of workers exposed to Western red cedar and other wood dust. Chest. 1981;80(Suppl):30–2.

28. Vedal S, Chan-Yeung M, Enarson D, et al. Symptoms and pulmonary function in Western red cedar workers related to duration of employment and dust exposure. Arch Environ Health. 1986;41:179–83.

29. Chan-Yeung M, Desjardins A. Bronchial hyperresponsiveness and level of exposure in occupational asthma due to Western red cedar (*Thuja plicata*): serial observations before and after development of symptoms. Am Rev Respir Dis. 1992;146:1606–9.

30. Balboni A, Baricordi OR, Fabbri LM, et al. Association between toluene diisocyanate-induced asthma and DQB1 markers: a possible role for aspartic acid at position 57. Eur Respir J. 1996;9:207–10.

31. Schlünssen V, Sigsgaard T, Raulf-Heimsoth M, et al. Workplace exposure to wood dust and the prevalence of wood-specific sensitization. Allergol Select. 2018;2:101–10.

32. Jacobsen G, Schaumburg I, Sigsgaard T, et al. Non-malignant respiratory diseases and occupational exposure to wood dust. Part I. Fresh wood and mixed wood industry. Ann Agric Environ Med 2010;17:15–28.

33. Jacobsen G, Schaumburg I, Sigsgaard T, et al. Non-malignant respiratory diseases and occupational exposure to wood dust. Part II. Dry wood industry. Ann Agric Environ Med. 2010;17:29–44.

34. Pérez-Ríos M, Ruano-Ravina A, Etminan M, et al. A meta-analysis on wood dust exposure and risk of asthma. Allergy. 2010;65:467–73.

35. Wiggans RE, Evans G, Fishwick D, et al. Asthma in furniture and wood processing workers: a systematic review. Occup Med (Lond). 2016;66:193–201.

36. Heikkilä P, Martikainen R, Kurppa K, et al. Asthma incidence in wood-processing industries in Finland in a register-based population study. Scand J Work Environ Health. 2008;34:66–72.

37. Tagiyeva N, Teo E, Fielding S, et al. Occupational exposure to asthmagens and adult onset wheeze and lung function in people who did not have childhood wheeze: a 50-year cohort study. Environ Int. 2016;94:60–8.

38. Burton C, Bradshaw L, Agius R, et al. Medium-density fibreboard and occupational asthma. A case series. Occup Med. 2011;61:357–63.

39. Fransman W, McLean D, Douwes J, et al. Respiratory symptoms and occupational exposures in New Zealand plywood mill workers. Ann Occup Hyg. 2003;47:287–95.

40. Wilhelmsson B, Jernudd Y, Ripe E, et al. Nasal hypersensitivity in wood furniture workers. An allergological and immunological investigation with special reference to mould and wood. Allergy. 1984;39:586–95.

41. Rongo LMB, Beselink A, Fouwes J, et al. Respiratory symptoms and dust exposure among male workers in small-scale wood industries in Tanzania. J Occup Environ Med. 2002;44:1153–60.

42. Shamssain MH. Pulmonary function and symptoms in workers exposed to wood dust. Thorax. 1992;47:84–7.

43. Priha E, Pennanen S, Rantio T, et al. Exposure to and acute effects of medium-density fiber board dust. J Occup Environ Hyg. 2004;1:738–44.

44. Mandryk J, Alwis KU, Hocking AD. Work-related symptoms and dose-response relationships for personal exposures and pulmonary function among woodworkers. Am J Ind Med. 1999;35:481–90.

45. Pisaniello DL, Tkaczuk MN, Owen N. Occupational wood dust exposures, lifestyle variables, and respiratory symptoms. J Occup Med. 1992;34:788–92.

46. Ahman M, Holmström M. Nasal histamine reactivity in woodwork teachers. Rhinology. 2000;38:114–9.

47. Schlünssen V, Schaumburg I, Andersen NT, et al. Nasal patency is related to dust exposure in woodworkers. Occup Environ Med. 2002;59:23–9.

48. Schlünssen V, Schaumburg I, Taudorf E, et al. Respiratory symptoms and lung function among Danish woodworkers. J Occup Env Med. 2002;44:82–98.

49. Holmström M, Rosén G, Wilhelmsson B. Symptoms, airway physiology and histology of workers exposed to medium-density fiber board. Scand J Work Environ Health. 1991;17:409–13.

50. Paraskevaidou K, Porpodis K, Kontakiotis T, et al. Asthma and rhinitis in Greek furniture workers. J Asthma. 2019;17:1–10.

51. Jacobsen G, Schlünssen V, Schaumburg I, et al. Increased incidence of respiratory symptoms among female woodworkers exposed to dry wood. Eur Respir J. 2009;33:1268–76.

52. Mackiewicz B, Dutkiewicz J, Siwiec J, et al. Acute hypersensitivity pneumonitis in woodworkers caused by inhalation of birch dust contaminated with *Pantoea agglomerans* and *Microbacterium barkeri*. Ann Agric Environ Med. 2019 Dec 19;26(4):644–55.

53. Færden K, Lund MB, Mogens Aaløkken T, et al. Hypersensitivity pneumonitis in a cluster of sawmill workers: a 10-year follow-up of exposure, symptoms, and lung function. Int J Occup Environ Health. 2014;20:167–73.

54. Rohr AC, Campleman SL, Long CM, et al. Potential occupational exposures and health risks associated with biomass-based power generation. Int J Environ Res Public Health. 2015;12:8542–605.

55. Hubbard R, Lewis S, Richards K, et al. Occupational exposure to metal or wood dust and aetiology of cryptogenic fibrosing alveolitis. Lancet. 1996;347:284–9.

56. Taskar VS, Coultas DB. Is idiopathic pulmonary fibrosis an environmental disease? Proc Am Thorac Soc. 2006;3:293–8.

57. Bislimovska D, Petrovska S, Minov J. Respiratory symptoms and lung function in never-smoking male workers exposed to hardwood dust. Open Access Maced J Med Sci. 2015;3:500–5.

58. Löfstedt H, Hagström K, Bryngelsson IL, et al. Respiratory symptoms and lung function in relation to wood dust and monoterpene exposure in the wood pellet industry. Ups J Med Sci. 2017;122:78–84.

59. Knight D, Lopata AL, Nieuwenhuizen N, et al. Occupational asthma associated with bleached chlorine-free cellulose dust in a sanitary pad production plant. Am J Ind Med. 2018;61:952–8.

60. Asgedom AA, Bråtveit M, Moen BE. High prevalence of respiratory symptoms among particleboard workers in Ethiopia: a cross-sectional study. Int J Environ Res Public Health. 2019;16(12):2158.

61. Carosso A, Ruffino C, Bugiani M. Respiratory diseases in wood workers. Br J Ind Med. 1987;44:53–6.

62. Skórska C, Krysińska-Traczyk E, Milanowski J, et al. Response of furniture factory workers to work-related airborne allergens. Ann Agric Environ Med. 2002;9:91–7.

63. Skovsted TA, Schlunssen V, Schaumburg I, et al. Only few workers exposed to wood dust are detected with specific IgE against pine wood. Allergy. 2003;58:772–9.

64. Ricciardi L, Fedele R, Saitta S, et al. Occupational asthma due to exposure to iroko wood dust. Ann Allergy Asthma Immunol. 2003;91:393–7.

65. Campo P, Aranda A, Rondon C, et al. Work-related sensitization and respiratory symptoms in carpentry apprentices exposed to wood dust and diisocyanates. Ann Allergy Asthma Immunol. 2010;105:24–30.

66. Schlünssen V, Kespohl S, Jacobsen G, et al. Immunoglobulin E-mediated sensitization to pine and beech dust in relation to wood dust exposure levels and respiratory symptoms in the furniture industry. Scand J Work Environ Health. 2011;37:159–67.

67. Kespohl S, Schlünssen V, Jacobsen G, et al. Impact of cross-reactive carbohydrate determinants on wood dust sensitization. Clin Exp Allergy. 2010;40:1099–106.

68. Kespohl S, Kotschy-Lang N, Tomm JM, et al. Occupational IgE-mediated softwood allergy: characterization of the causative allergen. Int Arch Allergy Immunol. 2012;157:202–8.

69. Krawczyk-Szulc P, Wiszniewska M, Pałczyński C, et al. Occupational asthma caused by samba (Triplochiton scleroxylon) wood dust in a professional maker of wooden models of airplanes: a case study. Int J Occup Med Environ Health. 2014;27:512–9.

70. Lytras T, Kogevinas M, Kromhout H, et al. Occupational exposures and incidence of chronic bronchitis and related symptoms over two decades: the European Community Respiratory Health Survey. Occup Environ Med. 2019;76:222–9.

71. Vested A, Basinas I, Burdorf A, et al. A nationwide follow-up study of occupational organic dust exposure and risk of chronic obstructive pulmonary disease (COPD). Occup Environ Med. 2019;76:105–13.

72. Li P, Wang X, Li ML, et al. Meta-analysis study on occupational wood dust exposure association with chronic obstructive pulmonary disease. Zhonghua Lao Dong Wei Sheng Zhi Ye Bing Za Zhi. 2019;37:764–7.

73. Bang KM, Syamlal G, Mazurek JM. Prevalence of chronic obstructive pulmonary disease in the U.S. working population: an analysis of data from the 1997–2004 National Health Interview Survey. Copd. 2009;6:380–7.

74. Holness DL, Sass-Kortsak AM, Pilger CW, et al. Respiratory function and exposure-effect relationships in wood dust-exposed and control workers. JOM. 1985;27:501–6.

75. Milanowski J, Góra A, Skórska C, et al. Work-related symptoms among furniture factory workers in Lublin region (eastern Poland). Ann Agric Environ Med. 2002;9:99–103.

76. Jacobsen GH, Schlünssen V, Schaumburg I, et al. Cross-shift and longitudinal changes in FEV1 among wood dust exposed workers. Occup Environ Med. 2013;70:22–8.

77. Noertjojo HK, Dimich-Ward H, Peelen S, et al. Western red cedar dust exposure and lung function: a dose-response relationship. Am J Respir Crit Care Med. 1996;154:968–73.

78. Glindmeyer HW, Rando RJ, Lefante JJ, et al. Longitudinal respiratory health study of the wood processing industry. Am J Ind Med. 2008;51:595–609.

79. Jacobsen G, Schlünssen V, Schaumburg I, et al. Longitudinal lung function decline and wood dust exposure in the furniture industry. Eur Respir J. 2008;31:334–42.

80. Bolund AC, Miller MR, Sigsgaard T, et al. The effect of organic dust exposure on long-term change in lung function: a systematic review and meta-analysis. Occup Environ Med. 2017;74:531–42.

16

METALS

Rolf Merget,[1] Vera van Kampen,[2] Denyse Gautrin,[3] Gareth I. Walters,[4] and Jean-Luc Malo[5]
[1]*Institute for Prevention and Occupational Medicine of the German Social Accident
Insurance (IPA), Institute of the Ruhr University, Bochum, Germany*
[2]*Institut für Prävention und Arbeitsmedizin, der Deutschen Gesetzlichen Unfallversicherung,
Institut der Ruhr-Universität-Bochum (IPA), Bochum, Germany*
[3]*(Formerly) Department of Medicine, Faculté de Médecine, Université de Montréal, Montréal, Québec, Canada*
[4]*NHS Regional Occupational Lung Disease Service, Birmingham Chest Clinic, Birmingham, UK*
[5]*Hôpital du Sacré-Cœur de Montréal and Université de Montréal, Montréal, Québec, Canada*

Contents

Introduction

A kind of work-related asthma (WRA) induced by inhalation exposure to metals was probably first described by Georgius Agricola, who published *De Re Metallica* in 1556 (1). The author described the possible harmful effects of metallic dust as follows: "On the other hand, some mines are so dry that they are entirely devoid of water, and this dryness cause the workmen even greater harm, for the dust, which is stirred and beaten up by digging, penetrates into the windpipe and lungs and produces difficulty in breathing and the disease the Greeks call *asthma*." Admittedly, this excerpt is more likely to pertain to mineworkers' pneumoconiosis than to what would now be called asthma. Although many forms of pulmonary toxicity have been noted after exposure to metals, metalloids, and their respective oxides, salts, and coordination complexes, the occurrence of OA induced by these substances has only been recognized as a medical entity in the early part of the twentieth century. While the numerical contribution of metal-induced asthma to the overall prevalence of OA appears to be relatively small, OA due to some metals, platinum salts in particular, poses an important health problem in precious metals refineries and catalyst production.

Differential diagnosis of metal-induced asthma

The spectrum of pulmonary toxicity due to inhalation of metallic compounds encompasses a wide range of acute and chronic obstructive syndromes, which in some instances may mimic asthma. Inhalation of fumes or dusts from many metallic salts and hydrides may cause chemical tracheobronchitis or chemical pneumonitis with a picture resembling the adult respiratory distress syndrome. Similarly, chronic exposure to cobalt, aluminum, manganese, titanium dioxide, and cadmium is associated with chronic obstructive lung diseases such as chronic bronchitis and pulmonary emphysema. Small airway involvement in these diseases may at times be confused with asthma. In the case of

CASE PRESENTATION

A 19-year-old man started his apprenticeship in a precious metals refinery. Two years later, when he was working in the silver refining department, he developed work-related sneezing and shortness of breath. A positive skin-prick test (SPT) with platinum salt was recorded by his plant physician. He was transferred to the adjacent department of palladium refining, without apparent platinum salt exposure. During the next 8 years, the symptoms continued. Because of the ongoing work-relatedness of the symptoms (possibly due to indirect platinum salt exposure), he was transferred to another building without any potential contact to metal salts and referred for evaluation 3 months later.

The patient had been treated with on-demand short-acting beta-agonists. His FEV_1 was 72% predicted. An SPT with sodium hexachloroplatinate 1 mg/mL was negative. He had an elevated total IgE of 397 kU/L, but SPT with common aeroallergens was negative. Fractional exhaled nitric oxide (FeNO) was elevated at 140 ppb. A specific inhalation challenge (SIC) with platinum salt was deferred due to his degree of airways obstruction. A diagnosis of probable platinum salt allergy was made, and asthma therapy with inhaled steroids and long-acting beta-agonists was initiated. When the patient presented for a follow-up examination 2 years later, he had improved considerably with only minor symptoms and requiring only occasional use of a rescue inhaled short-acting beta-agonist. While his spirometry was normal, he exhibited nonspecific bronchial hyperresponsiveness (NSBH) (methacholine $PD_{20}FEV_1$: 40 µg) and FeNO had fallen to 20 ppb (normal). A controlled SIC with sodium hexachloroplatinate that was considered necessary for the confirmation of occupational asthma (OA) demonstrated a positive immediate reaction with a maximal fall of FEV_1 of 39% from baseline after a cumulative challenge dose of 235 ng. A diagnosis of platinum salt-induced allergy and OA was made. His current job without any exposure to platinum salts was considered safe. He receives $500 per month of workers' compensation and was advised to continue to use his short-acting beta-agonists on demand.

CONCLUSIONS

- SPT with platinum salt may convert from positive to negative after allergen avoidance.
- The diagnosis of platinum salt allergy may require SIC testing.
- Exposure reduction (in contrast to cessation of exposure) may be an ineffective mean in controlling symptoms of OA.

occupational exposure to cobalt, alveolitis and asthma may coexist. Although the pathogenesis of metal fume fever in welders is not entirely understood, there have been reports of associated or superimposed asthma with this condition. Finally, small airway disease may occur in pneumoconiosis, for example, hard metal lung disease or pneumoconiosis with sarcoid-like granuloma formations such as chronic berylliosis. This chapter focuses on immunologic asthma, potroom asthma, and—in view of its frequency—obstructive airways disease in welders.

Occupational exposure to metals

Asthma induced by metals may be immunologically mediated OA or due to irritation. It is important to know the industrial settings where OA occurs, because this has consequences in prevention. Whereas exposure reduction may be a rational approach to the management of subjects with irritant asthma, this is rarely effective for workers with OA caused by a sensitizer. There are few workplaces where irritant-induced asthma due to metal compounds has been described in the absence of other irritants. Concurrent exposure to other irritants including sulfur oxide, ozone, chlorine, or nitrogen dioxide may constitute as much as or even a greater risk for development of WRA than exposure to specific metallic compounds. In the cobalt and zinc metallurgic industry, it is often unknown which of these is the causative substance. Prior or current cigarette smoking may obfuscate the diagnosis of asthma in some workers. In foundries, for example, mixed exposures to metals and reactive chemicals, such as methylenediphenyl diisocyanate (MDI) used in some molding resins, occur. MDI is more likely to cause OA than metal oxides.

Exposure to metals is not necessarily confined to workers involved in metal mining or metallurgical industries. For example, cobalt-induced bronchial asthma has been described in diamond polishers who use cobalt-containing polishing discs (2). Metallic compounds are also used as pigments in the paint and ceramic industry, as catalysts in the chemical industry, or as additives in the plastics industry.

Immunologic OA

It is important to be familiar with those hazardous agents known to cause OA because specific diagnostic tools can be used to confirm the diagnosis. A few metals may cause OA via an immunologic mechanism. They all belong to the transition metals of the fourth (chromium, cobalt, nickel, zinc), fifth (rhodium, palladium), and sixth (platinum, iridium) period of the elements (Table 16.1).

OA due to precious metals including gold, iridium, mercury, osmium, palladium, platinum, rhenium, rhodium, ruthenium, and silver is rare, with the exception of platinum salts, a well-known cause for OA. Platinum group metals (PGM) include

TABLE 16.1 The Periodic Table of the Elements/Transition Metals

Fourth period	SC	Ti	V	Cr	Mn	Fe	**Co**	**Ni**	Cu	**Zn**
Fifth period	Y	Zr	Nb	Mo	Tc	Ru	**Rh**	**Pd**	Ag	Cd
Sixth period	La	Hf	Ta	W	Re	Os	**Ir**	**Pt**	Au	Hg

Bold metals may induce immunologic occupational asthma. Platinum group metals (PGM) include platinum, palladium, rhodium, ruthenium, iridium and osmium.

platinum, palladium, rhodium, ruthenium, iridium, and osmium. A review on PGM has been published (3).

Traditionally, the primary route of exposure for the induction of sensitization to metals was considered via inhalation. However, a more recent publication has shown that allergy to platinum salts may be induced via skin application in a mouse model (4). According to this information it can be recommended to minimize skin contact to platinum salts in occupational settings.

Platinum

The main occupational exposure to platinum halide salts occurs in the primary and secondary refining of platinum. In the secondary refining processes, precious metals such as platinum, palladium, rhodium, and ruthenium are reclaimed from scrap metal and expended automobile exhaust catalysts. Platinum salt allergy has also been reported in catalyst production workers (5). The work processes in catalyst production are automated to a high degree in industrialized countries, thus exposure occurs mostly during operational disturbances, maintenance, and repair. The importance of chemical speciation has been shown because catalyst production workers exposed to tetraammine platinum dichloride do not develop platinum salt allergy (6).

Platinum salts induce symptoms in sensitized workers identical to those encountered in patients presenting with allergic rhinoconjunctivitis and asthma caused by common environmental aeroallergens. Symptoms at the time of SPT conversion from negative to positive were reported in 13 of 14 catalyst production workers in a prospective longitudinal study (28.6% asthma, 64.3% runny nose or sneezing, 35.7% burning or itching eyes, and 35.7% skin rash or itching). The corresponding numbers of work-related symptoms were 21.4%, 42.9%, 28.6%, and 35.7%, respectively (7). The number of symptoms was considerably higher in a group of 83 workers seen for compensation (100%, 86%, 63%, and 52%, respectively) (8). These workers had been exposed to platinum salts for longer periods despite having symptoms. Although this represents a highly selected group, the conclusion can be drawn that symptoms at the beginning of platinum salt allergy may vary somewhat, but sooner or later almost always include rhinitis and asthma. It has been demonstrated in many cross-sectional and longitudinal studies, as described below in the this section, that the prevalence or incidence of platinum salt skin sensitization correlates closely with OA.

SPT reactions in subjects sensitized to platinum salts are strongly dependent on the halide content of the platinum solution. SPT reactivity has been observed at platinum salt concentrations as low as 10^{-9} g/mL (9). There is general consensus that SPT is a useful technique for surveillance and early detection of platinum salt-sensitized workers.

A direct comparison between SPT and bronchial challenges revealed that SPT has excellent sensitivity and specificity (10). Sensitivity of SPT is difficult to assess, but it is clear that SPT may convert from positive to negative after exposure cessation (7, 11). SIC may be performed by direct inhalation of the platinum salt using a nebulizer. Due to the high specificity of SPT, SIC that present as immediate or, rarely, dual responses may be avoided if the SPT is positive. SPT and SIC with platinum salts should be performed with sodium hexachloroplatinate with a maximal concentration of 1 g/L. Although SPT may be performed with 10-fold dilutions of platinum salts in saline or phosphate-buffered saline, quadrupling doses in phosphate-buffered saline are recommended for SIC administered by a dosimeter in a cumulative dose range of about 3 pg to 60 µg (a parent solution of 1 mg/mL is diluted in 13 four-fold dilution steps to 60 pg/mL) (12).

Several radioallergosorbent test (RAST) procedures with platinum salts conjugated to different proteins or anion exchange resin have been used for the detection of platinum salt sensitivity. In all studies, a wide overlapping range between the amount of IgE binding to the solid phase was reported between SPT positive and negative subjects. One study found a high correlation between total IgE and RAST results; no difference was found for platinum salt-"specific" IgE between SPT positive subjects and nonexposed atopic controls (13).

It is estimated that only several thousand workers have significant exposure to platinum salts. Thus platinum salt allergy is not among the leading causes of WRA worldwide by number of affected workers, but it is a considerable health problem in some chemical plants with high risks for sensitization (Table 16.2). The occupational threshold limit value for soluble platinum in many countries is 2 µg/m³, although it is not known whether this threshold prevents sensitization. In a large retrospective cohort study with inclusion of more than 1000 refinery workers from five refineries and more than 1700 personal exposure measurements, a clear exposure-response (SPT positivity) relation was observed which was modified by atopy and smoking (14).

A longitudinal study in a catalyst production facility provided detailed measurements of airborne metallic and soluble platinum concentrations by area sampling during 2 consecutive years and by personal sampling during 1 year (5). Area sampling yielded soluble platinum salt air concentrations at the production lines (where cases were detected) within a range of 5 to 549 ng/m³, while personal sampling showed about 10-fold higher values within a range of 43 to 3697 ng/m³. Due to the limited number of exposure measurements and the high variability of the results the authors did not recommend to use their study for the derivation of an occupational exposure limit (Figure 16.1).

Secondary prevention by medical surveillance programs has a long tradition in precious metals refineries. It has been shown in a catalyst production that immediate removal from exposure after SPT conversion from negative to positive resulted in an excellent prognosis (7), and reversion of positive SPT to negative (Figure 16.2). In this study, a questionnaire and SPT with platinum salts have been recommended for surveillance. The importance of immediate removal from the workplace—preferably immediately after SPT conversion to positive—is also highlighted by a more recent retrospective longitudinal study of 96 German workers with sensitization to platinum salts. Although almost all subjects with platinum salt allergy had been removed from exposure, the percentage of subjects with asthma symptoms decreased only marginally after a median period of about 8 years between the two examinations from 91% to 77%. As the subjects were not removed from exposure until they complained of asthma, the authors recommend to remove workers to areas without any platinum salt exposure as early as possible, i.e. also SPT positive asymptomatic workers (15). These results were corroborated by an earlier cross-sectional study of US refinery workers who demonstrated a high prevalence of airway symptoms, abnormal spirometry, and positive cold air challenges despite the apparent lack of further exposure to platinum salts after an average of 5 years since their termination dates (16).

Several longitudinal studies addressed the question of risk factors for platinum salt allergy (Table 16.3). There is agreement that smoking is strongly associated with SPT reactivity to platinum salts. Atopy is probably a weak predictor, but results may be biased by preemployment screening in many plants which do not employ atopic subjects. NSBH was not a risk factor in the only prospective

TABLE 16.2 Prevalence and Incidence Rates of Positive Skin-Prick Tests with Platinum Salts in Epidemiological Studies of Subjects Exposed to Platinum Salts

References	Country	Exposed Subjects (n)	Prevalence of Positive SPT (%)	Workplace Airborne Soluble Platinum (microg/m³)
Cross-sectional studies				
1. Hunter, 1945	United Kingdom	16	25	0.9–1700
2. Murdoch, 1986	South Africa	306	28	nd
3. Merget, 1988	Germany	20	20	<0.08
4. Bolm-Audorff, 1992	Germany	64	19	<0.1
5. Baker, 1990	United States	107	14	>2 in 50%–75%
6. Merget, 1996	Italy	153	14	nd

References	Country	Exposed subjects (n)	Number of sensitized cases, duration of study and incidence		Workplace airborne soluble platinum concentration (microg/m³)
Longitudinal studies					
7. Venables, 1989	United Kingdom[a]	91	22 cases	Study of 4 years Incidence rate: 2.4%	nd
8. Calverly, 1995	South Africa[b]	78	22 cases	Study of 2 years Incidence/100 person-months: 1.9 %	>2 in 27%
9. Niezborala, 1996	France[a]	77	18 cases	Study of 4 years Incidence: 0.59%	nd
10. Linnett, 1999	United Kingdom	270 chemical process operators	106 cases	Study of 20 years Rate of 1.4 cases per 100 person-months during the first 5 yrs	>2 in 2.4% 0.005–3.7 (<2 in 4%)[d]
11. Merget, 2000	Germany[c]	159	36 cases; 79 cases in newly employed	Study of 5 years Incidence per 100 person-yrs: 2.1 for already employed and 5.9 for newly employed	
12. Heederik, 2016	South Africa, United Kingdom, United States[a]	1040	98 cases	Study of 11 years Incidence rate /100 person-yrs: 2.4	

[a] Retrospective cohort study, refinery, preemployment screening for atop.
[b] Prospective study, refinery, preemployment screening for atopy.
[c] Prospective study; catalyst plant, no preemployment screening for atopy.
[d] Different exposure metrics and categories.

Abbreviations: nd, no data; SPT, skin-prick test.

References: **1.** Hunter D, et al. *Br J Ind Med.* 1945;2:92–8; **2.** Murdoch RD, et al. *Br J Ind Med.* 1986 Jan;43(1):37–43; **3.** Merget R, et al. *Clin Allergy.* 1988;18:569–80; **4.** Bolm-Audorff U, et al. *Int Arch Occup Environ Health.* 1992;64(4):257–60; **5.** Baker DB, et al. *Am J Ind Med.* 1990;18(6):653–64; **6.** Merget R, et al. *Occup Env Med.* 1996;53:422–6; **7.** Venables KM, et al. *Br Med J* 1989;299:939-42; **8.** Calverley AE, et al. *Occup Environ Med.* 1995;52:661–6; **9.** Niezborala M, et al. *Occup Environ Med.* 1996;53:252–7; **10.** Linnett PJ, et al. *Occup Environ Med.* 1999;56:191–6; **11.** Merget R, et al. *J Allergy Clin Immunol.* 2000;105:364–70; **12.** Heederik D, et al. *J Allergy Clin Immunol.* 2016;137:922–9.

study that included serial testing for NSBH. However, the number of subjects with NSBH in the total cohort was low (8 positive tests in 115 [7%] highly exposed subjects at the initial visit) (5).

Other precious metals

There is only one case report of iridium-induced OA in a worker of an electrochemical factory producing titanium anodes (17). Sensitization to iridium chloride was reported in three catalyst workers and was explained by allergenic cross-reactivity between iridium and platinum salts (18).

There is only one case report of OA due to palladium salt that was related to fumes of an electrolysis bath (19) in a worker with an isolated positive SPT to tetrammine palladium dichloride (1 µg/mL) and a positive SIC to this salt.

A case of OA due to rhodium salt in an electroplater exposed to rhodium and platinum salts has been described (20). The worker showed positive SPT reactions and bronchial immediate-type reactions separately with rhodium and platinum salts. Sensitivity to rhodium salt was much higher than to platinum salt.

Chromium

Chromium exists in a number of valence states from −2 to +6. Trivalent (e.g. chromium sulfate) and hexavalent compounds (e.g. chromium trioxide, sodium dichromate) are both of commercial value, and widely used for electroplating, leather tanning, paint and ceramic pigment, and timber preservation. Despite high numbers of workers exposed to chromium compounds in these industries, few subjects with OA have been

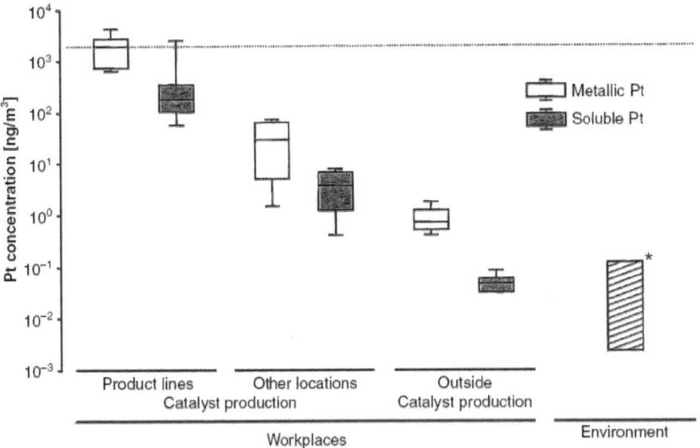

FIGURE 16.1 Metallic and soluble platinum (Pt) workplace air concentrations at the production lines, at other locations in the catalyst production, as well as outside the catalyst production. *As a reference, the concentrations of total platinum in the air at roadsides are presented (literature data). The dotted line represents the threshold limit value (TLV) for soluble platinum compounds of 2 $\mu g/m^3$. (Graph derived from data in Reference [5].)

described, and only one small-scale workforce epidemiological study has been performed (21). Case reports about OA due to welding of chromium-containing materials or welding with chromium-containing electrodes are sparse in the literature and are covered in the section on welding.

Although asthma after inhalation of chromium dust was mentioned in earlier reports, detailed information about an allergic disease and OA was not given before the 1930s (22, 23). Five subjects from different workplaces with WRA and dermatitis were described (24). A similar case series of four subjects from different professions was later reported (25).

Three toolmakers at a manufacturer of aerospace parts made from nimonic alloy, were diagnosed with OA following exposure

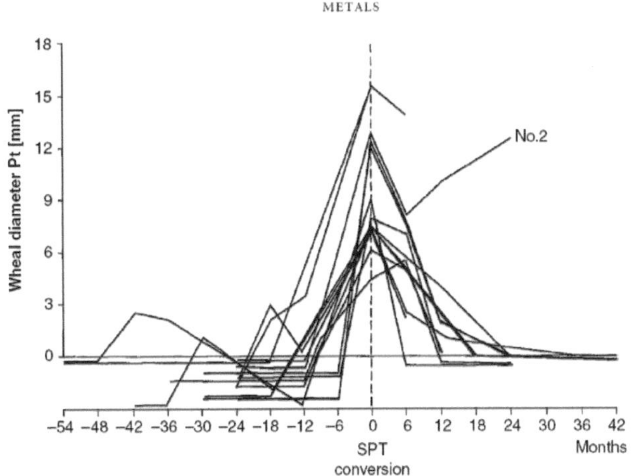

FIGURE 16.2 SPT results with platinum salts of 14 SPT converters in a prospective longitudinal survey. (Merget R, et al. *J Allergy Clin Immunol.* 2001;107:707–12. With permission.) SPT conversion was set to time "zero." Subjects were removed completely from exposure soon after conversion, with the exception of subject No. 2, who continued to be exposed to small amounts of platinum salts as a workman by contaminated material from the catalyst production.

to chromium in used metalworking fluid (26). Computer numerical controlled machining was undertaken using cobalt-containing hard metal tools. All three had negative SPTs to 1–2 mg/mL potassium dichromate, but two of them had positive SPTs to cobalt chloride. All three had positive SIC to 2 mg/mL potassium dichromate, with one dual and two immediate bronchial reactions; SIC to cobalt chloride was negative in all three. A subsequent workforce survey (n=62; 95% of workforce) identified no further cases of OA, but those with significant occupational rhinitis symptoms had significantly more chromium exposure and higher urine chromium levels than unexposed controls. One additional case of OA with positive SIC to 10 mg/mL cobalt chloride (but not chromium) was also identified.

Nickel

Occupational exposure to nickel and nickel compounds occurs in electroplating, metal grinding, and welding. Nickel ions bind to a Cu^{2+}/Ni^{2+} binding site of human serum albumin (HSA) and specific IgE antibodies to nickel-HSA have been demonstrated in several studies (27, 28). Positive SPTs, specific IgE antibodies, and lymphocyte proliferation tests with nickel have been described in subjects with hard metal asthma (29).

Due to the overlapping applications of nickel, chromium, and cobalt in the workplace, employees are often exposed to several metals, and some with OA to one or another metal (26).

Cobalt

OA due to cobalt has been reported in hard metal production workers, diamond polishers, and metalworkers. Epidemiologic studies that included immunologic testing are sparse, and most data stem from case studies and series. In one study, 18 out of 319 hard metal workers suffered from WRA. All of the nine asthmatics who underwent immunologic and challenge testing had positive SIC reactions to cobalt chloride, but only two of the nine subjects showed skin reactivity (30). Twenty-two cases of cobalt asthma were described in a cobalt plant in Finland between 1967 and 2003 (31). SPTs with cobalt chloride were negative; the diagnosis of OA was based on SIC with different cobalt compounds.

Subjects showing a positive SIC with hard metal dust generally demonstrate positive skin prick reactions and elevated specific IgE to cobalt chloride. Of eight subjects with OA due to hard metal, six showed positive skin reactions (32). In addition, 11 of 12 cases of OA had elevated cobalt-specific IgE. In a case series of 14 metalworkers with serial peak flow-confirmed OA, there were seven positive SIC tests using 1–10 mg/mL cobalt chloride, including three immediate, three dual, and one late reaction (26). Workers were exposed to cobalt in used metalworking fluid, primarily through grinding or machine setting using hard metal tools. In this study six out of eight workers with confirmed OA had positive SPTs to 10 mg/mL cobalt chloride.

Hard metal lung disease is a well-known interstitial lung disease, the hazardous agent being probably cobalt. Although the pathogenesis of hard metal lung disease is not well understood, it is distinct from OA. Workers presenting with both alveolitis and asthma have been described.

Zinc

There are reported cases of OA caused by zinc (33, 34).

Manganese

Manganese is a hard metal with multiple oxidation states, but most stable in its bivalent form. Manganese compounds are added to alloys to improve strength, used for manufacture of welding

TABLE 16.3 Host Risk Factors (Modifiers) for Sensitization to Platinum Salts as Assessed by Longitudinal Studies

		Risk Factors (OR)		
References	**Location**	**Smoking**	**Atopy**	**BHR**
1. Venables, 1989	Refinery	5.1 (1.68–15.2)	2.3 (0.9–6.0)	nd
2. Calverley, 1995	Refinery	8.0 (2.6–25.0)	nd	nd
3. Niezborala, 1996	Refinery	5.5 (1.56–19.7)	nd	nd
4. Merget, 2000	Catalyst production	3.9 (1.6–9.7)	1.1 (0.9–1.4)	1.1 (0.9–1.3)
5. Heederik, 2016	Refinery	1.7 (1.1–2.6)[a]	1.8 (1.2–2.7)[a]	nd

[a] Data for cumulative exposure.

Abbreviations: nd, no data; OR, odds ratio.

References: **1.** Venables KM, et al. *Br Med J.* 1989;299:939–42; **2.** Calverley AE, et al. *Occup Environ Med.* 1995;52:661–6; **3.** Niezborala M, et al. *Occup Environ Med.* 1996;53:252–7; **4.** Merget R, et al. *J Allergy Clin Immunol.* 2000;105:364–70; **5.** Heederik D, et al. *J Allergy Clin Immunol.* 2016;137:922–9.

electrodes, batteries, and pharmaceuticals, and in ceramics as a pigment. OA to manganese in a worker with negative skin test has been reported A single case of OA has been confirmed by SIC in a nonatopic welder with negative SPTs to 0.01%–1.0% manganese nitrate (35).

OA without known immunologic mechanism

Potroom asthma (asthma in aluminum production)

Asthma was first recognized as an occupational health hazard for workers in potrooms of Norwegian aluminum smelters in 1936 (36). Subsequently, the existence of asthma has also been reported in smelters of various countries as reviewed (37). The major components of the potroom environment include fluorides in particulate dust and gaseous forms. It was thought that an allergic reaction to fluoride could be the cause but SO_2 may also play a role (38). Whatever the cause, asthma occurring in aluminum smelter workers is now known as "potroom asthma," some aspects of the condition being related to OA (39) and others to COPD or the asthma-COPD overlap syndrome.

There is a large variation in the prevalence and incidence of OA in the aluminum industry. There is a lower prevalence of potroom asthma in North American compared to European studies (40). This could be related to different preemployment medical criteria, prevailing climatic conditions, high turnover of population at risk (healthy worker effect), or the degree of potroom environmental controls. The existence of potroom asthma in the US was demonstrated to occur at levels within regulatory guidelines (41). Workers in smelters have a greater decline in FEV_1 than controls, nonsmokers, and (more pronounced) smokers (42).

Atopic disorders at employment were reported as a significant host risk factor for OA (43). Genotyping for β2 adrenoreceptor, IgE receptor, or TNF alpha polymorphisms was not predictive of potroom asthma.

The asthmatic symptoms of potroom asthma are generally delayed, becoming more frequent and severe with repeated exposure. The prognosis of potroom asthma is variable. About 40% of workers may continue to have asthma after terminating exposure. NSBH may persist in many workers. An analogy between this type of persistent asthma and the reactive airways dysfunction syndrome (RADS) has also been suggested. Several reports suggest that early removal from exposure once symptoms are recognized may normalize both FEV_1 and NSBH (44).

Airway inflammation is a central feature of potroom asthma, and exposure to potroom emissions induces pathological alterations similar to those described in other types of asthma, including eosinophilic and neutrophilic infiltrates (45). Although allergy has been suggested as a possible cause, this association is not convincing. Immediate skin tests to aluminum and fluoride salts are uniformly negative.

FeNO may be a diagnostic adjunct in nonsmoking potroom workers as reviewed (37). Concentrations of FeNO were found to be significantly higher in exposed versus nonexposed workers, but they were also doubled in asthmatic compared to nonasthmatic workers (37).

Welding and respiratory illnesses

Welding includes several processes: gas metal, manual metal, flux cored, and gas tungsten arc. Welding produces aerosols and fumes of metals, metal oxides, and volatilized chemicals that originate from metal, soldering electrodes in stainless or mild steel, and flux. Fumes are made of particles of less than 1 micron in diameter that can reach bronchioles and alveoli. Welders are at high risk of metal fume fever, airway obstruction, OA, and occupational rhinitis.

Metal fume fever, asthma, and chronic bronchitis
Metal fume fever

This condition also known under various names has been identified in the nineteenth century (46). It is characterized by the occurrence of symptoms that include fever, metallic taste, myalgias, and a dry cough, mostly at the end of a workshift or some hours afterward, with complete recovery within 1 to 2 days. Symptoms are more pronounced after several days without exposure. Zinc oxide fumes and soldering on galvanized metal are often incriminated. Neutrophils and inflammatory cytokines are increased in blood and BAL. Slight impairment in lung function and hypoxemia with rapid recovery are rare. Metal fume fever was identified in 12% of 351 welders by El-Zein and coworkers (47) by comparison with 35% of 145 welders in an earlier study (48).

Chronic bronchitis, asthma, and occupational asthma

Welders show significant cross-shift decreases in FEV_1, this being greater for manual metal arc welding (49). Among welders who develop asthma, significant differences in frequency have been reported in those who were exposed to solid particles from stainless steel fumes as opposed to those engaged in welding on mild steel.

Surveillance scheme and registries of occupational diseases in the United States and in the United Kingdom have shown that welding is among the most frequent cause of WRA (50, 51). In a British study, NSBH in regular welders was twice that of welders with negligible exposure with the same duration of work (52). In a population-based study of more than 15,000 young adults living in Europe and other industrial countries, an excess asthma risk (more than 30%) was shown in welders when compared with professional, administrative, and clerical workers (53). Table 16.4 is a summary of major findings in longitudinal and cross-sectional studies. An excess of symptoms of chronic bronchitis was reported among more than 300 welders in the ECRHS study after a 9-year follow-up (54). Welding is also associated with airway obstruction (55), independently of smoking (56) and NSBH (52) in other studies. In the RHINE study, a subset of the ECRHS study, performed in more than 16,000 responders in Northern Europe, there was an excess of rhinitis in welders (hazard ratios [HR]:1.4, 95% confidence intervals (CI):1.3–1.6) and asthma (HR:1.4, 95% CI:1.0–2.0) (57). Occupational rhinitis in welders has been demonstrated by specific challenge (58).

El-Zein and coworkers carried out a 15-month prospective study in 203 welding apprentices (59) who were assessed at start, 8 months, and 15–18 months of apprenticeship. An average fall in FEV_1 (assessed in % pred) of 8.4% was found during the study period, 11.9% of subjects had a significant increase in NSBH, and the incidence of probable OA was 3%. The authors suggested that the observed decrease in FEV_1 could represent an acute effect that might be a predictor of chronic lung function impairment. Only 25% of subjects with increased NSBH had persistent welding-related respiratory symptoms suggestive of OA. The incidence of positive specific SPTs to metal salts increased by 12% over the training period, although remaining low, but were unrelated to welding-related respiratory symptoms (59). Apprentices with incident metal fume fever and no respiratory symptoms suggestive of OA at the 8-month follow-up had an increased risk of developing respiratory symptoms suggestive of OA (odds ratio [OR]:7.4, 95% confidence intervals [CI]:1.97–27.45) but not NSBH subsequently (60).

TABLE 16.4 Epidemiological Studies of Occupational Asthma in Welders

Authors Year Country	Studied Population	Controls	Confirmation of OA/ Adult-Onset Asthma	Risk/Prevalence/ Incidence
Longitudinal studies				
1. Wang, 1994 Sweden	137 welders in 4 vehicles assembling plants	26 assemblers nonwelders	Symptoms and NSBH	Incidence of 5% in welders exposed to inox, 7% in those exposed to mild metal per 1000 yrs of welding
2. Beckett, 1996 US	51 welders using manual arc in a shipyard	54 nonwelders	Symptoms, spirometry and NSBH	One identified case
3. El-Zein, 2003 Canada	194 welding apprentices		Symptoms and NSBH	Incidence of ~3% of probable OA
4. Storass, 2015 Seven countries in Northern Europe	2192 ever welded	13630 never welded	Symptoms of adult-onset asthma rhinitis	Incidence rate 1.8 Incidence rate 20.3 per 1000 years of welding
Cross-sectional studies				
5. Donoghue, 1994 *New Zealand*	20 electric arc welders	20 nonwelders	PEF reduction 12 hrs	No welder showed after beginning work 20% or more fall in PEF
6. Beach, 1996 UK	284 welders in a shipyard	75 persons who applied for a job at the same workplace (shipyard)	Symptoms, spirometry, and NSBH	~1% of symptoms after 5 yrs of work
7. El-Zein, 2003 Canada	351 welders		Respiratory symptoms on welding	~5.2%
8. Lillienberg, 2008 Sample of population of 10 European countries	316 men welding at work	2610 men not welding	Respiratory symptoms	Prevalence of asthma not significantly increased
9. Temel, 2010 Turkey	41 welders in a bicycle production plant	46 office workers in the same plant	Symptoms and fluctuation in PEF	9 welders (22%)

Modified and updated from: Gautrin D, Hannu T, El-Zein M. Asthme des soudeurs. In: Bessot JC, Pauli G, Vandenplas O, eds. L'Asthme professionnel. Paris: Margaux Orange; 2012:273–86.

References: **1.** Wang ZP, et al. *Am J Ind Med.* 1994;26:741–54; **2.** Beckett WS, et al. *J Occup Env Med.* 1996;38:1229–38; **3.** El-Zein M, et al. *Eur Respir J.* 2003;22:513–8; **4.** Storaas T, et al. *Eur Respir J.* 2015;46:1290–7; **5.** Donoghue AM, et al. *Occup Environ Med.* 1994; 58:553–6; **6.** Beach JR, et al. *Am J Respir Crit Care Med.* 1996;154:1394–400; **7.** El-Zein M, et al. *Occup Environ Med.* 2003;60:655–61; **8.** Lillienberg L, et al. *Ann Occup Hyg.* 2008;52:107–15; **9.** Temel O, et al. *Tuberkuloz ve toraks.* 2010;58:64–70.

Many well-documented case reports and case series of OA have been demonstrated by SICs in welders exposed to various metals: iron, aluminum, manganese, cobalt, nickel, and stainless steel in particular (61).

For a detailed list and evidence, see https://www.csst.qc.ca/en/prevention/reptox/occupational-asthma/Documents/AgentsAnglais.pdf. Contrary to platinum, IgE-mediated reactivity has not generally been demonstrated by skin testing, with the exception of chromium and nickel salts. However, 50 welders with metal-induced OA as confirmed by SIC had a significant increased risk of positive SPT results to metal salts as compared to 100 welders without suspicion of OA (62).

The mechanism of OA in welders remains unknown. Welders are at greater risk of pneumococcal infection (63). Welding on mild steel and stainless steel induces a systemic inflammatory response (increase in neutrophils and platelets) (64, 65). Symptoms are similar to those described with other causes of OA. The diagnosis is mainly based on serial PEF recording during periods at work and away from work or SICs. Protection from exposure to welding fumes (dedicated well-ventilated rooms, aspiration, and personal protection devices) is easier to apply in large industrial facilities. Welding is often carried out in small, poorly ventilated and equipped shops.

Exposure to steel-coating materials

Workers exposed to several processes unique to the steel manufacturing industry may develop OA. The coverings can contain sensitizing agents such as epoxy resins, formaldehyde, or polyisocyanates (66).

Other respiratory illnesses

Chest X-ray changes are common and reached 62% among 94 welders investigated, none of which had recognized OA due to metals (62). In welders' pneumoconiosis, small centrilobular nodules are frequently seen on high-resolution scans, representing siderosis. There are a few reports of welders who developed irritant-induced asthma in relation to welding exposure.

Summary

Halogenated platinum salts belong to the most prominent allergens that cause immunologic OA. In regards to exposure to platinum, the effectiveness of secondary prevention has been demonstrated. Cases of OA to chromium, nickel, and cobalt are found mainly in electroplating and hard metal industry, the causal mechanism being unidentified. Both cross-sectional and longitudinal studies indicate that working environments in aluminum smelters cause OA-like diseases. Surveillance systems as well as epidemiological and clinical studies have shown that exposure to welding fumes is associated with a significant risk of developing WRA and COPD.

Directions for future research

1. Delineation of host susceptibility factors and modifiers for sensitization and/or irritant responses to selected metallic salts in metal-exposed workers including welders.
2. Long-term studies comparing platinum-sensitized workers who continue to work in "low-exposure" areas after diagnosis.
3. Development of reasonable and valid exposure thresholds for platinum salts, potroom exposures, and welding constituents.

4. Assessment of the role of noninvasive methods after SIC, especially for asthma without immediate-type sensitizations (e.g. chromium, nickel, cobalt).

Acknowledgments

We greatly thank the late Leonard Bernstein who prepared the initial text of this chapter; some parts of it have been adopted in the present version.

References

1. Agricola G. De re metallica. The Mining Magazine (translated by HC Hoover and LH Hoover) (London). 1912:1556.
2. Gheysens B, Auxwerx J, Van Den Eeckhout A, Demedts M. Cobalt-induced bronchial asthma in diamond polishers. Chest. 1985;88:740–4.
3. Linde SJL, Franken A, du Plessis JL. Occupational respiratory exposure to platinum group metals: a review and recommendations. Chem Res Toxicol. 2017;30:1778–90.
4. Williams WC, Lehmann JR, Boykin E, et al. Lung function changes in mice sensitized to ammonium hexachloroplatinate. Inhal Toxicol. 2015;27:468–80.
5. Merget R, Kulzer R, Dierkes-Globisch A, et al. Exposure-effect relationship of platinum salt allergy in a catalyst production plant: conclusions from a 5-year prospective cohort study. J Allergy Clin Immunol. 2000;105:364–70.
6. Linnett PJ, Hughes EG. 20 years of medical surveillance on exposure to allergenic and non-allergenic platinum compounds: the importance of chemical speciation. Occup Environ Med. 1999;56:191–6.
7. Merget R, Caspari C, Kulzer SA, et al. Effectiveness of a medical surveillance program for the prevention of occupational asthma caused by platinum salts: a nested case-control study. J Allergy Clin Immunol. 2001;107:707–12.
8. Merget R, Schulte A, Gebler A, et al. Outcome of occupational asthma due to platinum salts after transferral to low-exposure areas. Int Arch Occup Environ Health. 1999;72:33–9.
9. Biagini RE, Bernstein IL, Gallagher JS, et al. The diversity of reaginic immune responses to platinum and palladium metallic salts. J Allergy Clin Immunol 1985;76:794–802.
10. Merget R, Schultze-Werninghaus G, Bode F, et al. Quantitative skin prick and bronchial provocation tests with platinum salt. Br J Ind Med. 1991;48:830–7.
11. Merget R, Reineke M, Rueckmann A, et al. Nonspecific and specific bronchial responsiveness in occupational asthma caused by platinum salts after allergen avoidance. Am J Respir Crit Care Med. 1994;150:1146–9.
12. Merget R, Fartasch M, Sander I, et al. Eosinophilic airway disease in a patient with a negative skin prick test, but a positive patch test with platinum salts–implications for medical surveillance. Am J Ind Med. 2015;58:1008–11.
13. Merget R, Schultze-Werninghaus G, Muthorst T, et al. Asthma due to the complex salts of platinum—a cross-sectional survey of workers in a platinum refinery. Clin Allergy. 1988;18:569–80.
14. Heederik D, Jacobs J, Samadi S, et al. Exposure-response analyses for platinum salt-exposed workers and sensitization: a retrospective cohort study among newly exposed workers using routinely collected surveillance data. J Allergy Clin Immunol. 2016;137:922–9.
15. Merget R, Pham N, Schmidtke M, et al. Medical surveillance and long-term prognosis of occupational allergy due to platinum salts. Int Arch Occup Environ Health. 2017;90:73–81.
16. Baker DB, Gann PH, Brooks SM, et al. Cross-sectional study of platinum salts sensitization among precious metals refinery workers. Am J Ind Med. 1990;18:653–64.
17. Bergman A, Svedberg U, Nilsson E. Contact urticaria with anaphylactic reactions caused by occupational exposure to iridium salt. Contact Dermatitis. 1995;32:14–7.
18. Cristaudo A, Sera F, Severino V, et al. Occupational hypersensitivity to metal salts, including platinum, in the secondary industry. Allergy. 2005;60:159–64.
19. Daenen M, Rogiers P, Van de Walle C et al. Occupational asthma caused by palladium. Eur Respir J. 1999;13:213–6.
20. Merget R, Sander I, van Kampen V et al. Occupational immediate-type asthma and rhinitis due to rhodium salts. Amer J Ind Med. 2010;53:42–6.
21. Walters GI, Burge PS, Moore VC, Robertson AS. Normal nonspecific bronchial reactivity excludes occupational asthma? J Allergy Clin Immunol. 2016;138:1238–9.

22. Smith AR. Chrome poisoning with manifestations of sensitization. JAMA. 1931;94:95–8.
23. Joules H. Asthma from sensitization to chromium. Lancet. 1932;2:182–3.
24. Olaguibel JM, Basomba A. Occupational asthma induced by chromium salts. Allergol Immunopathol. 1989;17:133–6.
25. Park HS, Yu HJ, Jung KS. Occupational asthma caused by chromium. Clin Exp Allergy. 1994;24:676–81.
26. Walters GI, Moore VC, Robertson AS, et al. An outbreak of occupational asthma due to chromium and cobalt. Occup Med (Lond). 2012;62:533–40.
27. Malo JL, Cartier A, Doepner M, et al. Occupational asthma caused by nickel sulfate. J Allergy Clin Immunol. 1982;69:55–9.
28. Shirakawa T, Kusaka Y, Morimoto K. Specific IgE antibodies to nickel in workers with known reactivity to cobalt. Clin Exper Allergy. 1992;22:213–8.
29. Kusaka Y, Nakano Y, Shirakawa T, et al. Lymphocyte transformation test with nickel in hard metal asthma: another sensitizing component of hard metal. Ind Health. 1991;29:153–60.
30. Kusaka Y, Yokoyama K, Sera Y, et al. Respiratory diseases in hard metal workers: an occupational hygiene study in a factory. Br J Ind Med. 1986;43:474–85.
31. Sauni R, Linna A, Oksa P, et al. Cobalt asthma–a case series from a cobalt plant. Occup Med (Lond). 2010;60:301–6.
32. Shirakawa T, Kusaka Y, Fujimura N, et al. Occupational asthma from cobalt sensitivity in workers exposed to hard metal dust. Chest. 1989;95:29–37.
33. Malo JL, Cartier A, Dolovich J. Occupational asthma due to zinc. Eur Respir J. 1993;6:447–50.
34. Leal A, Caselles I, Rodriguez-Bayarri MJ, Munoz X. Non-IgE-mediated asthma after zinc exposure. Arch Bronconeumol. 2017;53:346–7.
35. Wittczak T, Dudek W, Krakowiak A, et al. Occupational asthma due to manganese exposure: a case report. Int J Occup Med Environ Health. 2008;21:81–3.
36. Frostad EW. Fluorine intoxication in Norwegian aluminum plant workers. Tidsskr Nor Laegeforen. 1936;56:179–82.
37. Kongerud J, Soyseth V. Respiratory disorders in aluminum smelter workers. J Occup Environ Med. 2014 May;56(5 Suppl):S60–70.
38. Abramson MJ, Benke GP, Cui J, et al. Is potroom asthma due more to sulphur dioxide than fluoride? An inception cohort study in the Australian aluminum industry. Occup Environ Med. 2010;67:679–85.
39. Desjardins A, Bergeron JP, Ghezzo H, et al. Aluminum potroom asthma confirmed by monitoring of forced expiratory volume in one second. Am J Respir Crit Care Med. 1994;150:1714–7.
40. Søyseth V, Johnsen HL, Henneberger PK, Kongerud J. The incidence of work-related asthma-like symptoms and dust exposure in Norwegian smelters. Am J Respir Crit Care Med. 2012;185:1280–5.
41. Taiwo OA, Sircar KD, Slade MD, et al. Incidence of asthma among aluminum workers. J Occup Environ Med. 2006;48:275–82.
42. Soyseth V, Henneberger PK, Einvik G, et al. Annual decline in forced expiratory volume is steeper in aluminum potroom workers than in workers without exposure to potroom fumes. Am J Ind Med. 2016;59:322–9.
43. Sorgdrager B, deLooff AJA, deMonchy JGR, et al. Occurrence of occupational asthma in aluminum potroom workers in relation to preventive measures. Int Arch Occup Environ Health. 1998;71:53–9.
44. Sorgdrager B, de Looff AJ, Pal TM, et al. Factors affecting FEV1 in workers with potroom asthma after their removal from exposure. Int Arch Occup Environ Health. 2001;74:55–8.
45. Sjåheim T, Halstensen TS, Lund MB, et al. Airway inflammation in aluminum potroom asthma. Occup Environ Med. 2004;61:779–85.
46. Gordon T, Fine JM. Metal fume fever. Occup Med. 1993;8:505–17.
47. El-Zein M, Malo JL, Infante-Rivard C, Gautrin D. Prevalence and association of welding related systemic and respiratory symptoms in welders. Occup Environ Med. 2003;60:655–61.
48. Kilburn KH, Warshaw RH, Boylen CT, Thornton JC. Respiratory symptoms and functional impairment from acute (cross-shift) exposure to welding gases and fumes. Am J Med Sc. 1989;298:314–9.
49. Sobaszek A, Boulenguez C, Frimat P, et al. Acute respiratory effects of exposure to stainless steel and mild steel welding fumes. J Occup Environ Med. 2000;42:923–31.
50. Banga A, Reilly MJ, Rosenman KD. A study of characteristics of Michigan workers with work-related asthma exposed to welding. J Occup Environ Med. 2011;53:415–9.
51. Zhou AY, Seed M, Carder M, et al. Sentinel approach to detect emerging causes of work-related respiratory diseases. Occup Med (Lond). 2020;70:52–9.
52. Beach JR, Dennis JH, Avery AJ, et al. An epidemiologic investigation of asthma in welders. Am J Respir Crit Care Med. 1996;154:1394–400.
53. Kogevinas M, Anto JM, Sunyer J, et al. Group and the European Community Respiratory Health Survey Study. Occupational asthma in Europe and other industrialised areas: a population-based study. Lancet. 1999;353:1750–4.
54 Lillienberg L, Zock JP, Kromhout H, et al. A population-based study on welding exposures at work and respiratory symptoms. Ann Occup Hyg. 2008;52:107–15.
55. Cotes JE, Feinmann E, Male VJ, et al. Respiratory symptoms and impairment in shipyard welders and caulker/burners. Br J Ind Med. 1989;46:292–301.
56. Bradshaw LM, Fishwick D, Slater T, Pearce N. Chronic bronchitis, work related respiratory symptoms, and pulmonary function in welders in New Zealand. Occup Environ Med. 1998;55:150–4.
57. Storaas T, Zock JP, Morano AE, et al. Incidence of rhinitis and asthma related to welding in Northern Europe. Eur Respir J. 2015;46:1290–7.
58. Castano R, Suarthana E. Occupational rhinitis due to steel welding fumes. Am J Ind Med. 2014;57:1299–302.
59. El-Zein M, Malo JL, Infante-Rivard C, Gautrin D. Incidence of probable occupational asthma and of changes in airway calibre and responsiveness in apprentice welders. Eur Respir J. 2003;22:513–8.
60. El-Zein M, Infante-Rivard C, Malo JL, Gautrin D. Is metal fume fever a determinant of welding related respiratory symptoms and/or increased bronchial responsiveness? A longitudinal study. Occup Environ Med. 2005;62:688–94.
61. Hannu T, Piipari R, Tuppurainen M, et al. Occupational asthma caused by stainless steel welding fumes: a clinical study. Eur Respir J. 2007;29:85–90.
62. Wittczak T, Dudek W, Walusiak-Skorupa J, et al. Metal-induced asthma and chest X-ray changes in welders. Int J Occup Med Environ Health. 2012;25:242–50.
63. Toren K, Blanc PD, Naido RN et al. Occupational exposure to dust and to fumes, work as a welder and invasive pneumococcal disease risk. Occup Environ Med. 2020;77:57–63.
64. Kauppi P, Jarvela M, Tuomi T, et al. Systemic inflammatory responses following welding inhalation challenge test. Toxicol Rep. 2015;2:357–64.
65. Riccelli MG, Goldoni M, Poli D, et al. Welding fumes, a risk factor for lung diseases. Int J Environ Res Public Health. 2020;17:2552.
66. Venables KM, Dally MB, Burge PS, et al. Occupational asthma in a steel coating plant. Br J Ind Med. 1985;42:517–24.

17

CLEANING AGENTS

**Jolanta M. Walusiak-Skorupa,[1] Jonathan A. Bernstein,[2] Frédéric de Blay,[3]
Orianne Dumas,[4] Carole Ederle,[5] Ilenia Folletti,[6] and Susan M. Tarlo[7]**

[1]*Department of Occupational Diseases and Environmental Health, Nofer Institute of Occupational Medicine, Lodz, Poland*
[2]*Department of Internal Medicine, Division of Immunology/Allergy Section, Cincinnati, Ohio, USA*
[3]*Service de pneumologie, Les Hôpitaux universitaires de Strasbourg, University of Strasbourg, Strasbourg, France*
[4]*Université Paris-Saclay, UVSQ, Univ. Paris-Sud, Inserm, Equipe d'Epidémiologie Respiratoire Intégrative, CESP, Villejuif, France*
[5]*Service de Pneumologie, Les Hôpitaux universitaires de Strasbourg, University of Strasbourg, Strasbourg, France*
[6]*Department of Medicine and Surgery, Section of Occupational Medicine, University of Perugia, Terni Hospital, Terni, Italy*
[7]*University Health Network and St Michael's Hospital, Toronto, Department of
Medicine, University of Toronto, Toronto, Ontario, Canada*

Contents

CASE HISTORY

A 49-year-old ward attendant worked at a surgery unit for 5 years. After 2 years she developed respiratory symptoms i.e. first cough, then wheezing and dyspnea. The patient had spent the last 6 months on sick-leave for this and was administered long-lasting betamimetics and inhaled glucocorticosteroids.

History-derived data indicated a strong positive relationship of respiratory symptom occurrence and work exposure. Symptoms appeared 2 hours after starting work and exacerbated by the end of her shift. Symptoms significantly improved on weekends and holidays, however did not totally disappear. Personal and family history of atopy was negative. Skin-prick tests (SPTs) to common allergens were negative. Total IgE level was 32.74 ku/L and no specific IgE (sIgE) to mixed disinfectants (pax6: chloramine, formaldehyde, glutaraldehyde, phthalane anhydride) in blood serum were detected. The baseline values of resting spirometry were normal: FEV_1 87% of predictive values (PV), forced vital capacity (FVC) 84% PV, FEV_1/FVC ratio 82.76. Baseline methacholine challenge test revealed the presence of mild nonspecific BHR (PC20= 8 mg/mL). Then a single-blind, placebo-controlled (0.9% NaCl) work-like specific inhalation challenge (SIC) test with cleaning agents (benzalconium chloride) was performed. The patient applied cleaning liquids to a glass surface for 120 minutes in a chamber (6 m³). During 24 hours starting pre- and postexposure to specific inhalant agents, hourly spirometry and PEF measurements were noted. One hour after the SIC the patient reported cough; 3 hours later she developed dyspnea. She had a late-phase asthmatic reaction with 17% fall in FEV_1 at the 4th hour post-challenge and 19% at 5 hours post challenge. BHR significantly increased to PC20 = 0.9 mg/mL. Due to respiratory symptoms and an increase of BHR after exposure to the cleaning agent, with a late-phase asthmatic reaction, the diagnosis of occupational asthma was established.

Introduction

The role of cleaning and sterilizing agents in work-related asthma (WRA) has been increasingly recognized since early case reports of occupational asthma (OA) over 30 years ago from formaldehyde (in two hemodialysis nurses) (1–3), glutaraldehyde in endoscopy units (4), a sulfonate in a laboratory technician (5), glutaraldehyde (4), and chlorhexidine (6). While OA from recognized chemical sensitizers such as diisocyanates, has fallen over time as reported from several centers (7, 8), cleaning agents have become a bigger causative factor in reported series of recognized WRA (8, 9). The exposures leading to asthma-like symptoms have been reported from among domestic cleaners (10), and among healthcare workers both among those with primary use of cleaning/disinfecting agents, and among those with likely bystander exposure (10). In many cases the exposures have included multiple chemical agents in various cleaning products. Apart from select carefully documented case reports, the causative chemical(s) have often been difficult to determine and in addition, in epidemiologic studies it is often unclear as to whether symptoms have been due to sensitization or an airway irritant response with production of OA, or due to work-exacerbated asthma (WEA) (11), or in some cases to another disorder such as a laryngeal syndrome or chronic obstructive pulmonary disease (COPD) (12), mimicking asthma from questionnaire responses.

Although cleaning agents have been reported to cause sensitizer-induced OA many cleaning products are potential respiratory irritants, especially when sprayed in poorly ventilated areas. In addition, the inappropriate mixing of cleaning products such as bleach and ammonia can result in more irritant chemicals such as chlorones. Even without such mixing of cleaning products, a detailed case investigation showed that the addition of urine to a bleach product (mimicking the common real-life usage in healthcare facilities) induced asthma changes on challenge testing when the individual exposures caused no response (13). Similarly concurrent use of peracetic acid and hydrogen peroxide to disinfect endoscopes caused asthma with a late positive response on specific challenge, which was interpreted as an immunologic response (14).

While exposure to these chemicals in the occupational setting is important, additional concern relates to the fact that many of these agents are used in the home and in public buildings including schools, and therefore exposure occurs not only in workers but also in children, pregnant women, and the elderly. Greater exposure to cleaning products in homes has also been linked to increased rates of early childhood asthma (15), and exposure to presumed chlorones from swimming pools has also been linked to asthma both for lifeguards and possibly for children (16, 17). Due to these ubiquitous exposures, there is a strong need to clearly understand the response to these various cleaning agents and mechanisms for the responses.

Epidemiology

Epidemiological studies reporting associations between occupational exposure to specific cleaning or disinfecting agents and asthma outcomes are summarized in Table 17.1. Although some studies have reported associations with agents for which a sensitizing mechanism has been identified, most cleaning agents reported to be associated with asthma are airway irritants. Bleach (chlorine) and ammonia were among the first specific agents identified (18, 19), and bleach remains the most frequently reported

(20–22). An increasing number of studies have reported a role of high-level disinfectants, used more commonly in healthcare settings (20, 21, 23). Among them, aldehydes (formaldehyde, glutaraldehyde) have long been known as causative agents for OA (24). However, high-level disinfectants proposed as alternative to aldehydes, such as hydrogen peroxide or hydrogen peroxide/peracetic acid mixtures, also appear associated with asthma outcomes (20, 23). Although it is difficult to disentangle chronic from high peak exposure effects for these irritant agents, in most of these studies, workers were likely to experience chronic, low-to-moderate exposure levels. Consistently with findings from epidemiological studies, among cases of WRA attributed to cleaning agents reported to The Health and Occupation Research (THOR) network (UK, 1989–2017), the most frequent chemical categories for causing agents were aldehydes (30%), with a tendency to decrease over time, and chlorine/chlorine releasers (26%), which maintained their contribution over the reporting period (11).

In studies reported in Table 17.1, many cleaning products and disinfectants were investigated, and several were associated with asthma outcomes (21, 22, 25, 26). Beyond easily identified chemicals such as bleach or ammonia, associations were found with products with complex composition (e.g. sprays, multipurpose products) which may contain both irritants and sensitizers. Disentangling the mutual effect of the numerous chemicals contained in cleaning products, as well as their mixture is challenging. In the study by Su et al. (22), in addition to individual agents, several exposure clusters identified by hierarchical clustering such as "housekeeping/chlorine," "general cleaning/laboratory," or "disinfection products" were associated with different asthma outcomes. Overall, results from epidemiological studies suggest that adverse respiratory effects associated with cleaning products are not imputable to a single or a few agent(s) but may result from the frequent use of a multitude of products. Nonetheless, studies examining specific asthma phenotypes such as allergic vs nonallergic asthma are generally consistent with a predominant role of irritant exposures and the hypothesis of nonallergic mechanisms for workplace exposure to most cleaning products (27–29). Several large population-based studies have reported associations between occupational exposure to cleaning products and nonallergic/nonatopic asthma (28–30). In a Polish study of 142 cleaners (31), although many workers had work-related upper respiratory symptoms (e.g. 35% had work-related rhinitis), relatively few had positive skin-prick tests (SPTs) (19% for common allergens) or total IgE>100 IU/mL (16%). None of the cleaners had positive SPTs or specific IgE to disinfectants. In a 2-week panel study among cleaners in Spain, the association between use of cleaning products and lower respiratory tract symptoms was stronger among nonatopic participants (32). Inhalation of irritant cleaning products is likely to cause injury of the airway epithelium, and oxidative stress has been suggested as one of the underlying mechanisms (24). A few studies have examined the association between occupational exposure to cleaning agents and oxidative stress markers in humans. In a study of 92 Spanish cleaning workers, levels of exhaled breath condensate 8-isoprostanes, a specific marker of lipid peroxidation, were not associated with occupational exposure to cleaning products (33). In contrast, in a French study of 723 adults without asthma, exposure to cleaning products was associated with higher levels of plasma fluorescent oxidation products, a global marker of damage due to oxidative stress, although this association was significant in men only (34). Two studies in Italy reported that potential biomarkers of oxidative stress in exhaled breath condensate were higher in hospital

TABLE 17.1 Epidemiological Studies Reporting Associations between Occupational Exposure to Specific Cleaning or Disinfecting Agents and Asthma Outcomes

References	Study Design (Country, Year)	Outcome	Irritant Agents	Sensitizers	Agents Identified as Both Sensitizers and Irritants	Results[a] (Associations with Specific Agents)
18. Medina-Ramon et al., 2005	Case-control study, cleaners, 40 cases 155 controls (Spain, 2000–2002)	Current asthma/ chronic bronchitis	Bleach, ammonia			Bleach associated with asthma/ chronic bronchitis (OR 4.9; 95% CI:1.5–15)
19. Mirabelli et al., 2007	Cohort study, n=2813 (Europe, 1998–2003)	New-onset asthma	Bleach, ammonia			Ammonia/bleach among healthcare workers associated with new-onset asthma (RR 2.16; 95% CI:1.03–4.53)
26. Vizcaya et al., 2011	Cross-sectional study, cleaners, n=917 (Spain, 2007–2008)	Current asthma, asthma symptom score	Hydrochloric acid, ammonia			Hydrochloric acid and ammonia (mean ratio 1.6; 95% CI:1.0–2.5) associated with asthma symptom score (1.7; 1.1–2.6)
21. Arif et al., 2012	Cross-sectional study, healthcare workers, n=3650 (US, 2003–2004)	Work-related asthma symptoms, work-exacerbated asthma, occupational asthma	Bleach, ammonia		Formaldehyde, glutaraldehyde/ orthophthalaldehyde, ethylene oxide	Bleach, ammonia, glutaraldehyde/ orthophtalaldehyde, chloramines, ethylene oxide associated with work-related asthma symptoms (ORs>2); bleach and formaldehyde associated with work-exacerbated asthma (adjusted ORs>2.5); chloramines associated with occupational asthma (OR=4.81)
117. Dumas et al., 2012	Case-control and family-based study on asthma, n=724 (France, 2003–2007)	Current asthma	Decalcifiers (acids), ammonia			In women, exposure to decalcifiers (OR 2.38; 95% CI:1.06–5.33) and ammonia (3.05; 1.19–7.82) among hospital workers associated with current asthma
42. Gonzalez et al., 2014	Cross-sectional study, healthcare workers, n=543 (France, 2006–2007)	Physician-diagnosed asthma			Quaternary ammonium compounds	Quaternary ammonium compounds associated with physician-diagnosed asthma (OR 7.56; 95% CI:1.84–31.05)
20. Dumas et al., 2017	Cross-sectional study, female nurses with asthma, n=4102 (US, 2014–2015)	Asthma control	Bleach, hydrogen peroxide	Enzymatic cleaners	Formaldehyde, glutaraldehyde	Formaldehyde, glutaraldehyde, hypochlorite bleach, hydrogen peroxide and enzymatic cleaners associated with poor asthma control
23. Casey et al., 2017	Cross-sectional study (health hazard evaluation), hospital workers, n=163 (US, 2015)	Current asthma	Disinfectant containing hydrogen peroxide, peracetic acid, and acetic acid			Workers in the department with the highest air measurements had higher risk of current asthma (SMR 3.47; 95% CI:1.48–8.13) compared with the US population

(Continued)

TABLE 17.1 Epidemiological Studies Reporting Associations between Occupational Exposure to Specific Cleaning or Disinfecting Agents and Asthma Outcomes (*Continued*)

References	Study Design (Country, Year)	Outcome	Irritant Agents	Sensitizers	Agents Identified as Both Sensitizers and Irritants	Results[a] (Associations with Specific Agents)
22. Su et al., 2019	Cross-sectional study, healthcare workers, n=2030 (US, 2014)	Asthma health clusters, e.g. "undiagnosed/untreated asthma," "asthma attacks/exacerbations"	Alcohols, bleach	Enzymatic cleaners		Alcohols associated with "mild asthma symptoms" and "asthma attacks/exacerbations." Bleach associated with "mild asthma symptoms," "undiagnosed/untreated asthma," and "asthma attacks/exacerbations." Enzymes associated with "undiagnosed/untreated asthma" and "asthma attacks/exacerbations".
25. Brooks et al., 2020	Cross-sectional study, 425 cleaners and 281 reference workers (New Zealand, 2008–2010)	Current asthma, lung function	Bleach, decalcifiers (acids)			Bleach (OR 1.87; 95%:CI 1.12–3.14) and decalcifiers (2.77; 1.11–6.92) associated with current asthma; use of bleach associated with lower FEV_1 % predicted, compared to reference workers

[a] Results presented only for chemicals significantly associated with asthma outcomes. Products with mixed composition (e.g. detergents, cleaning sprays, multipurpose products) not reported in this table.

cleaners compared to control workers, while fractional exhaled nitric oxide (FeNO) levels were similar in both groups (35, 36).

Most epidemiological studies examining the role of occupational exposure to specific cleaning agents in asthma are cross-sectional and cannot distinguish risk factors for OA and WEA. It is likely that irritant cleaning agents play a role in both forms of WRA. For instance, in a study among US nurses, the association between use of disinfectants (mostly irritants) and poor asthma control was similar among nurses with childhood-onset asthma (i.e. preexisting but potentially exacerbated by occupational exposure) and adult-onset asthma (i.e. potentially caused by occupational exposures) (20). Although several longitudinal studies have reported associations between general occupational exposure to cleaning agents overall and asthma development (30, 37, 38) only one longitudinal study has examined specific agents (39). In this population of late-career nurses, no association was observed between exposure to disinfectants and asthma incidence, potentially because of a healthy worker effect. Additional longitudinal studies with detailed assessment of specific agents are needed to better understand their roles in occupational asthma vs WEA.

The irritant properties of many chemicals contained in cleaning products have prompted research on lung function outcomes. In a longitudinal analysis of the European Community Respiratory Health Survey (ECRHS), based on data collected over 20 years of follow-up, exposure to cleaning activities either at work or at home was associated with accelerated FEV_1 and forced vital capacity (FVC) decline (40). This result was observed in women only and independent of asthma. Similar results were found in a cross-sectional study in New Zealand, suggesting that cleaning, and specifically long-term exposure to irritants, was associated with lung function deficits and poorer overall lung health (25). In the British 1958 birth cohort, occupational exposure to cleaning products was associated with adult-onset asthma, with stronger associations for patients with airflow limitation (38). These

findings are also consistent with the recently reported association of exposure to cleaning agents and disinfectants with incidence of COPD, which has been found in both asthmatics and nonasthmatics (12, 41).

Cleaning agents have also been reported to cause sensitizer-induced OA. In a French cross-sectional study performed in 543 individuals employed in different healthcare settings, an association between quaternary ammonium compounds (quaternary amines)/latex IgE sensitization and prevalence of physician-diagnosed asthma was found (42). Recently, the application of the "quantitative structure activity relationship" (QSAR) model in asthma cases showed an IRR (95% CI) of 20.5 (15.4–27.3) for occupational and work-related respiratory symptoms in cleaners (43). The QSAR model identified 15 cleaning-related low-molecular-weight (LMW) chemicals, seven of which had a QSAR index consistent with being a sensitizer in asthma genesis (11). Chemicals identified were chlorhexidine, formaldehyde, diethanolamine, glutaraldehyde, ethanolamine, and dichloroisocyanurate. The same study observed an increased risk of work-related respiratory symptoms in healthcare workers in relation to glutaraldehyde and chlorine exposure with a QSAR index supporting the sensitizing mechanism.

In cleaners, few data are available for sensitizer OA diagnosed by specific inhalation challenge (SIC) tests, suggesting an immunologic response (44). A few clinical studies in patients affected by OA showed a positive SIC to agents, such as quaternary amines, glutaraldehyde, ethanolamines, and orthophthalaldehydes, although the exact mechanism was unclear (45). Among 975 patients diagnosed with OA, 80 patients (8%) with OA related to cleaning agents were identified; in 84% of asthma cases due to cleaning agents the suggested mechanism was sensitization and the median latency period from the first exposure to the diagnosis was 73 months (46). However, it seems that this finding should be interpreted with caution as it is likely that irritant-induced asthma is largely underestimated among OA cases reported by physicians in surveillance studies/case series, as for this type of OA the causal agent cannot be identified with certainty in a specific worker. In a clinical study, Vandenplas et al. demonstrated that 17 of 44 subjects who completed the SIC with cleaning/disinfecting agents had a fall of FEV_1 ≥20%, and in 11 there was an increase ≥2% of sputum eosinophils and/or > three-fold decrease in postchallenge histamine PC_{20} value; the aforementioned changes were mostly related to exposure to quaternary amines (44). The highest risk of reported asthma due to cleaning agents was associated with tasks involving dilution of disinfection products by manual mixing, suggesting possible repeated exposure to irritant/sensitizing agents such as quaternary amines (42). Even though there is a clear evidence linking cleaning agents and OA it is often difficult to identify specific causative agents and an immunologic mechanism probably because of exposure to a multitude of chemicals (47).

Agents and mechanisms

In cleaning professionals, new-onset asthma can be seen with or without a latency period (24, 48, 49). The main exposure location seems to be the upper and lower respiratory tract, even if dermal exposure may be important as well (50, 51). Nowadays, more than 400 agents have been described, being able to cause OA and WEA (52). Cleaning chemicals are defined as any material used for cleaning surfaces in general work environments. These chemicals are often mixed together, creating inappropriate mixtures of irritants and sensitizers (53). Many of these agents are actually used for disinfection i.e. to inactivate or destroy microorganisms on inert surfaces not for cleaning per se.

Cleaning products are divided into substances that can evaporate into the air as a gas or vapor (volatile) and those that cannot (nonvolatile). The most toxicologically significant fraction of cleaning agents are volatile organic compounds (VOCs) defined as organic compounds with boiling points between 0–400 °C (54). Chemical VOCs (cVOCs) are ubiquitous in the indoor air and there are many different sources in the workplace including building products, machinery, and cleaning products (54). In addition to cVOCs, microbial VOCs (mVOCs) may be present indoors released by molds that can cause similar symptoms as cVOCs. Therefore, it is important to identify risk factors for indoor mVOCs which have been attributed, in part, as causative to sick building syndrome (55). Researchers from NIOSH have developed personal exposure indices that can reliably determine if mold exposure is a problem in the workplace (56). Questions related to the presence of visible mold, mildew odors, freestanding water, condensation on windows, and water-stained ceiling tiles or wallboard indicate a greater likelihood for the presence of indoor mold often negating the need for environmental testing (56).

It is also important to appreciate that semivolatile compounds (>200 °C) often have a delayed emission over time, thereby increasing the probability of chronic exposure (54). In addition, cleaning agents contain (1) surfactants which can cause a range of skin and eye problems as well as mucous membrane irritation; (2) acidic and alkaline substances which are caustic and irritating; (3) complexing agents or water softeners; (4) disinfectants such as quaternary amines which can be both irritating and sensitizing in addition to a range of other components such as perfumes, scents, film formers, and polishers (54).

TABLE 17.2 Main Sensitizer and Irritant Cleaning Agents

Sensitizer	Irritants	Both Sensitizers and Irritants
• Scents containing terpenes	• Chlorine bleach	• Quaternary ammonium compounds
• Pinene	• Ammonia	
• D-limonene	• Hydrochloric acid	• Benzalkonium chloride
• Eugenol	• Sodium hydroxide	
• Isothiazolinones		• Lauryl dimethyl benzyl ammonium chloride
• Aldehydes		
• Formaldehyde		• Ethanolamines
• Glutaraldehyde		• Chloramines
• Latex		• Other amine compounds

Sources: Listed from References (10, 57, 67, 118).

Most cleaning products seem to be irritants, like chlorine bleach, hydrochloric acid, alkaline agents, or ammonia. However, an important number of these cleaning products can be sensitizers (e.g. amine compounds, disinfectants, quaternary ammonium compounds, pinene, limonene, latex) or both irritants and sensitizers (10). New chemical components are discovered each year with the development of new industrialized processes and better diagnosis by physicians (52, 57). The main sensitizer and irritant cleaning agents are summarized in Table 17.2.

A large number of studies have been conducted in the past years to understand the pathophysiology of OA in cleaning professionals but the consequences of an exposure to cleaning chemicals remains largely unclear. Many factors seem to be crucial in the development of the disease, such as genetic, environmental, or behavioral factors.

Immune response to cleaning chemicals

WRA due to cleaning products can be induced by both allergic and irritant mechanisms (10, 42, 58–60). Most of the cleaning products are LMW agents (<1000 Da), but some of them can be classified as high-molecular-weight (HMW) agents (>10 kDa). Some cleaning products, such as quaternary ammonium compounds, even have both irritant and sensitizer properties (42). The immune mechanisms of WRA due to cleaning agents are still unclear. Some authors found a sensitizing mechanism with Th2 immune responses through the synthesis of IgE and increased sputum eosinophil counts, especially for quaternary ammoniums, glutaraldehyde, and ethanolamines (44, 61). However, some other studies did not find an IgE-dependent mechanism. The immune response to LMW agents could be Th2, Th1, or/and Th17. For example, Zock and al. (27) described cleaning professionals with OA as less atopic than office workers, and atopy didn't seem to play a role in the mechanisms of asthma in cleaning professionals or people exposed to LMW agents. The pathophysiological pattern in this population also seems to sometimes include low eosinophilic counts (12, 29, 32, 44), and sometimes high neutrophilic counts in venous blood and sputum (29) with rare bronchial reversibility after ß2-mimetics (12). Other authors found some airway patterns with eosinophilic or neutrophilic infiltration or some with neither (62, 63). Women using bleach for home cleaning are at increased risk of nonallergic asthma (64, 65). A possible limitation of these studies could be the difficulty in distinguishing asthma-like symptoms from asthma.

Epithelial response

Inhalation of irritant or toxic components is likely to induce epithelial damage, promoting allergic sensitization, increased immune response, neurogenic inflammation, increased epithelial and capillary permeability, and airway remodelling (66, 67). Some authors described an altered secretion of relaxing epithelial factors, an increased secretion of epithelial growth factors, a release of inflammatory mediators and proinflammatory cytokines (53). The increased epithelial permeability enables the penetration of allergens, virus, and toxins, permitting new sensitizations (58, 66). Epithelial cells seem to play a central role in the immune response by a cross-talk with immune cells (68).

Toxicity

Cleaning professionals are exposed to a large variety of cleaning products and chemicals, often mixed together. Most of the allergenic components posing a risk for WRA can be cytotoxic even if patients are exposed to low concentrations. Irritants can induce a "danger signal," such as danger associated molecular patterns (DAMPs), leading to an increased systemic and local inflammation (58, 69). This increased inflammation due to toxic mechanisms can be accountable for epithelial cell damage with an increased epithelial barrier permeability, extracellular matrix modification (haemorrhagic exudate, fibrin, and edema), and oxidative damages (53, 70, 71). Immune cell infiltrates are also seen, as well as an enhanced secretion of cytokine, proinflammatory mediators, and growth factors (72, 73).

Oxidative stress

In asthma, an increased production of reactive oxygen species (ROS), reactive nitrogen species (RNS), and other pro-oxidant factors are seen (74, 75). This phenomenon leads to an imbalance between oxidant and antioxidant systems (75–77). Local epithelial injuries also seem to cause oxidative damage to epithelial cells, smooth muscle cells, and immune cells. A nitration of amino acids and the synthesis of nitrotyrosine are some of the ways to produce ROS after exposure to chlorine (36). The production of ROS could take place in damaged epithelial cells as well as in inflammatory immune cells (macrophages, neutrophils), due to an imbalance between oxidizing and reducing systems (34, 74). Mechanisms of increased local and systemic oxidative stress have been studied in mice but we still lack studies in humans (74, 76, 78). Oxidative stress seems to be the consequence of an exposure to an irritant or a sensitizer rather than its cause (79), but induces a worsening of the bronchial and systemic immune response (34, 80). Rava et al. (81) recently studied the interactions between genetic polymorphisms of genes involved in oxidative stress and an exposure to LMW molecules on new-onset asthma. Eight single nucleotide polymorphisms (SNPs) by exposure interactions at five loci were positively associated with new-onset asthma. These genes are likely to play a role in the NF-κB pathway that is known to be involved in the general inflammatory process. A few of these SNPs may also be involved in regulatory mechanisms. Air pollution, diesel, tobacco smoke, and other toxics can also aggravate local oxidative stress (58).

Neurogenic inflammation

Neuronal fibers tangle together near the bronchial epithelium, and appear to be able to penetrate the basal membrane and to come in contact with epithelial cells (82). These fibres are able to recognize external signals via TRP channels, inducing the synthesis and secretion of various proinflammatory molecules and, by this way, bronchoconstriction when they are overstimulated

(83). TRPA1 is a neuronal receptor found in lung cells and mast cells, able to recognize a large variety of toxic stimuli such as occupational allergens, environmental irritants (tobacco smoke, air pollution, chlorine), and endogenous components (ROS, RNS, and arachidonic acid derivative) (84). Drake et al. (85) recently showed that the increased innervation and nerve dysfunction was associated with a lack of bronchodilator responsiveness and an increased sensitivity to irritants. There is a cross-talk between the immune system and nervous system, in particular via the epithelial-derived enzyme neutral endopeptidase (NEP) that breaks down proinflammatory neuropeptides (86). The NEP's activity can be influenced by professional and environmental exposures (87, 88).

Genetics

Susceptibility genes involved in WRA can be categorized in four different subtypes. Type II HLA genes, genes involved in Th2 inflammation, genes coding for antioxidant enzymes (NADPH-dehydrogenase, superoxide dismutase, glutathion S-transferase, heme-oxygenase 1, catalase), genes associated with epithelial function, catenines, mucosal immunity, bronchial and pulmonary function (58, 81, 89, 90). Gene-gene and gene-environment interactions seem to play a substantial role (81). Further studies on genetics in OA, especially in cleaning professionals, are needed in order to get a better understanding of the disease.

Associated factors

Interactions have been described between inflammation due to an allergen (sensitizer, irritant, or both) and inflammation due to other stimuli like air pollution, VOC, formaldehyde, nitrogen dioxide, sulphur dioxide, chlorine, diesel, or tobacco smoke (91, 92). Physical factors such as cold or dry air, physical activity, acute or chronic respiratory infections might aggravate the inflammatory response (68, 91). Studies on animal models showed that an exposure to these associated factors seemed to lead to an increased immune response due to allergens, and aggravation of asthma (93–95).

In conclusion, OA in cleaning professionals seems to depend on an immunological non-IgE-dependent mechanism and at least a part of airway irritation. There is still much to learn on the underlying mechanisms of asthma in cleaning professionals, to determine specific risk factors and biomarkers.

Diagnosis

Diagnosis of patients with cleaning agent induced OA and differentiating it from WEA requires a thorough history of the work process as well as home exposures since many cleaning agents can be found in both locations (11, 20, 40, 96–98). The initial approach to diagnosis requires querying the worker about her/his upper and lower respiratory symptoms in relationship to product use. Often occupational rhinitis (OR) symptoms (nasal congestion, post nasal drainage, rhinorrhea, sneezing, itching of the eyes, ears, nose, throat) precede asthma symptoms (chest tightness, cough, shortness of breath, wheezing), so a careful history is important to differentiate between allergic (AR), nonallergic (NAR), and mixed rhinitis (MR) subtypes. Brandt et al. previously reported risk stratification factors for accurately differentiating NAR from AR which included onset of symptoms later in life (>30 years), no family history of atopy, no seasonality, no symptoms around furry pets, and trouble around perfumes and fragrances (99). Since patients with NAR or MR frequently have irritant-induced symptoms after exposure to cleaning agents, it is difficult to separate nonspecific environmental irritants from work-related cleaning agent induced symptoms. Further confounding the history is that many workers may not use these agents directly but work near where they are being used. Thus, it can be very challenging to establish a temporal relationship between cleaning agent exposure and symptoms to establish a diagnosis of OR and/or OA. Other demographic characteristics such as smoking history, personal home cleaning activities, and home environmental exposures in addition to a thorough past medical history should be obtained.

Like any workplace assessment, material safety data sheets should be requested and reviewed. The clinician should be knowledgeable about cleaning agent ingredients and their level of irritation and toxicity. The NIH has developed a rating scale for cleaning agents where 0 = minimal toxicity (including dish soaps or Fantastik cleaning agent); 1 = slight toxicity (including Pledge, Windex, Glass Plus, Mr. Clean, Formula 409, or Murphy's Oil Soap); 2 = moderate toxicity (including chlorine-based products); and 3 = serious toxicity (including Lysol, ceramic countertop cleaners, or oven cleaners) (98). It is also important for the clinician to be familiar with cleaning product classification.

Once suspected agents are identified, it is important to objectively assess for the presence of airway hyperresponsiveness, a central feature of asthma, to help confirm an objective diagnosis of asthma. Spirometry with flow volume loops is the first step for assessing the presence and severity of airflow obstruction. It also helps in the differential diagnosis of work-related OA as it can identify obstructive versus possible restrictive lung disease (Figure 17.1). A 12% or greater reversibility in FEV_1 postbronchodilators is consistent with a diagnosis of asthma. For patients that have normal lung function and/or no significant reversibility postbronchodilator medication, a methacholine challenge or some comparable provocation method should be performed near or at the end of the work week and repeated one or more weeks away from work to confirm airway hyperresponsiveness (97). In some cases, vocal cord dysfunction can obfuscate the diagnosis of cleaning agent induced OA and therefore, video stroboscopic examination may be necessary to identify or exclude this condition (100). In addition, exercise-induced bronchospasm has to be differentiated from cleaning agent induced OA as workers are often overexerting themselves while cleaning (40, 98).

It is important to emphasize that confirmation of asthma does not confirm a diagnosis of OA. To determine a direct relationship between OA induced by cleaning agents, serial PEF rates can be useful for monitoring changes in airflow related to exposures in and out of the workplace. They should be performed every 1–2 hours at work and at home while awake to determine if they correlate with airway reactivity in proximity to a specific exposure (Figure 17.2) (52). However, the gold standard to establish a definitive diagnosis of OA requires provocation to the specific agent. This can be challenging as many of the cleaning agents are irritating chemicals and there are no well-standardized protocols. Exceptions are certain chemicals such as quaternary amines which have been demonstrated to be sensitizing and safe provocation protocols have been established (101, 102). Provocation, if performed, should be conducted in a center with experienced personnel and readily available rescue medications.

Routine SPT or serum-specific IgE (sIgE) to aeroallergens is useful to assess the worker's atopic status as a potential underlying risk factor for cleaning agent induced OA as preexisting allergic airway inflammation may predispose individuals to enhanced airway hyperresponsiveness to nonspecific irritants (103). However, Zock et al. reported that nonatopic workers who were exposed to LMW chemicals were at a higher risk for asthma than atopic workers and a similar trend, although not statistically significant, was seen for cleaning workers (27). In addition, a large questionnaire survey found no difference in the association between cleaning agents and poor asthma control according to atopy (20). Other supportive diagnostic tests include SPT to the chemical agent(s) or ingredient(s) in question. In contrast to HMW asthmagens, only a handful of LMW chemicals like chloramine T, chlorhexidine, formaldehyde, glutaraldehyde, quaternary amines like benzalkonium chloride, and acid anhydrides like trimellitic anhydride, have been found to be potentially sensitizing (104). A study by Lipinska-Ojrzanowska and colleagues performed SPT to chloramine T, chlorhexidine, formaldehyde, glutaraldehyde, and benzalkonium chloride in 142 cleaning workers and found no positive skin test responses (31). Similarly, in vitro testing of chemical constituents in cleaning agents is limited as there are no commercially standardized or validated assays (31, 105, 106). This is largely because most LMW chemicals, with the exceptions cited above, are not structurally capable of binding to endogenous proteins to form new antigenic determinants capable of eliciting a specific IgE mediated response. The study by Lipinska-Ojrzanowska et al. also found no sIgE responses to the chemicals used for testing in their population (31). In addition, patch testing may be useful in selected cases using nonirritating dilutions of chemical cleaning agents especially in patients presenting with occupational dermatitis (107). For example, with delayed respiratory reactions associated with skin eruptions, patch testing may be useful to help confirm a T-cell mediated response for some preservatives like quaternary amines (101).

In summary, the diagnosis of cleaning agent induced OA is similar to other forms of HMW and LMW induced OA with the exception that chemical cleaning agents cannot always be used as skin test reagents or as antigens for eliciting specific IgE immune responses by in vitro assay testing. Therefore, the diagnosis relies on clinical suspicion and a thorough medical history that includes careful assessment of chemical exposures. Material safety data sheets should be obtained to identify potential causative agents. Establishing an objective diagnosis of asthma is essential and whenever possible a temporal relationship between exposure and symptoms strengthens the diagnosis. Specific provocation is often challenging due to the irritant nature of these agents and therefore when performed should incorporate control days with a nonirritating agent(s) to qualify the challenge results.

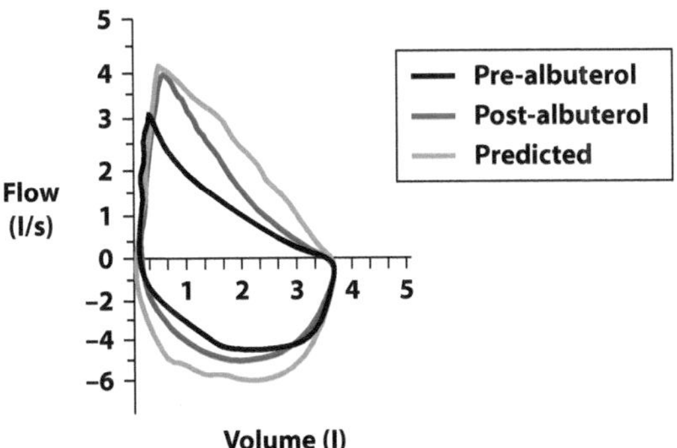

FIGURE 17.1 Flow-volume loops in asthma demonstrating nonobstructed pattern and reversal of airflow obstruction following administration of a beta-agonist agent (albuterol).

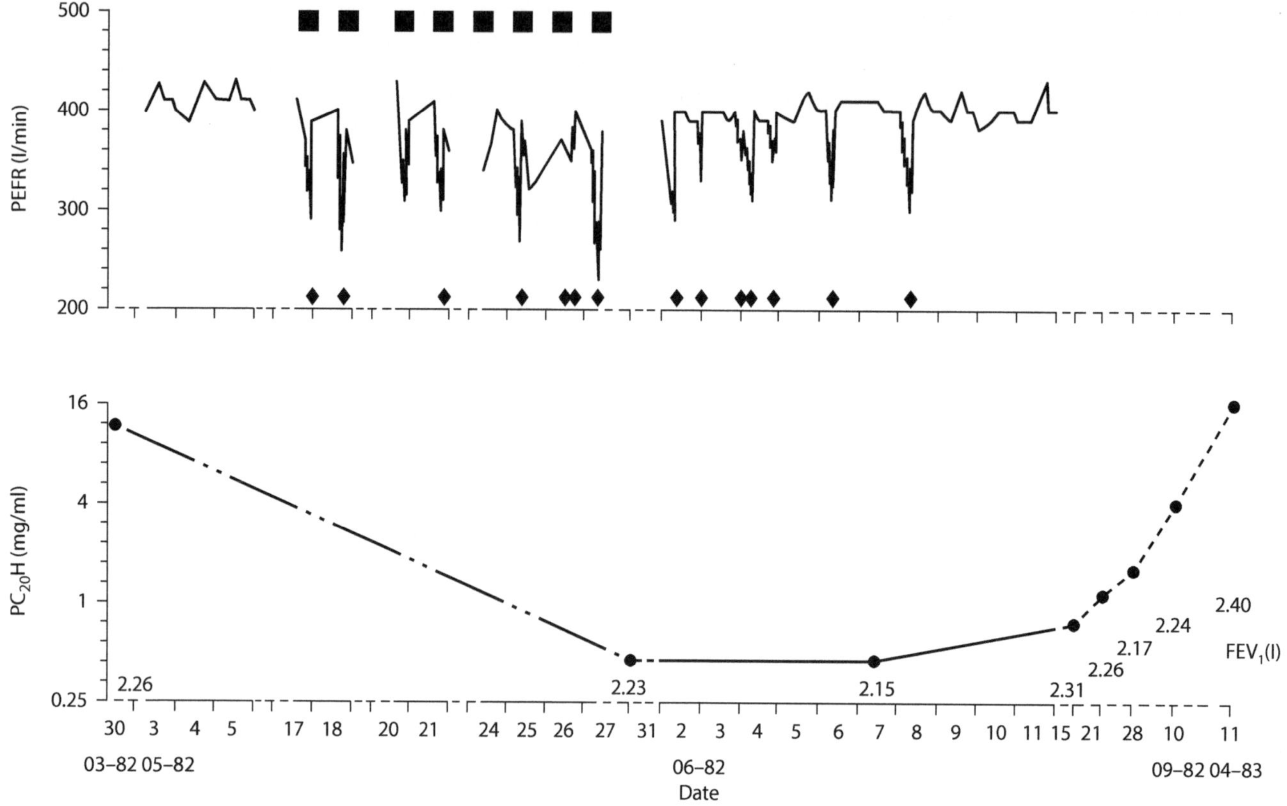

FIGURE 17.2 Serial PEFR and PC20 histamine measurements at work and away from work over weeks and months (52). (By permission.)

Treatment

Treatment of asthma induced by cleaning agents should be in accordance with GINA asthma guidelines 2020. Treatment should be implemented based on disease severity and control. Patient response to treatment should be monitored using validated patient-reported outcome instruments and medications should be stepped up or down based on the level of control. Comorbid conditions that impact asthma control such as chronic rhinosinusitis, gastroesophageal reflux, vocal cord dysfunction, psychosocial issues, obstructive sleep apnea, and obesity should be identified and managed to optimize treatment outcomes. Relevant environmental avoidance measures should be addressed to reduce further exposure burden to inciting agents in and out of the workplace. Patients should be educated about medication adherence and all patients should have an asthma action plan to follow in case of an exacerbation. It is essential to monitor patients regularly in the outpatient setting. The frequency of visits will depend on the disease severity and control (108).

Prevention

Agents used for cleaning activities display potential ability to induce or aggravate a clinical course of preexisting asthma in exposed workers (109), thus preventive measures must be undertaken. Work-related respiratory diseases in cleaners can be prevented in three stages: primary, secondary, and tertiary ones.

Primary prevention aims to reduce disease incidence, which means preventing exposure to hazards that cause disease. Therefore minimizing, avoiding, or substitution of cleaning

agents, seem to be the most needed actions. The incidence of asthma is higher among cleaners who often use sprays (110): although similar components of cleaning products were present, this increase was not observed among cleaners who usually used liquid chemicals (54). It is possible that using liquid (wiped, not sprayed) forms of cleaning chemicals is connected with minor occurrence of asthma-like symptoms due to dust particle hydration and decreased risk of inhalation through the airways (18).

The American Lung Association recommends using only cleaning products without VOCs, fragrances, irritants, or flammable ingredients, as well as avoidance of air fresheners (111). In the European Union it is required that labels on cleaning products must warn consumers about possible toxic ingredients within these products (EU decision). Using less volatile ortho-phthalaldehyde instead of glutaraldehyde is also recommended (67).

Moreover, there is a need for emerging nonchemical technologies for disinfection (e.g. steam, ultraviolet light) as a potential alternative to chemical disinfection (20). Furthermore, green cleaning, which comprises an interdisciplinary, systemic approach and aims at balancing and addressing multiple needs (environmental cleanliness for infection prevention and control, environmental impact, human health effects) is a chance for improving occupational exposure for cleaners; however, it requires evaluation by using sound and standard methods to examine effects on multiple outcomes.

Although the use of personal protective equipment (PPE) such as various forms of respirator, occupies the lowest tier of the hierarchy of control measures for airborne contaminants (112) and is reserved for situations where other methods have failed adequately to control airborne exposures, in the case of cleaners it is worth mentioning (113). However, long-term wearing of respiratory PPE may be intolerable and difficult to enforce. It was documented in different studies that low compliance rates had been associated with PPE discomfort and lack of awareness of safety precautions, whereas increased compliance rates were associated with receiving reminders of safety protocols, high PPE availability within the workplace, coworker usage, and positive social norms, adequate training, concerns about the risks of workplace exposures, and having workplace fit testing available (114).

The above associations emphasize the problem of workers' education concerning health and safety, which is the employer's responsibility. However to make it effective and long-lasting, training must change workers' behavior by informing of risks, teaching how to minimize risks through the implementation of safety protocols, and convincing workers that the benefits of these protocols outweigh their drawbacks (114).

Secondary prevention aims to reduce the impact of a disease that has already occurred. This is done by detecting and treating disease as soon as possible to halt or slow its progress, which may be achieved by regular examinations and screening tests. As the mechanism of developing cleaners' asthma is very often irritative, questionnaire and pulmonary function tests are the main tools that can be used in employees' health monitoring. Reporting any work-related respiratory symptoms by a worker or decrease in spirometry parameters should start the diagnostic procedure of suspected occupational disease.

In a Brazilian study, the estimated risk of occupational allergic rhinitis and asthma development increased in conjunction with the period of employment as a professional cleaning worker (115). This fact imposes adequate monitoring of workers' health conditions during periodical examinations. Early recognition enables exposed workers' recognition of the necessity of workplace agents' avoidance and beginning of treatment, which are some of the most important factors preventing occupational disability.

Additionally, a healthy worker effect, i.e. a tendency of employees with an asthma history or more severe asthma to quit jobs with exposure to disinfectants, is a way of prevention applied by workers themselves.

Tertiary prevention aims to soften the impact of an ongoing illness and is done by helping people manage long-term health problems in order to improve as much as possible their ability to function, their quality of life, and their life expectancy, e.g. by vocational rehabilitation programs to retrain workers for new jobs when they have recovered as much as possible. In the case of cleaners' asthma continuation of exposure to cleaning products is not recommended unless full control of asthma is possible. For the same reasons, nonoccupational asthmatics are not advised to enter these jobs since exposures to cleaning sprays, ammonia, bleach, and disinfectants have been identified as specific causes of exacerbation of asthma (19, 67, 116). In Dumas et al. study of 4102 US nurses with asthma, disinfections tasks, especially disinfection of medical instruments, were associated with poor asthma control (20). In particular increased risks of poor asthma control were associated with exposure to glutaraldehyde, formaldehyde, enzymatic cleaners, hypochlorite bleach, and hydrogen peroxide, while exposure to quaternary amines and alcohol did not result in worsening of asthma.

Conclusions and research needs

Cleaning and disinfecting products are essential for the prevention of infection, especially in healthcare facilities and in public areas. Understanding the extent of risk for asthma associated with these products, and the relative risk from each chemical agent is essential for the planning of measures to reduce risks of WRA as well as public health risks. In general, it appears that sprayed products carry more risk than the same product used as a solution for wiping with a cloth, but further studies are needed to confirm whether this simple change is effective in risk-reduction. Understanding risks of interactions between chemicals should also be further studied as this can also provide relatively simple measures such as washing of urine-soiled bedding and other hospital contents before wiping with chlorinated products (97). A recent study of nurses who were followed from 2009–2015, unlike previous reports, did not show an increased risk of asthma (39) associated with disinfectants, possibly due to a healthy worker effect, or perhaps a difference in exposures from other studies. However, the same group reported an association with COPD incidence from questionnaire (41). Currently there are relatively few chemical cleaning agents that are recognized to be sensitizers (aldehydes, quaternary ammonium compounds, enzymes, chlorhexidine, and less commonly sulfones and other agents) and alternative agents to these should be developed to further restrict the use of these. Further objective investigations are needed to determine the true role of low-level chlorinated products and hydrogen peroxide in contributing to asthma or to laryngeal syndromes. Additional epidemiologic studies such as those performed in nurses (20, 39, 117) will be helpful to assess effectiveness of intervention measures, and potentially may also be relevant for use of household cleaning products.

References

1. Hendrick DJ, Lane DJ. Formalin asthma in hospital staff. Br Med J. 1975;5958(1):607–8.
2. Hendrick DJ, Lane DJ. Occupational formalin asthma. Br J Ind Med. 1977;34:11–8.
3. Hendrick DJ, Rando RJ, Lane DJ, Morris MJ. Formaldehyde asthma: challenge exposure levels and fate after five years. JOM. 1982;24:893–7.
4. Corrado OJ, Osman J, Davies RJ. Asthma and rhinitis after exposure to glutaraldehyde in endoscopy units. Human Toxicol. 198;5:325–7.
5. Hendrick DJ, Connolly MJ, Stenton SC, et al. Occupational asthma due to sodium iso-nonanoyl oxybenzene sulphonate, a newly developed detergent ingredient. Thorax. 1988;43:501–2.
6. Waclawski ER, McAlpine LG, Thomson NC. Occupational asthma in nurses caused by chlorhexidine and alcohol aerosols. Br Med J. 1989;298:929–30.
7. Ribeiro M, Tarlo SM, Czyrka A, et al. Diisocyanate and non-diisocyanate sensitizer-induced occupational asthma frequency during 2003 to 2007 in Ontario, Canada. JOM. 2014;56(9):1001–7.
8. Walters GI, Kirkham A, McGrath EE, et al. Twenty years of SHIELD: decreasing incidence of occupational asthma in the West Midlands, UK? Occup Environ Med. 2015;72(4):304–10.
9. Gotzev S, Lipszyc JC, Connor D, Tarlo SM. Trends in occupations and work sectors among patients with work-related asthma at a Canadian tertiary care clinic. Chest. 2016;150(4):811–8.
10. Folletti I, Siracusa A, Paolocci G. Update on asthma and cleaning agents. Curr Opin Allergy Clin Immunol. 2017;17(2):90–5.
11. Carder M, Seed MJ, Money A, et al. Occupational and work-related respiratory disease attributed to cleaning products. Occup Environ Med. 2019;76(8):530–6.
12. De Matteis S, Jarvis D, Hutchings S, et al. Occupations associated with COPD risk in the large population-based UK Biobank cohort study. Occup Env Med. 2016;73:378–84.
13. Moore VC, Burge PS, Robertson AS, Walters GI. What causes occupational asthma in cleaners? Thorax. 2017;72(6):581–3.
14. Walters GI, Burge PS, Moore VC, et al. Occupational asthma caused by peracetic acid-hydrogen peroxide mixture. Occup Med (Lond). 2019;69(4):294–7.
15. Parks J, McCandless L, Dharma C, et al. Association of use of cleaning products with respiratory health in a Canadian birth cohort. CMAJ. 2020;192(7):E154–E61.

16. Rosenman KD, Millerick-May M, Reilly MJ, et al. Swimming facilities and work-related asthma. J Asthma. 2015;52(1):52–8.
17. Weisel CP, Richardson SD, Nemery B, et al. Childhood asthma and environmental exposures at swimming pools: state of the science and research recommendations. Environ Health Perspect. 2009;117(4):500–7.
18. Medina-Ramon M, Zock JP, Kogevinas M, et al. Asthma, chronic bronchitis, and exposure to irritant agents in occupational domestic cleaning: a nested case-control study. Occup Environ Med. 2005;62(9):598–606.
19. Mirabelli MC, Zock JP, Plana E, et al. Occupational risk factors for asthma among nurses and related healthcare professionals in an international study. Occup Environ Med. 2007;64(7):474–9.
20. Dumas O, Wiley AS, Quinot C, et al. Occupational exposure to disinfectants and asthma control in US nurses. Eur Respir J. 2017;50(4):1700237.
21. Arif AA, Delclos GL. Association between cleaning-related chemicals and work-related asthma and asthma symptoms among healthcare professionals. Occup Environ Med. 2012;69(1):35–40.
22. Su FC, Friesen MC, Humann M, et al. Clustering asthma symptoms and cleaning and disinfecting activities and evaluating their associations among healthcare workers. Int J Hyg Environ Health. 2019;222(5):873–83.
23. Casey ML, Hawley B, Edwards N, et al. Health problems and disinfectant product exposure among staff at a large multispecialty hospital. Am J Infect Control. 2017;45(10):1133–8.
24. Tarlo SM, Lemiere C. Occupational asthma. N Engl J Med. 2014;370(7):640–9.
25. Brooks C, Slater T, Corbin M, et al. Respiratory health in professional cleaners: symptoms, lung function, and risk factors. Clin Exp Allergy. 2020;50(5):567–76.
26. Vizcaya D, Mirabelli MC, Anto JM, et al. A workforce-based study of occupational exposures and asthma symptoms in cleaning workers. Occup Environ Med. 2011;68(12):914–9.
27. Zock JP, Kogevinas M, Sunyer J, et al. Asthma characteristics in cleaning workers, workers in other risk jobs and office workers. Eur Respir J. 2002;20(3):679–85.
28. Wang TN, Lin MC, Wu CC, et al. Risks of exposure to occupational asthmogens in atopic and nonatopic asthma: a case-control study in Taiwan. Am J Respir Crit Care Med. 2010;182(11):1369–76.
29. Dumas O, Siroux V, Luu F, et al. Cleaning and asthma characteristics in women. Am J Ind Med. 2014;57(3):303–11.
30. Lillienberg L, Andersson E, Janson C, et al. Occupational exposure and new-onset asthma in a population-based study in Northern Europe (RHINE). Ann Occup Hyg. 2013;57(4):482–92.
31. Lipinska-Ojrzanowska A, Wiszniewska M, Swierczynska-Machura D, et al. Work-related respiratory symptoms among health centres cleaners: a cross-sectional study. Int J Occup Med Environ Health. 2014;27(3):460–6.
32. Vizcaya D, Mirabelli MC, Gimeno D, et al. Cleaning products and short-term respiratory effects among female cleaners with asthma. Occup Environ Med. 2015;72(11):757–63.
33. Vizcaya D, Mirabelli MC, Orriols R, et al. Functional and biological characteristics of asthma in cleaning workers. Respir Med. 2013;107(5):673–83.
34. Dumas O, Matran R, Zerimech F, et al. Occupational exposures and fluorescent oxidation products in 723 adults of the EGEA study. Eur Respir J. 2015;46(1):258–61.
35. Casimirri E, Stendardo M, Bonci M, et al. Biomarkers of oxidative-stress and inflammation in exhaled breath condensate from hospital cleaners. Biomarkers. 2016;21(2):115–22.
36. Corradi M, Gergelova P, Di Pilato E, et al. Effect of exposure to detergents and other chemicals on biomarkers of pulmonary response in exhaled breath from hospital cleaners: a pilot study. Int Arch Occup Environ Health. 2012;85(4):389–96.
37. Kogevinas M, Zock JP, Jarvis D, et al. Exposure to substances in the workplace and new-onset asthma: an international prospective population-based study (ECRHS-II). Lancet. 2007;370(9584):336–41.
38. Ghosh RE, Cullinan P, Fishwick D, et al. Asthma and occupation in the 1958 birth cohort. Thorax. 2013;68(4):365–71.
39. Dumas O, Boggs KM, Quinot C, et al. Occupational exposure to disinfectants and asthma incidence in U.S. nurses: a prospective cohort study. Am J Ind Med. 2020;63(1):44–50.
40. Svanes O, Bertelsen RJ, Lygre SHL, et al. Cleaning at home and at work in relation to lung function decline and airway obstruction. Am J Respir Crit Care Med. 2018;197(9):1157–63.
41. Dumas O, Varraso R, Boggs KM, et al. Association of occupational exposure to disinfectants with incidence of chronic obstructive pulmonary disease among US female nurses. JAMA Netw Open. 2019;2(10):e1913563.
42. Gonzalez M, Jegu J, Kopferschmitt MC, et al. Asthma among workers in healthcare settings: role of disinfection with quaternary ammonium compounds. Clin Exp Allergy. 2014;44(3):393–406.
43. Jarvis J, Seed MJ, Stocks SJ, Agius RM. A refined QSAR model for prediction of chemical asthma hazard. Occup Med (Lond). 2015;65(8):659–66.
44. Vandenplas O, D'Alpaos V, Evrard G, et al. Asthma related to cleaning agents: a clinical insight. BMJ Open. 2013;3(9):e003568.
45. Tarlo SM, Arif AA, Delclos GL, et al. Opportunities and obstacles in translating evidence to policy in occupational asthma. Ann Epidemiol. 2018;28(6):392–400.
46. Walters GI, Burge PS, Moore VC, Robertson AS. Cleaning agent occupational asthma in the West Midlands, UK: 2000–16. Occup Med (Lond). 2018;68(8):530–6.
47. Tarlo SM, Quirce S. Impact of identification of clinical phenotypes in occupational asthma. J Allergy Clin Immunol Pract. 2020;8:3277–82.
48. Malo JL, Vandenplas O. Definitions and classification of work-related asthma. Immunol Allergy Clin North Am. 2011;31(4):645–62, v.
49. Munoz X, Cruz MJ, Bustamante V, et al. Work-related asthma: diagnosis and prognosis of immunological occupational asthma and work-exacerbated asthma. J Investig Allergol Clin Immunol. 2014;24(6):396–405.
50. Redlich CA, Herrick CA. Lung/skin connections in occupational lung disease. Curr Opin Allergy Clin Immunol. 2008;8(2):115–9.
51. Lynde CB, Obadia M, Liss GM, et al. Cutaneous and respiratory symptoms among professional cleaners. Occup Med (Lond). 2009;59(4):249–54.
52. Cartier A, Malo JL, Forest F, et al. Occupational asthma in snow crab-processing workers. J Allergy Clin Immunol. 1984;74(3 Pt 1):261–9.
53. Ederle C, Donnay C, Khayath N, et al. Asthma and cleaning: what's new? Current Treatment Options in Allergy. 2018;5(1):29–40.
54. Wolkoff P, Schneider T, Kildeso J, et al. Risk in cleaning: chemical and physical exposure. Sci Total Environ. 1998;215(1–2):135–56.
55. Saijo Y, Kishi R, Sata F, et al. Symptoms in relation to chemicals and dampness in newly built dwellings. Int Arch Occup Environ Health. 2004;77(7):461–70.
56. Park JH, Schleiff PL, Attfield MD, et al. Building-related respiratory symptoms can be predicted with semi-quantitative indices of exposure to dampness and mold. Indoor Air. 2004;14(6):425–33.
57. Rosenman K, Reilly MJ, Pechter E, et al. Cleaning products and work-related asthma, 10 year update. J Occup Environ Med. 2020;62(2):130–7.
58. Lummus ZL, Wisnewski AV, Bernstein DI. Pathogenesis and disease mechanisms of occupational asthma. Immunol Allergy Clin North Am. 2011;31(4):699–716, vi.
59. Malo JL, Tarlo SM, Sastre J, et al. An official American Thoracic Society Workshop Report: presentations and discussion of the fifth Jack Pepys Workshop on Asthma in the Workplace. Comparisons between asthma in the workplace and non-work-related asthma. Ann Am Thorac Soc. 2015;12(7):S99–S110.
60. De Vooght V, Cruz MJ, Haenen S, et al. Ammonium persulfate can initiate an asthmatic response in mice. Thorax. 2010;65(3):252–7.
61. Lipinska-Ojrzanowska AA, Wiszniewska M, Walusiak-Skorupa JM. Work-related asthma among professional cleaning women. Arch Environ Occup Health. 2017;72(1):53–60.
62. Quirce S, Sastre J. Occupational asthma: clinical phenotypes, biomarkers, and management. Curr Opin Pulm Med. 2019;25(1):59–63.
63. Sadakane K, Ichinose T. Effect of the hand antiseptic agents benzalkonium chloride, povidone-iodine, ethanol, and chlorhexidine gluconate on atopic dermatitis in NC/Nga mice. Int J Med Sci. 2015;12(2):116–25.
64. Matulonga B, Rava M, Siroux V, et al. Women using bleach for home cleaning are at increased risk of non-allergic asthma. Respir Med. 2016;117:264–71.
65. Miszkiel KA, Beasley R, Holgate ST. The influence of ipratropium bromide and sodium cromoglycate on benzalkonium chloride-induced bronchoconstriction in asthma. Br J Clin Pharmacol. 1988;26(3):295–301.
66. Van Den Broucke S, Pollaris L, Vande Velde G, et al. Irritant-induced asthma to hypochlorite in mice due to impairment of the airway barrier. Arch Toxicol. 2018;92(4):1551–61.
67. Siracusa A, De Blay F, Folletti I, et al. Asthma and exposure to cleaning products—a European Academy of Allergy and Clinical Immunology task force consensus statement. Allergy. 2013;68(12):1532–45.
68. Lambrecht BN, Hammad H. The immunology of asthma. Nat Immunol. 2015;16(1):45–56.
69. Patel S. Danger-Associated Molecular Patterns (DAMPs): the derivatives and triggers of inflammation. Curr Allergy Asthma Rep. 2018;18(11):63.
70. Castano R, Miedinger D, Maghni K, et al. Matrix metalloproteinase-9 increases in the sputum from allergic occupational asthma patients after specific inhalation challenge. Int Arch Allergy Immunol. 2013;160(2):161–4.

71. Maghni K, Malo JL, L'Archeveque J, et al. Matrix metalloproteinases, IL-8 and glutathione in the prognosis of workers exposed to chlorine. Allergy. 2010;65(6):722–30.
72. Friedman-Jimenez G, Harrison D, Luo H. Occupational asthma and work-exacerbated asthma. Semin Respir Crit Care Med. 2015;36(3):388–407.
73. Tarlo SM. Update on work-exacerbated asthma. Int J Occup Med Environ Health. 2016;29(3):369–74.
74. Ederle C, Charles AL, Khayath N, et al. Mitochondrial function in peripheral blood mononuclear cells (PBMC) is enhanced, together with increased reactive oxygen species, in severe asthmatic patients in exacerbation. J Clin Med. 2019;8(10):1613.
75. Aldakheel FM, Thomas PS, Bourke JE, et al. Relationships between adult asthma and oxidative stress markers and pH in exhaled breath condensate: a systematic review. Allergy. 2016;71(6):741–57.
76. Sahiner UM, Birben E, Erzurum S, et al. Oxidative stress in asthma. World Allergy Organ J. 2011;4(10):151–8.
77. Louhelainen N, Myllarniemi M, Rahman I, Kinnula VL. Airway biomarkers of the oxidant burden in asthma and chronic obstructive pulmonary disease: current and future perspectives. Int J Chron Obstruct Pulmon Dis. 2008;3(4):585–603.
78. Antus B. Oxidative stress markers in sputum. Oxid Med Cell Longev. 2016:2930434.
79. Pignatti P, Frossi B, Pala G, et al. Oxidative activity of ammonium persulfate salt on mast cells and basophils: implication in hairdressers' asthma. Int Arch Allergy Immunol. 2013;160(4):409–19.
80. Mittal M, Siddiqui MR, Tran K, et al. Reactive oxygen species in inflammation and tissue injury. Antioxid Redox Signal. 2014;20(7):1126–67.
81. Rava M, Ahmed I, Kogevinas M, et al. Genes interacting with occupational exposures to low molecular weight agents and irritants on adult-onset asthma in three European studies. Environ Health Perspect. 2017;125(2):207–14.
82. Kabata H, Artis D. Neuro-immune crosstalk and allergic inflammation. J Clin Invest. 2019;129(4):1475–82.
83. van der Velden VH, Hulsmann AR. Autonomic innervation of human airways: structure, function, and pathophysiology in asthma. Neuroimmunomodulation. 1999;6(3):145–59.
84. Zholos AV. TRP channels in respiratory pathophysiology: the role of oxidative, chemical irritant and temperature stimuli. Curr Neuropharmacol. 2015;13(2):279–91.
85. Drake MG, Scott GD, Blum ED, et al. Eosinophils increase airway sensory nerve density in mice and in human asthma. Sci Transl Med. 2018;10(457).
86. Di Maria GU, Bellofiore S, Geppetti P. Regulation of airway neurogenic inflammation by neutral endopeptidase. Eur Respir J. 1998;12(6):1454–62.
87. Gagnaire F, Ban M, Cour C, et al. Role of tachykinins and neutral endopeptidase in toluene diisocyanate-induced bronchial hyperresponsiveness in guinea pigs. Toxicology. 1997;116(1–3):17–26.
88. Sheppard D, Thompson JE, Scypinski L, et al. Toluene diisocyanate increases airway responsiveness to substance P and decreases airway neutral endopeptidase. J Clin Invest. 1988;81(4):1111–5.
89. Acouetey DS, Zmirou-Navier D, Avogbe PH, et al. Genetic predictors of inflammation in the risk of occupational asthma in young apprentices. Ann Allergy Asthma Immunol. 2013;110(6):423–8, e5.
90. Bernstein DI, Wang N, Campo P, et al. Diisocyanate asthma and gene-environment interactions with IL4RA, CD-14, and IL-13 genes. Ann Allergy Asthma Immunol. 2006;97(6):800–6.
91. Henneberger PK, Redlich CA, Callahan DB, et al. An official American Thoracic Society statement: work-exacerbated asthma. Am J Respir Crit Care Med. 2011;184(3):368–78.
92. Casset A, Purohit A, Marchand C, et al. [The bronchial response to inhaled formaldehyde]. Rev Mal Respir. 2006;23(1 Suppl):3S25–34.
93. Depuydt PO, Lambrecht BN, Joos GF, Pauwels RA. Effect of ozone exposure on allergic sensitization and airway inflammation induced by dendritic cells. Clin Exp Allergy. 2002;32(3):391–6.
94. Hashimoto K, Ishii Y, Uchida Y, et al. Exposure to diesel exhaust exacerbates allergen-induced airway responses in guinea pigs. Am J Respir Crit Care Med. 2001;164(10 Pt 1):1957–63.
95. Hao M, Comier S, Wang M, et al. Diesel exhaust particles exert acute effects on airway inflammation and function in murine allergen provocation models. J Allergy Clin Immunol. 2003;112(5):905–14.
96. Hawley B, Casey M, Virji MA, et al. Respiratory symptoms in hospital cleaning staff exposed to a product containing hydrogen peroxide, peracetic acid, and acetic acid. Ann Work Expo Health. 2017;62(1):28–40.
97. Li RWH, Lipszyc JC, Prasad S, Tarlo SM. Work-related asthma from cleaning agents versus other agents. Occup Med (Lond). 2018;68(9):587–92.
98. Bernstein JA, Brandt D, Rezvani M, et al. Evaluation of cleaning activities on respiratory symptoms in asthmatic female homemakers. Ann Allergy Asthma Immunol. 2009;102(1):41–6.
99. Brandt D, Bernstein JA. Questionnaire evaluation and risk factor identification for nonallergic vasomotor rhinitis. Ann Allergy Asthma Immunol. 2006;96(4):526–32.
100. Tonini S, Dellabianca A, Costa C, et al. Irritant vocal cord dysfunction and occupational bronchial asthma: differential diagnosis in a health care worker. Int J Occup Med Environ Health. 2009;22(4):401–6.
101. Bernstein JA, Stauder T, Bernstein DI, Bernstein IL. A combined respiratory and cutaneous hypersensitivity syndrome induced by work exposure to quaternary amines. J Allergy Clin Immunol. 1994;94(2 Pt 1):257–9.
102. Purohit A, Kopferschmitt-Kubler MC, Moreau C, et al. Quaternary ammonium compounds and occupational asthma. Int Arch Occup Environ Health. 2000;73(6):423–7.
103. D'Amato G, Liccardi G, D'Amato M, Holgate S. Environmental risk factors and allergic bronchial asthma. Clin Exp Allergy. 2005;35(9):1113–24.
104. Quirce S, Bernstein JA. Old and new causes of occupational asthma. Immunol Allergy Clin North Am. 2011;31(4):677–98, v.
105. Blomqvist AM, Axelsson IG, Danielsson D, et al. Atopic allergy to chloramine-T and the demonstration of specific IgE antibodies by the radioallergosorbent test. Int Arch Occup Environ Health. 1991;63(5):363–5.
106. Kramps JA, van Toorenenbergen AW, Vooren PH, Dijkman JH. Occupational asthma due to inhalation of chloramine-T. II. Demonstration of specific IgE antibodies. Int Arch Allergy Appl Immunol. 1981;64(4):428–38.
107. Mirabelli MC, Vizcaya D, Marti Margarit A, et al. Occupational risk factors for hand dermatitis among professional cleaners in Spain. Contact Dermatitis. 2012;66(4):188–96.
108. GINA Full Report 2020 Front Cover ONLY - GINA-2020-report_20_06_04-1-wms.pdf 2020. https://ginasthma.org/wp-content/uploads/2020/06/GINA-2020-report_20_06_04-1-wms.pdf
109. Zock JP, Vizcaya D, Le Moual N. Update on asthma and cleaners. Curr Opin Allergy Clin Immunol. 2010;10(2):114–20.
110. Zock JP, Plana E, Jarvis D, et al. The use of household cleaning sprays and adult asthma: an international longitudinal study. Am J Respir Crit Care Med. 2007;176(8):735–41.
111. Abrams EM. Cleaning products and asthma risk: a potentially important public health concern. CMAJ. 2020;192(7):E164–E5.
112. Hierarchy of Controls | NIOSH | CDC 2020 updated 2020-06-17T11:54:25Z. https://www.cdc.gov/niosh/topics/hierarchy/default.html
113. Cullinan P, Munoz X, Suojalehto H, et al. Occupational lung diseases: from old and novel exposures to effective preventive strategies. Lancet Respir Med. 2017;5(5):445–55.
114. Fukakusa J, Rosenblat J, Jang B, et al. Factors influencing respirator use at work in respiratory patients. Occup Med (Lond). 2011;61(8):576–82.
115. de Fatima Macaira E, Algranti E, Medina Coeli Mendonca E, Antonio Bussacos M. Rhinitis and asthma symptoms in non-domestic cleaners from the Sao Paulo metropolitan area, Brazil. Occup Environ Med. 2007;64(7):446–53.
116. Massin N, Hecht G, Ambroise D, et al. Respiratory symptoms and bronchial responsiveness among cleaning and disinfecting workers in the food industry. Occup Environ Med. 2007;64(2):75–81.
117. Dumas O, Donnay C, Heederik DJ, et al. Occupational exposure to cleaning products and asthma in hospital workers. Occup Environ Med. 2012;69(12):883–9.
118. Cartier A. New causes of immunologic occupational asthma, 2012–2014. Curr Opin Allergy Clin Immunol. 2015;15(2):117–23.

18

VARIOUS HIGH- AND LOW-MOLECULAR-WEIGHT AGENTS

Paul Cullinan,[1] **Ilenia Folleti,**[2] **Xavier Munoz,**[3] **Hille Suojalehto,**[4] **Katri Suuronen,**[5]
Marta Wiszniewska,[6] **Jean-Luc Malo,**[7] **and Olivier Vandenplas**[8]

[1]*Department of Occupational and Environmental Lung Disease, Imperial College (NHLI) and Royal Brompton Hospital, London, UK*
[2]*Department of Medicine and Surgery, Section of Occupational Medicine, University of Perugia, Terni Hospital, Terni, Italy*
[3]*Pneumology Department, Hospital Vall d'Hebron, and Physiology and Immunology*
Department, Universidad Autonoma de Barcelona, Barcelona, Spain
[4]*Finnish Institute of Occupational Health, University of Helsinki, Helsinki, Finland*
[5]*Finnish Institute of Occupational Health, Helsinki, Finland*
[6]*Department of Occupational Diseases and Environmental Health; Nofer Institute of Occupational Medicine, Lodz, Poland*
[7]*Hôpital du Sacré-Cœur de Montréal and Université de Montréal, Montréal, Québec, Canada*
[8]*Department of Chest Medicine, Centre Hospitalier Universitaire UCL Namur, Université Catholique de Louvain, Yvoir, Belgium*

Contents

Introduction

Agents causing occupational asthma (OA) can be divided into two groups: high-molecular-weight (HMW) and low-molecular-weight (LMW) agents. HMW agents are protein-derived antigens that cause sensitization through an immunoglobulin E (IgE)-mediated mechanism. Some of the HMW agents are covered in specific chapters: flour and baking additives (Chapter 12) and animals, including laboratory animals, insects, and seafoods (Chapter 13). In this chapter, various proteinaceous agents derived from plants causing OA are described.

LMW agents include reactive chemicals, metals (Chapter 16), and wood dusts (Chapter 15). Polyisocyanates remain the most often implicated cause of OA and are addressed in Chapter 14. Some LMW agents (i.e. acid anhydrides, platinum salts, reactive

dyes, sulfonechloramide) have been documented as inducing the production of specific IgE antibodies, but the immunological mechanisms of asthma induction remain largely uncertain for most LMW agents (Chapters 4 and 7). LMW agents are incomplete antigens (i.e. haptens) that must bind to carrier macromolecules such as airway proteins to become immunogenic. The potential diversity of chemical interactions with airway proteins could explain heterogeneous pathophysiological responses and our inability to identify specific IgE in OA caused by LMW agents. Typically, LMW agents are reactive, electrophilic molecules. Structure-activity modeling suggests that isocyanate (N=C=O), amine (NH2), and carbonyl (C=O) groups are associated with a sensitization capability, especially when two or more of them are found in the same molecule (1). Quantitative structure-activity relationship models have been developed in order to estimate the "asthma hazard index" of organic LMW chemicals and so predict their potential to cause OA (2).

OA caused by HMW and LMW agents shows distinct clinical phenotypic profiles that further support the categorization of agents causing OA into HMW and LMW agents (3). OA caused by HMW agents is more often associated with atopy, work-related rhinitis, early asthmatic reactions, and a greater postchallenge increase in fractional nitric oxide (FeNO) compared to LMW agents. By contrast, OA due to LMW agents is more frequently associated with daily sputum production and late asthmatic reactions.

A comprehensive list of the chemical agents that have been reported to cause OA together with the diagnostic evidence can be found in

https://reptox.cnesst.gouv.qc.ca/en/occupational-asthma/Pages/occupational-asthma.aspx

High-molecular-weight agents

Enzymes

Enzymes are "biocatalysts," which usefully accelerate and enhance chemical reactions. They have a very wide range of applications in the detergent, food, brewing, paper, cleaning, and pharmaceutical industries, among others (4). Enzyme development has been rapid and, largely through recombinant gene expression and protein engineering, it is now possible to tailor-make enzymes for very specific processes. The result has been the introduction of a bewildering array of enzymes to a growing range of industries (Table 18.1).

All enzymes are proteins, of up to 20 different amino acids, and consequently all are potential sensitizing agents; it is perhaps surprising, then, that OA from enzyme sensitization is not more widespread. This apparent disparity has several possible explanations: enzymes tend to be potent and may be used in only small quantities; they may, as in brewing, be used in enclosed systems with limited potential for workers to be exposed; and they are often used in liquid form with relatively low bioavailability to the respiratory tract. Workers and employers may be unaware that the agents with which they work contain enzymes since it is not always a requirement that they be listed in safety data sheets (SDSs); even when they are listed, they may be so only generically ("contains enzymes") or by an uninformative trade name.

The mechanism of action is that of a type I hypersensitivity and the clinical features are accompanied, and probably preceded, by the production of specific IgE antibodies. An important caveat is that there are very few standardized and commercially available

TABLE 18.1 Array of Enzyme Use in Industry

Industry	Enzyme Class (Examples)	Purpose	References[a] (Nonexhaustive)
Textile and dishwasher detergents	Protease	Stain removal	*Numerous (see text)*
	Amylase	"De-balling"	
	Lipase		
	Cellulase		
Baking	α-amylase	Acceleration of "proving"	*Numerous (see text)*
	Maltogenic amylase	Crumb improvement	*1. Elms, 2003*
	Cellulase	Extension of shelf-life	*2. Jones, 2016*
	Xylanase		*3. Merget, 2001*
	Lipase		
	Glucose oxidase		
Food industry	Papain/bromelain	Meat tenderizing	*4. Tarlo, 1978*
	Lipase/peptidase	(Cheese) flavoring	*5. Baur, 1979*
	Protease/lactase	Dairy products	*6. Casper, 2008*
	Pectinase/cellulase/gluconase	Fruit and vegetable pulping	*7. Hartmann, 1983*
			8. Sen, 1998
Brewing/wine-making/fruit juice	Pectinase	Brewing	*9. Veza, 2015*
		Wine-making	
		Fruit juice	
Animal feedstuff	Xylanase	Enhanced digestion	*10. O'Connor, 2001*
	Cellulase		*11. Vanhanen, 1997*
	Phytase		
Cleaning	Protease	Stain removal	*12. Adisesh, 2011*
	Amylase	Decontamination	
Paper manufacture	Cellulase	Wood pulp processing	*None reported*
Pharmaceuticals	Glucose oxidase	Blood glucose monitoring	*None reported*
	Penicillin acylase/glucose isomerase	Penicillin manufacture	*None reported*
	Cellulase/lactase	Digestive aids	*13. Losada, 1986*
			14. Bernstein, 1999
	Empynase	Anti-inflammatory	*15. Bahn, 2006*

[a] Reference numbers refer to bibliographic references detailed in this table's footnote.

References: **1.** Elms J, et al. *Occup Environ Med.* 2003;60:802–4; **2.** Jones M, et al. *Allergy.* 2016;71:997–1000; **3.** Merget R, et al. *Int Arch Allergy Immunol.* 2001;124:502–5; **4.** Tarlo SM, et al. *Clin Allergy.* 1978;8:207–15; **5.** Baur X, et al. *Clin Allergy.* 1979;9:75–81; **6.** Casper R, et al. *Allergy Asthma Proc.* 2008;29:376–9; **7.** Hartmann AL, et al. *Schweiz Med Wochenschr.* 1983;113:265–7; **8.** Sen D, et al. *Clin Exp Allergy.* 1998;28:363–7; **9.** Veza S, et al. *Occup Environ Med.* 2015;72:237–8; **10.** O'Connor TM, et al. *Occup Environ Med.* 2001;58:417–9; **11.** Vanhanen M, et al. *Scand J Work Environ Health.* 1997;23:385–91; **12.** Adisesh A, et al. *Occup Med (Lond).* 2011;61:364–9; **13.** Losada E, et al. *J Allergy Clin Immunol.* 1986;77:635–9; **14.** Bernstein JA, et al. *J Allergy Clin Immunol.* 1999;103:1153–7; **15.** Bahn JW, et al. *Clin Exp Allergy.* 2006;36:352–8.

assay materials and most enzymes require the use of bespoke material and an experienced laboratory. Here it is worth noting that apparently different enzymes produced through recombinant technology may be immunologically indistinguishable, especially if they have been produced through gene editing of the same microbial "host."

Detergent industry

While the first enzyme-enhanced detergent ("Burnus") was produced in 1913, the widespread manufacture of "biological" detergents started in the 1960s. In a familiar tale (5), the introduction of powdered proteases (Alcalase and Maxatase) at that time was rapidly followed by the development of epidemic OA detected first by an occupational physician working in north west England and then by others elsewhere (6, 7). In 1970 Belin and colleagues reported cases of sensitization in those using the new detergent powders at home (8) and, as a consequence, biological powders were temporarily removed from the market. Improvements in workplace dust control and the formulation of encapsulated, non-respirable enzymes allowed their reintroduction; there is now a very large, global market in textile and dishwashing detergents that contain not only proteases but also combinations of amylases, lipases, and cellulases. The range of individual enzymes is expanding rapidly and producers frequently change the combinations making it increasingly difficult to know to which enzymes a patient is (and has been) exposed at work.

Atopy and the intensity of exposure are the chief risk factors for OA in the detergent sector. Except in factories with very high standards of dust control, workers in this industry are at high risk of OA (9). This is especially the case where powdered or tablet products are being manufactured; those working in liquid-only plants appear to be at lower risk (10).

Baking

In order to increase the speed of its production, almost all bread is made using a combination of enzymes; since these are classified as process improvers they seldom appear on ingredient lists. Enzymes are responsible for around 10% of cases of OA in bakers (11). Bakers (and indeed employers) rarely know that the concentrate or improver that they add to their dough mixes contains fungal α-amylase and up to a dozen other enzymes. Fortunately, sensitization to nonamylase enzymes in the absence of amylase sensitisation appears to be rare (12).

Other environments

While the great majority of cases of OA from enzymes occur in the detergent and baking sectors, the very wide variety of other workplaces where enzymes are commonly used is summarized in Table 18.1. Instances of OA have been reported in most, sometimes as single or few case reports from clinics but often in larger numbers following full workplace surveys, a reminder that cases of OA seldom occur in isolation. The list also includes one or two sectors where although conditions make it probable that OA would occur, no cases have (yet) been reported; an example is paper manufacture where cellulase, in a readily aerosolisable form, is often used. Taken together, these observations suggest that enzyme-induced OA is likely to be considerably more widespread than is recognized.

Latex

Natural rubber latex (NRL) refers specifically to the milky fluid produced by the laticifers of the tropical rubber tree *Hevea brasiliensis*. NRL is widely used in the manufacturing of medical devices (gloves, catheters, drainage tubes, anesthetic masks, tourniquets, dental dams, etc.) as well as in the production of a variety of everyday articles, such as household gloves, toys, balloons, and condoms (13). In the late 1980s, following the introduction of universal precautions against viral infections, NRL gloves became a major cause of immediate IgE-mediated allergy reactions ranging from localized urticaria to extensive angioedema and life-threatening anaphylaxis (13). In addition, it was demonstrated that NRL proteins bind onto glove powder particles and can then act as airborne allergens causing rhinoconjunctivitis and asthma (14, 15).

Epidemiological surveys of workforces exposed to NRL gloves, mainly healthcare workers (HCW), showed that about half of NRL-sensitized workers develop occupational rhinitis and OA due to airborne NRL allergens (i.e. ~3% of exposed workers) (16, 17). OA caused by NRL has also been described in workers manufacturing medical gloves (18) and in nonmedical occupations with NRL glove exposure, such as food processors, chemical and pharmaceutical workers, hairdressers, cleaners, and greenhouse workers (19). OA induced by exposure to NRL dust has also been occasionally reported in workers manufacturing NRL toys (20) and in in the textile industry (21).

Intense research efforts were made to identify the allergen sources and delineate preventive strategies. These efforts led to the characterization of 15 NRL allergens (Table 18.2) and the development of assays for measuring the allergen content of NRL materials. Strategies to prevent the development of NRL allergy have been implemented at the local, national, and international levels since the early 1990s (22, 23). The development of powder-free, low-protein/allergen NRL gloves and the widespread substitution of powdered NRL gloves by NRL-free gloves for nonsterile healthcare procedures were associated with a sharp decline in the incidence of NRL allergy and OA (24–28).

TABLE 18.2 Natural Rubber Latex Allergens

Allergen	Biochemical Name	Clinical Relevance
Hev b 1	Rubber elongation factor	Major allergen in SB
Hev b 2	β-1,3-Glucanase	Uncertain
Hev b 3	Small rubber particle proteins	Major allergen in SB
Hev b 4	Lecithinase homologue	Minor allergen
Hev b 5	Acidic structural protein	Major allergen in HCW and important in SB
Hev b 6.01/6.02	Prohevein/hevein	Major allergen in HCW
Hev b 7	Patatin-like protein (esterase) from latex-B- and C-serum	Minor allergen
Hev b 8	Profilin (actin-binding protein)	Minor allergen
Hev b 9	Enolase	Minor allergen
Hev b 10	Manganese superoxide dismutase	Minor allergen
Hev b 11	Class I chitinase	Minor allergen
Hev b 12	Nonspecific lipid transfer protein type 1	Minor allergen
Hev b 13	Esterase	Uncertain
Hev b 14	Hevamine	Minor allergen
Hev b 15	Serine protease inhibitor	Minor allergen

Abbreviations: HCW, healthcare workers; SB, spina bifida patients.

NRL allergy is instructive in many respects. The story of NRL allergy demonstrated that potent allergens such as NRL proteins can cause the rapid development of IgE-mediated sensitization and clinical allergy reaching epidemic proportions in highly exposed populations. Translation of research findings into preventive strategies markedly altered the course of the NRL allergy outbreak within about 15 years. NRL allergy should be regarded as one of the few conditions where reduced workplace exposure to allergens alone proved highly effective in the primary prevention and management of an occupational allergy. However, the evidence pertaining to the prevention of NRL allergy is prominently derived from studies conducted in HCWs in high-income countries. Thus, its generalizability to other workers exposed to NRL gloves and to HCWs in economically developing settings must be assumed with caution and recent studies outline the need for ongoing vigilance (29, 30).

Beans, flowers, and allergens in greenhouses

Workers are frequently exposed to plant-derived allergens. In an analysis of the Australian Work Exposures Study, el-Zaemey and colleagues found that 13% of nearly 5000 workers were exposed to HMW asthmagens derived from plants, mainly as female farmers/animal workers, education workers, and food-processing workers (31). Various components of plants are allergenic but pollens remain the most likely to cause symptoms.

Among beans, castor beans have been incriminated as early as in the beginning of the twentieth century (32) followed by coffee beans and soybeans (Table 18.3). Although both green and

TABLE 18.3 Selected Studies of Occupational Asthma Due to Beans and Flowers

Agent	Occupation/ Workplace	Type of Report and Number of Subjects	Prevalence of Asthma, Rhinitis, or Respiratory Symptoms	Positive Skin Test (%) or Otherwise Specified	Increased Specific IgE	Positive Broncho/ Nasal Provocation Tests	References
Beans							
Green coffee beans	Coffee factory	372 workers	Asthma after starting to work: 2% Rhinitis: 43%	Green coffee beans: 10%	Green coffee beans: 6%	ND	*1. Jones, 1982*
Green coffee bean	Coffee manufacturing plant	31 green coffee workers 37 roasted coffee workers 44 clerks	WRR: 13% WRA: 7% WRA: 3% WRR: 0% WR symptoms: 2%	10% 3% 5%	ND	ND	*2. Larese, 1988*
Green coffee bean and castor bean	Coffee manufacturing plant	211 workers	Asthma: 16% RC: 10%	Green coffee beans: 15% Castor beans: 22%	ND	ND	*3. Romano, 1995*
Roasted coffee bean	Roastery coffee factory	22 symptomatic workers	ND	GCB extract: 82%	50% (GCB)	Bronchial: 36%+ Nasal: 32%+	*4. Osterman, 1985*
Roasted coffee bean	17 coffee roasting and packaging facilities	384 participants	WR upper respiratory symptoms: 11% WRA symptoms: 10%	ND	ND	ND	*5. Harvey, 2020*
Green coffee dust	Coffee roasting plant	41 nonsmoking women	WRA: 9%	Green coffee extract: 18% Roasted coffee: 9%	ND	ND	*6. Zuskin, 1981*
Castor bean (*Ricinus communis*)	Agricultural workers in Rumania	3000 workers	WRR: 35% WRA: 40%	80% + to 17 specific allergens in symptomatic workers; 12% positive in asymptomatic	ND	ND	*7. Lupu, 1962*
Soybean	Soybean processing plants in South Africa	181 workers (75%–80% participation)	WR nasal symptoms: 11% WR lower respiratory symptoms: 21%:	ND	32%	ND	*8. Harris-Roberts, 2012*
Locust bean gum	Cheesemaker at a creamery	1 worker	NA	ND	+ Locust bean gum	Functional improvement off-work	*9. Hawley, 2017*

Flowers

Agent	Occupation	Population	Symptoms	Skin test	Specific IgE	Challenge	Reference
Flowers (general)	Florists	128 florists in Turkey	WRA: 14% WRR: 13%	Flower mix extract: 9%	ND	ND	*10. Akpinar-Elci, 2004*
Flowers (general)	Ornamental plant growers	39 growers (98% participation)	Asthma attacks in the past year: 12.5%; confirmed OA (SIC): 5%	Workplace molds: 18% Workplace flower: 21%	ND	ND	*11. Monso, 2002*
Pollen of flowers (general)	Flower growers	75/105 flower growers	45% with nasal, respiratory, ocular symptoms	52%	ND	ND	*12. Goldberg, 1998*
Gysophila panniculata	Indoor carnation cultivation	16 symptomatic referred in clinic	WRR: 94% WRA: 94%	94% 94%	69%	Nasal: 81%+ Bronchial (PEF changes>20%): 88% +	*13. Sanchez-Guerrero, 1999*
Bell pepper	Greenhouse workers	472	WRR: 40% WRA: 12%	38%	35%	ND	*14. Groenewoud, 2002*
Weeping fig	Plant keepers	84	WRR: 94% of 18 symptomatic WRA: 33% of 18 symptomatic	30% (likely)	30% (likely)	4/6 bronchial challenges + 9/10 nasoconjunctival challenges +	*15. Axelsson, 1987*
Flowers of saffron	Saffron workers	50 workers	WRR: 26% WRA: 12%	6%	22%	Bronchial: 2% + Nasoconjunctival: 4% +	*16. Feo, 1985*
Sunflower pollen (*Helianthus annuus* pollen)	Sunflower processing factories	102 directly exposed employees	WRR: 35% WR respiratory symptoms: 17%	24%	ND	ND	*17. Atis, 2002*
Broccoli and cauliflower	5 producing companies	54 employees	WR symptoms: 44%	50%	33%	ND	*18. Hermanides, 2006*
Strawberry	Greenhouse workers	75 employees	WRR: 31% WRA: 4%	3 with work-related symptoms +	2 with work-related symptoms +	Nasal + in 2 workers	*19. Patiwael, 2010*
Chrysantenum	Greenhouse workers	104 workers	WRR: 48% WR symptoms of the lower airways: 8%	20%	11%	ND	*20. Groenewoud, 2002*
Chamomile	Maintenance worker	1	Asthma and rhinoconjunctivitis	+	+	Bronchial +	*21. Vandenplas, 2008*
Easter lily (*Lilium longiflorum*)	Floral shop worker	1	Asthma and rhinoconjunctivitis	+	+	Bronchial +	*22. Piirila, 1999*
Wall rocket (*Diplotaxis erucoides*)	Farmers (wine growers)	2	WRR and WRA	+ in two	+ in two	Bronchial + in one, conjunctival + in two	*23. Brito, 2001*
Rose (*Rosa rugosa*)	Rose culture	290 villagers in Turkey	Rose-related wheeze: 8%	19%	20% (8/41 sera)	ND	*24. Demir, 2002*

Abbreviations: GCB, text; NA, text; ND, text; OA, occupational asthma; PEF, peak expiratory flow; RC, text; SIC, specific inhalation challenge; WR, work-related; WRA, work-related asthma; WRR, work-related rhinitis.

References: **1.** Jones RN, et al. *Am Rev Respir Dis.* 1982;125:199–202; **2.** Larese F, et al. *Am J Ind Med.* 1998;34(6):623–7; **3.** Romano C, et al. *Clin Exp Allergy.* 1995;25:643–50; **4.** Osterman K, et al. *Allergy.* 1985;40:336–43; **5.** Harvey RR, et al. *Front Public Health.* 2020;Jan 30, 8:5. doi:10.3389/fpubh.2020.00005. eCollection 2020; **6.** Zuskin E, et al. *Thorax.* 1981;36:9–13; **7.** Lupu NG, et al. *Concours Méd.* 1962;84:5843–6; **8.** Harris-Roberts J, et al. *Am J Ind Med.* 2012;55:458–64; **9.** Hawley B, et al. *Am J Ind Med.* 2017;60:658–63; **10.** Akpinar-Elci M, et al. *Chest.* 2004;125:2336–9; **11.** Monso E, et al. *Am J Respir Crit Care Med.* 2002;165:954–60; **12.** Goldberg A, et al. *J Allergy Clin Immunol.* 1998;102:210–4; **13.** Sanchez-Guerrero IM, et al. *J Allergy Clin Immunol.* 1999;104:181–5; **14.** Groenewoud GCM, et al. *Clin Exper Allergy.* 2002;32:434–40; **15.** Axelsson IGK, et al. *Allergy.* 1987;42:161–7; **16.** Feo F, et al. *Allergy.* 1997;52:633–41; **17.** Atis S, et al. *Allergy.* 2002;57:35–9; **18.** Hermanides HK, et al. *Allergy.* 2006;61:498–502; **19.** Patiwael JA, et al. *Int Arch Allergy Immunol.* 2010;152:58–65; **20.** Groenewoud GCM, et al. *Allergy.* 2002;57:835–40; **21.** Vandenplas O, et al. *Allergy.* 2008;63:1090–2; **22.** Piirila P, et al. *Allergy.* 1999;54(3):273–7; **23.** Brito FF, et al. *J Allergy Clin Immunol.* 2001;108:125–7; **24.** Demir AU, et al. *Allergy.* 2002;57:936–9.

roasted beans can cause OA, green coffee beans seem more allergenic probably due to their higher antigenic content (33). Three relevant recombinant allergens for the specific diagnosis and/or therapy of coffee allergy were identified in workers of a coffee industry with work-related skin and respiratory symptoms, Cof a 1 (Chitinase) (34), Cof a 2, and Cof a 3 (metallothioneins) (35). Castor bean is a relevant occupational allergen because it is a contaminant in green coffee sacks (36, 37). Soybean and locust bean gum have also been reported as causing sensitization (Table 18.3).

Many decorative or horticultural flowers have been shown to induce OR and OA, mostly through an IgE-dependent mechanism. Although various parts of flower plants can cause sensitization, pollens seem to put more workers at risk, with a frequency of sensitization reaching nearly 50% in a study of flower growers (38) (Table 18.3). As a relevant example, pollen from peach tree (PT) can induce sensitization to Pru p 9 both in subjects working in PT cultivars and subjects living near crops (39). It has been suggested that immunological cross-reactivity of several pollens to mugwort pollen extract may be of predictive value in the identification of occupational allergy to flowers (40, 41).

Greenhouse workers and farmers are not only at risk of OR and OA to various flower-derived allergens but also to mites (Table 18.4). In a meta-analysis, Zhou and co-workers reported on 23 studies, with 13 conducted in Korea, that have examined the prevalence of sensitization to spider mites (42). The authors found that the overall frequency of sensitization was 22% with 7% being monosensitized and T. urticae being the most often reported sensitizing mite (15 studies) (42).

Low-molecular-weight agents

Acrylates

Acrylates, or acrylic resins, are reactive starting materials of acrylic polymers. The generic term *acrylates* is often used for all acrylic resins, which can be divided into three main structural subgroups: (plain) acrylates, methacrylates, and cyanoacrylates. Plain acrylates (having no methyl- nor cyano-side group) are encountered e.g. in UV-hardened products such as special adhesives, printing emulsions, and parquet varnishes. Methacrylates are hardened with peroxides or UV-light and used in dental and prosthetic materials, acrylic and gel nails, adhesives, coatings, and lamination resins. Cyanoacrylates harden in humid surroundings and are used as instant glues in e.g. wound sealing, artificial lash and nail work, and assembly. Glues and coatings based on methacrylates and plain acrylates often contain not only one acrylate compound but a mixture of several kinds. The harmful effects of acrylates are coupled to unhardened resins in liquid or semiliquid form whereas fully hardened acrylic plastics are not hazardous to health. Respiratory exposure to acrylates is dependent on their volatility and the process. For example, methyl methacrylate (MMA) and hydroxyethyl methacrylate (HEMA) are highly volatile and reach the airways easily, while poorly volatile acrylates do not end up in the air unless spraying, heating, or other related process is used.

TABLE 18.4　Selected Studies of Occupational Asthma Due to Mites Growing on Farms and in Greenhouses

Agent	Occupation/ Workplace	Type of Report and Number of Subjects	Prevalence of Asthma, Rhinitis, or Respiratory Symptoms	Positive Skin Test (%) or Otherwise Specified	Increased Specific IgE	Positive Broncho/Nasal Provocation Tests	References
Various mites	Farmers	188 cattle workers	WRR: 16% Probable OR: 5% WRA: 6% Probable OA: 3%	18%	NA	NA	*1. Patussi, 1994*
Tetranychus urticae	Greenhouses	246 workers	Symptoms suggestive of allergic disease in the greenhouse: 29%	25%	24/61 (39%)	NA	*2. Navarro, 2000*
Amblyseius Cucumeris	Greenhouses	472 workers	WRR: 72% WRA: 26%	23%	63/109 (58%)	11/23 (48%) + nasal challenge	*3. Groenewoud, 2002*
Predatory mites *P. persimilis and H. miles*	Greenhouses	31 workers	Not mentioned	NA	52%	NA	*4. Johansson, 2003*
Storage mites *L. destructor, T. putrescentiae, A siro*	General population in the ECRHS study in Northern Europe	1180 participants	Sensitization significantly associated with asthma and rhinitis. No sensitization in workers exposed to storage mites.	10%	NA	NA	*5. Jogi, 2020*

Abbreviations:　ECRHS: European Community Respiratory Health Survey; NA, not available; ; OA, occupational asthma; OR, text; WRA, work-related asthma; WRR, work-related rhinitis.

References:　**1.** Patussi V, et al. *Med Lav.* 1994;85(5):402–11; **2.** Navarro AM, et al. *Clin Exp Allergy.* 2000;30:863–6; **3.** Groenewoud GCM, et al. *Allergy.* 2002;57:614–9; **4.** Johansson E, et al. *Allergy.* 2003;58:337–41; **5.** Jogi NO, et al. *Clin Exp Allergy.* 2020;50:372–82.

TABLE 18.5 Case Series Reporting on Occupational Asthma Caused by Acrylate Compounds

Agents	Occupation	Number of Subjects	SPT	sIgE	SIC	References
Metacrylates Cyanoacrylates Plain acrylates	Manufacturing workers; assemblers; mechanics; painters; various industrial workers Dental care personnel Beauticians and hairdressers	55	0/22	NA	55/55	*1. Suojalehto H, 2020*
Methyl methacrylate Cyanoacrylates	Manufacturing workers; assemblers; teacher or teaching assistant; nail technician; dentist; orthopedic theater worker	20	NA	NA	3/20[a]	*2. Walters GI, 2017*
Methacrylates	Dental personnel	9	0/9	NA	9/9	*3. Piirilä P, 1998*
Cyanoacrylates Methacrylates Other acrylates	Manufacturing workers; assemblers; dental technician	15	NA	NA	15/15	*4. Savonius B, 1993*
Methyl methacylate Cyanoacrylates	Manufacturing worker; assemblers; solderer; dental assistant	6	NA	NA	6/6	*5. Lozewicz S, 1985*

[a] The diagnosis of OA was confirmed by consistent pattern of peak expiratory flow rates at work and off work in the 20 reported subjects.

Abbreviations: NA, not assessed; SIC, specific inhalation challenge; sIgE, specific IgE antibodies; SPT, skin-prick test.

References: **1.** Suojalehto H, et al. *J Allergy Clin Immunol Pract.* 2020;8:971–9; **2.** Walters GI, et al. *Occup Med.* 2017;67:282–9; **3.** Piirilä P, et al. *Clin Exp Allergy.* 1998;28:1404–11; **4.** Savonius B, et al. *Clin Exp Allergy.* 1993;23:416–24; **5.** Lozewicz S, et al. *Thorax.* 1985;40:836–9.

In 1985 Lozewicz et al. (43) reported isolated late or dual reactions after exposure to methylmethacrylate and cyanoacrylates. Since then numerous reports have described OA to acrylates. The prevalence of acrylate-induced OA among exposed workforces has never been formally evaluated. Series reporting the highest numbers of cases verified with specific inhalation challenge (SIC) are detailed in Table 18.5. Recently Suojalehto et al. described 55 acrylate-induced OA cases from several European centers (44). Acrylate-containing glues were the most prevalent products and industrial manufacturing, dental work, and beauty care the most frequently involved occupations. Acrylate-induced OA cases had more concomitant work-related rhinitis that isocyanate-induced OA and showed greater increase in postchallenge FeNO than other LMW-induced OA suggesting that acrylates may induce OA through different immunological mechanisms than other LMW agents.

Epoxy resins and amines

Epoxy resin systems

Epoxy resins (ER) pose superior technical qualities such as workability, good adhesion, and endurance, which make them popular in varied applications such as coatings, adhesives, composites, and modern sewage relining materials. ER nearly always appear as two-component systems, in which liquid or semiliquid resin and hardener are mixed. The resin part is usually based on diglycidylether of bisphenol A (DGEBA-ER) or diglycidylether of bisphenol F (DGEBF-ER). Hardeners of two-component ER systems are based on organic polyamines and their mixtures (Table 18.6). They are not only reactive organic molecules but also alkaline having irritant effects. ER themselves are nonvolatile, whereas reactive diluents and polyamines may be more easily evaporated into the breathing zone. Solvents, spraying, and heating of the resin-hardener mixture upon polymerization may enhance respiratory exposure also to poorly volatile ER components. ER systems are the most common causes of allergic contact dermatitis. These systems and their components, ER and polyamines, have been identified as causing OA (Table 18.7). The mechanism

by which these agents cause asthma remains controversial; evidence of immediate skin reactivity has been identified only in few cases. In some special products the resin and the hardener are in a ready-made mixture, which starts to polymerize when heated up. These one-component products contain organic acid anhydrides as hardeners (see section "Acid Anhydrides").

Amines

The term *amines* refers to a very heterogeneous group of organic molecules carrying one or more amine groups. Thus, various amines may be chemically and toxicologically quite different. In addition to ER systems, these compounds have numerous occupational uses (Table 18.6). Several different types of amines have been recognized to cause asthma. Of these, paraphenylenediamine is discussed in "Hairdressing Chemicals," quaternary ammonium salts and Chloramine-T in the "Biocides" section, and ethanolamine in the "Metalworking fluids" section. Examples of OA caused by other amines are presented in Table 18.7. IgE-mediated sensitization has not been shown for most of the amines, with the exception of piperazine (45).

Hairdressing products

Several epidemiological surveys have documented an increased risk of asthma among hairdressers (Table 18.8). Two studies investigated the prevalence of work-related asthma (WRA) symptoms in large samples of hairdressers (Table 18.8) (46, 47). In a random sample of 335 female hairdressers working in the Helsinki metropolitan area, a structured interview of 130 workers with work-related skin or respiratory symptoms categorized 46 subjects (13%) as "suspected WRA," of whom 3 (0.8% of 355) subjects were confirmed as having OA after clinical investigations that included PEF and SIC (46). Using a symptom-based classification tree among 1334 hairdressers in the city of Barcelona, Espuga et al. (47) identified 72 out of 174 subjects with a physician-based diagnosis of asthma has having possible OA, yielding an overall estimated prevalence rate of 7.8% (95% CI:6.4%–9.4%).

TABLE 18.6 Amines: Examples of Specific Compounds Causing Occupational Asthma and Their Uses

Class of Amines	Examples	Product Types	Uses and Occupations
Polyamines in epoxy resin systems	Trimethylhexane diamine Isophoronediamine	• Hardeners of two-component epoxy resins	• Industrial coating • Construction coating • Plastic industry
Other polyamines Para-amino compounds	Ethylenediamine Paraphenylenediamine (PPD)	• Photograph developers • Hair dyes	• Photography laboratory • Hairdressing • Fur-dyeing
Piperazine derivatives	• Piperazine • Piperazine citrate • N-methylpiperazine	• Chemical reagent/intermediate • Pharmaceuticals	• Production of chemicals and pharmaceuticals
Ethanolamines	• Monoethanolamine • Trietanolamine • Methyldietanolamine	• Corrosion inhibitors in metalworking fluids • pH adjusters in wax removers and detergents	• Metalworking • Cleaners and hospital assistants
Morpholine derivatives	• N-Methylmorpholine • 4,4-methylene-bismorpholine	• Antimicrobials (formaldehyde releasers) in metalworking fluids	• Machining • Tool setting
Other water-soluble amine derivatives	Ethylenediamine tetra-acetic acid (EDTA)	• Chelating (metal binding) agent in disinfectants and pharmaceuticals • Photographing chemicals	• Healthcare workers • Laboratory workers and biochemists • Photographers
Quaternary ammonium salts	• Benzalkonium chloride • Dodecyl dimethyl ammonium chloride	• Disinfectants • Antimicrobial agents	Healthcare and cleaning
Chloramine-T	Chloramine-T (sodium-chloro-toluenesulphonamide)	Disinfectants	Healthcare and cleaning

Hairdressers are exposed to a variety of substances that may induce OA (Table 18.8). However, the two agents that are most frequently involved in the development of OA among hairdressers are persulphate salts used in hair-bleaching products, which account for more than 90% of cases (46), and paraphenylendiamine, which is contained in hair dyes.

Individual case reports of OA due to persulphate salts were published as early as 1957 (48). Persulphate salts accounted for 2% to 12% of all OA cases reported to voluntary surveillance programs and compensation boards in European countries during the period 1995–2002 (49), being the second most frequent causal agent of OA in some countries, such as Catalunia, Spain (50), and France (51).

TABLE 18.7 Examples of Occupational Asthma Caused by Epoxy Resins and Amines

Agents	Occupation	Number of Subjects	SPT	sIgE	SIC	Other Evidence	References
Epoxy resin systems							
Epoxy resin and polyamine hardeners	Windmill wing builder, floor layer, automotive industry worker	5	NA	NA	5/5	BAT positive in 1 of 4 tested	*1. Brock Jacobsen, 2019*
Epoxy resin and polyamine hardeners	Industrial painters, construction workers, plumber/sewage pipe reliner	15	NA	NA	15/15		*2. Suojalehto, 2019*
Epoxy resin	Construction worker	1	1/1	1/1	1/1		*3. Hannu, 2009*
Polyamine hardener	Epoxy floor layer	1	NA	NA	1/1		*4. Vandenplas, 2017*
Polyamine hardeners	Chemical factory workers	12 (33%)[a]	NA	NA	2/2		*5. Ng, 1995*
Polyamine hardeners	Floor coverer	1	NA	NA	1/1	Eosinophilia after SIC in BAL and blood	*6. Aleva, 1992*
Other amines							
Piperazine derivatives	Chemical factory worker	1	1/1	NA	1/1		*7. Quirce, 2006*
Piperazine and derivatives	Chemists	2	1/2	NA	2/2		*8. Pepys, 1972*
Ethylene diamine	Photograph developing worker	1	0/1	0/1	1/1		*9. Lam, 1980*

[a] Prevalence of occupational asthma.

Abbreviations: BAL, bronchoalveolar lavage; BAT, basophil activation test; NA, not assessed; sIgE, specific IgE antibodies; SIC, specific inhalation challenge; SPT, skin-prick test.

References: **1.** Brock Jacobsen I, et al. *Occup Med.* 2019;69:511–514; **2.** Suojalehto H, et al. *J Allergy Clin Immunol Pract.* 2019;7:191–198; **3.** Hannu T, et al. *Int Arch Allergy Immunol.* 2009;148:41–3; **4.** Vandenplas O, et al. *Occup Med.* 2017;67:722–4; **5.** Ng TP, et al. *Occup Med.* 1995;45:45–8; **6.** Aleva RM, et al. *Am Rev Respir Dis.* 1992;145:1217; **7.** Quirce S, et al. *J Investig Allergol Clin Immunol.* 2006;16:138–9; **8.** Pepys J, et al. *Clin Allergy.* 1972;2:189–96; **9.** Lam S, et al. *Am Rev Respir Dis.* 1980;121:151–5.

TABLE 18.8 Epidemiological Surveys of Asthma among Hairdressers

Study Settings	Population	Risk of Asthma	References
Retrospective incidence study, population-based random sample of hairdressers, Finland (1980–1995)	• 4433 female hairdressers vs shop workers • Postal questionnaire	Incidence of asthma Sx: OR = 1.7 (1.1–2.5)	*1. Leino, 1997*
CS of 26 hair salons, New Zealand	• 100 hairdressers vs 106 office and shop workers • Administered questionnaire	Prevalence of asthma Sx: 24% in hairdressers vs 20% in controls; OR = 1.1 (0.5–2.2)	*2. Slater, 2000*
CS sample of hairdressers (unknown mode of selection), Norway	• 91 hairdressers vs 95 office workers • Postal questionnaire	Prevalence of wheezing >40 yrs: 56% in hairdressers vs 24% in office workers OR = 3.3 (1.0–11.0)	*3. Hollund, 2001*
Hairdressers graduated between 1970–1995 from 29 vocational schools, Sweden	• 3957 hairdresser vs random population sample • Postal questionnaire	Incidence of asthma Sx: 3.9 person-years RR = 1.3 (1.0–1.6)	*4. Albin, 2002*
Register-based longitudinal population survey, Finland	• 372 male and 376 female hairdressers vs administrative workers • Reimbursement of asthma medication	Incidence of asthma: - Males: OR = 2.1 (1.1–3.9) - Females : OR = 1.6 (1.4–1.8)	*5. Karjalainen, 2002*
Longitudinal study of a subgroup of hairdressing apprentices from 1 vocational school (1994–1997), France	• 191 hairdressers apprentices vs 189 office apprentices • Physician-administered questionnaire	Incidence of wheezing: OR = 0.8 (0.4–1.7) Incidence of NSBH: OR = 1.4 (0.5–3.9)	*6. Iwatsubo, 2003*

Abbreviations: CS, cross-sectional survey; NSBH, nonspecific bronchial hyperresponsiveness; OR, odds ratio (95% confidence interval); RR, rate ratio (95% confidence interval); Sx, symptoms.

References: **1.** Leino T, et al. *J Occup Environ Med.* 1997;39:534–9; **2.** Slater T, et al. *Occup Med (Lond).* 2000;50:586–90; **3.** Hollund BE, et al. *Occup Environ Med.* 2001;58:780–5; **4.** Albin M, et al. *Occup Environ Med.* 2002;59:119–23; **5.** Karjalainen A, et al. *Scand J Work Environ Health.* 2002;28:49–57; **6.** Iwatsubo Y, et al. *Occup Environ Med.* 2003;60:831–40.

In a multicenter European cohort of subjects with OA ascertained by a positive SIC between 2006 and 2015, persulphate salts accounted for 6.6% of all cases (3). Persulphate-induced OA has also been investigated among production workers (52, 53). Wrbitzky et al. (52) found a positive SPT with ammonium salts associated with work-related respiratory symptoms in 4 of 52 production plant workers, while Merget et al. (53). failed to document any case of OA in 32 employees of a persulphate producing chemical plant.

The immunological mechanisms by which these substances induce airway sensitization and OA have not yet been established. SPTs with persulphate salts diluted in phosphate buffered serum were positive in 5 of 8 subjects with a positive SIC with persulphate (54), but were negative in another series of 21 subjects with persulphate-induced OA (55) (Table 18.9). Foss-Skiftesvik et al. (56) failed to document any association between work-related respiratory symptoms and the result of the histamine release test with persulphate solutions.

A mouse model of ammonium persulphate-induced asthma was able to elicit an asthma-like response after dermal sensitization and subsequent intranasal instillation of ammonium persulphate, including airway hyperresponsiveness to methacholine, neutrophilic inflammation, increased levels of total serum IgE as well as T and B cell proliferation and increased production of IL-4, IL-10, and IL-13 (57). Airway hyperresponsiveness appeared immediately after challenge exposure and persisted for 4 days, while neutrophils increased only transiently (58).

Biocides

Biocides are broadly defined as a diverse group of substances including disinfectants, preservatives, insecticides, and pesticides used for the control of organisms that are harmful to human or animal health or that cause damage to natural or manufactured products.

Chloramine-T (N-chloro-4-methylbenzenesulfonamide), a chlorine-releasing sterilizing agent, has been widely used in the food and beverage industry, in water disinfection, and as a topical antiseptic. Chloramine-T was first reported as a potential cause of OA and OR through "atopic sensitivity" in workers of a pharmaceutical company producing chloramine tablets by Feinberg and Watrous in 1945 (59). The role of chloramine-T in inducing OA was later convincingly demonstrated by SIC and the identification of sIgE against chloramine-T conjugated to HSA (Table 18.10).

Other chlorine-releasing agents (e.g. calcium or sodium hypochlorite) are widely used for the disinfection of water in swimming pools. The free chlorine may react with nitrogen from human sources to form chloramines, the most volatile being nitrogen trichloride (trichloramine). Three workers showed a positive SIC to gaseous nitrogen trichloride, while challenge exposures to chlorine released from sodium hypochlorite were negative (60). An increased risk of asthma has been reported in indoor swimming pool workers compared to the general population, although the mechanisms underlying the respiratory effects of chloramines remain unknown (61).

Glutaraldehyde and other aldehydes are highly effective antimicrobial agents against viruses, bacteria, and mycobacteria without causing damage to fiber-optic equipment. Glutaraldehyde has been widely used in the hospital setting for cold sterilization of endoscopes and other medical instruments. A substantial number of cases of OA due to glutaraldehyde have been reported among HCWs, mainly endoscopy nurses (Table 18.10). sIgE antibodies against glutaraldehyde-HAS conjugates have been inconsistently found in affected workers, but Palczynski et al. (62) documented

TABLE 18.9 Agents Causing Occupational Asthma in Hairdressers

Agent	Number of Subjects	Prevalence	SPT	sIgE	SIC	References
Persulphates (hair bleach)	1	NA	+ 1/1	NA	+ 1/1	1. Pepys, 1976
	23	WRA: 7/23 (WS)	+ 1/14	NA	+ 4/14	2. Blainey, 1986
	1	NA	− 1/1	NA	+ 1/1	3. Gamboa, 1989
	1	NA	+ 1/1	− 1/1	+ 1/1	4. Parra, 1992
	38	9/38 (CS)	+ 11/38	NA	+ 9/38	5. Schwaiblmair, 1997
	3	WRA: 46/335 (WS)	+ 4/107	NA	+ 3/10	6. Leino, 1998
	8	NA	+ 5/8	NA	+ 7/8	7. Munoz, 2003
	47	21/47 (CS)	+ 0/14	NA	+ 21/44	8. Moscato, 2005
	18/19	2/18 (CS)	+ 0/18	NA	+ 2/18	9. Foss-Skiftesvik, 2016
Paraphenylendiamine (PPD, hair dyes)	2	2/47 (CS)	NA	NA	+ 2/4	8. Moscato, 2005
Hair dyes containing PPD	5	5/52 (CS)	− 4/5	NA	+ 5/9	10. Helaskoski, 2014
Formaldehyde (hair straightening)	2	NA	NA	NA	NA	11. Dahlgren, 2018
Henna (hair dye)	1	NA	+ 1/1	NA	+ 1/1	1. Pepys, 1976
	2	NA	+ 2/2	+ 2/2	+ 2/2	12. Starr, 1982
	1	NA	+ 1/1	+ 1/1	NA	13. Bolhaar, 2001
	1	NA	+ 1/1	NA	1/1	14. Villalobos, 2020
Senna (plant-derived hair dye)	1	NA	+ 1/1	+ 1/1	1/1	15. Helin, 1996
Eugenol (fragrance)	1	NA	− 1/1	NA	+ 1/1	16. Quirce, 2008
Hydrolyzed wheat protein (hair conditioner spray)	1	NA	+ 1/1	NA	+ 1/1	17. Airaksinen, 2013

[a] Hair dye production.

Abbreviations: CS, case series; NA, not assessed; PPD, paraphenylendiamine; SIC, specific inhalation challenge; sIgE, specific IgE antibodies; SPT, skin-prick test; WS, workforce prevalence study; WRA, work-related asthma symptoms.

References: **1.** Pepys J, et al. *Clin Allergy.* 1976;6:399–404; **2.** Blainey AD, et al. *Thorax.* 1986;41:42–50; **3.** Gamboa PM, et al. *Allergol Immunopathol (Madr).* 1989;17:109–11; **4.** Parra FM, et al. *Allergy.* 1992;47:656–60; **5.** Schwaiblmair M, et al. *Int Arch Occup Environ Health.* 1997;70:419–23; **6.** Leino T, et al. *Scand J Work Environ Health.* 1998;24:398–406; **7.** Munoz X, et al. *Chest.* 2003;123:2124–9; **8.** Moscato G, et al. *Chest.* 2005;128:3590–8; **9.** Foss-Skiftesvik MH, et al. *Clin Translation Allergy.* 2016;6:26; **10.** Helaskoski E, et al. *Ann Allergy Asthma Immunol.* 2014;112:46–52; **11.** Dahlgren JG, et al. *Toxicol Ind Health.* 2018;34:262–9; **12.** Starr JC, et al. *Ann Allergy.* 1982;48:98–9; **13.** Bolhaar ST, et al. *Allergy.* 2001;56:248; **14.** Villalobos V, et al. *J Investig Allergol Clin Immunol.* 2020;30:133–4; **15.** Helin T, et al. *Allergy.* 1996;51:181–4; **16.** Quirce S, et al. *Allergy.* 2008;63:137–8; **17.** Airaksinen L, et al. *Ann Allergy Asthma Immunol.* 2013;111:577–9.

a significant increase in eosinophil counts in bronchoalveolar lavage fluid and nasal washing after challenge exposure to glutaraldehyde in HCWs with OA and OR due to this compound. Other aldehyde derivatives (ortho-phthalaldehyde, succinaldehyde) have been proposed as less irritating and faster-acting alternatives to glutaraldehyde, but these compounds also have a high "asthma hazard index" (63) and OA due to ortho-phthalaldehyde has been documented by SIC (64).

Quaternary ammonium compounds (QAC), mainly benzalkonium chloride (alkyldimethylbenzyl ammonium chloride) and didecyldimethylammonium, have been increasingly used as disinfectants in healthcare environments and food-processing industries. A questionnaire survey of a large sample of hospital employees in France demonstrated that exposure to QACs increased significantly the risk of reported physician-diagnosed asthma and nasal symptoms at work, whereas no significant association was found with exposure to chlorinated products/bleach or glutaraldehyde (65). A number of reports have ascertained the role of QACs in the development of OA through SIC (Table 18.10). In addition, there is some evidence that the incidence of OA caused by QACs has increased over the last two decades, probably due to the increasing use of QAC-containing products to clean medical and surgical instruments as well as floors and surfaces in hospitals and food-processing facilities (Chapter 17). The French national network of occupational health surveillance and prevention (Réseau National de Vigilance et de Prévention des Pathologies Professionnelles) reported a significant increase

in OA related to exposure to QACs from 1.4% of cases reported in 2001 to 8.3% in 2009 (27). In contrast, OA due to aldehydes decreased from 6.8% in 2001 to 1.6% in 2009. A retrospective review of 335 subjects with OA ascertained by a positive SIC during the period 1992–2011 in a tertiary center in Belgium identified 17 (5.1%) subjects with OA due to cleaning products and/or disinfectants (66). The majority of the products that induced a positive SIC contained QACs (10 of 17), while glutaraldehyde was involved in 3 cases and both QAC and glutaraldehyde in one case. Almost all cases (16 of 17) were diagnosed after the year 2000. In addition, this study provided evidence supporting a specific hypersensitivity mechanism rather than a nonspecific irritant effect as 11 of the 17 (65%) positive SICs were associated with a significant postchallenge increase in sputum eosinophils (n=6), NSBH (n=3), or both of these outcomes (n=2).

In recent years, aldehydes have been increasingly replaced by peracetic acid and hydrogen peroxide mixtures for the decontamination of medical equipment. However, two reports suggested that these oxidizing compounds may induce OA despite a very low "asthma hazard index" (Table 18.10). Other antimicrobial agents have also been documented as causing OA, including (Table 18.10): hexachlorophene and Triclosan (topical antiseptic agents), chlorhexidine (skin disinfection and surgical instruments sterilization), isothiazolinone derivatives (i.e. microbicide and fungicide used as preservative in detergents and many other industrial products). A few anecdotal reports described OA due to fungicides and the insecticide tetramethrin (Table 18.10).

TABLE 18.10 Occupational Asthma Caused by Biocides

Agents	Occupation	Number of Subjects	SPT	sIgE	SIC	References
Chloramine-T	Brewery workers	7	+ 7/7	NA	NA	1. Bourne, 1979
	Brewery workers	1	NA	NA	+ 1/1	2. Charles, 1979
	Food processors, lab technicians, nurse	5	+ 4/4	+ 4/4	+ 3/3	3. Dijkman, 1981 4. Kramps, 1981
	Milk quality control	1	+ 1/1	+ 1/1	NPT	5. Wass, 1989
	Swimming pool cleaner	1	+ 1/1	+ 1/1	+ 1/1	6. Kujala, 1995
	HCWs	6	+ 6/6	+ 4/6	+ 6/6	7. Palczynski, 2003
	Nurse	1	− 1/1	+ 1/1	EB	8. Krakowiak, 2005
Chlorinamines	Swimming pool workers	3	ND	ND	+ 3/3	9. Thickett, 2002
Formaldehyde	Nurse (dialysis)	1	NA	NA	+ 1/1	10. Hendrick, 1975
Glutaraldehyde	Nurses (endoscopy)	4	NA	NA	+ 2/4	11. Corrado, 1986
	Nurses	5	NA	NA	+ 5/5	12. Gannon, 1995
	Nurses (endoscopy, operating theater)	21	NA	+ 7/21	+ 8/8 13 PEF +	13. Di Stefano, 1999
Ortho-phthalaldehyde	Nurse (endoscopy)	1	NA	NA	+ 1/1	14. Robitaille, 2015
QAC	Laundry worker (BAC)	1	− 1/1	NA	+ 1/1	15. Innocenti, 1978
	Pharmacist (BAC)	1	NA	NA	+ 1/1	16. Burge, 1994
	Cleaning products manufacture (BAC)	1	+ 1/1	− 1/1	+ 1/1	17. Bernstein, 1994
	Nurses (BAC)	3	NA	− 3/3[a]	+ 3/3	18. Purohit, 2000
	HCWs, cleaners (DDC)	24	NA	NA	+ 12/24	19. Bellier, 2015
Hexachlorophene	Nurse	1	− 1/1	NA	+ 1/1	20. Nagy, 1984
	Nursery nurse (Triclosan)	1	NA	NA	+ 1/1	21. Walters, 2017
Chlorhexidine	Nurses	2	NA	NA	+ 2/2	22. Waclawski, 1989
Peracetic acid-hydrogen peroxide	Nurse (endoscopy)	2	NA	NA	+ 1/1 + PEF 1/1	23. Cristofari-Marquand, 2007
	Environmental microbiologist	1	NA	NA	+ 1/1	24. Walters, 2019
Isothiazolinones	Isothiazolinone production	1	NA	NA	+ 1/1	25. Bourke, 1997
	Detergent manufacture	1	NA	NA	+ 1/1	26. Moscato, 1997
Chlorothalonil	Farmer	1	NA	− 1/1	+ 1/1	27. Honda, 1992
	Fungicide production	1	NA	NA	+: 1	28. Draper, 2003
Tributyl tin oxide	Carpet fungicide	1	NA	- 1/1	+ 1/1	29. Shelton, 1992
Captafol (Difolatan)	Fungicide production	1	NA	NA	+ 1/1	30. Royce, 1993
Fluazinam	Fungicide production	1	NA	NA	+ 1/1	28. Draper, 2003
Tetramethrin	Insecticide applicator	1	1/1	NA	+ 1/1	31. Vandenplas, 2000

[a] Determination of sIgE levels against "quaternary ammonium reactive groups."

Abbreviations: BAC, benzalkonium chloride (alkyldimethylbenzylammonium chloride); DDC, didecyldimethylammonium chloride; EB, eosinophilic bronchitis; HCW, healthcare worker; NA, not assessed; NPT, nasal provocation test; PEF, peak expiratory flows at work and off work; QAC, quaternary ammonium compounds, sIgE, specific IgE antibodies; SIC, specific inhalation challenge; SPT, skin-prick test.

References: 1. Bourne MS, et al. *BMJ.* 1979;2:10–2; 2. Charles TJ. Br Med J 1979;2:334; 3. Dijkman JH, et al. *Int Arch Allergy Appl Immunol.* 1981;64:422–7; 4. Kramps JA, et al. *Int Arch Allergy Appl Immunol.* 1981;64:428–38; 5. Wass U, et al. *Clin Exp Allergy.* 1989;19:463–71; 6. Kujala VM, et al. *Respir Med.* 1995;89:693–5; 7. Palczynski C, et al. *Int J Occup Med Environ Health.* 2003;16:231–40; 8. Krakowiak AM, et al. *Occup Med (Lond).* 2005;55:396–8; 9. Thickett KM, et al. *Eur Respir J.* 2002;19:827–32; 10. Hendrick DJ, et al. *BMJ.* 1975;1:607–8; 11. Corrado OJ, et al. *Human Toxicol.* 1986;5:325–8; 12. Gannon PF, et al. *Thorax.* 1995;50:156–9; 13. Di Stefano F, et al. *Allergy.* 1999;54:1105–9; 14. Robitaille C, et al. *Occup Environ Med.* 2015;72:381; 15. Innocenti A. *Med Lav.* 1978;69:713–5; 16. Burge PS, et al. *Thorax.* 1994;49:842–3; 17. Bernstein JA, et al. *J Allergy Clin Immunol.* 1994;94:257–9; 18. Purohit A, et al. *Int Arch Occup Environ Health.* 2000;73:423–7; 19. Bellier M, et al. *J Allergy Clin Immunol Pract.* 2015;3:819–20; 20. Nagy L, et al. *Thorax.* 1984;39:630–1; 21. Walters GI, et al. *Ann Allergy Asthma Immunol.* 2017;118:370–1; 22. Waclawski ER, et al. *BMJ.* 1989;298:929–30; 23. Cristofari-Marquand E, et al. *J Occup Health.* 2007;49:155–8; 24. Walters GI, et al. *Occup Med (Lond).* 2019;69:294–7; 25. Bourke SJ, et al. *Thorax.* 1997;52:746–8; 26. Moscato G, et al. *Occup Med (Lond).* 1997;47:249–51; 27. Honda I, et al. *Thorax.* 1992;47:760–1; 28. Draper A, et al. *Occup Environ Med.* 2003;60:76–7; 29. Shelton D, et al. *J Allergy Clin Immunol.* 1992;90:274–5; 30. Royce S, et al. *Chest.* 1993;103:295–6; 31. Vandenplas O, et al. *Allergy.* 2000;55:417–8.

Pharmaceutical products

A large number of pharmaceutical products have been documented as causing OA among exposed workers, predominantly pharmaceutical industry and HCWs. Most of these products are LMW compounds (Table 18.11), while a few are HMW agents from plant origin (Table 18.12). The LMW pharmaceutical products that were most frequently involved in OA are antibiotics, mainly beta-lactams and related compounds and precursors, such as aminopenicillanic and aminocephalosporanic acids (Table 18.11) (67).

As with most other LMW causes of OA, the immunological mechanisms underlying the development of OA induced by LMW pharmaceutical agents remain uncertain. A systematic review of antibiotic-induced OA found that all implicated antibiotics show a very high "asthma hazard index" (0.99 to 1.00)

TABLE 18.11 Pharmaceutical Products Causing Occupational Asthma: Low-Molecular-Weight Compounds

Agent	Number of Subjects (Occupation)	SPT	sIgE	SIC	References
Antibiotics and related compounds					
Ampicillin, benzyl penicillin, 6-APA	3 (PIW)	—	NA	+ 3/3	*1. Davies, 1974*
6-APA	1 (PIW)	NA	NA	+ 1/1	*2. Diaz Angulo, 2011*
Amoxicillin	1 (PIW)	NA	NA	+ 1/1	*3. Vandenplas, 1997*
	1 (PIW)	– 1/1	+ 1/1	+ 1/1	*4. Jimenez, 1998*
	2 (PIW)	NA	+ 2/2	+ 2/2	*2. Diaz Angulo, 2011*
Piperacillin sodium	1 (PIW)	+ 1/1	NA	+ 1/1	*5. Moscato, 1995*
Cephalexin	1 (PIW)	+ 1/1	NA	+ 1/1	*6. Coutts, 1981*
Ceftazidime	1 (PIW)	NA	NA	+ 1/1	*7. Stenton, 1995*
Cefadroxil	1 (PIW)	– 1/1	– 1/1	+ 1/1	*8. Sastre, 1999*
Cefteram pivoxil	2 (PIW)	+ 2/2	+ 2/2	+ 2/2	*9. Suh, 2003*
7-ACA	1 (PIW)	+ 1/1	NA	+ 1/1	*6. Coutts, 1981*
	2 (PIW)	+ 1/2	– 2/2	+ 2/2	*10. Park, 2004*
7-TACA	1 (PIW)	NA	NA	+ 1/1	*11. Pala, 2009*
Spiramycin	1 (PIW)	+ 1/1	NA	+ 1/1	*12. Davies, 1975*
	2 (PIW)	– 2/2	NA	+ 2/2	*13. Moscato, 1984*
	51 (PIW)	NA	NA	+ 4/15	*14. Malo, 1988*
Erythromycine	1 (PIW)	NA	– 1/1	+ 1/1	*2. Diaz Angulo, 2011*
Clarithromycin	1 (PIW)	NA	NA	+ 1/1	*15. Valverde-Monge, 2019*
Tetracycline	1 (PIW)	+ 1/1	NA	+ 1/1	*16. Menon, 1977*
Isonicotinic acid hydrazide	1 (pharmacist)	+ 1/1 (ID)	NA	+ 1/1	*17. Asai, 1987*
Thiamphenicol	3 (PIW)	+ 2/3	+ 2/3	+ 3/3	*18. Ye, 2006*
Vancomycin	1 (PIW)	– 1/1	– 1/1	PEF	*19. Choi, 2009*
Colistin	1 (PIW)	NA	– 1/1	+ 1/1	*20. Gomez-Olles, 2010*
Other drugs					
Alpha-methyldopa	1 (PIW)	– 1/1	NA	+ 1/1	*21. Harries, 1979*
Cimetidine	4 (PIW)	– 4/4	NA	+ 1/4	*22. Coutts, 1984*
Penicillamine	1 (PIW)	– 1/1	NA	+ 1/1	*23. Lagier, 1989*
Hydralazine	1 (PIW)	– 1/1	– 1/1	+ 1/1	*24. Perrin, 1990*
Mitoxantrone	1 (HCW)	NA	NA	+ 1/1	*25. Walusiak, 2002*
Thiamine	1 (cereal production)	NA	– 1/1	+ 2/2	*26. Drought, 2005*
Aescin	1 (PIW)	NA	NA	+ 1/1	*27. Munoz, 2006*
Sevoflurane	2 (HCW)	NA	NA	+ 2/2	*28. Vellore, 2006*
5-aminosalicylic acid	1 (PIW)	– 1/1	NA	+ 1/1	*29. Sastre, 2010*
Tafenoquine	1 (PIW)	NA	– 1/1	+ 1/1	*30. Cannon, 2015*
Ranitidine	1 (PIW)	– 1/1	NA	+ 1/1	*31. Henriquez-Santana, 2016*
Minoxidil	1 (hair care)	– 1/1	NA	+ 1/1	*15. Valverde-Monge, 2019*
Glucosamine hydrochloride	1 (PIW)	NA	NA	+ 1/1	*15. Valverde-Monge, 2019*

Abbreviations: 6-APA, 6-aminopenicillanic acid; 7-ACA, 7-aminocephalosporanic acid; 7-TACA, 7-amino-3-thiomethyl-3-cephalosporanic acid; HCW, healthcare worker; ID, intradermal skin test; NA, not assessed; PEF, peak expiratory flow rates at work and off work; PIW, pharmaceutical industry worker; SIC, specific inhalation challenge; sIgE, specific IgE antibodies; SPT, skin-prick test.

References: **1.** Davies RJ, et al. *Clin Allergy.* 1974;4:227–47; **2.** Diaz Angulo S, et al. *J Allergy.* 2011;2011:365683; **3.** Vandenplas O, et al. *Allergy.* 1997;52:1147–9; **4.** Jimenez I, et al. *Allergy.* 1998;53:104–5; **5.** Moscato G, et al. *Eur Respir J.* 1995;8:467–9; **6.** Coutts, II, et al. *BMJ.* 1981;283:950; **7.** Stenton SC, et al. *Eur Respir J.* 1995;8:1421–3; **8.** Sastre J, et al. *Eur Respir J.* 1999;13:1189–91; **9.** Suh YJ, et al. *J Allergy Clin Immunol.* 2003;112:209–10; **10.** Park HS, et al. *J Allergy Clin Immunol.* 2004;113:785–7; **11.** Pala G, et al. *Allergy.* 2009;64:1390–1; **12.** Davies RJ, et al. *Clin Allergy.* 1975;5:99–107; **13.** Moscato G, et al. *Clin Allergy.* 1984;14:355–61; **14.** Malo JL, et al. *Thorax.* 1988;43:371–7; **15.** Valverde-Monge M, et al. *J Allergy Clin Immunol Pract.* 2019;7:740–2 e1; **16.** Menon MP, et al. *Clin Allergy.* 1977;7:285–90; **17.** Asai S, et al. *J Allergy Clin Immunol.* 1987;80:578–82; **18.** Ye YM, et al. *Allergy.* 2006;61:394–5; **19.** Choi GS, et al. *Allergy.* 2009;64:1391–2; **20.** Gomez-Olles S, et al. *Chest.* 2010;137:1200–2; **21.** Harries MG, et al. *BMJ.* 1979;1:1461; **22.** Coutts IL, et al. *BMJ.* 1984;288:1418; **23.** Lagier F, et al. *Thorax.* 1989;44:157–8; **24.** Perrin B, et al. *Thorax.* 1990;45:980–1; **25.** Walusiak J et al. *Allergy.* 2002;57:461; **26.** Drought VJ, et al. *Allergy.* 2005;60:1213–4; **27.** Munoz X, et al. *Ann Allergy Asthma Immunol.* 2006;96:494–6; **28.** Vellore AD, et al. *Allergy.* 2006;61:1485–6; **29.** Sastre J, et al. *Occup Environ Med.* 2010;67:798–9; **30.** Cannon J, et al. *Occup Med (Lond).* 2015;65:256–8; **31.** Henriquez-Santana A, et al. *Ann Allergy Asthma Immunol.* 2016;117:88–9.

TABLE 18.12 Pharmaceutical Products Causing Occupational Asthma: High-Molecular-Weight Agents

Agent	Number of Subjects (Occupation)	Prevalence According to Diagnostic Criteria	SPT	sIgE	SIC	References
Psyllium	3 (PIW)	NA	+ 3/3	NA	+ 2/3	*1. Busse, 1975*
	5 (HCW)	NA	+ 4/5	+ 5/5	+ 5/5	*2. Cartier, 1987*

	130/140 (PIW)	• Positive SIC: 3.8% (5/130)
		SIC performed in 18/21 workers with:
		  • NSBH and positive SPT (n=10) or
		  • Increase in NSBH at work (n=4) or
		  • Fall in FEV_1 >10% at work (n=13)
		  • WRA: 39/140 (28%)
		  • SPT and/or sIgE: 39/120 (32%)
			+ 23/120	+ 31/118	+ 5/18	*3. Bardy, 1987*

	198/248 (HCW)	• Positive SIC: 4.0% (8/198)[a] SIC performed in 10 subjects with: SPT and/or sIgE • WRA: 20/193 (10%)	+ 10/198	+ 24/164	+ 8/10	*4. Malo, 1990*
Ipecacuanha	42 (PIW)	• Work-related "asthma and/or rhinitis" and positive SPT or sIgE: 26.2% (11/42)	+ 12/39	+ 14/32	NA	*5. Luczynska, 1984*
Papaver somniferum	28/30 (PIW)	• Positive SIC: 14.3% (4/28) SIC: performed in 4 of 6 subjects with WRA and positive SPT or sIgE • WRA: 21.4% (6/28)	+ 4/26	+ 6/28	+ 4/6	*6. Moneo, 1993*
Ferrimanitol ovalbumin	1 (PIW)	NA	+ 1/1	+ 1/1[a]	+ 1/1	*7. Valverde-Monge, 2019*

[a] Western blot showing a single IgE-binding band of 200 kDa.

Abbreviations: HCW, healthcare worker; NA, not assessed; NSBH, nonspecific bronchial hyperresponsiveness; PIW, pharmaceutical industry worker; SIC, specific inhalation challenge; sIgE, specific IgE antibodies; SPT, skin-prick test; WRA, work-related asthma symptoms.

References: **1.** Busse WW, et al. *Ann Intern Med.* 1975;83:361–2; **2.** Cartier A, et al. *Clin Allergy.* 1987;17:1–6; **3.** Bardy JD et al. *Am Rev Respir Dis.* 1987;135:1033–8; **4.** Malo JL, et al. *Am Rev Respir Dis.* 1990;142:1359–66; **5.** Luczynska CM, et al. *Clin Allergy.* 1984;14:169–75; **6.** Moneo I, et al. *Allergol Immunopathol (Madr).* 1993;21:145–8; **7.** Valverde-Monge M, et al. *J Allergy Clin Immunol Pract.* 2019;7:740–2 e1.

using a quantitative structure-activity relationship analysis (67). The high prevalence of associated occupational rhinitis among subjects described in published case reports of OA caused by LMW pharmaceutical agents (55 of 76; 71%), suggests that these compounds may induce OA through an IgE-mediated mechanism similar to that involved in OA due to HMW agents (44) (see Chapter 22). An IgE-associated mechanism has been documented by SPT and/or sIgE against hapten-protein conjugates in about half of the reported cases evaluated by immunological tests (Table 18.11). However, a Korean survey of 161 HCWs found that 17.4% of the subjects showed sIgE against one of the three most frequently used cephalosporins conjugated to HSA, but the presence of sIgE antibodies did not correlate with work-related upper or lower respiratory symptoms (68). In the specific context of OA, the value of SPT and available sIgE assays for the investigation of immunological sensitization to LMW pharmaceuticals remains unclear. Notably, oral challenges with the antibiotic causing OA that also induced an asthmatic reaction and other systemic allergic symptoms have been reported in several case reports (67).

Very few informative surveys on the prevalence of OA caused by LMW pharmaceutical agents are available (67). In a survey of 51 employees of a pharmaceutical company producing spiramycin, Malo et al. reported a positive SIC in 4 of 15 workers who had WRA symptoms and baseline NSBH to methacholine or a significant increase in the level of NSBH during a spiramycin production period (Table 18.11). The investigators concluded that the prevalence estimate of OA caused by spiramycin was at least 7.8%. A survey of 33 opiates production workers (unknown participation rate) documented a variability in PEF >20% compared to a nonwork period in 10 of 32 workers and a cross-shift fall FEV_1 of more than 10% in 5 of 30 subjects (69). However, SIC with the suspected opiate dusts were not performed.

In contrast, cross-sectional workforce surveys investigated the prevalence of OA among workers exposed to HMW pharmaceuticals products, including psyllium (laxative), ipecacuanha (expectorant), and *Papaver somniferum* (Table 18.12). The three surveys that used SIC as a final confirmatory step found prevalence estimates of OA ranging from 3.8% to 14.3%.

Metalworking fluids

Metalworking fluids (MWFs) are a range of oils and other liquids that are used to cool and/or lubricate metal workpieces to reduce the heat and friction between the cutting tool and the workpiece, and help to prevent burning and smoking. There are four general classes of MWF: straight oils, soluble oils, synthetic, and semisynthetic (70). MWFs contain different substances, some of which are well-known as irritants or allergens, causing skin diseases, respiratory disorders, and asthma (Table 18.13), and in some cases intoxication or cancers.

Workers exposed to even low airborne concentrations of MWF significantly more likely reported asthma symptoms as well as WRA symptoms than unexposed participants (71, 72). Kennedy et al. concluded that exposure to water-based MWFs (especially synthetic fluids) is associated with increasing BHR during the first 2 years of exposure (73). A significant proportion of inhalable particles of MWF is represented by endotoxins (74).

TABLE 18.13 Occupational Asthma Caused by Metalworking Fluids

Agent	Occupation	Number of Subjects	Prevalence	SPT	sIgE	SIC	Other Evidence	References
Emulsified oils mist	Tool setter and machine operator	1	NA	NA	NA	+	Improvement off-work	1. Hendy MS et al., 1985
Metalworking fluid	Workers of an automobile parts engine manufacturing plant	12	1.5%	NA	NA	NA	PC20, FEV1	2. Zacharisen et al., 1998
Oil mists	Tool setter, machine tool operator	6	66%	NA	NA	+	Peak flow response is heterogeneous	3. Robertson et al., 1988
Triethalomanine	Metal-tooling using cutting fluid	1	NA	NA	NA	+		4. Savonius et al., 1994
Diethanolamine	Metal worker; cutting fluid	1	NA	NA	NA	+		5. Piipari et al., 1998
Biocide additive 4,4-methylene-bismorpholine present in clean MWF	Machine tool setter operator	1	NA	NA	NA	+		6. Walters et al., 2013
Metalworking fluids	Factory machinist assembling automobile parts	1	NA	NA	NA		In induced sputum the intense neutrophilic bronchitis without eosinophilia	7. Leigh R and Hargreave FE, 1999
Metalworking fluids (general)	Compensation in Switzerland (2004–2013)	96	Of 1385 workers exposed to MWF and compensated 7% were subjects with respiratory conditions, 2.2% with asthma	NA	NA	NA	NA	8. Koller MF et al., 2016

Abbreviations: FEV$_1$, forced expiratory volume in 1 second; NA, not assessed; ND: not doneMWF: metalworking fluid; SIC, specific inhalation challenge; sIgE, specific IgE antibodies; SPT, skin-prick test.

References: **1.** Hendy MS, et al. *Br J Ind Med.* 1985; 42:51–54; **2.** Zacharisen MC, et al. *J Occup Env Med.* 1998;40:640–7; **3.** Robertson AS, et al. *Thorax.* 1988; 43:200–205; **4.** Slavonius B. *Allergy.* 1994;49:877–81; **5.** Piipari R, et al. *Clin Exp Allergy.* 1998;28:358–62; **6.** Walters GI, Moore VC, et al. *Eur Respir J.* 2013 Oct;42(4):1137–9; 7. Leigh R, Hargreave FE. *Can Respir J.* 1999 Mar-Apr;6(2):194–6; **8.** Koller MF, et al. *Int J Occup Environ Health.* 2016;22:193–200.

Rosenman et al. reported that approximately 20% of the workers exposed to MWFs had daily or weekly respiratory symptoms suggestive of WRA. Workers exposed to emulsified, semisynthetic, or synthetic machining coolants were more likely to have chronic bronchitis; to have visited a doctor for shortness of breath or a sinus problem; and to have an increased prevalence of respiratory symptoms consistent with WRA, compared to workers exposed to mineral oil MWFs (75).

In an industrialized part of the United Kingdom the MWFs were responsible for 11% of OA (76). Burge et al. emphasize that serial PEF responses to MWF aerosols do not distinguish OA from alveolitis except in timing; PEF can be used to identify the workplace as the cause of asthma and also alveolitis (77). Ilgaz et al. tried to quantify the effectiveness of air-fed respiratory protective equipment (RPE) in workers with sensitizer-induced OA exposed to MWF aerosols in a car engine and transmission manufacturing facility, and they found that the RPE reduced falls in PEF associated with work exposure, but this was rarely complete. They suggest that RPE use cannot be relied on to replace source control in workers with OA, and that monitoring post-RPE introduction is needed (78).

Acid anhydrides

Organic dicarboxylic acid anhydrides (Table 18.14) are highly reactive chemicals that are widely used as cross-linking agents in the production of epoxy, alkyd, and polyester resins for the manufacture of coatings, adhesives, and thermoplastics (79). A halogen—chlorine or bromine—in the molecule confers flame-retardant properties. Exposure to anhydrides occurs either in powder form or as fumes when anhydrides are used at elevated temperatures during resin curing or when they are released as thermal degradation products (e.g. welding on resin-coated metal surfaces) (79).

Besides their irritant effects, acid anhydrides can cause different forms of immunologically mediated respiratory diseases (80): (i) a cytotoxic syndrome that results in pulmonary hemorrhage with hemoptysis and anemia, (ii) a hypersensitivity pneumonitis-like "late respiratory systemic syndrome," and (iii) OA associated with sIgE antibodies.

Kern (81) was the first to describe a case of OA due to PA and to suggest the IgE-mediated induction of the disease. Later, it was shown that acid anhydrides can act as haptens (82, 83), elicit the production of sIgE antibodies, and cause OA, usually preceded by OR (84–86). A number of studies have convincingly documented the role of various acid anhydrides in the development of OA among exposed workers (Table 18.14). Of note, most reports and epidemiological surveys of anhydride-induced OA were published more than 20 years ago, suggesting that the burden of the disease has decreased over time probably in relation to improved workplace exposure control (87).

IgE-mediated sensitization has been documented by SPTs with anhydrides conjugated to human serum albumin (HAS) and by

TABLE 18.14 Acid Anhydrides Causing Occupational Asthma

Agent	Occupation	Number of Subjects	Prevalence (%)	SPT	sIgE	SIC	References
Chorendic anhydride (CA)	Welding coated metal	1	NA	+ 1/1	+ 1/1	+ 1/1	*1. Keskinen, 2000*
Hexahydrophthalic anhydride (HHPA)	Electronic component coating	1	NA	NA	NA	+ 1/1 (PEF)	*2. Chee, 1991*
	Electronic component molding	27 (WS)	WRA: 4/27 (15%)	NA	+ 12/27 + 4/4 with WRA	NA	*3. Moller, 1985*
HHPA, Methyl-HHPA	Plants manufacturing electrical capacitors, ignition system, grenade barrels	163 (PC)	WRA: 12/144 (8.5%); Incidence: 31 per 1000 person-yr	13/163; Incidence: 3.0/1000 mo	21/163; Incidence: 4.1/1000 mo	NA	*4. Welinder, 2001* *5. Nielsen, 2006*
Himic anhydride (HA)	Flame-retardant manufacture	20 (WS)	WRA: 3/20 (15%)	NA	+ 3/3 with WRA	NA	*6. Rosenman, 1987*
Maleic anhydride (MA)	Polyester resin production	1	NA	NA	NA	+ 1/1	*7. Lee, 1991*
Methyltetrahydrophthalic anhydride (MTHPA)	Plastic products manufacture	164	WRA: 18/164 (11%)	+ 25/164	+ 28/164	NA	*8. Nielsen, 1992*
MTHPA+HHPA	Electrical plant	110 (WS)	WRA: 14/110 (13%) OA: 6/110 (5.5%)	15/110	+ 16/109	+ 6/8	*9. Drexler, 1994*
Phthalic anhydride (PA)	Plastic molding, coating manufacture	3	NA	NA	NA	+ 3/3	*10. Fawcett, 1977*
	Alkyd and polyester resin production	118 (WS)	WRA: 21/118 (18%)	+ 3/11 with WRA	NA	NA	*11. Wernfors, 1986*
	Alkyd resin production	60 (WS)	WRA: 5/60 (8%)	+ 1/5 with WRA	+ 4/57 + 1/5 with WRA	+ 1/1	*12. Nielsen, 1988*
Pyromellitic dianhydride (PMDA)	Plastic foil manufacture	3	NA	NA	+ 1/3	+ 3/3	*13. Madsen, 2019*
Tetrachlorophthalic anhydride (TCPA)	Epoxy resins production	5	NA	NA	NA	+ 5/5	*14. Schlueter, 1978*
	Electronic component encapsulation	7	NA	+ 7/7	+ 7/7	+ 4/4	*15. Howe, 1983*
	Epoxy resin coating	52 (WS)	WRA: 18/52 (35%)	NA	+ 15/49	NA	*16. Liss, 1993*
Trimellitic anhydride (TMA)	TMA production	4	NA	+ 4/4	+ 3/4	NA (> 50% change in FEV_1 at work + 1/1)	*17. Zeiss, 1977*
	TMA production	119 (PC)	10/119 (8.4%)	NA	9/10 with WRA	NA	*18. Grammer, 1998*
Various: PA, MA, TMA	3 alkyd resin manufacturing plants and 1 flooring manufacturer	401 (WS)	WRA: 34/401 (8.5%)	12/378	NA	NA	*19. Barker, 1998*

Abbreviations: NA, not assessed; OA, occupational asthma based on a positive specific inhalation challenge result; PEF, peak expiratory flow rates at work and off work; PC, prospective cohort study (mean follow-up of 32 months [ref. 4 and 5] and 5 years [ref. 18]); SIC, specific inhalation challenge; sIgE, specific IgE antibodies; SPT, skin-prick test; WRA, work-related asthma based on questionnaire; WS, workforce survey.

References: **1.** Keskinen H, et al. *Allergy.* 2000;55:98–9; **2.** Chee CB, et al. *Br J Ind Med.* 1991;48:643–5; **3.** Moller DR, et al. *J Allergy Clin Immunol.* 1985;75:663–72; **4.** Welinder H, et al. *Allergy.* 2001;56:506–11; **5.** Nielsen J, et al. *Allergy.* 2006;61:743–9; **6.** Rosenman KD, et al. *Scand J Work Environ Health.* 1987;13:150–4; **7.** Lee HS, et al. *Scand J Work Environ Health.* 1989;15:154–5; **8.** Nielsen J, et al. *Br J Ind Med.* 1992;49:769–75; **9.** Drexler H, et al. *Int Arch Occup Environ Health.* 1994;65:279–83; **10.** Fawcett IW, et al. *Clin Allergy.* 1977;7:1–14; **11.** Wernfors M, et al. *Int Arch Allergy Appl Immunol.* 1986;79:77–82; **12.** Nielsen J, et al. *J Allergy Clin Immunol.* 1988;82:126–33; **13.** Madsen MT, et al. *Occup Environ Med.* 2019;76:175–7; **14.** Schlueter DP, et al. *J Occup Med.* 1978;20:183–8; **15.** Howe W, et al. *J Allergy Clin Immunol.* 1983;71:5–11; **16.** Liss GM, et al. *J Allergy Clin Immunol.* 1993;92:237–47; **17.** Zeiss CR, et al. *J Allergy Clin Immunol.* 1977;60:96–103; **18.** Grammer L, et al. *Chest.* 1998;114:1199–202; **19.** Barker RD, et al. *Occup Environ Med.* 1998;55:684–91.

the determination of specific IgE (sIgE) antibodies (Table 18.14). Monitoring of trimellitic anhydride (TMA)-specific IgG and IgE antibodies has been used in surveillance programs of exposed workforces (88, 89). SPT with acid anhydrides and assessment of sIgE have a high sensitivity for diagnosing OA caused by these chemicals, but these tests may be positive in asymptomatic exposed workers (90). A recent pooled analysis of available studies provided an estimated sensitivity of 81% (95% CI:46–95) for the determination of sIgE against various anhydrides for diagnosing OA, this figure being derived from two studies with small numbers of subjects (91). Cross-reactivity among anhydrides has been shown, but is inconstant (92). After avoidance of exposure, the level of sIgE antibodies against TCPA declines slowly with a median half-life of 1 year (93).

High levels of exposure to acid anhydrides were associated with an increased prevalence of IgE sensitization (93, 94) and work-related respiratory symptoms (93, 95). Smoking and atopy have also been suggested as risk factors for the development of sIgE against acid anhydrides (94, 96, 97), but not for work-related symptoms (97). IgE sensitization to anhydrides has been associated with the presence of NSBH (98). Genetic susceptibility factors (i.e. human leukocyte antigens DR3 allele for TMA and TCPA; DQB1*05 allele for other acid anhydrides) have been involved in the development of IgE sensitization to acid anhydrides (Chapter 4).

Animal models of anhydride-induced IgE sensitization have been developed (99, 100) (Chapter 4). In sensitized animals, inhalation challenge with TMA elicited both early- and late-phase airway responses and eosinophilic airway inflammation. Specific airway responses to TMA were still elicited after a second TMA airway challenge performed 18–24 months after the initial airway challenge, although the sIgE response and eosinophilic inflammation were attenuated after the second TMA challenge (101).

Colophony and fluxes

Colophony is the resin obtained from pine trees, which mainly contains abietic acid and fumaric acid. This product is used as a flux in the electronics industry to prevent corrosion. Fawcett (102) and later Burge (103, 104) who worked with Jack Pepys described subjects who had developed asthmatic or alveolitis-type reactions (Table 18.15). Burge et al. as well as other authors have since thoroughly investigated and summarized several aspects of this form of OA (105, 106). The mechanism of the asthmatic reaction to colophony resin remains unknown and no specific antibodies have been found. Colophony first undergoes an oxidation process, yielding products that may interact with body proteins (107). Unheated colophony also causes OA (108). Dehydroabietic acid is a biomarker of exposure (109). Fluxes containing amino-ethyl-ethanolamine (110), zinc chloride and ammonium chloride (111), polyether alcohol-polypropylene glycol (112), adipic acid (113) and dodecanedioic acid (114), aluminium (110), and potassium aluminium tetrafluoride (115) have also been reported to cause OA (Table 18.15).

Other chemicals

Resins and their additives

Only few reports have presented OA due to other resins than those based on diisocyanate-containing polyurethane products, epoxy resins, and acrylates. These include furan resin in casting molds (116), aziridine cross-linker in water-based acrylate-binders (117) and azodicarbonamide blowing agent in the production of plastics and synthetic rubbers (118) (Table 18.16).

TABLE 18.15 Occupational Asthma Caused by Colophony and Other Fluxes

Agent	Occupation	Number of Subjects	Prevalence	SPT	sIgE	SIC	Other Evidence	References
Colophony	Electronic workers	4	NA	NA	NA	+		1. Fawcett IW, 1976
	Electronic workers	34	NA	NA	NA	100% +		2. Burge PS, 1980
	Manufacture of solder flux	68 low exposure	4%	NA	NA	ND	History+FEV$_1$	3. Burge PS, 1981
		14 medium exposure	21%	NA	NA	ND	History+FEV$_1$	
		6 high exposure	21%	NA	NA	ND	History+FEV$_1$	
Zinc chloride and ammonium chloride flux	Metal jointing	2	NA	NA	NA	+	NSBH	4. Weir DC, 1989
95% alkylaryl polyether alcohol + 5% polypropylene glycol	Electric assembler	1	NA	NA	NA	+		5. Stevens JJ, 1976
Adipic acid	Solderer	1	NA	NA	NA	+	PEF	6. Moore VC, 2010
Lipophilic resin	Aerospace plant	1	NA	NA	NA	+	Improvement off-work	7. Suresh K, 2016
Amino-ethyl-ethanolamine	Cable joiner	2	NA	-	NA	+		8. Sterling GM, 1967
Potassium aluminium tetrafluoride	Heat exchanger production	5	NA	NA	NA	+		9. Laštovková A, 2015

Abbreviations:　FEV$_1$, forced expiratory volume in 1 second; NA, not assessed; NSBH, nonspecific bronchial hyperresponsiveness; SIC, specific inhalation challenge; sIgE, specific IgE antibodies; SPT, skin-prick test.

References:　**1.** Fawcett IW, et al. *Clin Allergy.* 1976;6:577–85; **2.** Burge PS, et al. *Clin Allergy.* 1980;10:137–49; **3.** Burge PS, et al. *Thorax.* 1981;36:828–34; **4.** Weir DC, et al. *Thorax.* 1989;44:220–3; **5.** Stevens JJ. *Ann Allergy.* 1976;36:419–22; **6.** Moore VC, et al. *Eur Respir J.* 2010;36:962–3; **7.** Suresh K et al. *Lung.* 2016;194:787–9; **8.** Sterling GM. *Thorax.* 1967;22:533–7; **9.** Laštovková A, et al. *Ind Health.* 2015;53:562–8.

TABLE 18.16 Examples of Chemical Agents Identified as Causing Occupational Asthma, Verified by Specific Inhalation Challenge

	Occupation	Number of Subjects	Prevalence	SPT Positive/ Tested	Specific IgE Positive/ Tested	SIC Positive/ Tested	Other Evidence	References
Resins								
Triglycidyl isocyanurate (TGIC)	Gas fire factory workers Metal product factory workers	6	NA	NA	0/2	4/4	Positive PEF measurements	*1. Anees, 2011*
Triglycidyl isocyanurate (TGIC)	Powder paint shop workers Spray painter	3	NA	NA	NA	3/3		*2. Suojalehto, 2019*
Polyester powder paint	Spray painter	1	NA	NA	NA	1/1	Alveolar reaction	*3. Cùrtier, 1994*
Furan resin	Foundry mold making	1	NA	NA	NA	1/1		*4. Cockcroft, 1980*
Aziridine hardener	Parquet layers Fiberboard/spray painters	7	NA	4/7	0/5	7/7		*5. Kanerva, 1995*
Azodicarbonamide	Plastic industry workers	4	NA	NA	NA	2/4		*6. Malo, 1985*
Azodicarbonamide	Plastic industry workers	6	NA	0/6	NA	6/6		*7. Suojalehto, 201*
Dyes								
Reactive dyes	Textile industry workers	4	NA	4/4	4/4	4/4		*8. Alanko,1978*
Reactive dyes	Reactive dye industry workers	309	4% (13/309)	25/309	23/78	13/20		*9. Park,1991*
Reactive dyes	Textile industry worker	1	NA	1/1	1/1	1/1		*10. Jin,2011*
Reactive dyes	Textile dyer	1	NA	1/1	NA	1/1	Anaphylactic reaction during SIC	*11. Romano, 1992*
Methylene blue ink	Laboratory nurse	1	NA	NA	NA	1/1		*12. Keskinen, 1981*
Carmine	Butchers	2	NA	2/2	1/2	2/2		*13. Anibarro, 2003*
Carmine	Dye factory workers	24	8% (2/24)	10/24	4/24	2/7		*14. Tabar-Purroy, 2003*
Other								
Diazonium compound	Manufacturer of photocopy paper	1	NA	NA	NA	1/1		*15. Graham, 1981*
Diazonium compound	Manufacture of fluorine polymer precursor	45	4% (2/45)	NA	9/45	2/2		*16. Luczynska, 1990*
Benzoic acid derivative (BCMBA)	Chemical factory workers	87	2% (2/87)	9/87	NA	2/4		*17. Suojalehto, 2018*
Peptide coupling reagent (TBTU and HBTU)	Laboratory technician	1	NA	1/1	0/1	1/1	Increase in sputum eosinophils and NSBHR	*18. Vandenplas, 2008*

Abbreviations: NA, not assessed; SIC, specific inhalation challenge; SPT, skin-prick test; BCMBA, 3-(Bromomethyl)-2-chloro-4-(methylsulfonyl)-benzoic acid; HBTU, 2-(1H-benzotriazol-1-yl)-1,1,3,3-tetramethyluronium hexafluorophosphate; TBTU, 2-(1H-benzotriazol-1-yl)-1,1,3,3-tetramethyluronium tetrafluoroborate; NSBHR, nonspecific bronchial hyperresponsiveness.

References: 1. Anees W, et al. *Occup Med.* 2011;61:65–7; 2. Suojalehto H, et al. *J Allergy Clin Immunol Pract.* 2019 Jan;7:191-8; 3. Cartier A, et al. *Eur Respir J.* 1994;7:608–11; 4. Cockcroft DW, et al. *J Allergy Clin Immunol.* 1980;66:458–63; 5. Kanerva L, et al. *Clin Exp Allergy.* 1995;25:432–9; 6. Malo JL, et al. *Clin Allergy.* 1985;15:261–4; 7. Suojalehto H, et al. *Regul Toxicol Pharmacol.* 2018;94:330–1; 8. Alanko K, et al. *Clin Allergy.* 1978;8:25–3; 9. Park H, et al. *J Allergy Clin Immunol.* 1991;87:639–49; 10. Jin H, et al. *Allergy Asthma Immunol Res.* 2011;3:212–4; 11. Romano C, et al. *Am J Ind Med.* 1992;21:209–16; 12. Keskinen H, et al. *Allergy.* 1981;36:275–6; 13. Añíbarro B, et al. *Int J Occup Environ Health.* 2003;16:133–7; 14. Tabar-Purroy AI, et al. *J Allergy Clin Immunol.* 2003;111:415–9; 15. Graham V, et al. *Thorax.* 1981;36:950–1; 16. Luczynska C, et al. *J Allergy Clin Immunol.* 1990;85:1076–82; 17. Suojalehto H, et al. *Occup Environ Med.* 2018;75:277–82; 18. Vandenplas O, et al. *Occup Environ Med.* 2008;65:715–6.

Triglycidyl isocyanurate (TGIC) is a reactive plastic chemical used as a cross-linking agent in powder paints based on epoxy resins or polyesters (119).

Reactive dyes

Reactive dyes are organic color molecules that are able to react rapidly and permanently with natural textile fibers, which produces durable and bright colors. When handled in powder form, they reach the airways easily. Cross-sectional surveys among textile plant (120) and dye-producing plant workers (121) have demonstrated sensitization to various reactive dyes in 3%–17% of the subjects. Several case series have reported OA to these agents, with IgE-mediated sensitization in most cases (121). Other asthma-inducing dyes include carmine, collected from *Cochinella* insects and used as a coloring agent in foodstuffs, drinks, and medicaments (122), and methylene blue in electrocardiogram (ECG) inks (123). Hair dyes are discussed in "Hairdressing Products" section.

Other agents

A few reports have described OA to diazonium compounds used as light couplers in photocopying. Specific IgE antibodies to diazonium tetrafluoroborate-human serum albumin conjugates were found in 20% of 45 workers in polymer industry using diazonium intermediate (124). OA to another intermediate in a chemical synthesis, 3-(Bromomethyl)-2-chloro-4-(methylsulfonyl)-benzoic acid (BCMBA), has also been described: 8% of all exposed workers and 25% of highest exposure group had positive SPTs to that agent, sensitized suspects reported airway and/or urticaria symptoms (125). Peptide-coupling agent in laboratory work caused asthma, rhinitis, and/or urticarial/eczema reaction in four workers (126). Case reports and workplace surveys have identified also various other chemical agents causing OA (https://reptox.cnesst.gouv. qc.ca/en/occupational-asthma/Pages/occupational-asthma.aspx).

The mechanisms of asthma induction are unknown.

Conclusion and research needs

With the increased use of new chemical products steadily appearing in workplace settings, it is highly probable that the list of agents categorized under the heading of miscellaneous chemical products causing OA will grow. It is also likely that the increased use of these products will result in not only more documentation of individual cases but also proper surveys of workplaces where the products are used. As for other LMW agents, more studies exploring the mechanism of sensitization are needed.

References

1. Enoch SJ, Seed MJ, Roberts DW, et al. Development of mechanism-based structural alerts for respiratory sensitization hazard identification. Chem Res Toxicol. 2012;25(11):2490–8.
2. Seed MJ, Agius RM. Progress with structure-activity relationship modelling of occupational chemical respiratory sensitizers. Curr Opin Allergy Clin Immunol. 2017;17:64–71.
3. Vandenplas O, Godet J, Hurdubaea L, et al. Are high- and low-molecular-weight sensitizing agents associated with different clinical phenotypes of occupational asthma? Allergy. 2019;74:261–72.
4. Lobedanz S, Damhus T, Borchert TV, et al. Enzymes in industrial biotechnology. In: Kirk-Othmer Encyclopedia of Chemical Technology, 1. John Wiley & Sons, Inc; 2016.
5. Flindt MLH. Pulmonary disease due to inhalation of derivatives of Bacillus subtilis containing protelolytic enzyme. Lancet. 1969;1:1177–81.
6. Newhouse ML, Tagg B, Pocock SJ, et al. An epidemiological study of workers producing enzyme washing powders. Lancet. 1970;1:689–93.
7. Weill H, Waddell LC, Ziskind M. A study of workers exposed to detergent enzymes. JAMA. 1971;217(4):425–33.
8. Belin L, Hoborn J, Falsen E, et al. Enzyme sensitization in consumers of enzyme-containing washing powder. Lancet. 1970;2:1153–7.
9. Cullinan P, Newman Taylor AJ, Hole AM, et al. An outbreak of asthma in a modern detergent factory. Lancet. 2000;356:1899–900.
10. van Rooy FG, Houba R, Palmen N, et al. A cross-sectional study among detergent workers exposed to liquid detergent enzymes. Occup Environ Med. 2009;66:759–65.
11. Brisman J, Lillienberg L, Belin L, et al. Sensitization to occupational allergens in bakers' asthma and rhinitis: a case-referent study. Int Arch Occup Environ Health. 2003;76:167–70.
12. Jones M, Welch J, Turvey J, et al. Prevalence of sensitization to 'improver' enzymes in UK supermarket bakers. Allergy. 2016;71(7):997–1000.
13. Raulf M. The latex story. Chem Immunol Allergy. 2014;100:248–55.
14. Baur X, Jäger D. Airborne antigens from latex gloves. Lancet. 1990;335(8694):912.
15. Lagier F, Badier M, Charpin D, et al. Latex as aeroallergen. Lancet. 1990;2:516–7.
16. Vandenplas O, Delwich JP, Evrard G, et al. Prevalence of occupational asthma due to latex among hospital personnel. Am J Respir Crit Care Med. 1995;151:54–60.
17. Archambault S, Malo JL, Infante-Rivard C, et al. Incidence of sensitization, symptoms and probable occupational rhinoconjunctivitis and asthma in apprentices starting exposure to latex. J Allergy Clin Immunol. 2001;107:921–3.
18. Tarlo SM, Wong L, Roos J, et al. Occupational asthma caused by latex in a surgical glove manufacturing plant. J Allergy Clin Immunol. 1990;85:626–31.
19. Carrillo T, Blanco C, Quiralte J, et al. Prevalence of latex allergy among greenhouse workers. J Allergy Clin Immunol. 1995;96:699–701.
20. Orfan NA, Reed R, Dykewicz MS, et al. Occupational asthma in a latex doll manufacturing plant. J Allergy Clin Immunol. 1994;94:826–30.
21. Lopata AL, Adams S, Kirstein F, et al. Occupational allergy to latex among loom tuners in a textile factory. Int Arch Allergy Immunol. 2007;144:64–8.
22. Palosuo T, Antoniadou I, Gottrup F, et al. Latex medical gloves: time for a reappraisal. Int Arch Allergy Immunol. 2011;156(3):234–46.
23. Wrangsjö K, Boman A, Lidén C, et al. Primary prevention of latex allergy in healthcare-spectrum of strategies including the European glove standardization. Contact Dermatitis. 2012;66:165–71.
24. LaMontagne AD, Radi S, Elder DS, et al. Primary prevention of latex related sensitisation and occupational asthma: a systematic review. Occup Environ Med. 2006;63:359–64.
25. Vandenplas O, Larbanois A, Vanassche F, et al. Latex-induced occupational asthma: time trend in incidence and relationship with hospital glove policies. Allergy. 2009;64:415–20.
26. Kelly KJ, Wang ML, Klancnik M, et al. Prevention of IgE sensitization to latex in health care workers after reduction of antigen exposures. J Occup Environ Med. 2011;53(8):934–40.
27. Paris C, Ngatchou-Wandji J, Luc A, et al. Work-related asthma in France: recent trends for the period 2001–2009. Occup Environ Med. 2012;69:391–7.
28. Walters GI, Kirkham A, McGrath EE, et al. Twenty years of SHIELD: decreasing incidence of occupational asthma in the West Midlands, UK? Occup Environ Med. 2015;72:304–10.
29. Vandenplas O, Raulf M. Occupational latex allergy: the current state of affairs. Curr Allergy Asthma Rep. 2017;17:14.
30. Raulf M. Current state of occupational latex allergy. Curr Opin Allergy Clin Immunol. 2020;20:112–116.
31. El-Zaemey S, Carey RN, Darcey E, et al. The prevalence of exposure to high molecular weight asthmagens derived from plants among workers in Australia. Am J Ind Med. 2018;61:824–30.
32. Bernton HS. On occupational sensitisation to the castor bean. Am J Med Sci. 1923;165:196–202.
33. Lemière C, Malo JL, McCants M, et al. Occupational asthma caused by roasted coffee: immunologic evidence that roasted coffee contains the same antigens as green coffee, but at a lower concentration. J Allergy Clin Immunol. 1996;98:464–6.
34. Manavski N, Peters U, Brettschneider R, et al. Cof a 1: identification, expression and immunoreactivity of the first coffee allergen. Int Arch Allergy Immunol. 2012;159(3):235–42.
35. Peters U, Frenzel K, Brettschneider R, et al. Identification of two metallothioneins as novel inhalative coffee allergens cof a 2 and cof a 3. PLOS ONE. 2015;10(5):e0126455.

36. Romano C, Sulotto F, Piolatto G, et al. Factors related to the development of sensitization to green coffee and castor bean allergens among coffee workers. Clin Exp Allergy. 1995;25:643–50.

37. Gasperazzo A, Toffanin P, Larese Filon F. Green coffee been exposure and symptoms in dock workers in Trieste (Italy). Med Lav. 2017;108(5):349–57.

38. Goldberg A, Confino-Cohen R, Waisel Y. Allergic responses to pollen of ornamental plants: high incidence in the general atopic population and especially among flower growers. J Allergy Clin Immunol. 1998;102:210–4.

39. Blanca M, Victorio Puche L, Garrido-Arandia M, et al. Pru p 9, a new allergen eliciting respiratory symptoms in subjects sensitized to peach tree pollen. PLOS ONE. 2020;15(3):e0230010.

40. van Toorenenbergen AW. Occupational allergy to flowers: immunoblot analysis of allergens in freesia, gerbera and chrysanthemum pollen. Scand J Immunol. 2014;80(4):293–7.

41. de Jong NW, Vermeulen AM, Gerth van Wijk R, et al. Occupational allergy caused by flowers. Allergy. 1998;53:204–9.

42. Zhou Y, Jia H, Zhou X, et al. Epidemiology of spider mite sensitivity: a meta-analysis and systematic review. Clin Transl Allergy. 2018;8:21.

43. Lozewicz S, Davison AG, Hopkirk A, et al. Occupational asthma due to methyl methacrylate and cyanoacrylates. Thorax. 1985;40:836–9.

44. Suojalehto H, Suuronen K, Cullinan P, et al. Phenotyping occupational asthma caused by acrylates in a multicenter cohort study. J Allergy Clin Immunol Pract. 2020;8(3):971–9.e1.

45. Hagmar L, Welinder H. Prevalence of specific IgE antibodies against piperazine in employees of a chemical plant. Int Arch Allergy Appl Immunol. 1986;81:12–6.

46. Leino T, Tammilehto L, Hytönen M, et al. Occupational skin and respiratory diseases among hairdressers. Scand J Work Environ Health. 1998;24:398–406.

47. Espuga M, Muñoz X, Plana E, et al. Prevalence of possible occupational asthma in hairdressers working in hair salons for women. Int Arch Allergy Immunol. 2011;155:379–88.

48. Pichat R, Chatanay R. A propos d'un asthme au persulfate d'ammonium. Arch Mal Prof. 1957;18:280–2.

49. Vandenplas O. Occupational asthma: etiologies and risk factors. Allergy Asthma Immunol Res. 2011;3:157–67.

50. Orriols R, Costa R, Albanell M, et al. Reported occupational respiratory diseases in Catalonia. Occup Environ Med. 2006;63:255–60.

51. Ameille J, Pauli G, Calastreng-Crinquand A, et al. Reported incidence of occupational asthma in France, 1996–99. Occup Environ Med. 2003;60:136–42.

52. Wrbitzky R, Drexler H, Letzel S. Early reaction type allergies and diseases of the respiratory passages in employees from persulphate production. Int Arch Occup Environ Health. 1995;67:413–7.

53. Merget R, Buenemann A, Kulzer R, et al. A cross sectional study of chemical industry workers with occupational exposure to persulphates. Occup Env Med. 1996;53:422–6.

54. Munoz X, Cruz MJ, Orriols R, et al. Validation of specific inhalation challenge for the diagnosis of occupational asthma due to persulphate salts. Occup Environ Med. 2004;61:861–6.

55. Moscato G, Pignatti P, Yacoub MR, et al. Occupational asthma and occupational rhinitis in hairdressers. Chest. 2005;128:3590–8.

56. Foss-Skiftesvik MH, Winther L, Mosbech HF, et al. Optimizing diagnostic tests for persulphate-induced respiratory diseases. Clin Transl Allergy. 2016;6:26.

57. de Vooght V, Cruz MJ, Haenen S, et al. Ammonium persulfate can initiate an asthmatic response in mice. Thorax. 2010;65:252–7.

58. Ollé-Monge M, Muñoz X, Vanoirbeek JA, et al. Persistence of asthmatic response after ammonium persulfate-induced occupational asthma in mice. PLOS ONE. 2014;9(10):e109000.

59. Feinberg SM, Watrous RM. Atopy to simple chemical compounds-sulfone-chloramides. J Allergy. 1945;16:209–20.

60. Thickett KM, McCoach JS, Gerber JM, et al. Occupational asthma caused by chloramines in indoor swimming-pool air. Eur Respir J. 2002;19:827–32.

61. Bureau G, Lévesque B, Dubé M, et al. Indoor swimming pool environments and self-reported irritative and respiratory symptoms among lifeguards. Int J Environ Health Res. 2017;27:306–22.

62. Palczynski C, Walusiak J, Krakowiak A, et al. Glutaraldehyde-induced occupational asthma: BALF components and BALF and serum Clara cell protein (CC16) changes due to specific inhalatory provocation test. Occup Med (Lond). 2005;55:572–4.

63. Seed MJ, Hussey LJ, Lines SK, et al. Prediction of asthma hazard of glutaraldehyde substitutes. Occup Med (Lond). 2006;56(4):284–5.

64. Robitaille C, Boulet LP. Occupational asthma after exposure to ortho-phthalaldehyde (OPA). Occup Environ Med. 2015;72:381.

65. Gonzalez M, Jegu J, Kopferschmitt MC, et al. Asthma among workers in healthcare settings: role of disinfection with quaternary ammonium compounds. Clin Exp Allergy. 2014;44:393–406.

66. Vandenplas O, D'Alpaos V, Evrard G, et al. Asthma related to cleaning agents: a clinical insight. BMJ Open. 2013;3:e003568.

67. Díaz Angulo S, Szram J, Welch J, et al. Occupational asthma in antibiotic manufacturing workers: case reports and systematic review. J Allergy (Cairo). 2011;2011:365683.

68. Kim JE, Kim SH, Jin HJ, et al. IgE sensitization to cephalosporins in health care workers. Allergy Asthma Immunol Res. 2012;4:85–91.

69. Biagini RE, Bernstein DM, Klincewicz SL, et al. Evaluation of cutaneous responses and lung function from exposure to opiate compounds among ethical narcotics-manufacturing workers. J Allergy Clin Immunol. 1992;89:108–17.

70. Massawe E, Geiser K. The dilemma of promoting green products: what we know and don't know about bio-based metalworking fluids. J Environ Health. 2012;74(8):8–16.

71. Meza F, Chen L, Hudson N. Investigation of respiratory and dermal symptoms associated with metal working fluids at an aircraft engine manufacturing facility. Am J Ind Med. 2013;56(12):1394–401.

72. Jaakkola MS, Suuronen K, Luukkonen R, et al. Respiratory symptoms and conditions related to occupational exposures in machine shops. Scand J Work Environ Health. 2009;35:64–73.

73. Kennedy SM, Chan-Yeung M, Teschke K, et al. Change in airway responsiveness among apprentices exposed to metalworking fluids. Am J Respir Crit Care Med. 1999;159:87–93.

74. Dahlman-Höglund A, Lindgren Å, Mattsby-Baltzer I. Endotoxin in size-separated metal working fluid aerosol particles. Ann Occup Hyg. 2016;60(7):836–44.

75. Rosenman K. Occupational diseases in individuals exposed to metal working fluids. Curr Opin Allergy Clin Immunol. 2015;15(2):131–6.

76. Bakerly ND, Moore VC, Vellore AD, et al. Fifteen-year trends in occupational asthma: data from the Shield surveillance scheme. Occup Med (Lond). 2008;58:169–74.

77. Burge PS, Moore VC, Burge CB, et al. Can serial PEF measurements separate occupational asthma from allergic alveolitis? Occup Med (Lond). 2015;65:251–5.

78. Ilgaz A, Moore VC, Robertson AS, et al. Occupational asthma; the limited role of air-fed respiratory protective equipment. Occup Med (Lond). 2019;69:329–35.

79. Keskinen H. 136. Cyclic acid anhydrides. The Nordic Expert Group for Criteria Documentation of Health Risk from Chemicals and the Dutch Expert Committee on Occupational Standards. 2004; Stockholm.

80. Grammer LC, Shaughnessy MA, Zeiss CR, et al. Review of trimellitic anhydride (TMA) induced respiratory response. Allergy Asthma Proc Research Support, Non-US Gov't, Review. 1997;18:235–7.

81. Kern RA. Asthma and allergic rhinitis due to sensitisation to phthalic anhydride. Report of a case. J Allergy. 1939;10:164–5.

82. Johannesson G, Rosqvist S, Lindh CH, et al. Serum albumins are the major site for in vivo formation of hapten-carrier protein adducts in plasma from humans and guinea-pigs exposed to type-1 allergy inducing hexahydrophthalic anhydride. Clin Exp Allergy. 2001;31(7):1021–30.

83. Griffin P, Allan L, Beckett P, et al. The development of an antibody to trimellitic anhydride. Clin Exp Allergy. 2001;31:453–7.

84. Bernstein DI, Gallagher JS, D'Souza L, et al. Heterogeneity of specific-IgE responses in workers sensitized to acid anhydride compounds. J Allergy Clin Immunol. 1984;74:794–801.

85. Topping MD, Venables KM, Luczynska CM, et al. Specificity of the human IgE response to inhaled acid anhydrides. J Allergy Clin Immunol. 1986;77:834–42.

86. Grammer LC, Ditto AM, Tripathi A, et al. Prevalence and onset of rhinitis and conjunctivitis in subjects with occupational asthma caused by trimellitic anhydride. J Occup Environ Med. 2002;44:1179–81.

87. Liss GM, Bernstein D, Genesove L, et al. Assessment of risk factors for IgE-mediated sensitization to tetrachlorophthalic anhydride. J Allergy Clin Immunol. 1993;92:237–47.

88. Bernstein JA, Ghosh D, Sublett WJ, et al. Is trimellitic anhydride skin testing a sufficient screening tool for selectively identifying TMA-exposed workers with TMA-specific serum IgE antibodies? J Occup Environ Med. 2011;53:1122–7.

89. Ghosh D, Clay C, Bernstein JA. The utility of monitoring trimellitic anhydride (TMA)-specific IgG to predict IgE-mediated sensitization in an immunosurveillance program. Allergy. 2018;73:1075–83.

90. Baur X, Czuppon A. Diagnostic validation of specific IgE antibody concentrations, skin prick testing, and challenge tests in chemical workers with symptoms of sensitivity to different anhydrides. J Allergy Clin Immunol. 1995;96:489–94.

91. Lux H, Lenz K, Budnik LT, et al. Performance of specific immunoglobulin E tests for diagnosing occupational asthma: a systematic review and meta-analysis. Occup Environ Med. 2019;76(4):269–78.

92. Madsen MT, Skadhauge LR, Nielsen AD, et al. Pyromellitic dianhydride (PMDA) may cause occupational asthma. Occup Environ Med. 2019;76:175–7.

93. Barker RD, Harris JM, Welch JA, et al. Occupational asthma caused by tetrachlorophthalic anhydride: a 12-year follow-up. J Allergy Clin Immunol. 1998;101:717–9.

94. Welinder H, Nielsen J, Rylander L, et al. A prospective study of the relationship between exposure and specific antibodies in workers exposed to organic acid anhydrides. Allergy. 2001;56(6):506–11.

95. Nielsen J, Welinder H, Bensryd I, et al. Ocular and airway symptoms related to organic acid anhydride exposure–a prospective study. Allergy. 2006;61(6):743–9.

96. Venables KM, Topping MD, Howe W, et al. Interaction of smoking and atopy in producing specific IgE antibody against a hapten protein conjugate. Br Med J. 1985;290:201–4.

97. Barker RD, van Tongeren MJA, Harris JM, et al. Risk factors for sensitisation and respiratory symptoms among workers exposed to acid anhydrides: a cohort study. Occup Environ Med. 1998;55:684–91.

98. Barker RD, van Tongeren MJ, Harris JM, et al. Risk factors for bronchial hyperresponsiveness in workers exposed to acid anhydrides. Eur Respir J. 2000;15(4):710–5.

99. Vanoirbeek JA, Tarkowski M, Vanhooren HM, et al. Validation of a mouse model of chemical-induced asthma using trimellitic anhydride, a respiratory sensitizer, and dinitrochlorobenzene, a dermal sensitizer. J Allergy Clin Immunol. 2006;117(5):1090–7.

100. Zhang XD, Andrew ME, Hubbs AF, et al. Airway responses in Brown Norway rats following inhalation sensitization and challenge with trimellitic anhydride. Toxicol Sci. 2006;94:322–9.

101. Zhang XD, Hubbs AF, Siegel PD. Changes in asthma-like responses after extended removal from exposure to trimellitic anhydride in the Brown Norway rat model. Clin Exp Allergy. 2009;39:1746–53.

102. Fawcett IW, Newman Taylor AJ, Pepys J. Asthma due to inhaled chemical agents—fumes from "Multicore" soldering flux and colophony resin. Clin Allergy. 1976;6:577–85.

103. Burge PS, Harries MG, O'Brien I, et al. Bronchial provocation studies in workers exposed to the fumes of electronic soldering fluxes. Clin Allergy. 1980;10:137–49.

104. Burge PS, Edge G, Hawkins R, et al. Occupational asthma in a factory making flux-cored solder containing colophony. Thorax. 1981;36:828–34.

105. Innocenti A, Loi F. Occupational allergic asthma due to colophony. Med Lavoro. 1978;69:720–2.

106. So SY, Lam WK, Yu D. Colophony-induced asthma in a poultry vender. Clin Allergy. 1981;11:395–9.

107. Elms J, Allan LJ, Pengelly I, et al. Colophony: an in vitro model for the induction of sensitization. Clin Exp Allergy. 2000;30:209–13.

108. Burge PS, Wieland A, Robertson AS, et al. Occupational asthma due to unheated colophony. Br J Ind Med. 1986;43:559–60.

109. Baldwin PE, Cain JR, Fletcher R, et al. Dehydroabietic acid as a biomarker for exposure to colophony. Occup Med (Lond). 2007;57:362–6.

110. Sterling GM. Asthma due to aluminium soldering flux. Thorax. 1967;22:533–7.

111. Weir DC, Robertson AS, Jones S, et al. Occupational asthma due to soft corrosive soldering fluxes containing zinc chloride and ammonium chloride. Thorax. 1989;44:220–3.

112. Stevens JJ. Asthma due to soldering flux: a polyether alcohol-polypropylene glycol mixture. Ann Allergy. 1976;36:419–22.

113. Moore VC, Burge PS. Occupational asthma to solder wire containing an adipic acid flux. Eur Respir J. 2010;36:962–3.

114. Suresh K, Belchis D, Askin F, et al. Occupational asthma due to inhalation of aerosolized lipophilic coating materials. Lung. 2016;194:787–9.

115. Laštovková A, Klusáčková P, Fenclová Z, et al. Asthma caused by potassium aluminium tetrafluoride: a case series. Ind Health. 2015;53:562–8.

116. Cockcroft DW, Cartier A, Jones G, et al. Asthma caused by occupational exposure to a furan-based binder system. J Allergy Clin Immunol. 1980;66:458–63.

117. Kanerva L, Keskinen H, Autio P, et al. Occupational respiratory and skin sensitization caused by polyfunctional aziridine hardener. Clin Exp Allergy. 1995;25:432–9.

118. Suojalehto H, Malo JL, Cullinan P. The classification of azodicarbonamide (ADCA) as a respiratory sensitiser; adding to the weight of evidence. Regul Toxicol Pharmacol. 2018;94:330–1.

119. Anees W, Moore VC, Croft JS, et al. Occupational asthma caused by heated triglycidyl isocyanurate. Occup Med (Lond). 2011;61:65–7.

120. Nilsson R, Nordlinder R, Wass U, et al. Asthma, rhinitis, and dermatitis in workers exposed to reactive dyes. Br J Ind Med. 1993;50:65–70.

121. Park HS, Hong CS. The significance of specific IgG and IgG4 antibodies to a reactive dye in exposed workers. Clin Exp Allergy. 1991;21:357–62.

122. Tabar-Purroy AI, Alvarez-Puebla MJ, Acero-Sainz S, et al. Carmine (E-120)–induced occupational asthma revisited. J Allergy Clin Immunol. 2003;111:415–9.

123. Keskinen H, Nordman H, Terho EO. ECG ink as a cause of asthma. Allergy. 1981;36:275–6.

124. Luczynska CM, Hutchcroft BJ, Harrison MA, et al. Occupational asthma and specific IgE to diazonium salt intermediate used in the polymer industry. J Allergy Clin Immunol. 1990;85:1076–82.

125. Suojalehto H, Karvala K, Ahonen S, et al. 3-(Bromomethyl)-2-chloro-4-(methylsulfonyl)-benzoic acid: a new cause of sensitiser induced occupational asthma, rhinitis and urticaria. Occup Environ Med. 2018;75:277–82.

126. Vandenplas O, Hereng MP, Heymans J, et al. Respiratory and skin hypersensitivity reactions caused by a peptide coupling reagent. Occup Environ Med. 2008;65:715–6.

Part V
Specific Disease Entities and Variants

19

IRRITANT-INDUCED ASTHMA AND REACTIVE AIRWAYS DYSFUNCTION SYNDROME

Jonathan A. Bernstein,[1] Orianne Dumas,[2] Frédéric de Blay,[3] Carole Ederlé,[4] and Jean-Luc Malo[5]

[1]*Department of Internal Medicine, Division of Immunology/Allergy Section, University of Cincinnati College of Medecine, Cincinnati, OH, USA*

[2]*Université Paris-Saclay, UVSQ, Univ. Paris-Sud, Inserm, Equipe d'Epidémiologie Respiratoire Intégrative, CESP, Villejuif, France*

[3]*Service de pneumologie, Les Hôpitaux universitaires de Strasbourg, University of Strasbourg, Strasbourg, France*

[4]*Service de pneumologie, Les Hôpitaux universitaires de Strasbourg, University of Strasbourg, Strasbourg, France*

[5]*Hôpital du Sacré-Cœur de Montréal and Université de Montréal, Montréal, Québec, Canada*

Contents

An accidental workplace leak of chlorine gas affects 20 workers at a magnesium production plant.

1. On their arrival 10 minutes after the leak, the emergency responders observe two employees who are unconscious and immediately take them to a nearby hospital. Four conscious workers are transferred to the plant's first aid station where they are provided a few hours of oxygen therapy and sent home after clinical improvement. However, several hours later they experience persistent coughing and shortness of breath. Several other workers report nasal mucosal burning and severe coughing. These workers left the plant facility and went outside for "fresh air."

2. Two workers transported to the local hospital recover consciousness but their chest radiographs reveal noncardiac pulmonary edema. They remain in the hospital for 2 days and are discharged home taking 50 mg of oral prednisone daily over 5 days. These two workers are assessed by a pulmonary specialist 6 weeks after the accident and report persistent coughing following the accident. Their methacholine challenge tests are "positive." They are prescribed inhaled corticosteroids.

3. The four nonhospitalized workers taken to the first aid station return to work the following day after the accident. Two of the four report coughing during strenuous exercises persisting for 1 year.

4. Two asymptomatic workers note impaired sense of smell for 2 years after the accidental inhalation.

5. By questioning and examining all workers of the same work plant, many of them regularly underwent episodes of lower exposure accidents in which they had to leave the premises for a few minutes after experiencing burning of the nose and eyes as well as coughing without necessarily reporting to the first aid unit. They currently report being more easily short of breath and coughing on exercise.

Introduction

Acute inhalational injuries comprise a spectrum of respiratory disorders with clinical manifestations mainly determined by the part of respiratory tract that becomes damaged. Outcomes from acute inhalational injuries to upper (RUDS) and/or lower airways (RADS) depend mainly on the degree of exposure and/or the proximity of the irritant emission.

In contrast to the acute course of RADS, a second type of irritant-induced asthma develops after repeated, nonmassive irritant exposures (1, 2). Low-intensity chronic exposure to irritants (LICEDS), even at acceptable concentrations, can lead to airway obstruction and hyperresponsiveness, especially in subjects exposed to cleaning agents (see Chapter 17).

An irritant induces a nonimmunologic, inflammatory reaction upon direct contact with the respiratory system and has acute and chronic effects. Features that characterize sensitizer-induced occupational asthma (OA) and non-sensitizer-induced OA (i.e. irritant-induced asthma) are summarized in Table 19.1.

TABLE 19.1 Similarities and Differences between Sensitizer and Nonsensitizer (Irritant-Induced) Occupational Asthma

	Sensitizer-Induced	Non-Sensitizer-Induced
Latency period	Present	Absent (RADS) or present (chronic form)
Diagnosis	Multiple tools	History, assessment of airway caliber and responsiveness
Pathology	Like nonoccupational asthma	Acute: epithelial damage Chronic: inflammation and airway remodeling
Functional	+++ Reversibility of airway obstruction	++ Reversibility of airway obstruction
Treatment	Steroids useful	Steroids useful

Irritants and irritancy, sensitizers and sensitization

Whereas sensitizers are products that can induce inflammatory responses through innate immunity or by production of IgE and IgG through adaptive immunity, irritants are considered as "noncorrosive substances that cause temporary inflammation on direct contact with the skin, eyes, nose, or respiratory system by a chemical action at the point of contact" (3, 4). Irritant agents are in most instances low-molecular-weight (LMW) agents that may contain reactive nitrogen or oxygen functional groups. Some LMW chemicals are also able to bind to self-macromolecules (airway proteins, serum albumin) causing structural changes that can become antigenic. Three variables seem crucial in inducing a biologic reaction: the intrinsic sensitizing and/or irritant nature of the chemical, the condition of exposure (concentration, intensity, and duration), and personal susceptibility. The majority of respiratory allergens can elicit positive responses in one or more standard tests used for the identification of skin-sensitizing potential including the local lymph node assay (5), considered as the reference standard, that can be associated with gene expression analysis, as thoroughly reviewed (6). Exposing epithelial cells at the air-liquid interface and other in vitro methods are also discussed in the aforementioned article (6). Chemical agents causing contact dermatitis are also in the list of agents causing OA. Although the T cell response diverges in regards to dermal or respiratory sensitization, it is generally accepted that LMW chemicals that do not induce skin sensitization using in vivo assays should not be considered as a potential respiratory sensitizer (6).

Many LMW agents, like cleaning agents or disinfectants, can act as sensitizers and as irritants. Some irritants can induce IgE-mediated responses along with an eosinophilic infiltrate (7). The different mechanisms that can be involved in the immunological response to irritants are summarized in Table 19.2. Sensitizers are often high-molecular-weight (HMW) agents, commonly airborne proteins or complex polysaccharides that can be from animal, vegetal, or microbial origin (Chapter 3).

Upper airways responses to irritants

RADS may be accompanied by RUDS (reactive upper airways dysfunction syndrome) (8) (see Workplace Scenario). Symptoms of RADS are often preceded by an impression of intense burning in the nose (9). Furthermore, symptoms of chronic rhinitis, related to "puffs" experienced by workers exposed to chlorine, were found to be associated with lower respiratory symptoms (9).

TABLE 19.2 Possible Mechanisms of Irritation

Mechanism	Description	References
Effect on "airway "barrier" (epithelium)	Intraperitoneal preinjection of the airway damaging agent naphthalene renders the airways and alveoli of mice more sensitive to subsequent inhalation of chlorine (increase in alveolar protein exudate and in plasma surfactant protein [SPD]; eosinophilic and neutrophilic infiltration)	*1. Van Den Broucke, 2018*
	Increased epithelial permeability enables penetration of allergens, virus, and toxins, possibly causing new sensitizations	*1. Van Den Broucke, 2018*
	Onset of immune response by a "cross-talk" with immune cells (interaction of epithelial and dendritic cells, conventional and plasmacytoid, induces TH2 and TH17 adaptive immunity	*2. Lambrecht, 2015*
	Epithelial cells fuel airway inflammation, monocytes adopting an immunologic phenotype and chemokines + cytokines activating eosinophils and neutrophils	*2. Lambrecht, 2015*
	Altered secretion of relaxing epithelial and growth factors, release of inflammatory mediators, and proinflammatory cytokines	*3. Ederlé, 2018*
Toxicity	Induction of a danger signal (danger-associated molecular patterns [DAMPs]) leading to an increased systemic and local inflammation, immune cell infiltrates and damage to epithelial cells	*4. Patel, 2018*
Oxidative stress	Increased production of reactive oxygen, nitrogen, and pro-oxidant factors accompany inflammation and asthma	*5. Mittal, 2014* *6. Ederlé, 2019*
	Imbalance between oxidant and antioxidant reducing systems with production of amino acids and nitrotyrosine (assessment of human breath condensate in cleaners exposed to detergents and other chemicals)	*7. Aldakheel, 2016* *8. Corradi, 2012*
	Production of reactive oxygen products can take place in damaged epithelial cells and in inflammatory immune cells (macrophages, neutrophils) (increase in peripheral mononuclear mitochondrial function of subjects with severe asthma vs controls)	*6. Ederlé, 2019*
	Causes a worsening of the bronchial and systemic immune response	*5. Mittal, 2014*
Gene–environment interaction	Eight single nucleotide polymorphisms (SNPs) at five loci significantly associated with current asthma in 3 European cohorts (> 2500 adults) by exposure interactions with low-molecular-weight and irritant occupational agents (these genes play a role in the NF-kB pathway of inflammation)	*9. Rava, 2019*
Neurogenic inflammation	Neuronal fibers close to the bronchial epithelium penetrate the basal membrane and are in contact with epithelial cells via transient receptor potential (TRP) channels, TRPA1 being found in lung cells and mast cells	*10. Kabata, 2019* *11. Zholos, 2015*
	Neuroimmune cross-talk: a variety of stimulants, including inflammatory mediators, lead to stimulation of nociceptors via the epithelial-derived enzyme neutral endopeptidase (NEP) that breaks down proinflammatory neuropeptides	*12. di Maria, 1998*
	NEP activity is lower after exposure to diisocyanates	*13. Gagnaire, 1997* *14. Sheppard, 1988*
Interactions between various types of inflammation	Exposure to pollutants enhances airway response and inflammation due to a sensitizing agent	*15. Carlsten, 2016* *16. Wu, 2018*
	As an etiologic factor of work-exacerbated asthma	*17. Henneberger, 2011* *18. Harber, 2018*

References: 1. Van Den Broucke S, et al. Arch Toxicol. 2018;92:1551–61; 2. Lambrecht BN, et al. Nat Immunol. 2015;16:45–56; 3. Ederlé C, et al. Curr Treat Options Allergy. 2018;5:29–40; 4. Patel S. Curr Allergy Asthma Rep. 2018;18:63; 5. Mittal M, et al. Antioxid Redox Signal. 2014;20:1126–67; 6. Ederle C, et al. J Clin Med. 2019;8:10.3390/jcm8101613; 7. Aldakheel FM, et al. Allergy. 2016;71:741–57; 8. Corradi M, et al. Int Arch Occup Environ Health. 2012;85:389–96; 9. Rava M, et al. Environ Health Perspect. 2017;125:207–14; 10. Kabata H, et al. J Clin Invest. 2019;130:1475–82; 11. Zholos AV. Curr Neuropharmacol. 2015;13:279–91; 12. di Maria GU, et al. Eur Respir J. 1998;12:1454–62; 13. Gagnaire F, et al.Toxicology. 1997;116(1–3):17–26; 14. Sheppard D, et al. J Clin Invest. 1988;81:1111–5; 15. Carlsten C, et al. Thorax. 2016;71:35–44; 16. Wu W, et al. J Allergy Clin Immunol. 2018;141:833–44; 17. Henneberger PK, et al. Am J Respir Crit Care Med. 2011;184:368–78; 18. Harber P, et al. Am J Respir Crit Care Med. 2018;197(2):P1-P2. doi:10.1164/rccm.972P1.*

Olfactive dysfunction

Although the consequences of RADS and RUDS on olfaction have not been examined, several occupational exposures are associated with olfactory impairment. This includes chronic exposure to metals and various chemicals (acrylates, styrene, and solvent mixtures) (10).

Irritable larynx syndrome

Work-induced and work-exacerbated irritable larynx syndromes have been described in several workers, including teachers, World Trade Center rescuers, and all those exposed to airborne chemicals with irritant properties in various workplaces (11). Irritable larynx syndrome happens more frequently in women after exposure to odorant LMW chemicals and occurs without much delay upon exposure (12). The diagnosis is based on clinical features that are unspecific and associated with different degrees of severity: dysphonia, cough, dyspnea, wheezing, and *globus pharyngeus*.

Lower airways responses to irritants

Inhalation of irritants can cause modification in the breathing rate in an exposed mice model (13). Cough is the most important and frequent symptom that occurs after irritant inhalation (14) (see Workplace Scenario).

Both acute and chronic exposure to irritants result in functional (airway caliber and responsiveness) and inflammatory changes documented by exhaled nitric oxide (FeNO), inflammatory cells, and mediators in induced sputum. These aspects are discussed in detail in Chapter 17 in the context of cleaning agents and summarized in Table 19.2 with regards to their effects on airway barrier (epithelium), and other considerations related to toxicity, oxidative stress, gene-environment interaction, neurogenic inflammation, and interactions.

Specific inhalation challenges (SICs) (see Chapter 8) can clarify the type of reaction (sensitizing or irritant), as shown by Vandenplas and coworkers who identified 17/44 (39%) workers exposed to cleaning and disinfectant "irritant" agents and experienced "sensitizer-induced" asthmatic reactions (15).

Causative agents of RADS

Theoretically, all agents generated as particles and mostly as vapors, at sufficiently high concentrations, can cause RADS (16).

Pathogenesis

Factors that can play a role on the intensity of the irritant reaction are mainly related to intensity and proximity of exposure (17) and not to such factors as odors (3). Vapors can reach distal airways more readily than aerosols that mainly deposit in the proximal airways.

Animal models of RADS have been developed. In rats exposed to 1500 ppm of chlorine for 5 minutes, the maximum functional and pathological effects occur within 1–3 days (18). The principal pathological changes include flattening, necrosis, and signs of regeneration of the epithelium, increase in smooth muscle mass, and influx of neutrophils. In a model of RADS in mice, dose-response exposure to chlorine showed pathological changes associated with oxidative stress manifested as increase in macrophages, granulocytes, epithelial cells, and nitrate/nitrite levels (19). Gamma delta T cells exert a different effect on the alteration of airway epithelium, airway hyperresponsiveness, and inflammatory response, and Nrf2 dependent phase II enzymes play a role in the resolution of the process. Maximum airway epithelial proliferation occurred after 5 days and muscle hyperplasia, after 10 days (20). Pretreatment with capsaicin reduced the effect on nasal obstruction, suggesting the involvement of sensory nerves.

Historical background

Industrial exposures

In 1970, Gandevia et al. (21) described four workers with new-onset asthma named "acute inflammatory bronchoconstriction" after exposures to high concentrations of various smoke and fumes from combustion of acids. Twenty-five of 35 firemen involved in a fire at a polyurethane factory experienced irritation of the eyes, nose, and throat, and 14 developed respiratory symptoms (22). A study by Kowitz et al. (23) reported on 115 longshoremen accidentally exposed to chlorine gas; 11 subjects subsequently developed respiratory distress and showed persistent airways obstruction over a 2- to 3-year period.

Civilian exposures

Civilians living in close proximity to railways appeared to be at greater risk of developing airflow obstruction and nonspecific airway hyperresponsiveness as a result of being exposed to accidental releases of chlorine gas (24).

Warfare

During World War I and the Iran–Iraq war, high-level exposures to mustard gas affected both soldiers and the civilian population.

Airway obstruction was shown in 21% of 603 patients who had been exposed to sulfur mustard and had visited a hospital in Iran from 1983 to 1988 (25).

Bhopal

Thousands of inhabitants of Bhopal, India, were exposed to toxic levels of methyl isocyanate as a result of an accidental leak in 1994. Medical surveys of survivors identified a variety of adverse respiratory outcomes including irritant-induced asthma among survivors (26).

World Trade Center

Six months following the World Trade Center (WTC) collapse on September 11, 2001, 28% of the highly exposed and 8% of the moderately exposed rescue workers and firefighters who were tested reported respiratory symptoms and demonstrated a positive methacholine challenge test (27). In more than 12,000 fire department rescue workers, an accelerated decline in forced expiratory volume in 1 second (FEV_1) was demonstrated in the year following the event (28). A 9-year follow-up in more than 27,000 rescue and recovery workers showed a 27% 9-year cumulative incidence for asthma, of 42% for sinusitis, and of 42% for spirometric abnormalities (29).

Single-exposure event: Acute irritant-induced asthma (RADS)

Definition

Reactive airways dysfunction also known as irritant-induced asthma was originally proposed in 1984 by Brooks and Bernstein as a variant form of OA, as based on satisfying the following criteria: (1) a documented absence of preceding respiratory disease; (2) the onset of symptoms occurred after a single specific exposure incident or accident; (3) the exposure was to a gas, smoke, fume, or vapor which was present in very high concentrations and had irritant qualities to its nature; (4) the onset of symptoms occurred within 24 hours after the exposure and persisted for at least 3 months; (5) symptoms simulated asthma with cough, wheezing, and dyspnea predominating; (6) pulmonary function tests may show airflow obstruction; (7) methacholine challenge testing was positive; and (8) other types of pulmonary diseases were ruled out (30). A more concise consensus definition of RADS is "asthma occurring after a single exposure to high levels of an irritating vapor, fume, or smoke." This form of OA is unique as it is not associated with a latency period. In susceptible individuals, persistent airway inflammation and airway remodeling develops and is associated with airway hyperresponsiveness manifesting as asthma symptoms.

Clinical features

RADS is typically diagnosed in adults and has several clinical characteristics, which are summarized in Table 19.3.

A review of reported cases has shown that the criteria listed in Table 19.3 are not uniformly met (31). The most classic feature is the onset of symptoms within 24 hours after irritant exposure. Immediate symptoms frequently manifest as burning of the eyes, nose, and throat after the acute exposure but subsequently workers develop a cough often associated with chest tightness and shortness of breath. The severity of the symptoms often warrants emergency treatment. In contrast to classic forms of OA, symptoms are less likely to improve away from work. Pulmonary

TABLE 19.3 Characteristics of RADS[a]

1. Identification of the date, time(s), frequency, and magnitude of exposure although the latter may be difficult to quantify
2. Onset of symptoms within the first 24 hours
3. No latency period between initial exposure and onset of symptoms
4. Symptoms less likely to improve away from work
5. Pulmonary function testing demonstrating airway obstruction with or without reversibility after short-acting bronchodilators
6. Presence and persistence of nonspecific airway hyperresponsiveness

[a] *From*: Brooks S, Malo JL, Gautrin, D. Irritant induced asthma and reactive airways dysfunction syndrome. In: Malo JL, Chan-Yeung, M, Bernstein, D.I., eds. *Asthma in the Workplace*. 4th ed. Boca Raton, FL: CRC Press; 2013:305–22.

function testing may show airway obstruction with reversibility postbronchodilators but could be normal, thus requiring nonspecific provocation testing such as a methacholine challenge to document airway hyperresponsiveness, a central feature of asthma. As this is a retrospective diagnosis, it is essential to obtain an accurate history of the work process including the materials involved, the duration of exposure, magnitude of exposure, and time to onset of symptoms.

Atypical RADS

The term *atypical RADS* refers to a condition in which workers experience a single massive exposure to an irritant vapor, gas, or fume, but, in contrast to typical RADS, do not experience the onset of asthma symptoms until days, weeks, or months after additional exposures in the workplace. Among a small group of workers (n=25) with atypical, not-so-sudden RADS described by Brooks and coworkers, 88% were atopic and 40% had a previous history of asymptomatic asthma, at least 1 year before the development of atypical RADS (32).

Frequency

The frequency of RADS has generally been evaluated based on data from work-related asthma (WRA) surveillance programs. Data collected since the 1980s indicate that RADS represent ˜5%–20% of OA cases. In 2003, Henneberger et al. (33) summarized reports from a surveillance program of WRA in the United States over different periods (late 1980s to early 1990s) and different areas (one to four US states). The proportion of RADS among all cases of new-onset WRA varied from 8% to 14% (33). The most recent report based on data collected in Michigan over 31 years (1988–2018) indicates a proportion of 14% (407 of 2905 cases) (34). In the United Kingdom (35) and in Catalonia (Spain) (36), surveillance systems for work-related respiratory diseases distinguish "inhalation accidents" (including RADS) and "occupational asthma." Inhalation accidents represented 19% of all potential OA cases (i.e. cases labeled *occupational asthma* and *inhalation accidents*) in the United Kingdom (1992–2001) and 21% in Catalonia (2002). A lower proportion of RADS was reported by the surveillance network for work-related diseases in France where RADS represented 4.7% of all OA cases in 1997 (37) and 3.9% in 2008–2010 (38).

Risk factors

Few studies have examined the environmental and host factors that may modify the risk of RADS (3). Studies have mainly focused on smoking and atopy, and did not show strong modifications by these factors. In a cohort of sulfite mill workers in Sweden, repeated peak exposures to sulfur dioxide giving rise to respiratory symptoms were associated with asthma incidence, and this association was slightly more pronounced in atopic workers (39).

In bleachery workers in a sulfate mill, participants who reported repeated peak exposures to irritant gases had increased risk of adult-onset asthma and/or wheeze, and a positive association was observed in both never and ever smokers, as well as in participants with and without hay fever (40). In the RHINE population-based study in Northern Europe (41) an association between accidental peak exposures to irritant at work and new-onset asthma was reported in men and was of similar magnitude among atopic and nonatopic participants.

Pathology of RADS and irritant-induced asthma

In a few case reports, bronchoalveolar lavage (BAL) and bronchial biopsies carried out after an inhalation accident of moderate intensity showed epithelial desquamation and hemorrhagic exudate with lymphocytosis in the first few days with progressive regeneration of ciliated epithelium in the months after (42). In 10 subjects with RADS events at a mean interval of 10 years before evaluation, with normal spirometry but increased NSBH, BAL showed increased eosinophils, neutrophils, and various inflammatory mediators and biopsies, increased thickness of basement membrane (43).

Management and treatment of RADS

Management and treatment of RADS is similar to the treatment of asthma. Avoidance of further irritant exposures is essential so as not to aggravate the underlying condition. This may require work restrictions and/or use of personal protective equipment (PPE) depending on the work process. For acute symptoms, similar to non-OA, treatment with bronchodilators is indicated. However, as RADS tends to be chronic and persistent and is characterized by airway inflammation, treatment with an inhaled corticosteroid depending on the severity of NSBH and airway obstruction is indicated. Although likely equally effective as previous shown for non-OA, it is still unclear whether using a single maintenance and reliever therapy method or other agents such as anti-IgE, anti-IL5, anti-IL5R, or IL4α agents would be effective in the management of RADS, as there have yet to be any case reports or studies using therapeutic approaches.

Prognosis and outcome of RADS

The outcome for RADS is variable but tends to reflect the natural course of allergic OA where 25% of patients experience resolution of NSBH within 2 years after the initial exposure. A study by Malo et al. who evaluated workers with a diagnosis of RADS (due to chlorine in 20/35 subjects) on average almost 14 years after their initial inhalational accident, showed that they were still symptomatic of asthma and 68% required inhaled corticosteroids (44). Among the 35 workers, 23 underwent repeat methacholine challenge and almost 75% still exhibited NSBH (44). Those who improved tended to be younger and have a higher FEV_1 and PC20 shortly after the accidental inhalation event. A subsequent study investigating WTC rescue workers who developed RADS post-911 reported that smoking was a risk factor for lower respiratory disease (45). Furthermore, the authors found that atopy was a risk factor for upper but not lower airway disease and that upper airway disease contributed to poor symptom control and decreased quality of life (45).

Low-dose repeated exposures type of irritant-induced asthma (LICEDS)

Clinical description

There is little known about a variant form of RADS which has also been described to occur over time after repeated exposures to a chemical or an irritant, for example in pulp mills (1, 46). This condition, called LICEDS, has been described mainly in epidemiological studies (see below in this section) but its pathophysiological mechanism is still poorly elucidated. Table 19.4 summarizes the clinical features for LICEDS as proposed in an earlier version of this book.

Management and prognosis

There have been epidemiologic cross-sectional and longitudinal surveys that have reported on the outcomes of workers who developed irritant-induced symptoms after exposures to chlorine spills or gassing and pulp mill ozone fumes (2, 45, 46). There were significant associations between high exposures and decreased lung function, persistent lower respiratory symptoms, and in one study of metal workers exposed to chlorine, increased airway hyperresponsiveness, which were all more prominent in smokers (2, 45, 46). Management of LICEDS is similar to the treatment of RADS. Removal and prevention from further irritant exposures and treatment according to the GINA asthma guidelines is recommended. Patients should be monitored longitudinally to determine response to therapy and stepping up or down of medications should be based on symptoms and assessment of lung function (47, 48).

Epidemiological studies

Epidemiological studies are particularly important in the case of LICEDS. Indeed, evidence for a causal relationship between low-dose repeated exposure to irritants at the workplace and asthma cannot be established with certainty for a specific worker (3). However, an increasing number of epidemiological studies, either in the general population or among workers in specific industries, have suggested an association between chronic/repeated exposure to low to moderate dose of irritant agents on the one hand and evidence of LICEDS in others.

Population-based studies have used asthma-specific job exposure matrices to evaluate exposure to low to moderate levels of

TABLE 19.4 Characteristics of Low-Intensity Chronic Exposure Dysfunction Syndrome (LICEDS)[a]

1. No preceding latency period but asthma symptoms begin during repeated intermittent or continuous inhalational exposures to nonmassive, moderate- to low-intensity tolerable concentrations of an irritant gas, fume, or smoke.

2. Duration of repeated exposures is always longer than 24 hours but typically not longer than 4 months before onset of symptoms; rarely does the irritant exposure last longer than 1 year before the onset of asthma symptoms.

3. Absence of preexisting asthma symptoms for the previous 1 year or there was a history of childhood asthma that resolved or adult asthma that was in remission for at least 1 year. Atopy is frequent.

4. Typical symptoms include coughing, wheezing, airway irritability, and sometimes intermittent chest tightness and nocturnal asthma symptoms.

5. Spirometry may be normal, show airflow limitation, and/or demonstrate a positive response to an inhaled bronchodilator.

6. A positive methacholine challenge that confirms nonspecific airway hyperresponsiveness.

7. Exclusion of other conditions that mimic asthma including vocal cord dysfunction. OA caused by a workplace sensitizing agent must also be excluded.

[a] *From:* Brooks SM, Malo JL, Gautrin D. Irritant-induced asthma and reactive airways dysfunction syndrome. In: Malo JL, Chan-Yeung, M, Bernstein, DI, eds. *Asthma in the Workplace.* 4th ed. Boca Raton, FL: CRC Press; 2013:305–22.

irritants. Irritant exposures generally included chemicals, combustion particles/fumes, irritant gases/fumes, and/or environmental tobacco smoke. In the French Epidemiological study on the Genetics and Environment of Asthma, an analysis using longitudinal data showed significant associations between chronic exposure to irritants and asthma attacks (49). In a cross-sectional study in Estonia (n=34,015), an increased risk of current physician-diagnosed asthma was observed among workers with exposure to low level of irritants (50). Interestingly, in both studies, the associations observed for irritant exposures were of similar magnitude, or even stronger than those observed for known HMW or LMW sensitizers. In a cross-sectional study conducted in a historically industrialized region of Norway (n=16,099), occupational exposure to irritating agents was associated with increased risk of asthma symptoms (51). However, these studies could not determine whether associations were driven by irritant-induced OA (new-onset asthma) or work-exacerbated asthma. A longitudinal study in Northern Europe examining new-onset asthma in adulthood reported no significant association for irritant exposures overall. However, specific irritating agents, such as cleaning agents, were associated with increased risk of new-onset asthma (41).

Evidence for LICEDS comes largely from studies of specific work environments (3, 52). In the last two decades, a growing number of studies have reported increased risk of asthma among cleaners and healthcare workers, in relation to exposure to disinfectants and cleaning products (53). Although a sensitizing mechanism has been identified for some ingredients of cleaning products, most cleaning agents reported to be associated with asthma are airway irritants. The effects of cleaning agents on the onset of irritant-induced asthma are reported in detail in another chapter (Chapter 17). LICEDS has also been extensively investigated in the aluminum industry (54). So-called OA in aluminum smelters, thought to be mainly caused by exposure to irritant agents such as fluoride and dust, was first described as an asthma-like syndrome called "potroom asthma" (Chapter 16). No specific immunologic mechanism has been shown for this type of asthma (54). A literature review conducted in 2014 concluded, mostly on the basis of epidemiological studies, that there was substantial evidence of a higher risk of OA associated with work in aluminum production (54). In a longitudinal study of 12,002 male employees in 13 aluminum production facilities in the United States who were followed from 1996 to 2002, potroom workers had a significantly increased risk of asthma development compared to nonpotroom workers (55). Exposure concentrations were available for several agents through routine personal samples of chemical hazards, and only exposure to gaseous fluoride was associated with increased risk of asthma development (55). The clearest dose-response relationship was observed for SO2 exposure. In a longitudinal study in Norwegian smelters, Soyseth et al. (56) reported associations between dust exposure, mostly composed of nonspecific airway irritants, and the incidence of WRA symptoms as well as an increased decline in pulmonary function. Similar findings were reported in several cross-sectional or ecological studies (54).

LICEDS may also occur in work environments with simultaneous exposure to sensitizers. These "mixed environments" have been described in the welding, wood, or agriculture industry. Disentangling sensitizer-induced and irritant-induced asthma in these work environments is challenging. Welding fumes have long been suspected to be a cause of OA. In a longitudinal cohort of Canadian apprentices in welding, El-Zein et al. reported that

3% of the participants developed probable OA during 15 months of apprenticeship (57). Two large longitudinal population-based studies in Europe have reported contrasting results regarding the association between welding and asthma incidence. In the European Community Respiratory Health Survey (ECRHS), welding was not associated with increased asthma incidence but was associated with chronic bronchitis (58). In a study in Northern Europe (RHINE), welding was associated with asthma incidence among men (58). Several epidemiological studies have also reported increased risk of asthma associated with work in the wood industry (Chapter 15), as reviewed (59). Several potential causal agents have been suggested, including plicatic acid, terpenes, endotoxins, as well as formaldehyde (59). For some agents (e.g. terpene), both irritating and sensitizing effects have been suggested. Similarly, agricultural workers are exposed to many known sensitizers (e.g. animal protein, plant, insects, and mites), but also potentially to irritant gases and chemicals, including pesticides (60).

Frequency and risk factors

The proportion of LICEDS among OA cases is difficult to evaluate from surveillance data. In most of these studies, RADS is the only type of irritant-induced asthma reported. In a few studies, LICEDS and RADS are reported together or separately. The Korea Work-Related Asthma Surveillance program reported that irritant-induced asthma—potentially including RADS and LICEDS—represented 5.9% of new-onset WRA cases in 2004–2009 (61). In South Africa (1996–1998), the percentage of OA induced by irritants, not including inhalation accidents, was 13% (62). However, it is likely that the frequency of LICEDS is largely underestimated among OA cases reported by chest/occupational physicians in surveillance studies, as for this type of OA the causal agent cannot be identified with certainty in a specific worker (3). In the latest report from the Michigan surveillance system, a known sensitizer was identified as a causal agent in less than half (48%) of non-RADS OA cases (34). Chronic low-dose irritant exposures may represent a substantial proportion of the remaining cases.

Gene–environment interactions have been reported in studies for the association between occupational exposure to irritants and asthma or respiratory symptoms, suggesting potential host risk factors in LICEDS. In an analysis of adult-onset asthma in three large European cohorts, interactions between occupational exposure to irritants or LMW agents (mainly cleaning products and disinfectants) and genes playing a role in the NF-κB pathway, which is involved in inflammation, were reported (63). In another analysis of these European cohorts, four polymorphisms in a transient receptor potential (TRP) gene, *TRPV1*, were found to increase the risk of cough symptoms from occupational exposures to irritants in asthmatics and nonasthmatics (64).

Conditions simulating irritant-induced asthma

Vocal cord dysfunction and hyperventilation syndrome

Vocal cord dysfunction (VCD) has also been referred to as paradoxical vocal fold motion, Munchausen stridor, factitious asthma, and functional laryngeal stridor. In such conditions, the vocal cords typically adduct on inspiration but also adduct on expiration, thereby restricting air movement through the glottis (65, 66). Symptoms can manifest as wheezing, dyspnea, stridor, cough, and tightness in the throat, which gives the sensation of throat swelling or choking. The presence of VCD often obfuscates the diagnosis of asthma because of similar symptoms and triggers such as exercise, extreme temperatures, chemical irritants, and anxiety. As a result, subjects are often incorrectly treated for asthma (66, 67). In addition, other comorbidities such as chronic allergic or nonallergic rhinitis and gastroesophageal reflux disease (GERD) can further complicate this diagnosis (68). The differential diagnosis for VCD includes asthma, chronic rhinitis with or without sinusitis, acute or chronic irritant-induced asthma (RADS and LICEDS), GERD, and psychogenic. Criteria to establish the diagnosis of VCD include noisy breathing and dyspnea, laryngoscopic evidence of vocal cord adduction, and a pulmonary function inspiratory flow volume loop that ends prematurely (69). However, there are still no established consensus VCD guidelines due to the heterogeneous nature of this condition, the lack of pathogenic data, and the absence of any well-designed clinical trials demonstrating the best approach for diagnosis and treatment. There is a consensus that videostroboscopy, which visualizes the vocal cords in response to different maneuvers or triggers including irritants, is the reference standard for confirming VCD (69, 70). Li et al. investigated 55 patients suspected of having VCD and found a significant association between VCD and age, and between VCD and shortness of breath (SOB) (71). Furthermore, in VCD suspected patients who were less than 35 years old in which shortness of breath was the presenting symptom, the authors described that with every 5-year decrement in age, subjects were 1.3 times more likely to have VCD confirmed by videostroboscopy (71). Thus, in patients with RADS not responsive to conventional asthma therapy, a VCD evaluation should be pursued.

Metalworking fluids

Metalworking fluids (MWFs) are mixtures of oils and additives such as biocides, antifoaming agents, and anticorrosive agents used as coolants and lubricants (72). They are used during a number of work processes including metalworking, machining, and metal cutting operations to lower frictional heat, reduce tool wear, and distortion of metal materials (72, 73). There are four classes of MWF: (1) straight oils; (2) soluble oils; (3) synthetic oils and; (4) semisynthetic oils. Oil diluted in water is referred to as suds oil. Metalworking fluids are used to improve the efficiency of work processes as they negate the need to pause production lines necessary to allow tools to cool (72, 73). The use of these oils in the workplace results in aerosolized mists with different compositions depending on the type of oil used and the type of contamination that occurs based on the metal being cut or microbial contaminants. They have been associated with a spectrum of respiratory conditions including hypersensitivity pneumonitis (HP) (Chapter 24). Airborne emission of MWFs over time becomes very irritating because of the deleterious effect of various contaminants including metals, particulate matter from grinding and machining, hydraulic fluids, and additives such as odorants, corrosion inhibitors, antifoam agents, emulsifiers, antioxidants, detergents, viscosity index improvers, antiwear agents, bactericides, and endotoxins (72–74). The pungent smell that workers experience at the beginning of a work week, known as "Monday morning smell," is a sign of bacterial contamination that occurs when the fluid is not used for several days (74).

Exposure to oil mists results in a number of respiratory health conditions related to workplace inhalation including irritant-induced or allergen-induced OA and HP (Chapter 24) (74). Some reports suggest that HP comprises up to 50% of cases (74).

Swimming pools and asthma

Swimming pool workers and attendants may be exposed to elevated concentrations of disinfection by-products (DBPs) such as chloramines (mono-, di-, and tri-), trihalomethanes, and haloacetonitriles (75, 76). The production of DBPs results from the reaction between organic matter (e.g. sweat, urine, skin particles) in water and the disinfectant (most often, chlorine) used to treat the water (75). The impact of exposure to DBPs in swimming pools on asthma, both among children and adults, remains debated (75, 76). In adults, studies have mainly focused on competitive swimmers and swimming pool workers. Although several studies have reported a higher proportion of asthma cases among competitive swimmers compared to other athletes, a potential bias of this association is possible as swimming has long been a recommended activity for patients with asthma (75, 76). Epidemiological studies among swimming pool workers (e.g. lifeguards) have reported an increased risk of respiratory and irritative symptoms associated with exposure to DBPs, but results regarding asthma outcomes are not entirely consistent (76). In a recent cross-sectional study of 870 lifeguards in Quebec, duration of work in indoor swimming pools was not associated with physician-diagnosed asthma, but workers with longer duration of exposure in the past 12 months had increased risk of asthma attacks (77). Such results have raised the question whether occupational exposures in swimming pools may exacerbate/aggravate preexisting asthma rather than causing new-onset asthma. Nonetheless, among 44 WRA cases attributed to exposures in swimming pools or environments with similar exposures (spa venues, water parks) identified by surveillance systems in California, Michigan, and New Jersey (1990–2012), more than half (57%) of the cases were new-onset asthma, including both RADS and sensitizer-induced OA (78). These findings are consistent with the earlier report of a case series of three swimming pool workers with OA in 2002 (79).

Multiple chemical sensitivity syndrome (idiopathic environmental intolerance)

Multiple chemical sensitivity, now more commonly referred to as idiopathic environmental intolerance (IEI), is defined as a "chronic, recurring disease caused by a person's inability to tolerate an environmental chemical or class of foreign chemicals for unknown reasons" (80–82). A consensus expert report suggested six criteria for a diagnosis of IEI, which include: (1) symptoms reproducible with repeated (chemical) exposures; (2) chronic nature; (3) low levels of exposure, by comparison with previous exposure that was usually tolerated, resulting in symptoms; (4) improvement of symptoms with avoidance; (5) symptoms in response to multiple chemically unrelated substances; and (6) multiple-organ related symptoms (i.e. runny nose, itchy eyes, headache, scratchy throat, ear ache, scalp pain, mental confusion or sleepiness, palpitations, upset stomach, nausea and/or diarrhea, abdominal cramping, aching joints) (83). Patients with IEI almost always experience a precipitating event, usually associated with a chemical smell, which leads to a response involving one or more organ systems. Once the initiating event has passed, the same response or even an exaggerated response occurs each time the stimulus is reencountered. Because patients with this syndrome manifest symptoms similar to certain allergic, complex unexplained disorders (i.e. fibromyalgia, chronic fatigue syndrome, dysautonomia) and emotional conditions, IEI has often been confused with allergy (atopy) or psychiatric illnesses. Disagreement among physicians and medical researchers regarding whether IEI represents a clinical problem or a psychiatric

condition has hindered investigational research. In fact, many professional medical organizations have concluded that IEI is a psychiatric disorder (80, 81, 82). IEI shares many similar features to other related medical conditions including sick-building syndrome (Chapter 26), food intolerance syndrome, and the Gulf War Illness. In each of these conditions, chemical odors have been reported to precipitate one or more organ-system responses (83). It has been postulated that free radical/antioxidant homeostasis may be implicated in IEI by affecting the regulation of xenobiotic metabolizing enzymes and by causing increased levels of oxidative products resulting in cell and tissue damage leading to clinical symptoms (84). Gugliandolo and coworkers conducted a cross-sectional study in 34 symptomatic subjects in which they evaluated the nutritional status and the presence of single nucleotide polymorphisms previously reported to be associated with IEI and oxidative stress pathways. Statistically significant differences between patients and controls were found for rs1801133 (MTHFR), rs174546 (FADS1), and rs1801282 (PPARγ) polymorphisms (85). IEI is generally easy to differentiate from RADS as NSBH is not a defining characteristic of this condition.

Summary

Irritant-induced asthma represents a spectrum of presentations. In the most extreme case, a single massive exposure leads to the sudden onset of asthma, on occasion with a not-so-sudden onset, as epitomized by the RADS leading to persistent airway inflammation and NSBH. Also, chronic exposure to irritants, especially in cleaners, may lead to airway obstruction and hyperresponsiveness, as documented in epidemiological studies. Prevention measures for irritant-induced asthma should include the improved recognition of dangerous work, ongoing worker education, and employer commitment to environmental control strategies.

Research needs

Efforts should encompass the following:

- Identify the irritant potential on the airways of products regularly introduced in workplaces.
- Explain the predominant presence of coughing in irritant-induced asthma.
- Examine the nasal consequences (inflammation and smell) of exposure to irritants.
- Determine the role of preexisting NSBH in all forms of irritant-induced asthma.
- Design prospective epidemiologic studies of newly hired workers in industries with both high- and low-intensity exposure to irritants.

References

1. Chan-Yeung M, Lam S, Kennedy SM, et al. Persistent asthma after repeated exposure to high concentrations of gases in pulpmills. Am J Respir Crit Care Med. 1994;149:1676–80.
2. Henneberger PK, Olin AC, Andersson E, et al. The incidence of respiratory symptoms and diseases among pulp mill workers with peak exposures to ozone and other irritant gases. Chest. 2005;128:3028–37.
3. Vandenplas O, Wiszniewska M, Raulf M, et al. EAACI position paper: irritant-induced asthma. Allergy. 2014;69:1141–53.
4. OSHA. Appendix A 29 CFR 1910.1200. The Hazard Communication Standard. 2012. https://www.osha.gov/dsg/hazcom/standards.html

5. Dearman RJ, Basketter DA, Kimber I. Inter-relationships between different classes of chemical allergens. J Appl Toxicol. 2013;33:558–65.

6. Arts J. How to assess respiratory sensitization of low molecular weight chemicals? Int J Hyg Environ Health. 2020;225:113469.

7. de Genaro IS, de Almeida FM, Hizume-Kunzler DC, et al. Low dose of chlorine exposure exacerbates nasal and pulmonary allergic inflammation in mice. Sci Rep. 2018;8:12636.

8. Meggs WJ. RADS and RUDS—The toxic induction of asthma and rhinitis. J Toxicol and Clin Toxicol. 1994;32:487–501.

9. Leroyer C, Malo JL, Girard D, et al. Chronic rhinitis in workers at risk of RADS due to chlorine exposure. Occup Env Med. 1999;56:334–8.

10. Gobba F. Olfactory toxicity: long-term effects of occupational exposures. Int Arch Occup Environ Health. 2006;79:322–31.

11. Denton E, Hoy R. Occupational aspects of irritable larynx syndrome. Curr Opin Allergy Clin Immunol. 2020;20(2):90–5.

12. Halvorsen T, Walsted ES, Bucca C, et al. Inducible laryngeal obstruction: an official joint European Respiratory Society and European Laryngological Society statement. Eur Respir J. 2017;50(3):1602221.

13. Gagnaire F, Marignac B, Morel G, et al. Sensory irritation due to methyl-2-cyanoacrylate, ethyl-2-cyanoacrylate, isopropyl-2-cyanoacrylate and 2-methoxyethyl-2-cyanoacrylate in mice. Ann Occup Hyg. 2003;47:297–304.

14. Tarlo SM, Akkaya A. Cough: occupational and environmental considerations: ACCP evidence-based clinical practice guidelines. Chest. 2006;129 Suppl:186S–96S.

15. Vandenplas O, D'Alpaos V, Evrard G, et al. Asthma related to cleaning agents: a clinical insight. BMJ Open. 2013;3:e003568.

16. Baur X. A compendium of causative agents of occupational asthma. J Occup Med Toxicol. 2013;8(1):15.

17. Kern DG. Outbreak of the reactive airways dysfunction syndrome after a spill of glacial acetic acid. Am Rev Respir Dis. 1991;144:1058–64.

18. Demnati R, Fraser R, Ghezzo H, et al. Time-course of functional and pathological changes after a single high acute inhalation of chlorine in rats. Eur Respir J. 1998;11:922–8.

19. Martin JG, Campbell HR, Iijima H, et al. Chlorine-induced injury to the airways in the mouse. Am J Respir Crit Care Med. 2003;168:568–74.

20. Tuck SA, Ramos-Barbon D, Campbell H, et al. Time course of airway remodelling after an acute chlorine gas exposure in mice. Respir Res. 2008;9:61.

21. Gandevia B. Occupational asthma, part I. Med J Aust. 1970;2:332–5.

22. Axford AT, McKerrow CB, Jones A Parry, et al. Accidental exposure to isocyanate fumes in a group of firemen. Br J Ind Med. 1976;33:65–71.

23. Kowitz TA, Reba RC, Parker RT, et al. Effects of chlorine gas upon respiratory function. Arch Environ Health. 1967;14:545–58.

24. Soffer Y, Schwartz D, Goldberg A, et al. Population evacuations in industrial accidents: a review of the literature about four major events. Prehosp Disaster Med. 2008;23:276–81.

25. Ghanei M, Tazelaar HD, Chilosi M, et al. An international collaborative pathologic study of surgical lung biopsies from mustard gas-exposed patients. Respir Med. 2008;102:825–30.

26. Cullinan P, Acquilla S, Dhara V Ramana, et al. Respiratory morbidity 10 years after the Union Carbide gas leak at Bhopal: a cross sectional survey. Br Med J. 1997;314:338–43.

27. Banauch GL, Alleyne D, Sanchez R, et al. Persistent hyperreactivity and reactive airway dysfunction syndrome in firefighters at the World Trade Center. Am J Respir Crit Care Med. 2003;168:54–62.

28. Banauch GI, Hall C, Weiden M, et al. Pulmonary function after exposure to the World Trade Center collapse in the New York City Fire Department. Am J Respir Crit Care Med. 2006;174(3):312–9.

29. Wisnivesky JP, Teitelbaum SL, Todd AC, et al. Persistence of multiple illnesses in World Trade Center rescue and recovery workers: a cohort study. Lancet. 2011;378:888–97.

30. Brooks SM, Weiss MA, Bernstein IL. Reactive airways dysfunction syndrome (RADS). Persistent asthma syndrome after high level irritant exposures. Chest. 1985;88:376–84.

31. Walters GI, Huntley CC. Updated review of reported cases of reactive airways dysfunction syndrome. Occup Med. 2020;102:223–30.

32. Brooks SM, Hammad Y, Richards I, et al. The spectrum of irritant-induced asthma. Chest. 1998;113:42–9.

33. Henneberger PK, Derk SJ, Davis L, et al. Work-related reactive airways dysfunction syndrome cases from surveillance in selected US states. J Occup Environ Med. 2003;45:360–8.

34. Reilly MJ, Wang L, Rosenman KD. The burden of work-related asthma in Michigan, 1988–2018. Ann Am Thorac Soc. 2020;17(3):284–92.

35. McDonald JC, Chen Y, Zekveld C, et al. Incidence by occupation and industry of acute work related respiratory diseases in the UK, 1992–2001. Occup Environ Med. 2005;62:836–42.

36. Orriols R, Costa R, Albanell M, et al. Reported occupational respiratory diseases in Catalonia. Occup Environ Med. 2006;63:255–60.

37. Kopferschmitt-Kubler MC, Ameille J, Popin E, et al. Occupational asthma in France: a 1-yr report of the Observatoire National de Asthmes Professionnels project. Eur Respir J. 2002;19:84–9.

38. Ameille J, Hamelin K, Andujar P, et al. Occupational asthma and occupational rhinitis: the united airways disease model revisited. Occup Environ Med. 2013;70(7):471–5.

39. Andersson E, Knutsson A, Hagberg S, et al. Incidence of asthma among workers exposed to sulphur dioxide and other irritant gases. Eur Respir J. 2006;27:720–5.

40. Andersson E, Olin AC, Hagberg S, et al. Adult-onset asthma and wheeze among irritant-exposed bleachery workers. Am J Ind Med. 2003;43:532–8.

41. Lillienberg L, Andersson E, Janson C, et al. Occupational exposure and new-onset asthma in a population-based study in Northern Europe (RHINE). Ann Occup Hyg. 2013;57:482–92.

42. Lemiere C, Malo JL, Boutet M. Reactive airways dysfunction syndrome due to chlorine: sequential bronchial biopsies and functional assessment. Eur Respir J. 1997;10:241–4.

43. Takeda N, Maghni K, Daigle S, et al. Long-term pathologic consequences of acute irritant-induced asthma. J Allergy Clin Immunol. 2009;124:975–81.

44. Malo JL, L'Archevêque J, Castellanos L, et al. Long-term outcomes of acute irritant-induced asthma. Am J Respir Crit Care Med. 2009;179:923–8.

45. de la Hoz RE. Long-term outcomes of acute irritant-induced asthma and World Trade Center-related lower airway disease. Am J Respir Crit Care Med. 2010;181:95–6.

46. Gautrin D, Leroyer C, Infante-Rivard C, et al. Longitudinal assessment of airway caliber and responsiveness in workers exposed to chlorine. Am J Respir Crit Care Med. 1999;160:1232–7.

47. Kennedy SM, Enarson DA, Janssen RG, et al. Lung health consequences of reported accidental chlorine gas exposures among pulpmill workers. Am Rev Respir Dis. 1991;143:74–9.

48. Patel NJ, Jorgensen C, Kuhn J, et al. Concurrent laryngeal abnormalities in patients with paradoxical vocal fold dysfunction. Otolaryngol Head Neck Surg. 2004;130(6):686–9.

49. Dumas O, Le Moual N, Siroux V, et al. Work related asthma. A causal analysis controlling the healthy worker effect. Occup Environ Med. 2013;70(9):603–10.

50. Dumas O, Laurent E, Bousquet J, et al. Occupational irritants and asthma: an Estonian cross-sectional study of 34,000 adults. Eur Respir J. 2014;44:647–56.

51. Abrahamsen R, Fell AK, Svendsen MV, et al. Association of respiratory symptoms and asthma with occupational exposures: findings from a population-based cross-sectional survey in Telemark, Norway. BMJ Open. 2017;7:e014018.

52. Quinot C, Dumas O, Henneberger PK, et al. Development of a job-task-exposure matrix to assess occupational exposure to disinfectants among US nurses. Occup Env Med. 2016;Aug 26. pii: oemed-2016-103606. doi:10.1136/oemed-2016-103606

53. Folletti I, Siracusa A, Paolocci G. Update on asthma and cleaning agents. Curr Opin Allergy Clin Immunol. 2017;17:90–5.

54. Kongerud J, Soyseth V. Respiratory disorders in aluminum smelter workers. J Occup Environ Med. 2014;56(5 Suppl):S60–70.

55. Taiwo OA, Sircar KD, Slade MD, et al. Incidence of asthma among aluminum workers. J Occup Environ Med. 2006;48:275–82.

56. Søyseth V, Johnsen HL, Henneberger PK, et al. Increased decline in pulmonary function among employees in Norwegian smelters reporting work-related asthma-like symptoms. J Occup Environ Med. 2015;57(9):1004–8.

57. El-Zein M, Malo JL, Infante-Rivard C, et al. Incidence of probable occupational asthma and of changes in airway calibre and responsiveness in apprentice welders. Eur Respir J. 2003;22:513–8.

58. Lillienberg L, Zock JP, Kromhout H, et al. A population-based study on welding exposures at work and respiratory symptoms. Ann Occup Hyg. 2008;52:107–15.

59. Wiggans RE, Evans G, Fishwick D, et al. Asthma in furniture and wood processing workers: a systematic review. Occup Med (Lond). 2016;66:193–201.

60. Mamane A, Raherison C, Tessier JF, et al. Environmental exposure to pesticides and respiratory health. Eur Respir Rev. 2015;137:462–73.

61. Kwon SC, Song J, Kim YK, et al. Work-related asthma in Korea—findings from the Korea work-related asthma surveillance (KOWAS) program, 2004–2009. Allergy Asthma Immunol Res. 2015;7:51–9.

62. Hnizdo E, Esterhuizen TM, Rees D, et al. Occupational asthma as identified by the Surveillance of Work-related and Occupational Respiratory Diseases programme in South Africa. Clin Exp Allergy. 2001;31:32–9.

63. Rava M, Ahmed I, Kogevinas M, et al. Genes interacting with occupational exposures to low molecular weight agents and irritants on adult-onset asthma in three European studies. Environ Health Perspect. 2017;125:207–14.

64. Smit LA, Kogevinas M, Anto JM, et al. Transient receptor potential genes, smoking, occupational exposures and cough in adults. Respir Res. 2012;13:26.

65. Newman KB, Mason UG, Schmaling KB. Clinical features of vocal cord dysfunction. Am J Respir Crit Care Med. 1995;152:1382–6.

66. Mathers-Schmidt BA, Brilla LR. Inspiratory muscle training in exercise-induced paradoxical vocal fold motion. J Voice. 2005;19(4):635–44.

67. Gurevich-Uvena J, Parker JM, Fitzpatrick TM, et al. Medical comorbidities for paradoxical vocal fold motion (vocal cord dysfunction) in the military population. J Voice. 2010;24(6):728–31.

68. Morris MJ, Christopher KL. Diagnostic criteria for the classification of vocal cord dysfunction. Chest. 2010;138:1213–23.

69. Treole K, Trudeau MD, Forrest LA. Endoscopic and stroboscopic description of adults with paradoxical vocal fold dysfunction. J Voice. 1999;13(1):143–52.

70. Vertigan AE, Gibson PG. Chronic refractory cough as a sensory neuropathy: evidence from a reinterpretation of cough triggers. J Voice. 2011;25(5):596–601.

71. Li RC, Singh U, Windom HP, et al. Clinical associations in the diagnosis of vocal cord dysfunction. Ann Allergy Asthma Immunol. 2016;117(4):354–8.

72. Koller MF, Pletscher C, Scholz SM, et al. Metal working fluid exposure and diseases in Switzerland. Int J Occup Environ Health. 2016;22(3):193–200.

73. Park RM. Risk assessment for metalworking fluids and respiratory outcomes. Saf Health Work. 2019;10(4):428–36.

74. Kennedy SM, Chan-Yeung M, Teschke K, et al. Change in airway responsiveness among apprentices exposed to metalworking fluids. Am J Respir Crit Care Med. 1999;159:87–93.

75. Villanueva CM, Cordier S, Font-Ribera L, et al. Overview of disinfection by-products and associated health effects. Curr Environ Health Rep. 2015;2(1):107–15.

76. Wastensson G, Eriksson K. Inorganic chloramines: a critical review of the toxicological and epidemiological evidence as a basis for occupational exposure limit setting. Crit Rev Toxicol. 2020;50(3):219–71.

77. Bureau G, Lévesque B, Dubé M, et al. Indoor swimming pool environments and self-reported irritative and respiratory symptoms among lifeguards. Int J Environ Health Res. 2017;27:306–22.

78. Rosenman KD, Millerick-May M, Reilly MJ, et al. Swimming facilities and work-related asthma. J Asthma. 2015;52:52–8.

79. Thickett KM, McCoach JS, Gerber JM, et al. Occupational asthma caused by chloramines in indoor swimming-pool air. Eur Respir J. 2002;19:827–32.

80. Watanabe M, Tonori H, Aizawa Y. Multiple chemical sensitivity and idiopathic environmental intolerance (part one). Environ Health Prev Med. 2003;7(6):264–72.

81. Watanabe M, Tonori H, Aizawa Y. Multiple chemical sensitivity and idiopathic environmental intolerance (part two). Environ Health Prev Med. 2003;7(6):273–82.

82. Multiple chemical sensitivity: a 1999 consensus. Arch Environ Health. 1999;54(3):147–9.

83. De Luca C, Scordo G, Cesareo E, et al. Idiopathic environmental intolerances (IEI): from molecular epidemiology to molecular medicine. Indian J Exp Biol. 2010;48(7):625–35.

84. Loria-Kohen V, Marcos-Pasero H, de la Iglesia R, et al. Multiple chemical sensitivity: genotypic characterization, nutritional status and quality of life in 52 patients. Med Clin. 2017;149(4):141–6.

85. Gugliandolo A, Gangemi C, Calabrò C, et al. Assessment of glutathione peroxidase-1 polymorphisms, oxidative stress and DNA damage in sensitivity-related illnesses. Life Sci. 2016;145:27–33.

20

ASTHMA EXACERBATED AT WORK

Paul K. Henneberger,[1] Gregory R. Wagner,[2] Ambrose K. Lau,[3] Susan M. Tarlo,[4] and Catherine Lemière[5]

[1]Respiratory Health Division, National Institute for Occupational Safety and Health, CDC, Morgantown, WV, USA
[2]Department of Environmental Health, Harvard T.H. Chan School of Public Health, Boston, MA, USA
[3]Department of Medicine, University of Toronto, University Health Network, Toronto Western Hospital,
Toronto, ON, Canada
[4]University Health Network and St Michael's Hospital, Toronto, Department of Medicine, University of Toronto,
Toronto, ON, Canada
[5]CIUSSS du Nord de l'île de Montréal, Université de Montréal, Montréal, Québec, Canada

Contents

WORKPLACE SCENARIO

A hospital began renovating patient rooms in one wing of the surgical floor. The improvements included removing all interior walls, erecting and painting new walls, applying new floor coverings, and replacing the electrical wiring, plumbing, and ventilation ducts. Many staff members working nearby were upset by the noise, and the cleaning staff complained about the increased demand on them to remove dust and grime coming from the renovation activities.

1. Renovation work can result in exposures such as dusts, paint fumes, and cleaning products that may exacerbate asthma symptoms.
2. A nursing aide with stable asthma cared for postoperative patients in the hospital. He was normally able to conduct his duties without breathing difficulties and required only occasional (<1×/week) use of a quick-relief inhaler in addition to a low-dose inhaled corticosteroid. During the past month, he started to experience more symptoms that required additional uses of his inhaler during the day. At one point, he felt his symptoms were escalating in frequency and severity and scheduled an urgent appointment with his physician.
3. The nursing aide also noticed that new gloves had been introduced at his workstation 2 months ago. He was unsure whether those gloves were made of latex.
4. The physician was familiar with the patient's history of adolescent-onset, normally stable asthma, having previously performed a comprehensive work-up and periodic follow-up examinations. During the clinical interview, the physician asked about changes in the patient's environment or activities at home, work, and elsewhere. The patient described no changes at home or in daily activities but noted construction crews had recently started to renovate space on his floor of the hospital.
5. Lung function measurement with in-office spirometry confirmed the diagnosis of asthma and demonstrated a decline when compared to baseline.
6. The physician knew that identifying and minimizing workplace symptom triggers could help both her patient and other workers with asthma, as well as hospital inpatients and visitors. After obtaining permission from the patient, the physician contacted the hospital's director of health and safety, being careful to protect her patient's confidentiality, and asked the director to confirm that the area being renovated was adequately isolated from the rest of the hospital. Health and safety staff determined that shrouding and ventilation of the renovation area were inadequate and implemented changes to correct these problems. This greatly decreased the "bystander" exposures of staff working near the renovations, and the symptoms of the nursing aide returned to

baseline over the following week. Since construction activities and personnel can change frequently in the course of a project, the physician urged her patient to monitor the situation and offered to assist again if the exposures recurred.

Introduction

Exacerbation of asthma can result from exposures at home, at work, in the outdoor environment, and in public buildings. There is a general agreement in clinical practice that troublesome home environmental exposures should be avoided; physicians may advise asthma patients to rid their homes of sources of allergens (e.g. pets) and repositories for allergens (e.g. carpets). Asthma-related exposures in the work environment are less frequently addressed, because exposures are often beyond the control of employees and employers may or may not accept their responsibility or have the ability to control exposures. The issue of an affected employee's right to workplace accommodation or compensation further clouds the issue.

Work-related asthma (WRA) comprises occupational asthma (OA) that is caused by conditions at work and work-exacerbated asthma (WEA), in which preexisting or concurrent asthma is worsened by workplace conditions (1, 2). The number of articles that address WEA has increased considerably since the last version of this chapter was published in 2013. This chapter covers various topics related to WEA, including definitions, frequency, agents, characteristics of cases, clinical approach, prevention, and future research directions.

Definitions of WEA

A clear definition of WEA can help clinicians and policymakers refine approaches to prevention, treatment, and compensation, and is necessary for the continuing scientific investigation of the spectrum of WRA.

WEA describes a worsening from baseline respiratory health resulting from workplace exposures or conditions in any individual with asthma. WEA is the result of an interaction between an individual with asthma and the environment in which the individual works. As discussed in the 2011 statement from the American Thoracic Society (ATS) (1), the term WEA does not denote the underlying cause of the asthma or limit the candidate causes of exacerbation. The ATS appropriately defined WEA as a "worsening of asthma due to conditions at work ..." (1). For individuals with asthma at risk for WEA, their underlying asthma might have been caused by nonwork exposures or by work (either allergic or irritant-induced asthma). The etiology of the asthma is a separate and infrequently relevant consideration to understanding and responding effectively to WEA. As a rule, the triggers for the exacerbations are more relevant than the original asthma category or cause.

The ATS committee recognized the prime importance of temporality of symptom occurrence in their proposed case definition for WEA. The case definition includes the following considerations:

- Preexisting or concurrent asthma. Asthma onset may have either predated current work or may have first occurred while in the worksite of interest but was not caused by specific exposures in that workplace.

- Increased frequency of asthma symptoms, medication use, or healthcare utilization is temporally associated with work. Medical test results may document more frequent abnormality associated with work.
- Workplace exposures or conditions exist that can exacerbate asthma.
- OA (asthma caused by a specific, identified workplace exposure) is unlikely.

A somewhat similar case definition has been used in the United States since the 1990s for public health surveillance in the Sentinel Event Notification System for Occupational Risks (SENSOR) (3). The SENSOR criteria for work-aggravated asthma are (*i*) healthcare professional's diagnosis consistent with asthma, (*ii*) an association between symptoms and work, (*iii*) asthma symptoms or treatment with asthma medication within the 2 years before entering a new occupational setting, and (*iv*) increased asthma symptoms or increased asthma medication use upon entering a new occupational setting. There is a longitudinal component to this definition, stipulating that asthma onset and the presence of asthma symptoms or related medication use must come before entering the new occupational exposure setting, and the condition must worsen after entering. Thus, the clinician or researcher must obtain, either prospectively or retrospectively, the knowledge of asthma status before and after subjects enter a new occupational exposure setting. The SENSOR definition of work-aggravated asthma has a critical difference with definitions of WEA offered by the 2011 ATS statement and by a 2008 consensus document of the American College of Chest Physicians (ACCP) (2). Specifically, the later definitions include exacerbations of "concurrent" asthma, namely asthma that is first recognized after work begins in the workplace of interest but is not caused by conditions at work. The ATS and ACCP definitions recognize the reality that asthma may develop in working adults with or without documentation of specific workplace exposures and clinical testing that confirms OA, and may be exacerbated by exposures or conditions in that same workplace.

Of note, the definition of WEA does not specify a minimum frequency or duration of asthma exacerbation. Thus it can range from a single transient episode requiring 1 day or less off work (4), up to daily worsening of asthma at work and/or recurrent emergency visits/hospital admissions. The former, transient episodes are more common (5) and most likely to lead to primary care assessments with little or no objective documentation, while more frequent exacerbations are more likely to have greater individual impact and to lead to specialist investigations similar to those performed for OA (6).

Medical records may be useful to document an asthma patient's change in status. For example, in a study of recruits who entered the Israel Defense Force at the age of 18–21 years, baseline asthma status was established at the time of induction into the military and repeated clinical evaluations documented changes in asthma status over time (7). However, in the absence of medical records, determination of the progression of disease and of milder or transient exacerbations will often depend, at least in part, on subject or patient recall. This is evident in Section "Frequency of WEA", in which nearly all of the studies summarized in Table 20.1 used self-reported data gathered by questionnaire in clinical or population-based settings to determine WEA status. The specific definitions used in the literature reviewed in this chapter vary somewhat among different investigators, but reflect common efforts to understand the causes, consequences, and frequency

TABLE 20.1 Prevalence of Work-Exacerbated Asthma from Studies Conducted in the General Population or General Healthcare Settings

References	Location	Study Setting and Number of Participants (% of eligible)	Criteria for Asthma	Number of Asthma Cases	Age (Years)	Timeframe for WEA	Criteria for WEA (Self-Reported on Questionnaire Unless Indicated Otherwise)	WEA Prevalence In All Adults with Asthma	In Working Adults with Asthma
8. Abramson, 1995	Australia	FU 589 with asthma symptoms, from G Pop survey (74%)	SR asthma dx	159	mean 43	Ever	Respiratory symptoms at work associated with particular job	20%	NA
9. Blanc, 1999	Sweden	FU 1562 in G Pop study (ECRHS) (65%)	SR asthma and BHR	160	20–44	Ever	Being at work ever makes chest tight or wheezy	38%	NA
10. Bolen, 2007[a,b]	US (Massachusetts)	FU 95 employed asthma cases in HMO (25%)	Asthma dx by medical record	95	18–45, mean 34	Current, tested 3 weeks	Researchers judged pattern of serial peak expiratory flow rate consistent with WEA	NA	14%
11. Bradshaw, 2018	Great Britain	Surveyed adults with asthma treated in healthcare settings (13%)	Asthma dx by medical record and SR	199 (126 currently employed)	18–65, mean 48	Current	SR asthma symptoms are worse on days at work	NA	33%
12. Caldeira, 2006[a]	Brazil	FU 1922 in birth cohort (93%)	SR asthma symptoms and BHR	227	23–25	Ever	Preexisting asthma worsened by exposure at work, based on interview information	13%	NA
13. Goh, 1994	Singapore	802 asthma cases in large primary care clinics (63%)	Asthma dx by medical record	802	20–54	Current	Work environment is asthma trigger	27%	NA
16. Henneberger, 2002	US (Colorado)	1461 asthma cases enrolled in HMO (71%)	Asthma rx or care by medical record	1461	18–44	Current job	Current work environment makes asthma worse	25%	NA
14. Henneberger, 2003	US (Maine)	664 from random sample survey of G Pop (62%)	SR asthma dx and current rx	42 (28 employed)	18–65, mean 42	Last 12 months	Coughing or wheezing is worse at work than away from work	14%	21%
15. Henneberger, 2006[a,b]	US (Massachusetts)	598 asthma cases identified in HMO records (61%)	Asthma care and dx by medical record	598 (557 employed)	18–44	Last 12 months	Combination of relevant exposure as judged by researchers and SR work-related symptoms or medication use	23%, or 21% if more stringent criteria[c]	24%, or 22% if more stringent criteria[c]
17. Henneberger, 2010	11 European countries and US	FU 9812 in G Pop study (ECRHS) (59%)	SR asthma dx and current in past 12 months	966 (employed)	29–56, mean 42	Last 12 months	Job held in past 12 months made chest tight or wheezy	NA	22%
19. Johnson, 2000[a]	Canada	FU 2974 in G Pop study (ECRHS) (39%)	SR asthma dx	106 (adult onset)	20–44	Current job	Wheezing or dyspnea at or after work in current job	34% wheezing, 31% dyspnea	NA
18. Johnson, 2006[a]	Australia	5331 in G Pop study (ECRHS) (37%)	SR asthma dx	694 (employed)	18–49	Current	Asthma better on weekends or holidays	NA	18%

(Continued)

TABLE 20.1 Prevalence of Work-Exacerbated Asthma from Studies Conducted in the General Population or General Healthcare Settings (*Continued*)

References	Location	Study Setting and Number of Participants (% of eligible)	Criteria for Asthma	Number of Asthma Cases	Age (Years)	Timeframe for WEA	Criteria for WEA (Self-Reported on Questionnaire Unless Indicated Otherwise)	WEA Prevalence In All Adults with Asthma	In Working Adults with Asthma
20. Lutzker, 2010	US (Michigan, Minnesota, and Oregon)	G Pop study—2005 BRFSS Adult Asthma Call-Back Survey (MI=54%, MN=67%, and OR=63%)	SR asthma dx and SR current asthma	MI=642 MN=330 OR=694	18 and older	Current job	Asthma made worse by chemicals, smoke, fumes, or dust in current job	MI=21% MN=24% OR=18%	NA
21. Mancuso, 2003	US (New York)	Prospective study of 230 persistent asthma cases in primary care practice (39%)	Asthma dx by medical record	102 (employed)	18 and older, mean 39	Current job	Asthma made worse by workplace conditions	NA	58%
22. Saarinen, 2003[a]	Finland	1925 asthma cases in national health insurance system (74%)	Asthma dx by medical record	969 (employed)	20–65, mean 43	Past month	Asthma symptoms caused or worsened by work at least weekly in past month	NA	20%
23. Talini, 2017[a]	Italy (Tuscany)	893 adults with asthma identified in national healthcare records (69%)	Asthma dx by pulmonary specialist	684 (employed full-time)	15–46, mean 35	Current job	Answers "yes" to ≥1 of 7 questions about work-related asthma, and did not fulfill criteria for OA	NA	41%
24. Tice, 2010	US (New York)	G Pop study—2006 and 2007 BRFSS Adult Asthma Call-Back Survey (% of eligible not indicated)	SR asthma dx and SR current asthma	750	18 and older	Current job	Asthma made worse by chemicals, smoke, fumes, or dust in current job	16%	NA
25. Villa-Rigat, 2015[a]	Spain (Catalunya)	Surveyed 368 asthma patients with work history (87%) in 16 primary healthcare centers	Asthma dx in medical records	368	16–64	Ever	Investigators reviewed evidence and judged that preexisting asthma with increased symptoms or required more medication after starting new job or after exposure to new agents in workplace, and did not fulfill criteria for OA	NA	15%

[a] OA was determined unlikely when cases of WEA were identified.

[b] The participants in Bolen 2007 (10) were a subset of the study sample in Henneberger 2006 (15), but different methods were used to determine WEA status in the two studies.

[c] Thirteen study participants with asthma were judged not to have had relevant exposures at work but were still considered to have WEA because they had reported an association between asthma and work in three different items on the questionnaire. With the application of more stringent criteria that required evidence of exposure, the prevalence of WEA was 21% (instead of 23%) among all adults with asthma and 22% (instead of 24%) among working adults with asthma.

Abbreviations: BHR, bronchial hyperresponsiveness; BRFSS, Behavioral Risk Factor Surveillance System; dx, diagnosis; ECRHS, European Community Respiratory Health Survey; G Pop, general population; HMO, health maintenance organization; NA, not applicable; OA occupational asthma; rx, medications; SR, self-reported, US, United States; WEA, work-exacerbated asthma.

of workplace exposures and conditions that adversely affect the health of people with asthma.

Frequency of WEA

The search for published literature related to WEA was conducted using the same search strategy and database as completed for the last version of this chapter. Specifically, we used PubMed to conduct a systematic search for relevant literature that incorporated terms for several topics (i.e. asthma, occupation, and exacerbation), and covered the time period of January 2012 to March 2020. In this way, we extended the previous search of the time period January 1980–January 2012. The recent search added 1093 references to the 1511 of the past searches, for a total of 2604 references of potential interest. Review of titles and abstracts for all references and full-text articles for selected references provided information summarized in the current section on frequency of WEA and in the following section on exposures.

To arrive at an overall estimate of WEA frequency, the review of references published in peer-reviewed journals between January 1980 and March 2020 identified 18 articles reporting on studies that determined WEA status on a case-by-case basis, made it possible to express the frequency of WEA as a prevalence in adults with asthma or in working adults with asthma, and were conducted in general population or general healthcare settings (8–25).

Characteristics of the 18 studies with prevalence estimates are summarized in Table 20.1. One study was based on a common protocol implemented in 11 European countries and the United States (17), and each of the other studies was conducted in one of ten countries. Each reference provided one estimate of WEA prevalence except for the study by Lutzker and colleagues (20) in the United States, which reported three state-specific estimates. Few studies shared the same methods, but the definition of asthma was typically doctor-diagnosed asthma based on self-reports or review of medical records. Two studies included bronchial hyperresponsiveness (BHR) in the criteria for asthma (9, 12). WEA was usually defined as a self-reported association between asthma symptoms and work, but four studies used more objective criteria (10, 12, 15, 25). The 18 studies calculated prevalence as the percentage of all adults with asthma or all working adults with asthma. Since the second risk set was considered preferable for WEA, the prevalence estimate based on that denominator was used for two studies (14, 15) that calculated estimates using both types of denominators. The 20 estimates of WEA prevalence from the 18 studies had a minimum of 13%, maximum of 58%, median of 21.5%, and an interquartile range from 18% to 30%.

These summary estimates for WEA prevalence varied little by several characteristics. For example, the median value for the nine estimates from the United States was 21% (10, 14–16, 20, 21, 24), nearly the same as the median of 20% for all other countries (8, 9, 11–13, 17–19, 22, 23, 25). The median WEA frequency from nine studies conducted in general healthcare settings (10, 11, 13, 15, 16, 21–23, 25) was only somewhat greater than from the general population studies (8, 9, 12, 14, 17–20, 24) (25% vs 21%, respectively; p=0.32, Wilcoxon rank-sum test). The size of study cohort seemed to have little impact on the summary estimates, with medians of 21.5% for the ten samples with at least 500 asthma cases (13, 15–18, 20, 22–24) and 22.5% for the smaller samples (8–12, 14, 19–21, 25).

The four studies that used more objective criteria for WEA status yielded lower prevalence estimates (10, 12, 15, 25). The researchers in one investigation interviewed young adults and reviewed the data collected to decide which participants with preexisting asthma had experienced worsening of symptoms due to exposures at work (12). In another study, the criteria for WEA specified a work-related pattern of serial peak expiratory flow (PEF) (10). The third study defined WEA using a combination of self-reported work-related symptoms or medication use and a decision from an expert panel that the person had been exposed to workplace asthma agents (15). In the fourth study, investigators judged WEA status for each employed participant with asthma based on occurrence of clinical symptoms relative to likely occupational exposures in the working environment (25). The prevalence estimates for these four studies with more objective WEA criteria were 13% (12), 14% (10), 15% (25), and 22% (15), respectively. The median of these four values was 14.5%, which was less than that of 23% from the other 14 studies, and the difference was statistically significant (p=0.02, Wilcoxon rank-sum test).

Exposures associated with WEA

The medical literature was reviewed to identify the types of exposures most commonly associated with WEA (see Workplace Scenario item 1). The literature search for the last edition of this book (published in 2013) was extended to March 2020. Articles based on studies conducted in clinics or general population settings were selected with the goal of capturing the range of WEA triggers across different occupations and industries. Two types of investigations reported putative occupational agents for WEA or exacerbation of asthma. In one type, the authors compiled agents for individual WEA cases that had been identified in clinics, surveillance systems, or workers' compensation programs. In the other type of study, the authors used a risk set approach, modeling exacerbation or work-related exacerbation of asthma, and testing associations with occupational exposures while controlling for potential confounders.

Eleven articles from the literature search reported on studies based in clinical or general population settings and identified triggers for individual WEA cases. Nine of the investigations were conducted in North America in the following settings: a primary care practice in New York state in the United States (21); an asthma clinic in the province of Ontario in Canada (26); occupational health clinics in the US states of New York (27), Massachusetts (28), and Washington (29); WRA surveillance systems in Ontario (30); and workers' compensation programs in Ontario (5, 31) and Washington (32). The final two published investigations were based on WEA cases from a tertiary asthma referral clinic in Belgium (33, 34). In addition, we included data from two online government sources that reported putative agents for WEA cases identified by WRA surveillance systems in several US states: California, Massachusetts, Michigan, and New Jersey during 1993–2006 (35), and California, Massachusetts, Michigan, and New York during 2009–2012 (36). The 13 data sources reported on agents for 3628 WEA cases. Table 20.2 presents the 23 most common categories of agents among these cases, with each category noted at least 40 times. Taken together, the 23 agent categories in Table 20.2 account for approximately 97% of the 4746 agents attributed to the cases.

The WEA agents in Table 20.2 are arranged in descending frequency, and at the top of the list is a general category for miscellaneous chemicals and materials (n=824). The second most common agent is mineral and inorganic dusts (n=715), which includes dust from construction and renovations and dust not

TABLE 20.2 Distribution of 4746 Agents Associated with Work-Exacerbated Asthma (WEA) by Agent Category for 3628 WEA Cases[a]

Agent Category	n	% of 4746
Miscellaneous chemicals and materials	824	17.4
Mineral and inorganic dust[b]	715	15.1
Cleaning products[c]	535	11.3
Pyrolysis products	403	8.5
Indoor air	268	5.6
Plant/tree materials	236	5.0
Paints	231	4.9
Mold	227	4.8
Physical factors and ergonomics	213	4.5
Acids, bases, and oxidizing agents	101	2.1
Aliphatic and alicyclic hydrocarbons	99	2.1
Solvents, n.o.s.	94	2.0
Animal/insect materials	90	1.9
Cigarette smoke	79	1.7
Isocyanates	70	1.5
Hydrocarbons, n.o.s.	67	1.4
Polymers	62	1.3
Miscellaneous inorganic compounds	61	1.3
Welding	53	1.1
Aromatic hydrocarbons	43	0.9
Microorganisms	42	0.9
Metals and metalloids	41	0.9
Aldehydes and acetals	41	0.9
All other agents	151	3.2

[a] From 11 articles and two government documents. See text for details.

[b] Mineral and inorganic dust category includes dusts from construction and renovations, and dust n.o.s.

[c] Cleaning products include bleach, ammonia, disinfectant cleaners, floor strippers, and floor wax.

Abbreviation: n.o.s., not otherwise specified.

otherwise specified (n.o.s.). The third through fifth most frequent agents are cleaning products (n=535), pyrolysis products (n=403), and indoor air (n=268), respectively. A few of these top-five account for a higher percentage of all WEA agents as compared to the list published in the 2013 version of this chapter. Specifically, mineral and inorganic dust went from 9.7% (i.e. 114 of 1170 agents) in the earlier table to 15.1% with the current summary, cleaning products from 4.4% to 11.3%, pyrolysis products from 5.1% to 8.5%, and indoor air from 3.9% to 5.6%. Many of the exposures in Table 20.2 are respiratory irritants, but there are also several agents capable of causing sensitization, including plant/tree materials (n=236), mold (n=227), animal/insect materials (n=90), and isocyanates (n=70). However, exacerbation associated with these types of agents was not necessarily due to a sensitization response. Several nonchemical workplace factors such as exercise, stress, cold, heat, and humidity were reported as responsible for WEA and counted in the category of physical factors and ergonomics (n=213).

The review of references from the literature search yielded three articles that reported studies conducted in general population settings that used a risk set approach to identify occupational exposures associated with exacerbation or work-related exacerbation of asthma. Findings from these articles regarding agents are consistent with the findings for individual cases of WEA. In one of the three studies, the investigators used data from 969 working adults with asthma that were identified in the records of the national health insurance system in Finland (22). The outcome was the self-report that asthma symptoms were caused or made worse by work at least weekly in the past month. Workplace exposures were either self-reported or based on expert evaluations of occupational categories, and the regression models included covariates to control for age, sex, smoking, medication use, and adult versus childhood onset of asthma. Positive findings were reported for several self-reported exposures: dusts [odds ratio (OR) = 3.1, 95% confidence interval (CI) 1.9–4.9], poor indoor air quality or abnormal temperatures (OR=2.2, 95%CI:1.5–3.2), physically strenuous work (OR=2.0, 95%CI:1.4–2.8), and chemical agents or factors (OR=1.5, 95%CI:1.1–2.2) (22). Also, from expert evaluation of occupational exposure, workers with probable (OR=2.0, 95%CI:1.4–2.8) or possible (OR=1.5, 95%CI:1.1–2.1) daily occupational exposure to dusts, fumes, or gases had elevated risk for work-related exacerbation of asthma symptoms compared to those who were rated as unlikely to have such exposure.

The second study that used a risk set approach was an international population-based study of respiratory health, conducted in 11 countries in Europe and the United States (17). The 966 participants were working adults with current asthma, and the outcome was self-reported severe exacerbation of asthma in the past 12 months. Occupational exposures included in the regression models were based on a job-exposure matrix (JEM), and the covariates included to control for potential confounding were age, sex, and smoking status. An association with severe exacerbation of asthma was reported for high gas and fumes exposure [relative risk (RR) = 2.5, 95% CI:1.2–5.5], high exposure to mineral dust (RR=1.8, 95% CI:1.02–3.2), and both low (RR=1.7, 95% CI:1.1–2.6) and high exposures (RR=3.6, 95% CI:2.2–5.8) to biological dust (17). Severe exacerbation of asthma was also associated with a summary category of high dust, gas, or fumes exposure (RR=3.1, 95% CI:1.9–5.1).

The third risk-set study was based on data from five existing investigations conducted in Sweden (37). The 1356 subjects for this study had all reported that they currently or ever had asthma. Different levels of asthma exacerbation (severe, moderate, mild) were based on self-reported asthma care in the last 12 months, and occupational exposures were assessed with both self-reports and a JEM. The regression models of exacerbation adjusted for several potential confounders, including sex, age, current smoking, second-hand smoke exposure, and either self-reported history of allergies (with self-reported exposures) or atopy and allergy in childhood (with JEM-assigned exposures). Several self-reported work exposures in the last 12 months were associated with severe exacerbation of asthma: gas, smoke, or dust (OR=1.74, 95% CI:1.17–2.58), organic dust (OR=1.72, 95% CI:1.18–2.51), dampness and mold (OR=1.79, 95% CI:1.19–2.67), cold conditions (OR=1.74, 95% CI:1.12–2.69), and physically strenuous work (OR=1.55, 95% CI:1.03–2.32). Only mild exacerbation was associated with exposures assigned using a JEM, with statistically significant results for any asthmatic agent (OR=1.62, 95% CI:1.06–2.49), and low-molecular-weight (LMW) agents (OR=2.16, 95% CI:1.05–4.44).

The ATS Statement on WEA reviewed selected papers on the types of jobs and exposures associated with WEA and offered several observations (1). First, asthma can be exacerbated by a variety of workplace factors. Second, exposures capable of exacerbating asthma in nonoccupational settings may also be relevant in occupational settings. The contents of Table 20.2 are consistent with both observations. Examples in Table 20.2 of the second observation include dusts, cleaning products, plant materials, molds, and cigarette smoke. The final observation concerned the lack of information about quantitative exposures related to WEA and what workplace exposure levels are safe for workers with asthma, suggesting the need for further investigation (1).

Distinctive features of adults with WEA

Clinical characteristics

A few studies have compared workers with WEA to adults with non-WRA. The clinical characteristics of workers with WEA did not differ greatly from adults with non-WRA. Some studies reported that workers with WEA tended to be older (16, 22), and others found an increased proportion of smokers in subjects with WEA (16, 38).

Workers with WEA are often very difficult to differentiate from asthmatic subjects with OA, especially in cases who report a new onset of asthma while in the current workplace and who are exposed to known sensitizers (see Workplace Scenario item 3). The studies that compared subjects with WEA and OA report discrepant findings that can be explained by the different populations studied (general population vs tertiary clinics). Based on cases in the United States that fulfilled SENSOR surveillance case definitions, Goe et al. (39) found that subjects with WEA were more likely to be female, young, nonwhite, and nonsmokers compared with those with new-onset WRA. These findings were not confirmed in the studies where WEA cases were from a referral clinic and defined by a worsening of asthma symptoms when at work and a negative specific inhalation challenge (SIC) to the suspected agent(s) (33, 40).

Lemière et al. (41) found that after adjusting for age, asthma control, and forced expiratory volume in one second (FEV_1), the diagnosis of WEA was associated with more frequent prescriptions of inhaled corticosteroids, a noneosinophilic phenotype, and a trend toward a higher proportion of smokers than the diagnosis of OA. Psychological distress is prevalent in workers with WRA, and WEA cases tend to have even more anxiety than OA cases (44).

The timing of the onset of asthma with respect to the start of employment at the workplace of interest does not necessarily differentiate WEA from OA. For example, from a clinical investigation conducted in Belgium, Larbanois et al. defined WEA by the presence of WRA symptoms and a negative SIC, and showed that only 7% of the 71 WEA subjects had asthma before employment (33). Also, onset of asthma prior to employment in the workplace of interest does not preclude the diagnosis of OA. Workers with previously diagnosed asthma can become sensitized to a new agent at their workplace and develop OA. An increase in asthma symptoms or severity is usually noticed at this time.

In both cases of WEA and OA, the workers complain of a worsening of their asthma symptoms when at work with an improvement when removed from exposure. Serial PEF monitoring can show a greater variability during periods at work compared to periods away from work in both types of cases, and the PEF variability is greater in subjects with OA than with WEA (45). However, the difference in the magnitude of PEF variability does not allow differentiating WEA from OA in clinical practice.

SIC testing can be performed to diagnose OA, with a positive result considered indicative of OA. Although false-negative tests can occur, a negative SIC favors the diagnosis of WEA. In several clinical studies, the definition of OA and WEA relied on the positivity or negativity, respectively, of SIC (40). However, those tests are not available in the majority of settings. One study comparing clinical cases of WEA confirmed by negative SIC to those identified using an epidemiological case definition did identify significant differences in the clinical characteristics of the two populations (6). Clinical cases were more likely to have a history of asthma-related healthcare visits and be from manufacturing industries, while epidemiological cases were from education, healthcare, and retail environments.

An eosinophilic phenotype is more frequently found in subjects with OA compared with those with WEA. Workers with OA usually show an increase in eosinophilic inflammation when exposed to the agents to which they are sensitized. In contrast, workers with WEA had no increase in eosinophilic inflammation when at work compared with periods away from work or during exposure to the suspected agents in the laboratory (40). The presence of rhinitis has been reported to be more common in OA when compared to WEA (34).

Table 20.3 summarizes demographic, clinical, functional, and inflammatory differences between subjects with WEA and subjects with non-WRA or OA.

Some risk factors have been associated with the diagnosis of OA rather than with the diagnosis of WEA. Atopy has been shown to be associated with sensitization to high-molecular-weight (HMW) agents in subjects with OA (46, 47). Smoking may also play a role in association with atopy in the risk of developing OA to some specific agents such as laboratory animals (48) and tetrachlorophthalic anhydride (49). Although some predisposing factors have been suggested for OA, no specific risk factors have been clearly identified for WEA.

Socioeconomic impact

Data reporting the high costs of OA have been previously published (50, 51). The healthcare utilization of subjects with WRA has been previously reported and is much higher than the healthcare utilization of non-WRA (38, 52). Lemière et al. (41) investigated healthcare utilization by WEA and OA cases compared to asthmatic controls. The healthcare-related costs were similar between OA and WEA but were 10-fold greater than the costs related to non-WRA (41). Although the healthcare-related costs of the subjects with OA significantly decreased during the year following the diagnosis, this was not the case for the subjects with WEA. The decrease in the number of asthma exacerbations requiring emergency room visits or hospitalizations after removal from exposure compared with the year preceding removal from exposure seems greater in OA than in WEA; however, there is still a significant improvement in subjects with WEA after removal from exposure (42). Job changes occur very frequently in subjects affected with WRA, with the evidence primarily from studies of cases treated in specialty clinics. In a few studies in which the work disruption of subjects with WEA was evaluated, it was reported to be similar to OA (33, 53), though a more recent long-term follow-up study reported that OA patients are more likely to have changed their workplace and job (54) when compared to WEA patients. There is a high rate of unemployment in workers with persistent or recurrent WEA (30%–50%) (33, 55), which is equivalent to subjects with OA. The reduction in earnings seems to be similar in WEA and OA (33) but income loss may be partially offset for those who succeed in applying for workers' compensation.

Overall, WEA exerts a large socioeconomic impact on workers and society by using a large amount of healthcare resources and inducing substantial disruption of work.

TABLE 20.3 Distinctive Demographic, Clinical, Functional, and Inflammatory Characteristics of Subjects with Work-Exacerbated Asthma Compared to Those with Non-Work-Related Asthma or Occupational Asthma

Characteristics	Compared to Adults with Non-Work-Related Asthma	Compared to Adults with Occupational Asthma
Gender	Similar (16, 22) or predominance of men in subjects with WEA (38)	Similar (30, 38) or greater number of women in subjects with WEA (39)
Age	Older (16, 22)	Similar or younger (39)
Race	More nonwhite (16)	More nonwhite (39)
Education	Less (16)	NA
Smoking habits	More likely to have ever-smoked cigarettes (16)	More smokers (30, 38)
Asthma severity	More asthma exacerbations requiring ER visits or hospitalizations in workers with WEA (38)	Same or slightly lower number of asthma exacerbations requiring ER visits or hospitalizations (41, 42)
	More days with asthma symptoms; more severe asthma based on self-report (16)	Decrease in the number of exacerbations after removal from exposure in both groups (42)
		Greater need of ICS in subjects with WEA (41)
Functional characteristics	Similar FEV_1 and PC20 (38)	Higher PEF variability when at work in subjects with OA compared to those with WEA (41)
		PC20 may be lower in subjects with WEA (33)
Airway inflammation	Neutrophilic inflammation inconsistently found depending on the study (40, 43)	Eosinophilic airway inflammation in subjects with OA when at work (40, 41)

Abbreviations: ER, emergency room; FEV_1, forced expiratory volume in 1 second; ICS, inhaled corticosteroids; NA, not applicable; OA, occupational asthma; PC20, provocative concentration of methacholine causing a 20% fall in FEV_1; PEF, peak expiratory flow; WEA, work-exacerbated asthma.

Clinical approach to WEA

WEA should be suspected in all patients whose asthma is difficult to control and in patients who complain of a worsening of their symptoms or who require an increase of their asthma medication when at work (2) (see Workplace Scenario item 2).

Before establishing a diagnosis of WEA, the diagnosis of asthma needs to be confirmed by objective measures (see Workplace Scenario item 5). Most asthma guidelines recommend the performance of spirometry, including the measurement of FEV_1 both pre- and post-bronchodilator in order to show a FEV_1 reversibility of 12% with an absolute increase in FEV_1 of at least 200 mL (56). In the absence of a reversible airflow limitation, the measurement of airway hyperresponsiveness can confirm the diagnosis of asthma. The lack of objective confirmation of the diagnosis of asthma can lead to misdiagnosis in 30% of cases (57). Furthermore, nonspecific respiratory symptoms are frequent and can mimic asthma in workers exposed to a dusty or irritant environment (58).

The diagnosis of WEA relies on the demonstration of a relationship between occupational exposures and the occurrence of asthma exacerbations, or poor asthma control during periods at work, combined with the determination that OA is unlikely. Asthma exacerbations or loss of asthma control can be documented by a change in the frequency and severity of asthma symptoms or by the need for an increase in asthma medications. Asthma exacerbations can also be documented by the occurrence of emergency visits or hospitalizations or by changes in respiratory function at work. Serial PEF monitoring can show increased variability during periods at work compared to periods away from work (45). Identifying the factors that trigger asthma symptoms is important not only to confirm the diagnosis of WEA but also to decrease or remove the adverse environmental conditions at the workplace (see Workplace Scenario item 4). Identifying multiple triggers is common, since the workers are frequently exposed to several agents concomitantly.

Differentiating WEA from OA can be challenging when the prior history of asthma is not well established with objective testing. There is significant overdiagnosis and underdiagnosis of asthma in the population with estimates of underdiagnosis between 20% to 70% of cases, while overdiagnosis between 30%–35% of cases (59). This can make distinguishing new-onset WRA as compared to worsening of preexisting disease or new diagnosis of non-WRA difficult. When dealing with work environments with primarily irritant exposures, distinguishing a possible irritant-induced asthma case from WEA may not be possible with absolute certainty. Detailed assessment and review of prior medical documentation is helpful.

Although there is limited data concerning the management of WEA, professional organizations have advised minimizing exposures at work and optimizing standard medical management for asthma (e.g. pharmacologic treatment and avoidance of symptom triggers) (1, 2). Differentiating WEA from OA may be useful for asthma management. The approach used to differentiate one type of WRA case from the other should depend on the expected benefit to the patient and is likely to reflect the standards of practice where the patient resides. Although there is clear evidence that a persistent exposure to the occupational agent that caused their asthma is detrimental for workers with OA (60), the impact of continuing exposure to triggers for WEA has not been well studied. There is limited evidence that workers with OA may have a greater improvement in their lung function and asthma control than those with WEA when removed from exposure (41, 53).

Prevention of WEA

Exacerbations of asthma from workplace exposures or conditions can be prevented by modification of the work environment to reduce the frequency or intensity of exposure to triggers (see Workplace Scenario item 6). This requires an understanding of what the WRA triggers are, combined with the knowledge, motivation, and opportunity to make changes that result in improved control or elimination of WEA. Standard industrial hygiene practices should be employed to control exposures to offending agents such as dust, fumes, and vapors. There is a conceptual "hierarchy of controls" guiding workplace interventions that focus on environmental change (eliminating, containing, or diluting toxic exposures; temperature controls), administrative change (job rotation or redesign), and, least effectively, personal protective equipment (PPE) such as respirators.

In general, reduction of dusts, fumes, and vapors and other toxic exposures in the workplace, good housekeeping practices, control of ambient temperature and humidity, and maintaining a work organization that supports employee health and well-being and controls unnecessary stressors can benefit all workers, particularly those with asthma. A comprehensive respiratory protection program (involving proper selection, fit testing, and maintenance of respirators, as well as user training) is valuable where respirator use is a necessary or desirable supplement to environmental control of respiratory hazards.

Since WEA is the result of the interaction between the individual with asthma and their work environment, optimal medical management, including but not limited to pharmacologic management, is also appropriate. Unfortunately, the dearth of long-term outcome studies comparing different management strategies limits confidence in any single approach. In particular, use of bronchodilator and anti-inflammatory medications may control symptoms and enable exposure to higher levels of triggering agents, but the long-term consequences of symptom control without environmental control of triggers have not been investigated adequately.

In reality, specific approaches to prevention of exacerbations in an individual with asthma through environmental interventions at work are often easier to describe than to achieve in practice. Prevention relies upon the following:

- Recognition by the affected individual, the healthcare provider, and/or the employer that the work environment is triggering asthma in a susceptible individual.
- Belief that changes in the work environment are possible.
- Willingness of the affected individual to communicate health concerns to the employer and a pathway for this communication.
- The willingness and ability of an employer to make the changes in the work environment needed to control or eliminate triggers.
- The ability of clinicians to diagnose and document WEA and a willingness to assist the affected patient advocate for reduction or elimination of hazards triggering episodes.

Clinicians are often instrumental in helping patients with asthma to recognize the connection between workplace conditions and exposures, and exacerbations. Careful inquiry may identify specific triggers and the patient may be able to act on the possibility of eliminating or controlling them. Clinicians are also key to optimization of pharmacologic and nonpharmacologic management of asthma and adherence to recommended measures.

Employers in large measure, both legally and in reality, are responsible for workplace practices and exposures that may trigger asthma exacerbations. They may, however, lack the knowledge, resources, or motivation to make changes in work processes, job assignments, or workplace organization, or not believe or understand that it is their responsibility to do so. In some instances, especially for small employers, flexibility to reduce or eliminate triggers may be limited.

Patients, particularly the most economically vulnerable, may be reluctant to request changes in work assignments or exposures. While there may be some level of legal protection for a worker with asthma requesting accommodation through work reassignment or redesign, for example, by the Americans with Disabilities Act (ADA) in the United States, the results of ADA litigation are inconsistent. Legal consultation with an attorney familiar with this area may be useful. In some, but not all, jurisdictions there may be support available for people with OA through workers' compensation systems; however, compensation is rarely available for people with WEA.

Directions of future research

- Accurate exposure assessment is essential to estimating exposure-response relationships in clinical and epidemiologic studies. Improved methods are needed to characterize workplace exposures responsible for WEA. Identification of what exposure levels are safe for most workers with asthma would greatly assist prevention efforts.
- Additional research should elaborate whether subsets of people with asthma are at increased risk for workplace exacerbation. For example, are those who respond to specific identifiable triggers such as aeroallergens at increased risk for exacerbation in particular work environments, including those that do not include the specific triggers?
- Prospective surveillance of newly hired workers (preferably apprentices) with histories of currently controlled asthma or asthma in remission in workplaces where asthma triggers are likely to be encountered would contribute to understanding the development and natural history of WEA. Outcomes of interest would include (*i*) the number and frequency of asthma flares, (*ii*) the effects of workplace exposure on asthma control or severity both short term and long term, (*iii*) the extent of temporary or permanent time lost from work as a result of exposure, (*iv*) the health consequences of continuing employment at such worksites, (*v*) the responses to various interventions, and (*vi*) the amount of time required to resolve and reestablish control of asthma.
- General health surveillance programs should fine-tune annual incidence data by including the means to identify WEA among working participants with asthma.
- Additional studies are needed to examine the economic, social (e.g. family), and productivity impact of WEA over time.
- Evaluating the effectiveness of different interventions would help determine which strategies for reducing or eliminating exposures and for maximizing asthma care have the best chance of achieving primary prevention of WEA among those at risk and minimizing adverse outcomes among existing WEA cases.
- Further research is needed to determine whether having workers with persistent or recurrent WEA leave their workplace is more effective than maintaining workers with WEA at their workplace with optimal asthma care and reduction of exposures for achieving an adequate asthma control. Studies to advance understanding of the long-term pulmonary function consequences related to the frequency of exacerbations of WEA would be relevant. The socioeconomic consequences of both approaches should be assessed and compared.

Conclusions

Exacerbation of asthma can result from exposures at home, at work, in the outdoor environment, and in public buildings.

Asthma-related exposures in the work environment are less frequently addressed, because exposures are often beyond the control of the individual patient and an employer may or may not accept the responsibility or have the ability to control exposures. The issue of an affected employee's right to workplace accommodation or compensation further clouds the issue. Research demonstrates that WEA is an important source of work disability and economic loss and is an appropriate target for prevention. Additional outcomes research can help define how to address this problem more effectively.

Disclaimer

The findings and conclusions in this chapter are those of the authors and do not necessarily represent the views of the National Institute for Occupational Safety and Health.

References

1. Henneberger PK, Redlich CA, Callahan DB, et al. An official American Thoracic Society statement: work-exacerbated asthma. Am J Respir Crit Care Med. 201;184(3):368–78.
2. Tarlo SM, Balmes J, Balkissoon R, et al. Diagnosis and management of work-related asthma: American College of Chest Physicians consensus statement. Chest. 2008;134(3 Suppl):1S–41S.
3. Jajosky RA, Harrison R, Reinisch F, et al. Surveillance of work-related asthma in selected U.S. states using surveillance guidelines for state health departments–California, Massachusetts, Michigan, and New Jersey, 1993–1995. MMWR CDC Surveill Summ. 1999;48(3):1–20.
4. Ribeiro M, Buyantseva LV, Liss GM, et al. M. Impact of a cleaners' strike on compensation claims for asthma among teachers in Ontario. Can Respir J. [Research Support, Non-U.S. Gov't]. 2013;20(3):171–4.
5. Lim T, Liss GM, Vernich L, et al. Work-exacerbated asthma in a workers' compensation population. Occup Med (Lond). 2014;64:206–10.
6. Henneberger PK, Liang X, Lemière C. A comparison of work-exacerbated asthma cases from clinical and epidemiological settings. Can Respir J. 2013;20(3):159–64.
7. Katz I, Moshe S, Sosna J, et al. The occurrence, recrudescence, and worsening of asthma in a population of young adults—impact of varying types of occupation. Chest. 1999;116(3):614–8.
8. Abramson MJ, Kutin JJ, Rosier MJ, Bowes G. Morbidity, medication and trigger factors in a community sample of adults with asthma. Med J Aust.1995;162(2):78–81.
9. Blanc PD, Ellbjar S, Janson C, et al. Asthma-related work disability in Sweden. The impact of workplace exposures. Am J Respir Crit Care Med. 1999;160(6):2028–33.
10. Bolen AR, Henneberger PK, Liang X, et al. The validation of work-related self-reported asthma exacerbation. Occup Environ Med. 2007;64(5):343–8.
11. Bradshaw L, Sumner J, Delic J, et al. Work aggravated asthma in Great Britain: a cross-sectional postal survey. Prim Health Care Res Dev. 2018;19(6):561–9.
12. Caldeira RD, Bettiol H, Barbieri MA, et al. Prevalence and risk factors for work related asthma in young adults. Occup Environ Med. 2006;63(10):694–9.
13. Goh LG, Ng TP, Hong CY, et al. Outpatient adult bronchial asthma in Singapore. Singapore Med J. 1994;35(2):190–4.
14. Henneberger PK, Deprez RD, Asdigian N, et al. Workplace exacerbation of asthma symptoms: findings from a population-based study in Maine. Arch Environ Health. 2003;58(12):781–8.
15. Henneberger PK, Derk SJ, Sama SR, et al. The frequency of workplace exacerbation among health maintenance organisation members with asthma. Occup Environ Med. 2006;63(8):551–7.
16. Henneberger PK, Hoffman CD, Magid DJ, Lyons EE. Work-related exacerbation of asthma. Int J Occup Environ Health. 2002;8(4):291–6.
17. Henneberger PK, Mirabelli MC, Kogevinas M, et al. The occupational contribution to severe exacerbation of asthma. Eur Respir J. 2010;36(4):743–50.
18. Johnson A, Toelle BG, Yates D, et al. Occupational asthma in New South Wales (NSW): a population-based study. Occup Med (Lond). 2006;56(4):258–62.
19. Johnson AR, Dimich-Ward HD, Manfreda J, et al. Occupational asthma in adults in six Canadian communities. Am J Respir Crit Care Med. 2000;162(6):2058–62.
20. Lutzker LA, Rafferty AP, Brunner WM, et al. Prevalence of work-related asthma in Michigan, Minnesota, and Oregon. J Asthma. 2010;47(2):156–61.
21. Mancuso CA, Rincon M, Charlson ME. Adverse work outcomes and events attributed to asthma. Am J Ind Med. 2003;44(3):236–45.
22. Saarinen K, Karjalainen A, Martikainen R, et al. Prevalence of work-aggravated symptoms in clinically established asthma. Eur Respir J. 2003;22(2):305–9.
23. Talini D, Ciberti A, Bartoli D, et al. Work-related asthma in a sample of subjects with established asthma. Respir Med. 2017;130:85–91.
24. Tice CJ, Cummings KR, Gelberg KH. Surveillance of work-related asthma in New York state. J Asthma. 2010;47(3):310–6.
25. Vila-Rigat R, Panades Valls R, Hernandez Huet E, et al. Prevalence of work-related asthma and its impact in primary health care. Archivos de Bronconeumologia. 2015;51(9):449–55.
26. Tarlo SM, Leung K, Broder I, et al. Asthmatic subjects symptomatically worse at work: prevalence and characterization among a general asthma clinic population. Chest. 2000;118(5):1309–14.
27. Fletcher AM, London MA, Gelberg KH, Grey AJ. Characteristics of patients with work-related asthma seen in the New York State occupational health clinics. J Occup Environ Med. 2006;48(11):1203–11.
28. Gassert TH, Hu H, Kelsey KT, Christiani DC. Long-term health and employment outcomes of occupational asthma and their determinants. J Occup Environ Med. 1998;40(5):481–91.
29. Wheeler S, Rosenstock L, Barnhart S. A case series of 71 patients referred to a hospital-based occupational and environmental medicine clinic for occupational asthma. West J Med. 1998;168(2):98–104.
30. To T, Tarlo SM, McLimont S, et al. Feasibility of a provincial voluntary reporting system for work-related asthma in Ontario. Can Respir J. 2011;18(5):275–7.
31. Tarlo SM, Liss G, Corey P, Broder I. A workers' compensation claim population for occupational asthma. Comparison of subgroups. Chest. 1995;107(3):634–41.
32. Anderson NJ, Reeb-Whitaker CK, Bonauto DK, Rauser E. Work-related asthma in Washington state. J Asthma. 2011;48(8):773–82.
33. Larbanois A, Jamart J, Delwiche JP, Vandenplas O. Socioeconomic outcome of subjects experiencing asthma symptoms at work. Eur Respir J. 2002;19(6):1107–13.
34. Vandenplas O, Van Brussel P, D'Alpaos V, et al. Rhinitis in subjects with work-exacerbated asthma. Respir Med. 2010;104(4):497–503.
35. CDC. Work-related asthma: Most frequently reported agents associated with work-related asthma cases by asthma classification, 1993–2006. Atlanta: NIOSH; 2012.
36. CDC. Work-related asthma: Most frequently reported agents associated with work-related asthma cases by asthma classification, 2009–2012. 2017 [April 6, 2020]. https://wwwn.cdc.gov/eWorld/Grouping/Asthma/97#State-based
37. Kim JL, Henneberger PK, Lohman S, et al. Impact of occupational exposures on exacerbation of asthma: a population-based asthma cohort study. BMC Pulm Med. 2016;16(1):148.
38. Lemiere C, Forget A, Dufour MH, et al. Characteristics and medical resource use of asthmatic subjects with and without work-related asthma. J Allergy Clin Immunol. 2007;120(6):1354–9.
39. Goe SK, Henneberger PK, Reilly MJ, et al. A descriptive study of work aggravated asthma. Occup Environ Med. 2004;61(6):512–7.
40. Girard F, Chaboillez S, Cartier A, et al. An effective strategy for diagnosing occupational asthma: use of induced sputum. Am J Respir Crit Care Med. 2004;170(8):845–50.
41. Lemière C, Boulet LP, Chaboillez S, et al. Work-exacerbated asthma and occupational asthma: Do they really differ? J Allergy and Clin Immunol. 2013;131(3):704–10.
42. Lemiere C, To T, De Olim C, et al. Outcome of work-related asthma exacerbations in Quebec and Ontario. Eur Respir J. 2015;45(1):266–8.
43. Lemiere C, Pizzichini MM, Balkissoon R, et al. Diagnosing occupational asthma: use of induced sputum. Eur Respir J. 1999;13(3):482–8.
44. Lipszyc JC, Silverman F, Holness DL, et al. Comparison of psychological, quality of life, work-limitation, and socioeconomic status between patients with occupational asthma and work-exacerbated asthma. J Occup Environ Med. 2017;59(7):697–702.
45. Chiry S, Cartier A, Malo JL, et al. Comparison of peak expiratory flow variability between workers with work-exacerbated asthma and occupational asthma. Chest. 2007;132(2):483–8.
46. Archambault S, Malo JL, Infante-Rivard C, et al. Incidence of sensitization, symptoms, and probable occupational rhinoconjunctivitis and asthma in apprentices starting exposure to latex. J Allergy Clin Immunol. 2001;107(5 Suppl.):921–3.

47. Gautrin D, Ghezzo H, Infante-Rivard C, Malo JL. Incidence and determinants of IgE-mediated sensitization in apprentices: a prospective study. Am J Respir Crit Care Med. 2000;162(4 I):1222–8.

48. Venables KM, Upton JL, Hawkins ER, et al. Smoking, atopy, and laboratory animal allergy. Br J Ind Med. 1988;45(10):667–71.

49. Venables KM. Low molecular weight chemicals, hypersensitivity, and direct toxicity: the acid anhydrides. Br J Ind Med. 1989;46(4):222–32.

50. Ayres JG, Boyd R, Cowie H, Hurley JF. Costs of occupational asthma in the UK. Thorax. 2011;66(2):128–33.

51. Leigh JP, Romano PS, Schenker MB, Kreiss K. Costs of occupational COPD and asthma. Chest. 2002;121(1):264–72.

52. Breton CV, Zhang Z, Hunt PR, et al. Characteristics of work related asthma: results from a population based survey. Occup Environ Med. 2006;63(6):411–5.

53. Pelissier S, Chaboillez S, Teolis L, Lemiere C. Outcome of subjects diagnosed with occupational asthma and work-aggravated asthma after removal from exposure. J Occup Environ Med. 2006;48(7):656–9.

54. Moullec G, Lavoie KL, Malo JL, et al. Long-term socioprofessional and psychological status in workers investigated for occupational asthma in Quebec. J Occup Environ Med. 2013;55(9):1052–64.

55. Cannon J, Cullinan P, Newman Taylor A. Consequences of occupational asthma. BMJ. 1995;311(7005):602–3.

56. Lougheed DM, Lemière C, Dell SD, et al. Canadian Thoracic Society Asthma Management Continuum—2010 consensus summary for children six years of age and over, and adults. Can Respir J. 2010;17(1):15–24.

57. Aaron SD, Vandemheen KL, FitzGerald JM, et al. Reevaluation of diagnosis in adults with physician-diagnosed asthma. JAMA. 2017;317(3):269–79.

58. Chiry S, Boulet LP, Lepage J, et al. Frequency of work-related respiratory symptoms in workers without asthma. Am J Ind Med. 2009;52(6):447–54.

59. Aaron SD, Boulet LP, Reddel HK, Gershon AS. Underdiagnosis and overdiagnosis of asthma. Am J Respir Crit Care Med. 2018;198(8):1012–20.

60. Henneberger PK, Patel JR, de Groene GJ, et al. Workplace interventions for treatment of occupational asthma. Cochrane Database Syst Rev. 2019;10:Cd006308.

21

EOSINOPHILIC BRONCHITIS

Santiago Quirce,[1] Catherine Lemière,[2] Jolanta Walusiak-Skorupa,[3] Olivier Vandenplas,[4] and Joaquín Sastre[5]

[1]*Department of Allergy, La Paz University Hospital, IdiPAZ, Madrid, Spain*
[2]*CIUSSS du Nord de l'île de Montréal, Hôpital du Sacré-Coeur de Montréal and
Université de Montréal, Montréal, Québec QC, Canada*
[3]*Department of Occupational Diseases and Environmental Health, Nofer Institute of Occupational Medicine, Lodz, Poland*
[4]*Centre hospitalier Universitaire UCL Namur and Université Catholique de Louvain, Yvoir, Belgium*
[5]*Allergology Department. Fundacion Jimenez Diaz, Facultad de Medicina, Universidad Autonoma de Madrid, Madrid, Spain*

Contents

CASE HISTORY

1. A 51-year-old woman, in charge of a pastry/bakery shop for more than 14 years has experienced persistent cough, wheezing or dyspnea, over the last 8 years. Symptoms subsided during holidays and days off work and worsened during working days, especially when she was near to the pastry/bakery workroom.

2. Skin-prick testing (SPT) with allergen extracts was negative to wheat flour and positive to fungal α-amylase (12-mm wheal). Specific IgE (ImmunoCAP®, Thermo Fisher Scientific, Uppsala, Sweden) to fungal α-amylase was 3.83 kU/L and to wheat flour was <0.35 kU/L. SPTs and IgE determinations to soy flour and other baking additives were negative.

3. Spirometry revealed a forced vital capacity (FVC) of 3.7 L (106% predicted), FEV_1 of 3.2 L (108%), and FEV_1/FVC 87%. Methacholine inhalation test when at work was negative on three occasions, as was as bronchial challenge with adenosine. Fractional exhaled NO (FeNO) was measured at 82 ppb after a work shift. Peak expiratory flow (PEF) monitoring during 15 working days and 15 nonworking days revealed no significant daily variability.

4. Due to the high suspicion of eosinophilic bronchitis, induced sputum was assessed before and 24 hours after a specific bronchial challenge test with α-amylase. No asthmatic response was observed, and the methacholine inhalation test was negative both before and after the α-amylase bronchial challenge. However, sputum eosinophilia increased from 4.2% at baseline to 33.3% 24 hours after the α-amylase challenge.

5. The presence of sputum eosinophilia before specific challenge as well as the increase in sputum eosinophils after bronchial challenge with α-amylase, the worsening of respiratory symptoms during workdays, and the absence of airway hyperresponsiveness (AHR) to methacholine/adenosine strongly suggest the diagnosis of occupational eosinophilic bronchitis due to α-amylase. This patient was removed from exposure, and 1 month later, both respiratory symptoms and sputum eosinophilia waned up, which further supported the diagnosis.

6. Comment: Measuring sputum eosinophilia at work and away from work, along with monitorization of respiratory symptoms, is another way to confirm the diagnosis, and this approach is especially useful for centers that do not perform specific inhalation challenges.

Concept and definition

In 1989, Gibson et al. (1) described a series of seven patients with chronic cough and sputum eosinophilia (sputum eosinophil count >2.5%) but a normal spirometry, no evidence of airway hyperresponsiveness (AHR) to methacholine, and normal peak expiratory flow (PEF) variability. The functional features of this condition were thus different from those of asthma, and the authors suggested the term *nonasthmatic eosinophilic bronchitis* (NAEB) (1). Shortly afterward, these investigators reported that cough and sputum eosinophilia improved markedly with inhaled corticosteroid (ICS) treatment (2). NAEB has since been documented as a common cause of ICS-responsive cough, accounting for approximately 10%–33% of cases of chronic cough in tertiary referral clinics (3–5).

In the following two decades after the initial description of NAEB by Gibson et al., it became increasingly recognized that a similar condition could be caused by workplace sensitizing agents (6) and common allergens (7). Occupational eosinophilic bronchitis (OEB) does not fulfill the current definition of occupational asthma (OA) since variable airflow obstruction and AHR are lacking (Chapter 1). Nevertheless, OEB should be regarded as a variant syndrome of OA because respiratory symptoms, predominantly cough, are associated with changes in sputum eosinophil counts related to the exposure to a specific agent present at the workplace (8).

Eosinophils are the characteristic cells in asthma and OA (Chapters 4 and 7) and are useful in confirming the diagnosis and monitoring exacerbations and outcome. Eosinophils have been identified for long as a key cell in asthma. Curschmann (1846–1910) and Ernst von Leyden (1832–1910), respectively, discovered spirals and crystals in sputum of asthmatic subjects, derived from eosinophils (see Chapter 2). Although the initial proposal of definition of asthma made by the American Thoracic Society (9) did not mention the presence of eosinophils, later definitions refer to asthma and OA as conditions in which prevails "eosinophilic airway inflammation." Identification of eosinophils in bronchoalveolar lavage (BAL) and induced sputum were later proposed in the diagnosis and monitoring of the condition (10). Asthmatic reactions induced by occupational sensitizing agents are most often—but inconstantly—associated with eosinophilic airway inflammation (11).

Neutrophils are also involved in asthma. Increased sputum neutrophilia (40% to 60%) has been associated with a phenotype of asthma that reflects a more severe status and with a relative resistance to steroid treatment (12). Exposure to diisocyanates can cause asthmatic reactions with isolated increased sputum neutrophils or a combination of increased neutrophils and eosinophils, sometimes in the absence of changes in functional parameters (13). Anees and coworkers examined 38 subjects with OA to LMW agents (including six subjects with OA caused by diisocyanates) at the time they were still at work. More than one-third had increased sputum eosinophils, all subjects showing neutrophilia. Subjects with eosinophils had more severe asthma (14). There is only one case report suggesting that isocyanates may induce work-related cough associated with an isolated increase in sputum neutrophils in the absence of physiological evidence of asthma (15).

Pathogenesis

The pathophysiological mechanisms involved in the development of OEB remain largely uncertain. OEB and OA share common features. The workplace agents causing OEB have also been documented as potential sensitizers inducing OA. An IgE-mediated mechanism has been documented in all case reports of OEB related to HMW agents similar to what has been reported in OA (6, 16–18). However, OEB, like NAEB, is characterized by a dissociation between eosinophilic airway inflammation and AHR.

There has been intense research trying to explain why patients with NAEB do not demonstrate AHR despite similar degrees of eosinophilic airway inflammation and reticular basement membrane thickening as those observed in asthma (19, 20). One hypothesis was that NAEB might be associated with less active airway inflammation and a lower release of important proinflammatory mediators. This hypothesis, however, is not supported by studies that compared the concentration or gene expression of various inflammatory mediators in BAL fluid, induced sputum supernatants, and bronchial biopsies of patients with asthma,

patients with NAEB, and healthy individuals. Sputum eosinophil cationic protein and cysteinyl leukotriene concentrations were significantly higher both in NAEB and asthma than in control subjects (21). Gibson et al. (22) found that gene expression for interleukin (IL)-5 messenger RNA and granulocyte macrophage-colony-stimulating factor (GM-CSF) mRNA were expressed by BAL cells from asthmatic patients and individuals with chronic cough responsive to ICS while they were not detected in individuals with chronic cough nonresponsive to ICS. Brightling et al. (23) demonstrated that there were no differences between patients with asthma and NAEB in the expression of the T-helper type 2 (TH2) cytokines IL-4 and IL-5 in BAL CD4 T cells and bronchial submucosa suggesting that the release of TH2 cytokines is not directly responsible for the AHR that characterizes asthma. Overall, these findings in NAEB compared to asthma demonstrated that eosinophilic airway inflammation and basement membrane thickening are regulated independently from AHR (20). In addition, Siddiqui et al. (24) reported that vascular remodeling and increased expression of vascular endothelial growth factor (VEGF) are features of both NAEB and asthma, and are dissociated from AHR. These authors also showed that structural remodeling of the airway wall, notably increased airway smooth muscle mass, occurs to a similar degree in NAEB and asthma (25). However, the assessment of airway geometry by computed tomography imaging revealed airway wall thickening in asthma but not in OEB (26, 27). These results suggest that the absence of airway wall thickening in patients with NAEB may be involved in the absence of AHR in these patients.

The immunohistochemical analysis of bronchial biopsy specimens revealed that the number of mast cells in airway smooth muscle bundles was significantly higher in subjects with asthma than that in those with NAEB and in normal controls (19). In addition, the number of mast cells infiltrating the airway smooth muscle correlated with the degree of AHR to methacholine (25). These findings indicate that the interactions between mast cells and airway smooth muscle cells may be important in the pathogenesis of AHR. On the other hand, sputum IL-13 concentrations (28, 29) and IL-13 expression in eosinophils and mast cells in the bronchial submucosa were higher in patients with asthma than in patients with NAEB (29, 30). Sputum IL-13 concentration correlated with the level of AHR (28). Histamine and prostaglandin (PG) D2 sputum concentrations were significantly higher in NAEB than in asthma, suggesting that the activation of mast cells in superficial airway structures is a particular feature of this condition (21).

Sastre et al. (31) found that induced sputum PGE2 concentrations are strikingly increased in subjects with NAEB as compared with asthmatic and healthy subjects. These data suggest that the differences in airway function observed in subjects with NAEB and asthma might be due to differences in PGE2 production. In another investigation carried out by the same group, the authors showed that expression of two PGE2 receptors, EP2 and EP4, was increased in patients with NAEB (32). It was also shown that bronchial smooth muscle cell proliferation was inhibited to a greater extent with sputum supernatants from patients with NAEB than in those from asthmatic subjects and healthy controls, mostly due to PGE2 levels, a fact which was confirmed by employing synthetic EP2 and EP4 agonist and antagonist receptors (32). These findings suggest that PGE2 inhibits bronchial smooth muscle cell proliferation, entailing a reduction of smooth muscle hyperplasia and thus protecting against the onset of airflow obstruction (33).

TABLE 21.1 Causal Agents That Have Been Involved in Occupational Eosinophilic Bronchitis

Causal Agent/Occupation	Number of Workers	Diagnostic Procedure	References
Tetrahydrophthalic anhydride/epoxy resin handler	1	NA	(34)
Cyanoacrylate/methacrylate/glue handler	1	At/off work and SIC	(35)
Latex/nurse	1 (3.3%)[a]	SIC	(16)
Mushroom spores/mushroom workers	3 (7.1%)[a]	Sputum eosinophilia and absence of AHR at work	(42)
Lysozyme/confectioner	1 (4.7%)[a]	SIC	(6)
Welding fumes/welder	1	At/off work and SIC	(36)
Formaldehyde/laboratory technician	1	At/off work and SIC	(36)
Chloramine T/nurse	1	SIC	(37)
Isocyanate (MDI)/foundry worker	1	At/off work and SIC	(17)
Cereal flour/baker	1	At/off work and SIC	(17)
α-amylase and wheat flour/baker	1	At/off work and SIC	(18)
Styrene/auto body shop worker	1	At/off work (FeNO)[b]	(39)
Storage mites/baker	1	At/off work and SIC	(44)
Ammonium persulfate/hairdresser	1	SIC (FeNO[c])	(38)
Metalworking fluid/machine operator	1	At/off work (FeNO[c])	(40)

[a] Estimated prevalence in groups of subjects investigated for work-related respiratory symptoms; [b]Occupational eosinophilic bronchitis documented by work-related changes in sputum eosinophils and FeNO (no changes during SIC); [c]Exposure-related changes in eosinophilic airway inflammation documented using FeNO measurements.

Abbreviations: AHR, airway hyperresponsiveness; NA, not available (article in Japanese); FeNO, fractional exhaled nitric oxide; SIC, specific inhalation challenge (in the laboratory).

Causal agents

A number of HMW and LMW workplace sensitizing agents have been documented as causing OEB in case reports (6, 16–18, 34–40). These agents as well as the procedures used to establish a diagnosis of OEB are summarized in Table 21.1.

The prevalence of OEB remains largely unknown. Quirce et al. (16, 41) investigated 30 healthcare workers with possible OA caused by natural rubber latex. Specific inhalation challenge (SIC) with powdered latex gloves was performed in a 7-m^3 chamber. Twenty-seven patients (90%) had rhinoconjunctivitis; 19 patients (63%) had an asthmatic reaction; and 1 patient (3.3%) developed eosinophilic bronchitis after the challenge. These investigators (6) also evaluated 21 bakers or confectioners with possible OA through an SIC. OEB caused by egg lysozyme was documented in one worker (4.7%). Tanaka et al. (42) conducted a cross-sectional survey of 69 mushroom workers who produced *Hypsizigus marmoreus*. Participants completed a cross-sectional survey 2 years after starting work at the mushroom farm. Of the 63 workers included in the study, 42 workers (67%) reported chronic cough after starting to work in the farm. Three (7.1%) of these workers were diagnosed as having eosinophilic bronchitis based on a sputum eosinophil count >3% and the absence of AHR, although the work-relatedness of sputum eosinophilia was not demonstrated in these subjects. In a recent multicenter cohort study of 259 subjects with a negative SIC in terms of the changes in FEV$_1$ and AHR, 33 (13%) developed an isolated sputum eosinophilic response after challenge exposure to various workplace agents in the absence of demonstrable AHR both at baseline and postchallenge assessments (43). Among these 33 subjects with OEB documented through a SIC, the majority of causal agents were LMW compounds (n=24) and isocyanates accounted for half (n=13) of these LMW agents. HMW agents included predominantly wheat and rye flour (n=7). Some of the causal agents in this series have not been previously documented as inducing OEB (i.e. quaternary ammonium compounds, methylchloroisothiazolinone, paraphenylendiamine, and *Penicillium notatum*).

Diagnosis

The proposed criteria for establishing a diagnosis of OEB are presented below (same section, Diagnosis). OEB should be suspected in every adult with new-onset chronic cough or respiratory symptoms that are induced or worsened by their workplace (see Case History item 1). A comprehensive history detailing the employment history (current and past jobs) and the respiratory symptoms (nature, temporal relationship to work) should be collected (Chapter 5). In many cases, the patient may not be aware of the exact chemical exposures at work; material safety data sheets (SDSs) can be requested from the workplace and may be helpful in clarifying the presence of a workplace sensitizer. In addition to identifying potentially sensitizing agents, the exposure history should include the duration of exposure and the frequency and concentrations of exposure. As for OA, the diagnostic workup should include the performance of skin-prick tests (SPTs) and/or IgE measurements to HMW or LMW agents (if available) to which the patient may be exposed at work (see Case History item 2). It should be kept in mind, however, that a positive immunologic test indicates sensitization but not necessarily causality.

The patients suffering from OEB usually complain of a chronic cough when at work that resolves when they are removed from their workplace. Although isolated cough with or without sputum production is the predominant symptom associated with eosinophilic bronchitis and OEB, other asthma-like symptoms (i.e. wheezing, chest tightness, and breathlessness) have been reported in a substantial proportion of the subjects (5 of 12; 42%) described in published case reports of OEB (6, 35, 36, 39, 43). In contrast to patients with OA, there is no evidence of airflow obstruction, increased PEF variability, or AHR (see Case

History item 3). However, the performance of a spirometry and a methacholine/histamine challenge is an important part of the investigation since these tests allow for discarding the diagnosis of asthma. Indirect bronchial challenges with adenosine monophosphate and mannitol are dependent on the presence of airway inflammation, and may be positive in asthmatic subjects with a negative response to methacholine. It has been documented that subjects with NAEB are not responsive to either direct or indirect bronchial challenge (45) providing further evidence for a dissociation between airway inflammation and AHR.

The diagnosis of OEB relies on the demonstration of respiratory symptoms associated with an eosinophilic airway inflammation during periods at work that resolve or improve after a period away from work without treatment (see Case History items 1, 5, and 6). Eosinophilic inflammation can be assessed by performing an induced sputum analysis (see Case History item 4). A baseline sputum eosinophil count greater than 2.5% is considered significant compared to healthy subjects (Chapter 7), although the sputum eosinophil count may be less than 2.5% when the subjects are evaluated while removed from workplace exposure. The key diagnostic feature of OEB is the documentation of a significant (≥3%) increase in sputum eosinophil count while exposed to the offending agent at work as compared to a period away from exposure.

Another approach for diagnosing OEB is by performing SICs to the suspected agents and monitoring sputum eosinophil counts before and after challenge exposure to the offending agents (Chapter 8) (46). The exposure to the suspected occupational agent should reproduce the respiratory symptoms experienced by the patients at work and should induce a ≥3% increase in sputum eosinophil counts compared to baseline value without eliciting any change in FEV_1 or airway responsiveness (see Case History item 4). The performance of an SIC can be necessary to establish the diagnosing of OEB in patients who have already left their workplace and cannot be investigated at work and away from work. Furthermore, SIC allows for discarding the diagnosis of OA in subjects evaluated for work-related respiratory symptoms.

Measurement of FeNO concentration has been proposed as an easy and inexpensive alternative to induced sputum analysis in the assessment of eosinophilic airway inflammation because the induced sputum technique is not widely available and may be unsuccessful in a substantial proportion of patients (Chapter 7) (47, 48). Among individuals evaluated for chronic cough, the measurement of FeNO showed only a moderate diagnostic accuracy with an estimated sensitivity of 72% (95% CI:62%–80%) and a specificity of 83% (95% CI:73%–90%) in identifying NAEB (49). Currently, only three case reports have documented the usefulness of FeNO measurement for diagnosing OEB. These reports described subjects with work-related cough who failed to demonstrate AHR but showed an increase in FeNO after SIC or workplace exposure (38–40). In a multicenter cohort of 259 subjects with a negative SIC (43), the sensitivity of FeNO for detecting OEB was very low (24%) while the specificity was high (97%). These findings indicate that FeNO measurement should not be regarded as a suitable alternative to sputum analysis for detecting subjects with OEB because the test has a very low sensitivity (50). The criteria proposed for the diagnosis of occupational eosinophilic bronchitis as modified from reference (6) are as follows:

1. Isolated chronic cough ± productive of sputum that worsens at work and improves while away from work.
2. Normal lung function without variable airflow limitation and normal daily variability in PEF (<20%).

3. AHR to methacholine (and to indirect agents) absent at work and away from work.
4. Sputum eosinophilia (>2.5% eosinophils in sputum).
5. Increase in sputum eosinophils related to exposure to the offending agent (either at work or after SIC).
6. Other causes of chronic cough are ruled out.

Outcome and management

The recommendations of the American College of Chest Physicians for the treatment of NAEB are shown in Table 21.2 (51). ICS is recommended as the first-line therapy. The beneficial effect of ICSs on cough and sputum eosinophilia has been convincingly documented though in uncontrolled trials (2, 52, 53). Nevertheless, there is scarce information on the dose and duration of ICS treatment which is most often iterative and titrated according to symptoms and sputum eosinophil count. A recent randomized controlled trial among 101 patients with NAEB compared ICS treatment (budesonide 200 µg twice daily) for 1, 2, and 3 months and concluded that ICS should be administered for at least 2 months to decrease the risk of relapse (54). Two randomized controlled trials provided evidence supporting a beneficial effect of the cysteinyl leukotriene receptor antagonist montelukast as an add-on treatment to ICS (55, 56).

A number of observational studies have described the outcome of NAEB, but provided somewhat discordant information. Hancox et al. (57) re-assessed 6 of 12 patients with NAEB included in the original reports (1, 2) and concluded that the NAEB is generally a "benign and self-limiting disorder," although there was an early report of a patient who developed progressive chronic airflow limitation (58). A later publication by Park et al. (53) reported that 5 out of 24 patients (21%) with NAEB showed recurrent episodes of cough and sputum eosinophilia requiring iterative ICS treatment over a follow-up period of up to 48 months. A progressive FEV_1 reduction >20% was observed in three subjects (12%), including one patient who developed asthma. In this series, repeated episodes of NAEB were associated with the development of chronic airflow obstruction. Berry et al. (59) investigated prospectively 32 patients with NAEB for at least 1 year (mean 3.1 years), all of whom were treated with ICS. The majority of the patients (72%) had persistent eosinophilic airway inflammation and/or symptoms, whereas 16% of the patients developed fixed airflow obstruction and 9% of the patients developed AHR and symptoms consistent with asthma. In a cohort of 141 patients with NAEB followed for more than 1 year (median, 4.1 years) in

TABLE 21.2 Recommendations for Treatment of Eosinophilic Bronchitis

- In patients with chronic cough due to nonasthmatic eosinophilic bronchitis, the possibility of an occupation-related cause needs to be considered (level of evidence, expert opinion).
- When a causal allergen or occupational sensitizer is identified, avoidance is the best treatment (level of evidence, expert opinion).
- First-line treatment is inhaled corticosteroids, except when a causal allergen or sensitizer is identified (level of evidence, low).
- If symptoms are persistently troublesome and/or the natural history of eosinophilic airway inflammation progresses despite treatment with high-dose inhaled corticosteroids, oral corticosteroids should be given (level of evidence, expert opinion).

Source: Adapted from Brightling et al. (51) by permission.

China, Lai et al. (60) found that 60% of the patients had relapsing symptoms after withdrawal of ICS treatment. Eight subjects (6%) developed mild asthma, but there was no progressive decline in lung function parameters or chronic airway obstruction.

In patients with ascertained OEB, avoidance of exposure to the causal agent is by far the most sensible therapeutic option, although evidence supporting this approach is currently lacking. There are anecdotal reports of a short-term beneficial effect of treatment with ICS (16–18, 37), removal from exposure (17, 37), or reduced exposure associated with ICS (40) in subjects with OEB. However, the long-term outcome of OEB after environmental intervention and/or ICS has never been explored.

Clinical implications, research needs, and conclusions

It has been underlined that almost any patient presenting with cough may have an occupational or environmental cause or a workplace contributory factor to their symptoms (61, 62). The prevalence of OEB among of patients evaluated for work-related respiratory symptoms may be substantial but remain uncertain. The assessment of airway inflammation by noninvasive methods should thus be added as an important element of the investigation of work-related cough. The diagnosis of OEB should be substantiated by significant and reproducible work-related changes in sputum eosinophil counts. Once the diagnosis of this disorder has been established, a complete cessation of exposure to the offending agent seems the most appropriate treatment option. However, the outcome of OEB in terms of subsequent OA, airway remodeling, and the development of fixed airflow obstruction is basically unknown. Likewise, it is unknown whether avoidance of exposure to the causal agent is associated with a better prognosis than NAEB. Furthermore, controlled trials are needed to ascertain the efficacy of various drug interventions.

NAEB and OEB are intriguing diseases because their pathophysiological features challenge the conventional view of a direct relationship between eosinophilic airway inflammation and AHR, a hallmark feature of asthma. These conditions provided evidence that airflow obstruction, AHR, and eosinophilic airway inflammation can be dissociated and may occur independently. Nevertheless, NAEB has emerged as a useful model to study the structural and inflammatory mechanisms of AHR. Overexpression of IL-13 by mast cells and eosinophils in the bronchial submucosal and mast cell colocalization to airway smooth muscle are immunopathological features of asthma that are not shared by NAEB and have therefore been implicated in the pathogenesis of AHR. Finally, cough is a predominant symptom of this condition and it would be relevant to know how cough receptors are activated.

References

1. Gibson PG, Dolovich J, Denburg J, et al. Chronic cough: eosinophilic bronchitis without asthma. Lancet. 1989;1:1346–8.
2. Gibson PG, Hargreave FE, Girgis-Gabardo A, et al. Chronic cough with eosinophilic bronchitis: examination for variable airflow obstruction and response to corticosteroid. Clin Exp Allergy. 1995;25:127–32.
3. Brightling CE, Ward R, Goh KL, et al. Eosinophilic bronchitis is an important cause of chronic cough. Am J Respir Crit Care Med. 1999;160:406–10.
4. Ayik SO, Basoglu OK, Erdinc M, et al. Eosinophilic bronchitis as a cause of chronic cough. Respir Med. 2003;97:695–701.
5. Lai K, Chen R, Lin J, et al. A prospective, multicenter survey on causes of chronic cough in China. Chest. 2013;143:613–20.
6. Quirce S. Eosinophilic bronchitis in the workplace. Curr Opin Allergy Clin Immunol. 2004;4:87–91.
7. Bobolea I, Barranco P, Sastre B, et al. Seasonal eosinophilic bronchitis due to allergy to Cupressus arizonica pollen. Ann Allergy Asthma Immunol. 2011;106:448–9.
8. Malo JL, Vandenplas O. Definitions and classification of work-related asthma. Immunol Allergy Clin North Am. 2011;31:645–62.
9. American Thoracic Society. Chronic bronchitis, asthma, and pulmonary emphysema. Statement by the committee on diagnostic standards for nontuberculous respiratory disease. Am Rev Respir Dis. 1962;85:762–8.
10. Pizzichini E, Pizzichini MM, Efthimiadis A, et al. Measuring airway inflammation in asthma: eosinophils and eosinophilic cationic protein in induced sputum compared with peripheral blood. J Allergy Clin Immunol. 1997;99:539–44.
11. Prince P, Lemiere C, Dufour MH, et al. Airway inflammatory responses following exposure to occupational agents. Chest. 2012;141:1522–7.
12. Moore WC, Hastie AT, Li X, et al. Sputum neutrophil counts are associated with more severe asthma phenotypes using cluster analysis. J Allergy Clin Immunol. 2014;133:1557–63 e5.
13. Lemière C, Romeo P, Chaboillez S, et al. Airway inflammation and functional changes after exposure to different concentrations of isocyanates. J Allergy Clin Immunol. 2002;110:641–6.
14. Anees W, Huggins V, Pavord ID, et al. Occupational asthma due to low molecular weight agents: eosinophilic and non-eosinophilic variants. Thorax. 2002;57:231–6.
15. Pala G, Pignatti P, Moscato G. Occupational exposure to toluene diisocyanate and neutrophilic bronchitis without asthma. Clin Toxicol. 2011;49(6):506–7.
16. Quirce S, Fernandez-Nieto M, de Miguel J, Sastre J. Chronic cough due to latex-induced eosinophilic bronchitis. J Allergy Clin Immunol. 2001;108:143.
17. Di Stefano F, Di Giampaolo L, Verna N, Di Gioacchino M. Occupational eosinophilic bronchitis in a foundry worker exposed to isocyanate and a baker exposed to flour. Thorax. 2007;62:368–70.
18. Barranco P, Fernandez-Nieto M, del Pozo V, et al. Nonasthmatic eosinophilic bronchitis in a baker caused by fungal alpha-amylase and wheat flour. J Investig Allergol Clin Immunol. 2008;18:494–5.
19. Brightling CE, Bradding P, Symon FA, et al. Mast-cell infiltration of airway smooth muscle in asthma. N Engl J Med. 2002;346:1699–705.
20. Brightling CE, Symon FA, Birring SS, et al. Comparison of airway immunopathology of eosinophilic bronchitis and asthma. Thorax. 2003;58:528–32.
21. Brightling CE, Ward R, Woltmann G, et al. Induced sputum inflammatory mediator concentrations in eosinophilic bronchitis and asthma. Am J Respir Crit Care Med. 2000;162:878–82.
22. Gibson PG, Zlatic K, Scott J, et al. Chronic cough resembles asthma with IL-5 and granulocyte-macrophage colony-stimulating factor gene expression in bronchoalveolar cells. J Allergy Clin Immunol. 1998;101:320–6.
23. Brightling CE, Symon FA, Birring SS, et al. TH2 cytokine expression in bronchoalveolar lavage fluid T lymphocytes and bronchial submucosa is a feature of asthma and eosinophilic bronchitis. J Allergy Clin Immunol. 2002;110:899–905.
24. Siddiqui S, Sutcliffe A, Shikotra A, et al. Vascular remodeling is a feature of asthma and nonasthmatic eosinophilic bronchitis. J Allergy Clin Immunol. 2007;120:813–9.
25. Siddiqui S, Mistry V, Doe C, et al. Airway hyperresponsiveness is dissociated from airway wall structural remodeling. J Allergy Clin Immunol. 2008;122:335–41, e1-3.
26. Park SW, Park JS, Lee YM, et al. Differences in radiological/HRCT findings in eosinophilic bronchitis and asthma: implication for bronchial responsiveness. Thorax. 2006;61:41–7.
27. Siddiqui S, Gupta S, Cruse G, et al. Airway wall geometry in asthma and nonasthmatic eosinophilic bronchitis. Allergy. 2009;64:951–8.
28. Park SW, Jangm HK, An MH, et al. Interleukin-13 and interleukin-5 in induced sputum of eosinophilic bronchitis: comparison with asthma. Chest. 2005;128:1921–7.
29. Berry MA, Parker D, Neale N, et al. Sputum and bronchial submucosal IL-13 expression in asthma and eosinophilic bronchitis. J Allergy Clin Immunol. 2004;114:1106–9.
30. Brightling CE, Symon FA, Holgate ST, et al. Interleukin-4 and -13 expression is co-localized to mast cells within the airway smooth muscle in asthma. Clin Exp Allergy. 2003;33:1711–6.
31. Sastre B, Fernandez-Nieto M, Molla R, et al. Increased prostaglandin E2 levels in the airway of patients with eosinophilic bronchitis. Allergy. 2008;63:58–66.

32. Sastre B, Fernandez-Nieto M, Lopez E, et al. PGE(2) decreases muscle cell proliferation in patients with non-asthmatic eosinophilic bronchitis. Prostaglandins Other Lipid Mediat. 2011;95:11–8.

33. Sastre B, del Pozo V. Role of PGE2 in asthma and nonasthmatic eosinophilic bronchitis. Mediators Inflamm. 2012;2012:645383.

34. Kobayashi O. A case of eosinophilic bronchitis due to epoxy resin system hardener, methle endo methylene tetrahydro phthalic anhydride. Arerugi. 1994;43:660–2.

35. Lemiere C, Efthimiadis A, Hargreave FE. Occupational eosinophilic bronchitis without asthma: an unknown occupational airway disease. J Allergy Clin Immunol. 1997;100:852–3.

36. Yacoub MR, Malo JL, Labrecque M, et al. Occupational eosinophilic bronchitis. Allergy. 2005;60:1542–4.

37. Krakowiak AM, Dudek W, Ruta U, Palczynski C. Occupational eosinophilic bronchitis without asthma due to chloramine exposure. Occup Med (Lond). 2005;55:396–8.

38. Pala G, Pignatti P, Moscato G. The use of fractional exhaled nitric oxide in investigation of work-related cough in a hairdresser. Am J Ind Med. 2011;54:565–8.

39. Arochena L, Fernandez-Nieto M, Aguado E, et al. Eosinophilic bronchitis caused by styrene. J Investig Allergol Clin Immunol. 2014;24:68–9.

40. Wiggans RE, Barber CM. Metalworking fluids: a new cause of occupational non-asthmatic eosinophilic bronchitis. Thorax. 2017;72:579–80.

41. Quirce S, Swanson MC, Fernandez-Nieto M, et al. Quantified environmental challenge with absorbable dusting powder aerosol from natural rubber latex gloves. J Allergy Clin Immunol. 2003;111:788–94.

42. Tanaka H, Saikai T, Sugawara H, et al. Workplace-related chronic cough on a mushroom farm. Chest. 2002;122:1080–5.

43. Wiszniewska M, Dellis P, van Kampen V, et al. Characterization of occupational eosinophilic bronchitis in a multicenter cohort of subjects with work-related asthma symptoms. J Allergy Clin Immunol In Pract. 2020 Sep 10;S2213–2198(20):30942–9.

44. Pala G, Pignatti P, Gentile E, et al. Professional eosinophilic bronchitis: considerations and new diagnostic methods in a clinical case. G Ital Med Lav Ergon. 2010;32:145–8.

45. Singapuri A, McKenna S, Brightling CE, Bradding P. Mannitol and AMP do not induce bronchoconstriction in eosinophilic bronchitis: further evidence for dissociation between airway inflammation and bronchial hyperresponsiveness. Respirology (Carlton, Vic). 2010;15:510–5.

46. Vandenplas O, Suojalehto H, Aasen TB, et al. Specific inhalation challenge in the diagnosis of occupational asthma: consensus statement. Eur Respir J. 2014;43:1573–87.

47. Quirce S, Lemiere C, de Blay F, et al. Noninvasive methods for assessment of airway inflammation in occupational settings. Allergy. 2010;65:445–59.

48. Dweik RA, Boggs PB, Erzurum SC, et al. An official ATS clinical practice guideline: interpretation of exhaled nitric oxide levels (FeNO) for clinical applications. Am J Respir Crit Care Med. 2011;184:602–15.

49. Song WJ, Kim HJ, Shim JS, et al. Diagnostic accuracy of fractional exhaled nitric oxide measurement in predicting cough-variant asthma and eosinophilic bronchitis in adults with chronic cough: a systematic review and meta-analysis. J Allergy Clin Immunol. 2017;140:701–9.

50. Lemiere C, NGuyen S, Sava F, et al. Occupational asthma phenotypes identified by increased fractional exhaled nitric oxide after exposure to causal agents. J Allergy Clin Immunol. 2014;134:1063–7.

51. Brightling CE. Chronic cough due to nonasthmatic eosinophilic bronchitis: ACCP evidence-based clinical practice guidelines. Chest. 2006;129:116S–21S.

52. Brightling CE, Ward R, Wardlaw AJ, Pavord ID. Airway inflammation, airway responsiveness and cough before and after inhaled budesonide in patients with eosinophilic bronchitis. Eur Respir J. 2000;15:682–6.

53. Park SW, Lee YM, Jang AS, et al. Development of chronic airway obstruction in patients with eosinophilic bronchitis: a prospective follow-up study. Chest. 2004;125:1998–2004.

54. Zhan W, Tang J, Chen X, et al. Duration of treatment with inhaled corticosteroids in nonasthmatic eosinophilic bronchitis: a randomized open label trial. Ther Adv Respir Dis. 2019;13:1753466619891520.

55. Cai C, He MZ, Zhong SQ, et al. Add-on montelukast vs double-dose budesonide in nonasthmatic eosinophilic bronchitis: a pilot study. Respir Med. 2012;106:1369–75.

56. Bao W, Liu P, Qiu Z, et al. Efficacy of add-on montelukast in nonasthmatic eosinophilic bronchitis: the additive effect on airway inflammation, cough and life quality. Chin Med J (Engl). 2015;128:39–45.

57. Hancox RJ, Leigh R, Kelly MM, Hargreave FE. Eosinophilic bronchitis. Lancet. 2001;358:1104.

58. Brightling CE, Woltmann G, Wardlaw AJ, Pavord ID. Development of irreversible airflow obstruction in a patient with eosinophilic bronchitis without asthma. Eur Respir J. 1999;14:1228–30.

59. Berry MA, Hargadon B, McKenna S, et al. Observational study of the natural history of eosinophilic bronchitis. Clin Exp Allergy. 2005;35:598–601.

60. Lai K, Liu B, Xu D, et al. Will nonasthmatic eosinophilic bronchitis develop into chronic airway obstruction?: a prospective, observational study. Chest. 2015;148:887–94.

61. Tarlo SM. Cough: occupational and environmental considerations: ACCP evidence-based clinical practice guidelines. Chest. 2006;129:186S–96S.

62. Moscato G, Pala G, Cullinan P, et al. EAACI position paper on assessment of cough in the workplace. Allergy. 2014;69:292–304.

22

OCCUPATIONAL RHINITIS

Andrea Siracusa,[1] Dennis Shusterman,[2] and Olivier Vandenplas[3]
[1](Formerly) University of Perugia, Perugia, Italy
[2]Division of Occupational and Environmental Medicine, School of Medicine, University of California, San Francisco, California, USA
[3]Department of Chest Medicine, Centre hospitalier Universitaire UCL Namur, Université Catholique de Louvain, Yvoir, Belgium

Contents

CASE STUDY

IDENTIFICATION/CHIEF COMPLAINT

A 21-year-old male boat builder with nasal congestion, decreased sense of smell, wheezing, and skin rash.

HISTORY OF PRESENTING ILLNESS

1. The patient began employment as a fiberglass laminator and boat painter in a private boat works at age 19 years. He was a nonsmoker had no history of allergic disorders.
2. His job duties involved: (a) mixing epoxy putty and applying it to defects in boat hulls; (b) spraying epoxy primer on hulls; and (c) sanding hulls. He began experiencing nasal congestion and rhinorrhea while at work, along with an impaired sense of smell.
3. Over several months, he began experiencing chest symptoms, including chest tightness, wheezing, cough, and exertional dyspnea. After about 18 months of employment, he developed a skin rash involving his hands, forearms, and face, and he sought medical attention.
4. His general practitioner diagnosed "dermatitis" and prescribed both topical and oral corticosteroids. Respiratory symptoms were not investigated. When skin symptoms recurred, the patient was referred to a university occupational medicine clinic.

CONSULTATION

5. A detailed occupational history was obtained—now at 21 years of age. He wore latex or nitrile gloves when laminating or priming, although the gloves frequently failed, allowing visible entry of epoxy liquids. He also wore a half-face cartridge respirator when sanding, and a full-face cartridge respirator when spraying.
6. On examination, the patient had mild tap tenderness over his maxillary sinuses bilaterally and showed

inferior turbinate swelling with an increase in nasal mucus. His chest exam was normal.

7. The skin examination showed patchy erythema, lichenification, and scaling on the dorsa of both hands, as well as widespread erythema and scaling of facial skin, with a line of demarcation at the collar line.

DIAGNOSTIC TESTS

8. Spirometry showed normal values.

9. The patient returned to work equipped with a peak expiratory flowmeter (PEF) and logged a 22% across-shift decrease in PEF on the first working day, with incomplete recovery on the next day. Given his respiratory symptoms and pending medical follow-up, he was placed on sick leave.

10. On return to the outpatient clinic 1 week later, methacholine challenge showed marked bronchial hyperresponsiveness with a PC20 (concentration producing a 20% decrease in FEV_1) value of 0.025 mg/mL (normal ≥16 mg/mL).

11. Computerized tomography of the sinuses showed mild bilateral maxillary, ethmoid and sphenoid mucosal thickening, with opacification of the left ostiomeatal complex and contiguous nasal airway, suggestive of possible polyposis.

12. Consultation with an otorhinolaryngologist, however, established that the above opacification was due to nasal mucosal swelling rather than polyposis, and considered the case as nonsurgical.

13. Consultation with an occupational dermatologist—including patch testing—verified the diagnosis of allergic contact dermatitis due to phenyl glycidyl ether (an epoxy resin component).

DIFFERENTIAL DIAGNOSIS, MANAGEMENT, AND CLINICAL COURSE

14. The diagnoses rendered included occupational allergic rhinitis, occupational asthma (OA), and occupational contact dermatitis. The putative sensitizer for all three conditions was phenyl glycidyl ether. Since an alternative assignment to an uncontaminated workspace was not available, the patient was placed on total temporary disability under workers' compensation.

15. In addition to his albuterol rescue inhaler, the patient was started on anti-inflammatory medications, including nasal, inhaled, and topical corticosteroids.

16. Over a 6-month period, the patient's symptoms significantly improved. His skin cleared and his PC20 rose from 0.025 to 5.0 mg/mL. Residual symptoms included nasal congestion, reduced exercise tolerance, and triggering of respiratory symptoms by secondhand tobacco smoke and strong odors. He was deemed to have achieved maximum medical improvement and given a permanent disability rating with provision for future medical care, as well as a work preclusion from exposure to strong sensitizers or respiratory irritants.

Introduction

Rhinitis is an inflammation of the inner lining of the nose and is clinically defined by the presence of two or more of the following nasal symptoms: nasal congestion, rhinorrhea, sneezing, and itching (1). Up to 30 years ago, rhinitis was granted little attention because it was considered a trivial condition. Since then, both allergic rhinitis (AR) and nonallergic rhinitis (NAR) have been increasingly acknowledged as a public health concern due to their high prevalence and their adverse impacts on quality of life (QOL), work productivity, and associated comorbid conditions, especially asthma and sinusitis (2). There is accumulating evidence that workplace exposures account for a substantial—though still poorly quantified—fraction of rhinitis in adults (3–8). Indeed, a variety of dusts, gases, fumes, and vapors present in the workplace environment can induce or trigger different phenotypes of rhinitis that are grouped under the label "work-related rhinitis" (WRR), a broad term indicating that rhinitis symptoms are caused or worsened by the workplace.

The concept of "united airway disease" has been introduced to outline the tight interactions between upper and lower airways (1). Considering that this concept also applies in the context of the workplace, a task force of the European Academy of Allergy and Clinical Immunology proposed a nosological approach for disentangling subphenotypes within the spectrum of WRR (Figure 22.1) (4) similar to that used for work-related asthma (WRA) (9, 10). Thus, WRR encompasses both rhinitis caused by work (i.e. occupational rhinitis) and preexisting or coincident rhinitis exacerbated by nonspecific stimuli at work, referred to as *work-exacerbated rhinitis* (WER) (Figure 22.1). Occupational rhinitis has been defined as "an inflammatory disease of the nose, which is characterized by intermittent or persistent symptoms (i.e. nasal congestion, rhinorrhea, sneezing, and itching), and/or variable nasal airflow obstruction due to causes and conditions attributable to a particular work environment and not to stimuli encountered outside the workplace" (4). The term *occupational rhinitis* refers to the inception of rhinitis induced by either immunologically mediated sensitization to a specific substance at the workplace (i.e. sensitizer-induced occupational rhinitis or allergic occupational rhinitis—hereafter referred to as OR) or by exposure to an inhaled irritant at work, which is termed irritant-induced occupational rhinitis (IIR).

Phenotypes of work-related rhinitis

A number of subphenotypes can be discerned within the spectrum of WRR based on clinical features, nature of causal agents, underlying pathophysiological mechanisms, and strength of the evidence supporting the causal relationship (Figure 22.1).

Sensitizer-induced occupational rhinitis (OR)

OR is characterized clinically by the development of nasal hypersensitivity to a specific occupational agent after an asymptomatic period of exposure, the so-called latency period, which is necessary to acquire immunological sensitization to the causal agent (4). Once initiated, the symptoms recur on re-exposure to the sensitizing agent at concentrations not affecting other similarly exposed nonsensitized workers. The nasal symptoms can be intermittent or persistent according to the frequency and intensity of exposure to the causal agent, and are most often associated with conjunctivitis symptoms.

The workplace agents capable of causing OR are the same as those identified as inducing sensitizer-induced OA. These agents are traditionally distinguished into two broad categories: (1) high-molecular-weight (HMW) agents (>1 kDa) and (2)

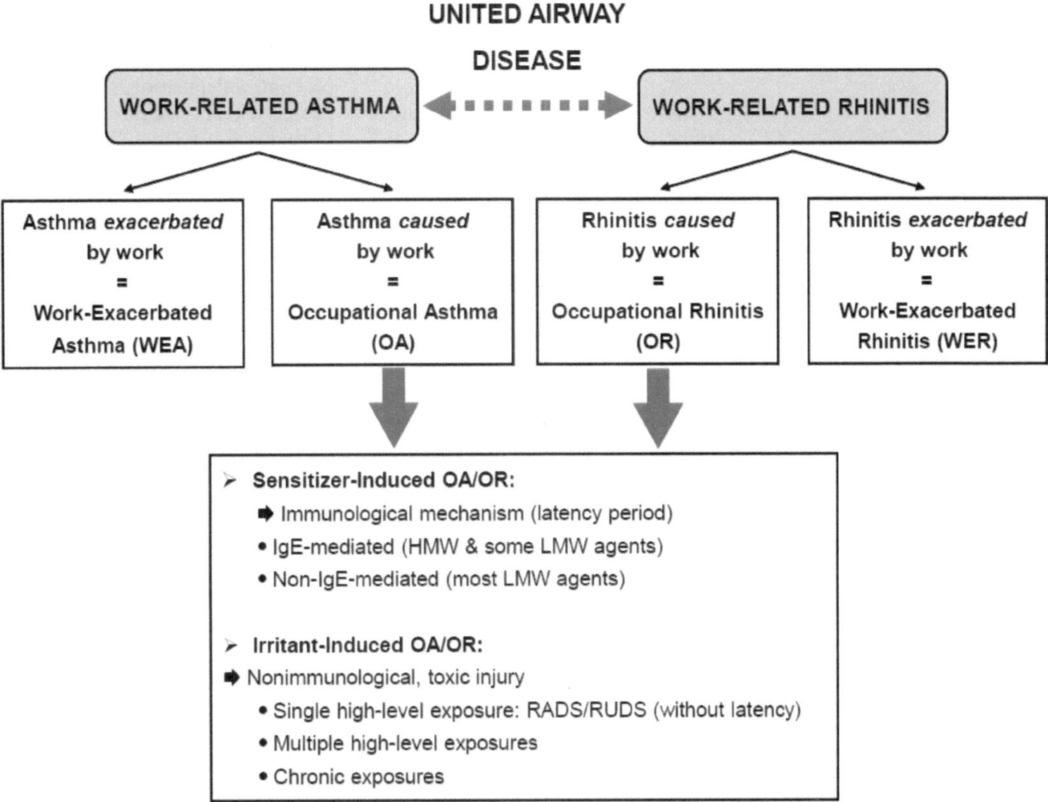

FIGURE 22.1 Phenotypes of work-related rhinitis. (*Abbreviations:* HMW, high-molecular-weight agent; LMW, low-molecular-weight agent; RADS, reactive airways dysfunction syndrome; RUDS, reactive upper airways dysfunction syndrome.)

low-molecular-weight (LMW) agents. HMW agents are biological substances derived from plants or animals, and enzymes produced from various sources. LMW agents include reactive chemicals, metals, and wood dusts.

HMW proteins and a few LMW compounds (i.e. acid anhydrides, platinum salts, reactive dyes, sulfonechloramide, and some wood species) act through the production of sIgE antibodies and induce a Th2 immune response. By contrast, for most LMW agents, sIgE antibodies have not been demonstrated and the immunological mechanisms leading to upper airway sensitization remain largely uncertain. LMW agents are incomplete antigens (i.e. haptens) that must bind to carrier macromolecules to become immunogenic. These LMW agents causing OA and OR are typically highly reactive electrophilic compounds that are capable of combining with amino acid residues on human airway proteins (11).

The resulting airway inflammatory process seems similar for both IgE- and non-IgE-inducing agents, and is predominantly characterized by the presence of eosinophils (12). An influx of eosinophils in the nasal mucosa has been demonstrated in nasal lavage fluid or nasal blown secretions after challenge exposure to both HMW (13–15) and LMW (16–19) agents in subjects with OR. Interestingly, eosinophilic inflammation of the nasal mucosa has been documented in subjects with OA due to persulfate salts who did not experience clinical manifestations of rhinitis, further supporting the concept of united airway disease in the occupational setting (19).

Irritant-induced occupational rhinitis (IIR)

Transient or persistent nasal symptoms may occur within a few hours after a single (20) or repeated (21, 22) exposure to very high concentrations of irritant compounds, such as chlorine, chlorine dioxide, sulfur dioxide, ozone, and hydrogen sulfide. By analogy with the reactive airways dysfunction syndrome (RADS) (10, 23), this entity has been termed *reactive upper airways dysfunction syndrome* (RUDS) (20) and is similarly characterized by the absence of a latency period. In contrast to the situation for RADS (or acute-onset irritant-induced asthma), the diagnostic criteria for RUDS do not include objective physiologic testing; consequently, the number of published case reports documenting RUDS is limited.

The nasal turbinates and septum present a relatively large surface area with which inhaled pollutants can interact, with functional consequences for heat exchange, humidification, particle "filtration," and "scrubbing" of soluble gases/vapors. In general, the upper respiratory tract tends to be most markedly impacted when an inhaled irritant gas or vapor has high water solubility and chemical reactivity (6). As a consequence, long-term exposure to irritants, at times in concentrations within occupational exposure limits (OELs), may also induce a chronic form of IIR (4–7). To the extent that chronic IIR resembles perennial nonallergic rhinitis, it would be expected to show greater neutrophilic inflammation—and fewer degranulated eosinophils—than does perennial allergic rhinitis (24). In addition, at least in the case of exposure to photochemical oxidants, IIR may be accompanied by squamous metaplasia of the pseudostratified epithelium lining the nasal cavity (25). At its extreme, irritant rhinitis is termed *corrosive rhinitis,* with the finding of mucosal ulceration, potentially progressing to nasal septal perforation, particularly in the metal-plating industry (26, 27).

A wide variety of occupational exposures have been associated with IIR (Table 22.1). Documentation ranges from case reports to epidemiologic studies. In addition to observational data, selected

TABLE 22.1 Examples of Occupations and Exposures Involved in Irritant-Induced Rhinitis

Occupation	Irritant Exposure(s)	Study Design	Prevalence of Rhinitis Symptoms	Excess Risk of Rhinitis vs Control Population, Odds Ratio (95% CI) When Available	References
Agriculture (crop farmers)	Dust, bioaerosols, agricultural chemicals	WS	117/178 (66%)	NA	*1. Akpinar-Elci, 2016 (32)[a]*
Agriculture (animals)	Ammonia, hydrogen sulfide, bioaerosols	PS	Pig farmers: 248/853 (29.1%)	1.5 (1.2–1.9)	*2. Radon, 2001*
		WS	Swine veterinarians: 81/122 (69%)	NA	*3. Andersen, 2004*
Agriculture (grape farmers)	Bipyridyl herbicides, dithiocarbamate fungicides, carbamate insecticides	WS	40/78 (51%) pesticide users vs 17/42 (40%) nonusers	Allergic rhinitis in pesticide users: 3.0 (1.4–6.2)	*4. Chatzi, 2007*
Agriculture (pesticide applicators)	Herbicides (petroleum oil, 2,4-D, glyphosate), insecticide (diazinon), fungicide (benomyl)	WS	1664/2245 (74%)	Significant associations of rhinitis Sx with specific pesticides	*5. Slager, 2009*
Auto parts manufacturing	Metalworking fluids, fungi, endotoxins	WS	115/187 (61%) workers	NA	*6. Park, 2008*
		WS	Runny or plugged nose: 995/2368 (42%)	2.38 (1.42–3.97) high vs low average aerosol exposure	*7. Oudyk, 2003*
Beverage processing	Hydrogen peroxide	WS	Higher VAS rhinitis symptom scores in 64 exposed workers vs 69 unexposed	NA	*8. Mastrangelo, 2009*
Boilermakers	Fuel oil ash, vanadium	WS	12/18 (67%) during boiler overhaul vs 4/11 (36%) in control utility workers	NA	*9. Woodin, 2000 (33)[a]*
Cleaners	Ammonia, bleach (hypochlorite), chloramines, dust	PS	NA	Men: 2.1 (1.1–4.0)	*10. Hellgren, 2002 (34)[a]*
		PS	291/4.853 (5.9%)	1.4 (1.0–2.1)	*11. Radon, 2008 (35)[a]*
		WS	118/341 (35%)	Women: 2.1 (1.2–3.7)	*12. de Fatima, 2007 (36)[a]*
Firefighters	Smoke, hazardous materials releases, alkaline dust (WTC)	WS	45%–48% at 1–2 years post-WTC	NA	*13. de la Hoz, 2010*
	Fire fumes	PS	NA	Men: 2.3 (1.2–4.4)	*10. Hellgren 2002 (34)[a]*
Health care	Glutaraldehyde	WS	Endoscopy nurses: 63/318 (20%)	NA	*11. Vyas 2000 (37)[a]*
Painters	Solvent vapors; sanding dusts	WS	129/288 (45%) vs 159/505 (31%) in carpenters	Indoor painters: 1.7 (1.2–2.5) compared to carpenters	*12. Kaukianinen, 2008 (38)[a]*
Pulp mill workers	Chlorine, chlorine dioxide, hydrogen sulfide	WS	89/211 (42%)	≥1 accidental exposure: 3.1 (1.3–7.5)	*13. Leroyer, 1999*
Swimming pool workers	Chlorine, chloramines	WS	NA	Range: 2.0–3.7 for rhinitis Sx in swimming instructors and attendants	*14. Jacobs, 2007*
Various	Paper dust	PS	NA	Women: 1.9 (1.2–3.2)	*10. Hellgren, 2002*
Waste handlers	Bioaerosols	WS	30/96 (31%) vs 12/90 (13%) controls	2.95 (1.4–6.2)	*15. Ray, 2005*
Welders	Metallic oxide fumes, nitrogen oxides, ozone	WS	26/44 (59%) in welders vs 0% in controls	NA	*16. Erhabor, 2001*
		WS	Rhinitis + low nasal patency: 15/90 (17%)	6.5 (1.4–30.0)	*17. Taghiakbari, 2018*
		PS	1132/2192 (53%)	1.4 (1.3–1.6)	*18. Storaas, 2015*
Woodworkers		SR	NA	Range: 2.3–5.0 (4/6 studies)	*19. Jacobsen, 2010*

[a] Refers to the order of references in the text (see list at the end of the chapter).

Abbreviations: NIR, noninfectious rhinitis; PS, population survey; SR, systematic review; Sx, symptoms; VAS, visual analogue scale; WS, workforce survey; WTC, World Trade Center.

References: **1.** Akpinar-Elci M, et al. *J Agromedicine.* 2016;21:217–23; **2.** Radon K, et al. *Eur Respir J.* 2001;17:747–54; **3.** Andersen CI, et al. *Am J Ind Med.* 2004;46:386–92; **4.** Chatzi L, et al. *Occup Environ Med.* 2007;64:417–21; **5.** Slager RE, et al. *Occup Environ Med.* 2009;66:718–24; **6.** Park DU, et al. *Industrial Health.* 2008;46:397–403; **7.** Oudyk J, et al. *Appl Occup Environ Hyg.* 2003;18:939–46; **8.** Mastrangelo G, et al. *Ann Occup Hyg.* 2009;53:161–5; **9.** Woodin MA, et al. *Am J Ind Med.* 2000;37:353–63; **10.** Hellgren J, et al. *Am J Ind Med.* 2002;42:23–8; **11.** Radon K, et al. *Occup Environ Med.* 2008;65:38–43; **12.** de Fatima Macaira E, et al. *Occup Environ Med.* 2007;64:446–53; **13.** de la Hoz RE, et al. *Curr Allergy Asthma Rep.* 2010;10:77–83; **14.** Vyas A, et al. *Occup Environ Med.* 2000;57:752–9; **15.** Kaukiainen A, et al. *Am J Ind Med.* 2008;51:1–8; **16.** Leroyer C, et al. *Occup Environ Med.* 1999;56:334–8; **17.** Jacobs JH, et al. *Eur Respir J.* 2007;29:690–8; **18.** Ray MR. *Int J Hyg Environ Health.* 2005;208:255–62; **19.** Erhabor GE, et al. *East Afr Med J.* 2001;78:461–4.

irritants, including ammonia, chlorine gas, ozone, formaldehyde (and other volatile organic compound vapors), sidestream tobacco smoke, and sulfur dioxide, have been studied in controlled human exposure studies. Endpoints examined postexposure have included changes in nasal patency, nasal mucociliary clearance, and influx of inflammatory cells and mediators in nasal lavage fluid (28). Complicating the picture, some LMW agents, such as diisocyanates, persulfate salts, cyanoacrylates, and trimellitic anhydride, can act as both irritants and sensitizers, with differing mechanisms of action between individuals (and over time, within individuals) (5).

Work-exacerbated rhinitis (WER)

By analogy with work-exacerbated asthma (29), work-exacerbated rhinitis (WER) has been defined as preexisting or concurrent (allergic or nonallergic) rhinitis that is worsened by workplace exposures, while the disease itself was not initiated by the work environment (4). A wide variety of conditions at work, including irritant agents (e.g. chemicals, dusts, and fumes), physical factors (e.g. temperature changes), emotions, secondhand smoke, and strong smells (e.g. perfumes) may trigger rhinitis symptoms in subjects with nasal hyperreactivity (30, 31).

Relationships with work-related asthma

The majority of well-conducted studies show a significant association between OR and OA in individual workers, and that OR often precedes the onset of OA (Table 22.2) (39–43). These associations between OR and OA are more frequent when HMW agents are involved (39–42). A prospective study of patients referred to tertiary care clinics for possible OA found that nasal itching, nasal secretions, and ocular itching were satisfactory predictors of OA caused by HMW but not LMW sensitizers (44).

Interestingly, in workers with OA induced by trimellitic anhydride, a LMW agent associated with the production of sIgE, the majority of patients (88%) also reported OR and in 77% of these cases, rhinitis symptoms preceded asthma symptoms (45). This observation indicates that the relationship between OR and OA is closely associated with an IgE-mediated mechanism rather than the category of causal agents.

There is also an association between WER and WEA, further supporting the concept of "united airway disease" (41, 46). However, in subjects with WEA, WRR symptoms seemed to be less frequent, less severe, and less often preceded the onset of asthma than in those with sensitizer-induced OA (40). Sneezing/itching and rhinorrhea were slightly less frequent, while postnasal discharge was more common in subjects with WER than in those with OR.

Available longitudinal cohort studies have convincingly demonstrated that OR is a strong risk factor for the subsequent development of OA (Table 22.3) (47–49), similar to what has been documented for nonoccupational rhinitis and asthma (50,51). However, only 11.4% of the apprentices in animal health technology with OR subsequently developed OA over a 44-month observation period (47).

Epidemiology

Prevalence and incidence

The contribution of workplace exposure to the global burden of rhinitis in the general population remains unknown (4). A systematic review of cross-sectional studies conducted among various workforces concluded that OR is two to three times more frequent than OA (3). An analysis of OR cases documented by immunological tests and/or specific nasal provocation tests (NPT) reported to the Finnish Register of Occupational Diseases (1986–1991) failed to provide incidence estimates in the general population but identified occupations at increased risk (i.e. bakers, livestock breeders, food-processing workers, veterinarians, farmers, electronic/electrical products assemblers, and boat builders) (52). A questionnaire survey of a large sample of workers employed in various industrial sectors in the French-speaking part of Belgium found that a substantial proportion (6.3%) of the workers (i.e. 28% of those with current rhinitis) experience WRR defined by the presence of two or more nasal symptoms at work (53). However, inherent to its questionnaire-based design, this survey failed to distinguish between OR and WER. In addition, this random sample of workers might not have been accurately representative of the whole workforce and the full spectrum of occupations with a high risk of OR.

TABLE 22.2 Association between Occupational Rhinitis and Asthma

	Work-Related Rhinitis in Subjects with Occupational Asthma		
Causal Agents	Prevalence (%)	Onset before Asthma (%)	References
HMW agents (n=24)	**92[a]**	58	(39)
LMW agents (n=14)	71[a]	25	
HMW agents (n=110)	92[a]	48	(40)
LMW agents (n=62)	55[a]	28	
HMW agents (n=174)	74[b]	52	(41)
LMW agents (n=381)	51[b]	39	
HMW agents (n=22)	20[c]	NA	(42)
LMW agents (n=21)	10[c]	NA	

[a] Occupational rhinitis defined by at least two nasal symptoms at work.

[b] Physician-based diagnosis of OR.

[c] Among 43 subjects with work-related asthma symptoms who completed specific inhalation challenge, concomitant positive nasal and bronchial responses were more frequent in subjects challenged with HMW agents than with LMW agents (n=2/21).

Abbreviations: HMW, high-molecular-weight agent; LMW, low-molecular-weight agent; NA, not available.

TABLE 22.3 Risk of Asthma in Subjects with Occupational Rhinitis

Causal Agent	Population	Study Design	Outcome	References
Laboratory animals	Animal health technology apprentices (n=417)	• Prospective cohort study • FU: 2.7–3.3 yr • OR defined by questionnaire + positive SPT	Positive predictive value for OA[a]: 11.4%	(46)
Various occupations	Compensated OR (Finnish Register of Occupational Diseases, 1988–1999; n=3637) vs other occupational diseases	• Linkage with national health insurance register (reimbursement of asthma medication) • Mean FU: 6 yr	Adjusted RR for asthma or OA[b]: 5.4 (4.8–6.2)	(47)
Laboratory animals	• Laboratory workers in a pharmaceutical company (n=603; 2527 person-years)	• Surveillance program by annual questionnaire • FU: 12.3 yr • OR defined by questionnaire	Adjusted HR for work-related asthma symptoms: 7.4 (3.3–16.6)	(48)

[a] Occupational asthma based on questionnaire, positive skin-prick tests for occupational allergens, and presence of nonspecific bronchial hyperresponsiveness to methacholine.

[b] Among incident cases of asthma, 37% of the subjects developed ascertained and compensated occupational asthma.

Abbreviations: FU, follow-up duration; OA, occupational asthma; OR, occupational rhinitis; RR, risk ratio with 95% confidence interval between brackets; HR, hazard ratio with 95% confidence interval between brackets; SPT: skin-prick test.

Cross-sectional surveys of workforces exposed to various agents documented high prevalence rates of WRR symptoms, ranging from 2% to 76% for HMW sensitizers and from 2% to 78% for LMW sensitizers (Table 22.4). However, the rates of OR documented by SPT or sIgE antibodies were usually much lower (3, 4). For instance, a sytematic review of cross-sectional studies of workers exposed to laboratory animals found that the prevalence of WRR symptoms ranged from 7% to 42%, while OR documented by immunological tests was approximately two-fold lower, ranging from 3% to 19% (54).

The incidence of OR has been investigated in a few prospective cohort studies of subjects exposed to HMW agents (i.e. laboratory animals, wheat flour, pepper bell pollen, and latex) that are summarized in Table 22.5 (55–64). The incidence of OR in laboratory workers ranged from 2.0 to 10.3 cases per 100 person-years and from 6.3 to 22.1 cases per 100 person-years in workers exposed to flour. Of note, the incidence of OR was three to four times higher than that of OA. In these longitudinal studies, sensitization to laboratory animals and rhinoconjunctivitis symptoms typically developed during the first 2 years of exposure (47, 56),

TABLE 22.4 Prevalence of Occupational Rhinitis Compared to Occupational Asthma

Occupation	Agents	Prevalence of WRR Symptoms % (Range)	Prevalence of WRA Symptoms % (Range)	Prevalence of OR[a] % (Range)	Prevalence of OA[a] % (Range)	References
High-Molecular-Weight Agents						
Laboratory workers	Laboratory animals	7–42	2–12	3–19	1–10	*1. Folletti, 2008[b]*
Insects	Sheep blowfly (*Lucilia cuprina*)	24	11	NA	NA	*2. Kaufman, 1989*
	Storage mites	15	21	7	11	*3. Blainey, 1988*
	Fish feed (*C. thummi thummi*)	24	16	21	15	*4. Liebers, 1993*
Fish and seafood processors	Clam/shrimp	7	4	9	4	*5. Desjardins, 1995*
Greenhouse workers/fruit growing	Bell pepper pollen	49	13	NA	NA	*6. Groenewoud, 2002*
	Chrysanthemum pollen	48	8	NA	NA	*7. Groenewoud, 2002*
	Spider mites (*Tetranychus urticae*)	13–30	7–26	3–18	2–8	*8. Siracusa 2000[b]*
	Predatory mite (*Amblyseius cucumeris*)	NA	NA	17	6	*9. Groenewoud, 2002*
Bird keepers	Birds	17	14	15	14	*10. Swiderska-Kielbik, 2011*
Grain elevators	Grain dust	28–64	15–42	NA	NA	*8. Siracusa, 2000[b]*
Bakers	Flour	14–25	6–8	NA	6	*8. Siracusa, 2000[b]*
	Flour and α-amylase					*11. De Zotti, 1994*
		14	5	NA	NA	*12. Houba, 1996*
		15	5	NA	NA	
Health care, glove manufacture	Latex	9–76	2–60	4–10	2–20	*8. Siracusa, 2000[b]*

Plant processing	Spices	43	17	NA	4–8	*13. van der Walt, 2013*
	Green coffee, castor beans	10	16	NA	NA	*14. Romano 1994*
	Guar gum	36	23	5	2	*15. Malo, 1990*
	Saffron flower	16	6	4	2	*16. Feo, 1997*
Pharmaceutical and detergent industry workers	Alpha-amylase	59	30	8	8	*17. Losada, 1992*
	Lactase	16	10	8	4	*18. Muir, 1997*
		10	7	7	6	*19. Bernstein, 1999*
	Psyllium	32	6	4	3	*20. Nelson, 1987*
Low-Molecular-Weight Agents						
Painters and urethane mold workers	Diisocyanates	36	18	<1	4	*21. Bernstein, 1993*
Epoxy resin workers, chemical workers, and electric condenser workers	Anhydrides	48	20	12	8	*22. Baur, 1995*
		43	0	39	0	*23. Yokota, 1998*
Carpenters and furniture makers	Wood dust: various	78	7	NA	NA	*24. Aguwa, 2007*
	Wood dust: obeche	NA	NA	11	8	*25. Aranda, 2013*
Metalworkers	Metals (Cr, Co)	57	8	29	8	*26. Walters, 2012*
Healthcare and pharmaceutical workers	Psyllium	9–29	3–20	5	4	*8. Siracusa, 2000*
	Spiramycin	31–41	12–19	NA	6	*27. Malo, 1988[c]*
Reactive dye workers	Reactive dyes	20	25	5	4	*28. Park, 1991*
	Carmine	30	20	30	20	*29. Quirce, 1994*
Hairdressers	Persulphate salts	3	0	NA	NA	*30. Merget, 1996*

[a] Prevalence of OR and OA documented by SPT and/or sIgE.

[b] Review of several studies.

[c] Two assessments.

Abbreviations: NA, not available; OA, occupational asthma; OR, occupational rhinitis; sIgE, specific IgE antibodies; SPT, skin-prick test; WRA, work-related asthma; WRR, work-related rhinitis.

References: **1.** Folletti I, et al. *Allergy.* 2008;63:834–41; **2.** Kaufman GL, et al. *Br J Indust Med.* 1989;46:473–8; **3.** Blainey AD, et al. *Thorax.* 1988;43:697–702; **4.** Liebers V, et al. *Allergy.* 1993;48:236–9; **5.** Desjardins A, et al. *J Allergy Clin Immunol.* 1995;96:608–17; **6.** Groenewoud GCM, et al. *Clin Exper Allergy.* 2002;32:434–40; **7.** Groenewoud GCM, et al. *Allergy.* 2002;57:835–40; **8.** Siracusa A, et al. *Clin Exp Allergy.* 2000;30:1519–34; **9.** Groenewoud GCM, et al. *Allergy.* 2002;57:614–9; **10.** Swiderska-Kiełbik S, et al. *Int J Occup Med Environ Health.* 2011;24:292–303; **11.** DeZotti R, et al. *Occup Environ Med.* 1994;51:548–52; **12.** Houba R, et al. *Am J Respir Crit Care Med.* 1996;154:130–6; **13.** Romano C, et al. *Clin Exp Allergy.* 1995;25:643–50; **14.** van der Walt A, et al. *Occup Environ Med.* 2013;70(7):446–52; **15.** Malo JL, et al. *J Allergy Clin Immunol.* 1990;86:562–9; **16.** Feo F, et al. *Allergy.* 1997;52:633–41; **17.** Losada E, et al. *J Allergy Clin Immunol.* 1992;89:118–25; **18.** Muir DCF, et al. *Am J Ind Med.* 1997;31:570–1; **19.** Bernstein JA, et al. *J Allergy Clin Immunol.* 1999;103:1153–7; **20.** Nelson WL. *J Occup Med.* 1987;29:497–9; **21.** Bernstein DI, et al. *J Allergy Clin Immunol.* 1993;92:387–96; **22.** Baur X, et al. *Int Arch Occup Environ Health.* 1995;67(6):395–403; **23.** Yokota K, et al. *Allergy.* 1998;53(8):803–7; **24.** Aguwa EN, et al. *Tanzan Health Res Bull.* 2007;9:52–5; **25.** Aranda A, et al. *PLOS ONE.* 2013;8(1):e53926; **26.** Walters GI, et al. *Occup Med (Lond).* 2012;62:533–40; **27.** Malo JL, et al. *Thorax.* 1988;43:371–7; **28.** Park HS, et al. *J Allergy Clin Immunol.* 1991;87:639–49; **29.** Quirce S, et al. *J Allergy Clin Immunol.* 1994;93:44–52; **30.** Merget R, et al. *Occup Env Med.* 1996;53:422–6.

TABLE 22.5 Incidence of Occupational Rhinitis and Asthma

Agents	Occupation (Number of Subjects)	Duration of Follow-Up (Yrs)	Incidence of OA (Per 100 Person-Years)	Incidence of OR (Per 100 Person-Years)	References
Laboratory animals	Laboratory workers (n=148)	1.0	2.0	7.4	(54)
Laboratory animals	Laboratory workers (n=342)	2.7	3.5	7.3	(55)
Laboratory animals	Animal-health apprentices (n=373)	3.7	2.0	10.3	(56)
Laboratory animals	Laboratory workers (n=495)	12	0.4	2.0	(57)
Flour	Bakery and flour mill workers (n=300)	3.3	4.1	11.8	(58)
Flour	Apprentices pastry-makers (n=188)	1.4	1.3	13.1	(59)
Flour	Apprentices pastry-makers (n=287)	2.0	4.3	6.3	(60)
Flour	Apprentices pastry-makers (n=114)	1.7	10.0	22.1	(61)
Bell pepper pollen	Greenhouse workers (n=280)	8.0	0.4	1.6	(62)
Latex	Dental hygiene apprentices (n=110)	2.7	1.8	0.7	(63)

Abbreviations: OA, occupational asthma; OR, occupational rhinitis.

whereas WRA symptoms occurred later, during the second and third years of exposure.

Risk factors

The level of exposure to the sensitizing agent is the most important determinant of the development of IgE-mediated sensitization and OR due to HMW agents (3). Atopy is a risk factor for sensitization due to HMW agents while the association with OR is controversial. The relationship between smoking and OR/occupational sensitization due to HMW agents is also controversial. The determinants of OR due to LMW agents have not yet been identified.

Diagnosis

An accurate diagnosis is crucial for a cost-effective management of WRR since advising avoidance of exposure or other environmental interventions are associated with substantial professional, psychosocial, and financial consequences. The different steps involved in the investigation of WRR are the clinical history, nasal examination, immunological testing, and nasal provocation test (NPT) in the laboratory or assessment of nasal parameters at the workplace (Figure 22.2).

Medical and occupational history

A detailed medical and occupational history is a key step for diagnosing OR. The purpose of the clinical history is to confirm the existence of rhinitis and to evaluate its temporal relationship with work exposure by carefully gathering information on the important items that are summarized in Table 22.6. However, the clinical history is not specific enough to establish a diagnosis of sensitizer-induced OR. Indeed, epidemiological surveys found that IgE sensitization to specific workplace agents could be usually documented in less than half of the subjects reporting WRR symptoms (56, 59, 60) (Table 22.4). Hence, objective tests confirming the causal relationship between WRR symptoms and exposure to a specific agent at the workplace are necessary for establishing a definite diagnosis of OR.

Examination of the nose

Inspection of endonasal cavities, preferably through nasal endoscopy, should be performed in order to document signs of rhinitis and exclude other nasal conditions that can interfere with the nasal function (e.g. atrophic rhinitis, crusting, septal deviation, chronic rhinosinusitis, nasal polyps, septal perforation) (66).

Immunological testing

IgE-mediated sensitization to occupational agents can be assessed by skin-prick testing (SPT) and/or assessment of sIgE (Chapter 7). The major limitation of in vivo and in vitro immunological tests results from the unavailability of standardized antigens for SPT and serum sIgE determination for most occupational allergens (67, 68).

By extrapolating data from OA, it may be expected that, when standardized extracts are available, immunological tests would yield a high sensitivity for diagnosing OR caused by HMW agents and a few LMW agents (i.e. platinum salts, reactive dyes, and acid anhydrides). However, there is only scarce evidence-based information on the sensitivity and specificity of immunological tests compared to NPTs. Among 47 bakery apprentices who developed WRR symptoms over a 2-year period, NPT was positive in the 36 subjects with IgE sensitization to flour, but also in two subjects with negative immunological tests (61). On the other hand,

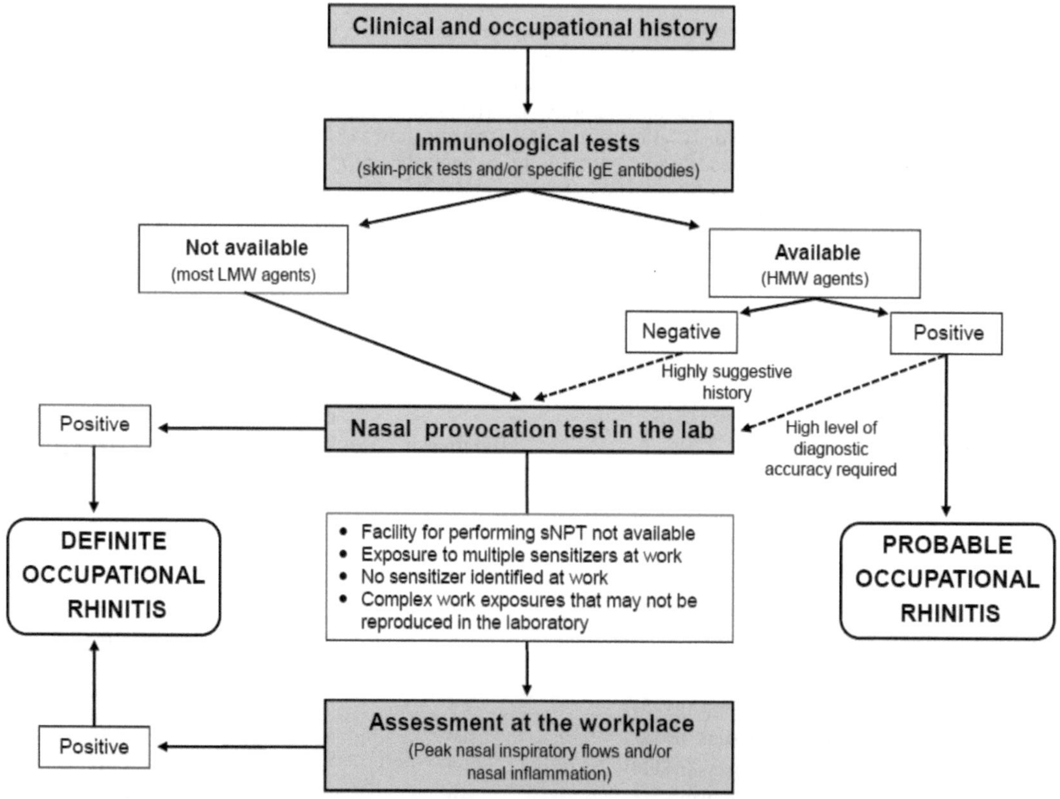

FIGURE 22.2 Proposed algorithm for diagnosing occupational rhinitis. (*Abbreviations:* HMW, high-molecular-weight; LMW, low-molecular-weight; sNPT: specific nasal provocation test.) (From Reference [8]. With permission.)

TABLE 22.6 Important Items of the Clinical History

Personal and/or familial history of allergy to ubiquitous allergens

Nature of nasal symptoms: Rhinorrhea, nasal blockage, sneezing, itching

Relationship between nasal symptoms and occupational exposure:

Duration of exposure at current job before onset of symptoms (latency period)

Pattern of symptoms in relation to daily work: Improvement after the work shift, during weekends, or prolonged periods off work

Identification of a specific product or task inducing nasal symptoms

Associated disorders and their temporal relationship with work exposure:

Conjunctivitis: Itching, redness, watery eyes

Asthma: Wheezing, cough, chest tightness, breathlessness, phlegm

Rhinosinusitis: Postnasal drip, facial pressure, reduction or loss of smell

Severity of nasal/ocular symptoms and their impact on daily life and sleep

Occupational history:

Detailed description of current job tasks and processes in adjacent work areas

Identification of direct and indirect exposures using safety data sheets

Recent changes in work processes or materials

Workplace hygiene conditions: Ventilation, personal protective equipment

Accidental high-level exposure(s)

---

a positive immunological test does not always indicate clinically relevant nasal hypersensitivity. For instance, only 10 out of 24 (42%) subjects with WRR symptoms and positive SPT to laboratory animals showed a positive nasal response to the handling of laboratory animals and litter (65).

Of note, the recent concept of "local allergic rhinitis" characterized by a local, IgE-mediated mucosal response in the absence of a positive SPT or serum sIgE, has emphasized the importance of considering NPT in the Section "Diagnostic algorithm." However, local allergic rhinitis due to occupational agents has not yet been formally demonstrated (69).

Nasal provocation tests

The NPT in the laboratory aims at reproducing the nasal reaction occurring at the workplace under controlled conditions and as such, is regarded as the reference standard procedure for establishing the causal relationship between WRR symptoms and exposure to a specific occupational agent (4, 66, 70–72).

NPT with nonoccupational allergens is considered a simple and safe technique, and has been established in many countries as a standard procedure for diagnosing allergic rhinitis caused by common allergens (73). However, NPTs with occupational agents are still poorly standardized and the technical details are largely variable among centers (4, 66, 70, 74). The reader is referred to published guidelines and reviews for general considerations on NPT procedures (71, 73).

Before challenging the subject with the suspected occupational agent, a sham provocation test is recommended to exclude nonspecific irritant responses to occupational agents in subjects with nasal hyperreactivity (74). NPT with common allergens are usually performed by the spray application of a known amount of a standardized allergen solution into the nostrils. In contrast, the method for delivering occupational agents should be adapted to

their chemical and physical properties (i.e. gas, liquid, particles, or aerosol) as well as the mode of usage at the workplace (74–76).

Unlike bronchial provocation tests (Chapter 8) (75), the criteria for defining a positive nasal response have been seldom compared nor validated (70, 77). There is general agreement that both subjective and objective indices must be considered in the assessment of nasal responses during NPT (70, 71, 73). The nasal response can be assessed by various subjective and objectives indices (4, 66, 73, 78), including: (1) symptom scores or visual analogue scales; (2) rhinoscopic examination; (3) weighting of nasal secretions; (4) measurements of nasal patency using nasal inspiratory flow, anterior or posterior rhinomanometry, and/or acoustic rhinometry; (5) assessment of nasal inflammation through the analysis of nasal blown secretions, nasal lavage fluid, nasal scraping/brushing, or the assessment of nasal nitric oxide (nNO) concentration. Available studies provided conflicting results regarding the correlation between objective measurements of nasal patency using rhinomanometry and acoustic rhinometry and the subjective sensation of nasal blockage (79). There is accumulating evidence that assessment of eosinophilic inflammation in nasal secretions could increase the specificity of nasal responses during NPT (19). A 4% increase in eosinophils recovered in nasal lavage or nasal blown secretions has been consistently documented as an adequate cut-off value for defining a significant inflammatory response (80, 81). nNO has been considered as a potential clinical biomarker of inflammation in allergic rhinitis (82). However, the usefulness of measuring nNO in the investigation of WRR still remains uncertain.

In a large series of 1229 NPTs with occupational agents, 13% elicited an asthmatic reaction (74). Accordingly, the subjects should be carefully evaluated for the possibility of associated asthma, and if this is confirmed, lung function parameters should be monitored for at least 6 hours after the NPT in order to detect an asthmatic reaction (74).

Differential diagnosis

The diagnosis of acute-onset IIR can be established with a reasonable level of confidence based on the retrospective documentation of a close temporal relationship between an inhalation incident and the development of persistent rhinitis symptoms (or other objective indices of the disease). By contrast, establishing a causal relationship between chronic workplace irritant exposures and the development of IIR is elusive on an individual basis since it can be supported only by epidemiological data demonstrating an increased risk of rhinitis in certain occupations.

The most challenging aspect of the differential diagnosis for OR is to distinguish this condition from WER. Epidemiological and clinical studies have consistently found that a high proportion of subjects who report WRR failed to demonstrate IgE-mediated sensitization to work-specific HMW agents (83, 84) or a positive nasal response to NPT (64) and actually should be considered as having WER. Overall, the clinical features of WER are similar to those of OR. Hence, a diagnosis of WER should be considered only after careful exclusion of OR through appropriate diagnostic procedures (see section "Diagnostic Algorithm"). Assessing nonspecific nasal hyperreactivity might be relevant, since WRR symptoms may result, at least in part, from nasal reactions to irritants. Nasal airway hyperactivity can be documented using nasal provocation tests, preferably with cold dry air (31). However, these tests are only available in specialized centers and their clinical relevance in diagnosing WER has not yet been explored.

Diagnostic algorithm

In everyday clinical practice, documentation of IgE-mediated sensitization by SPT or elevated sIgE should be considered sufficient to establish a diagnosis of probable OR in subjects with a consistent history while a positive NPT in a controlled laboratory setting is deemed to establish a diagnosis of definite OR. Alternatively, a workplace challenge demonstrating work-related nasal symptoms associated with increased nasal obstruction and/or enhanced nasal inflammation while exposed to the suspect causal agent may provide strong evidence supporting a diagnosis of definite OR. Workplace challenges should be considered in the following settings: (1) facility and expertise for performing NPT is not available; (2) the subject is exposed to multiple potential sensitizers at work; (3) no potential airway sensitizer has been identified at work; and (4) the conditions of exposure at work cannot be reliably reproduced in the laboratory in case of complex industrial processes. The measurement of peak nasal inspiratory flow (PNIF) has been proposed as a simple tool for evaluating nasal airway patency in the same individual over time at the workplace (78). The method is, however, effort-dependent and yields substantial variability (85). Assessment of eosinophilic inflammation in nasal secretions at work and away from work could be a suitable method for investigating of nasal responses during workplace challenges, although the role of such approach in clinical practice has not yet been validated.

Health and socioeconomic impact

In contrast to the significant literature on the burden of allergic and nonallergic rhinitis on QOL and work productivity (86–88), there is only limited information on the specific impact of WRR on these outcomes.

Quality of life

Studies of workers with IgE-mediated OR reported either a greater (89) or a similar level of impairment (90) in rhinitis-specific QOL as compared to adults with nonoccupational rhinitis. On the other hand, a Finnish study reported a worse general health-related QOL in workers with OR due to protein allergens compared to control subjects with allergic rhinitis and healthy controls without rhinitis (90). A cross-sectional questionnaire survey of a large sample of the general workforce in Belgium demonstrated that WRR, defined by the presence of at least two rhinitis symptoms at work, is associated with an incremental adverse impact on both rhinitis-specific and general health-related QOL as compared to rhinitis unrelated to work (53).

Work productivity

Follow-up studies of bakers and greenhouse workers showed that WRR was associated with a higher rate of job changes compared to asymptomatic workers (83, 91, 92). In a clinical series of patients diagnosed with allergic OR in Tunisia (92), the mean work time missed and mean impairment while working due to OR assessed using the Work Productivity and Activity Impairment questionnaire were similar (10±21% and 47±33%, respectively) to the estimates provided by a systematic review of nonoccupational rhinitis (88). By contrast, the aforementioned Belgian workforce survey found that the overall work productivity was more impacted in WRR than in rhinitis unrelated to work. Of note, the financial consequences resulting from either avoiding or reducing exposure to causal agents have never been investigated in workers suffering from OR alone.

Outcome

The major adverse outcome in workers with OR is the development of OA. Thus, longitudinal cohort studies provided consistent evidence that OR is a strong risk factor for the subsequent development of OA in workers who remain exposed to the sensitizing agent (Table 22.2) (47–49), similar to what has been documented for nonoccupational rhinitis and asthma (50, 51). These cohort studies identified individual risk factors for the development of OA, including female gender (48, 49) and a familial history of allergy or asthma (49), which were associated with a three times higher risk of subsequent OA. However, atopy (especially polysensitization to common allergens), severe OR symptoms, and the presence of asymptomatic nonspecific bronchial hyperresponsiveness might also be associated with an increased risk of OA since these characteristics were important cofactors in determining the risk of developing asthma among individuals with nonoccupational rhinitis (51, 94–96).

The outcome of workers with isolated OR has been scarcely investigated. A Finnish study assessed 119 patients with IgE-mediated OR due to a variety of agents at an average of 10 years after the diagnosis (90). Health-related QOL scores were impaired among workers with persistent workplace exposure, while among those removed from exposure, QOL was similar to healthy controls. Two other follow-up studies also showed a significant improvement in nasal symptom score and/or QOL (92, 97). Of note, repeated NPT in patients with allergic OR demonstrated that specific nasal reactivity to the sensitizing agent persists years after removal from exposure (98).

Management

The management of OR aims not only to minimize nasal symptoms and their impact on patients' QOL but may also offer the opportunity to prevent the development of OA. Complete avoidance of exposure to the sensitizing agent is considered the most rational and efficient management approach. However, complete avoidance of exposure to the causal agent is likely to require considerable professional changes for affected workers, which is most often associated with substantial socioeconomic consequences. On the other hand, reduction of exposure to the causal agent is often considered a pragmatic alternative to complete avoidance because of its presumably lower socioeconomic impact (99).

Reduction of exposure has been documented as resulting in a substantial improvement in the severity of OR symptoms due to laboratory animal allergens (100), platinum salts (101), and latex (102, 103), but the long-term efficacy of this approach has not yet been evaluated. In addition, reducing exposure to safe levels remains quite difficult in practice, because the threshold level (or dose) of an agent that can elicit respiratory reactions varies widely among sensitized workers (104, 105) and methods for measuring airborne levels of biological agents are not yet easily available (106).

Hence, it is currently difficult to decide whether a worker suffering from OR should be immediately and completely removed from the causal exposure due to the lack of quantitative estimates of the long-term risk of asthma. The beneficial effects of complete avoidance of exposure to the sensitizing occupational agent must be balanced against the potential socioeconomic consequences. There is a need to further identify the individual risk factors for the development of OA that could be considered for a more personalized management approach in order to minimize the socioeconomic impact of the disease. In patients with a high risk of OA, complete removal from exposure should be more strongly recommended. Workers with OR who remain exposed to "lower levels" of the sensitizing agent, must be medically monitored for the development of OA that would then dictate more aggressive interventions.

Pharmacological treatment of OR (i.e. intranasal corticosteroids; intranasal, ocular, or oral antihistamines) should be adapted to the severity of symptoms according to international guidelines issued for the management of rhinitis in general. However, information on the long-term efficacy of these medications is lacking since work-related rhinitis/conjunctivitis symptoms are currently not specifically assessed in treatment trials. Specific allergen immunotherapy has been evaluated for a few occupational agents, such as latex, flour, and laboratory animals (107), but it remains unknown whether this approach can alter the long-term course of the disease and reduce the risk of OA when workers with OR remain exposed to the causal agent. In addition, allergen immunotherapy is currently limited by the unavailability of standardized extracts (107).

Prevention

Prevention can target different stages of the development of OR. Primary preventive strategies aimed at reducing the development of immunological sensitization to occupational agents and subsequent OR should focus on reducing or eliminating exposure to potentially sensitizing agents using the same hierarchical approach as in OA (4, 5, 7). Another proposed approach is to identify susceptible individuals at the time of a pre-employment examination and exclude them from employment or from high-risk jobs. However, this strategy is unduly discriminating since currently identified markers of individual susceptibility offer only a low predictive value for the development of OA, especially when these markers, such as atopy, are highly prevalent in the general population.

Secondary prevention of OR implies the detection of the disease at an early, and preferably preclinical, stage to prevent progression through surveillance programs based on periodic administration of questionnaires and immunological tests when available. Observational studies and historical data provided evidence that prevention strategies, most often multicomponent programs targeting education, control of exposure, and medical surveillance, were effective in reducing the incidence of IgE-mediated sensitization to various occupational agents, including natural rubber latex in healthcare workers (108, 109), enzymes (110, 111), flour (112), and laboratory animals (113).

Conclusion and research needs

Available data indicate that OR is still often unrecognized and its contribution to the global burden of rhinitis remains largely unknown. An accurate diagnosis of OR is crucial for improving the management and minimizing the adverse socioeconomic impact of this prevalent work-related condition. Consensus algorithms for diagnosing OR need to be developed and validated. Complete avoidance of further exposure to the sensitizing occupational agent should still be recommended as the most effective treatment, although the beneficial effects of this option must be weighed against its potential adverse socioeconomic impact. There is a need to further identify the individual risk factors for the development of OA that would allow for a more personalized and cost-effective management of OR.

References

1. Bousquet J, Khaltaev N, Cruz AA, et al. Allergic rhinitis and its impact on asthma (ARIA) 2008 update (in collaboration with the World Health Organization, GA(2)LEN and AllerGen). Allergy. 2008;63 Suppl 86:8–160.
2. Greiner AN, Hellings PW, Rotiroti G, Scadding GK. Allergic rhinitis. Lancet. 2011;378:2112–22.
3. Siracusa A, Desrosiers M, Marabini A. Epidemiology of occupational rhinitis: prevalence, aetiology and determinants. Clin Exp Allergy. 2000;30:1519–34.
4. Moscato G, Vandenplas O, Gerth Van Wijk R, et al. Occupational rhinitis. Allergy. 2008;63:969–80.
5. Siracusa A, Folletti I, Moscato G. Non-IgE-mediated and irritant-induced work-related rhinitis. Curr Opin Allergy Clin Immunol. 2013;13:159–66.
6. Shusterman D. Occupational irritant and allergic rhinitis. Curr Allergy Asthma Rep. 2014;14:425.
7. Hox V, Steelant B, Fokkens W, et al. Occupational upper airway disease: How work affects the nose. Allergy. 2014;69:282–91.
8. Vandenplas O, Hox V, Bernstein DI. Occupational rhinitis. J Allergy Clin Immunol Pract. 2020;8:3311–21.
9. Malo JL, Vandenplas O. Definitions and classification of work-related asthma. Immunol Allergy Clin North Am. 2011;31:645–62.
10. Tarlo SM, Balmes J, Balkissoon R, et al. Diagnosis and management of work-related asthma: American College of Chest Physicians Consensus Statement. Chest. 2008;134:1S–41S.
11. Seed MJ, Agius RM. Progress with structure-activity relationship modelling of occupational chemical respiratory sensitizers. Curr Opin Allergy Clin Immunol. 2017;17:64–71.
12. Prince P, Lemiere C, Dufour MH, et al. Airway inflammatory responses following exposure to occupational agents. Chest. 2012;141:1522–7.
13. Palczynski C, Walusiak J, Ruta U, Gorski P. Nasal provocation test in the diagnosis of natural rubber latex allergy. Allergy. 2000;55:34–41.
14. Krakowiak A, Ruta U, Gorski P, et al. Nasal lavage fluid examination and rhinomanometry in the diagnostics of occupational airway allergy to laboratory animals. Int J Occup Med Environ Health. 2003;16:125–32.
15. Walusiak J, Wiszniewska M, Krawczyk-Adamus P, Palczynski C. Occupational allergy to wheat flour. Nasal response to specific inhalative challenge in asthma and rhinitis vs. isolated rhinitis: a comparative study. Int J Occup Med Environ Health. 2004;17:433–40.
16. Nielsen J, Welinder H, Ottosson H, et al. Nasal challenge shows pathogenetic relevance of specific IgE serum antibodies for nasal symptoms caused by hexahydrophthalic anhydride. Clin Exp Allergy. 1994;24:440–9.
17. Palczynski C, Walusiak J, Ruta U, Gorski P. Occupational asthma and rhinitis due to glutaraldehyde: changes in nasal lavage fluid after specific inhalatory challenge test. Allergy. 2001;56:1186–91.
18. Palczynski C, Walusiak J, Krakowiak A, et al. Nasal lavage fluid examination in diagnostics of occupational allergy to chloramine. Int J Occup Med Environ Health. 2003;16:231–40.
19. Moscato G, Pala G, Perfetti L, et al. Clinical and inflammatory features of occupational asthma caused by persulphate salts in comparison with asthma associated with occupational rhinitis. Allergy. 2010;65:784–90.
20. Meggs WJ, Elsheik T, Metzger WJ, et al. Nasal pathology and ultrastructure in patients with chronic airway inflammation (RADS and RUDS) following an irritant exposure. J Toxicol Clin Toxicol. 1996;34:383–96.
21. Leroyer C, Malo JL, Girard D, et al. Chronic rhinitis in workers at risk of reactive airways dysfunction syndrome due to exposure to chlorine. Occup Environ Med. 1999;56:334–8.
22. Hoffman CD, Henneberger PK, Olin AC, et al. Exposure to ozone gases in pulp mills and the onset of rhinitis. Scand J Work Environ Health. 2004;30:445–9.
23. Brooks SM, Weiss MA, Bernstein IL. Reactive airways dysfunction syndrome (RADS). Persistent asthma syndrome after high level irritant exposures. Chest. 1985;88:376–84.
24. Amin K, Rinne J, Haahtela T, et al. Inflammatory cell and epithelial characteristics of perennial allergic and nonallergic rhinitis with a symptom history of 1 to 3 years' duration. J Allergy Clin Immunol. 2001;107:249–57.
25. Fortoul TI, Rodriguez-Lara V, Lopez-Valdez N, et al. Biomarkers of nasal toxicity in humans. In: Morris J, Shusterman D, eds. Toxicology of the Nose and Upper Airway. New York: Informa Healthcare; 2010:167–73.
26. Castano R, Theriault G, Gautrin D. Categorizing nasal septal perforations of occupational origin as cases of corrosive rhinitis. Am J Ind Med. 2007;50:150–3.
27. Bolek EC, Erden A, Kulekci C, et al. Rare occupational cause of nasal septum perforation: nickel exposure. Int J Occup Med Environ Health. 2017;30:963–7.

28. Shusterman D. Nonallergic rhinitis: environmental determinants. Immunol Allergy Clin North Am. 2016;36:379–99.

29. Henneberger PK, Redlich CA, Callahan DB, et al. An official American Thoracic Society statement: work-exacerbated asthma. Am J Respir Crit Care Med. 2011;184:368–78.

30. Bernstein JA, Levin LS, Al-Shuik E, Martin VT. Clinical characteristics of chronic rhinitis patients with high vs low irritant trigger burdens. Ann Allergy Asthma Immunol. 2012;109:173–8.

31. Van Gerven L, Steelant B, Hellings PW. Nasal hyperreactivity in rhinitis: a diagnostic and therapeutic challenge. Allergy. 2018;73:1784–91.

32. Akpinar-Elci M, Pasquale DK, Abrokwah M, et al. United Airway Disease Among Crop Farmers. J Agromedicine. 2016;21:217–23.

33. Woodin MA, Liu Y, Neuberg D, et al. Acute respiratory symptoms in workers exposed to vanadium-rich fuel-oil ash. Am J Ind Med. 2000;37:353–63.

34. Hellgren J, Lillienberg L, Jarlstedt J, et al. Population-based study of non-infectious rhinitis in relation to occupational exposure, age, sex, and smoking. Am J Ind Med. 2002;42:23–8.

35. Radon K, Gerhardinger U, Schulze A, et al. Occupation and adult onset of rhinitis in the general population. Occup Environ Med. 2008;65:38–43.

36. de Fatima Macaira E, Algranti E, Medina Coeli Mendonca E, Antonio Bussacos M. Rhinitis and asthma symptoms in non-domestic cleaners from the Sao Paulo metropolitan area, Brazil. Occup Environ Med. 2007;64:446–53.

37. Vyas A, Pickering CA, Oldham LA, et al. Survey of symptoms, respiratory function, and immunology and their relation to glutaraldehyde and other occupational exposures among endoscopy nursing staff. Occup Environ Med. 2000;57:752–9.

38. Kaukiainen A, Martikainen R, Riala R, et al. Work tasks, chemical exposure and respiratory health in construction painting. Am J Ind Med. 2008;51:1–8.

39. Malo JL, Lemière C, Desjardins A, Cartier A. Prevalence and intensity of rhinoconjunctivitis in subjects with occupational asthma. Eur Respir J. 1997;10:1513–5.

40. Vandenplas O, Van Brussel P, D'Alpaos V, et al. Rhinitis in subjects with work-exacerbated asthma. Respir Med. 2010;104:497–503.

41. Ameille J, Hamelin K, Andujar P, et al. Occupational asthma and occupational rhinitis: the united airways disease model revisited. Occup Environ Med. 2013;70:471–5.

42. Castano R, Gautrin D, Theriault G, et al. Occupational rhinitis in workers investigated for occupational asthma. Thorax. 2009;64:50–4.

43. Balogun RA, Siracusa A, Shusterman D. Occupational rhinitis and occupational asthma: Association or progression? Am J Ind Med. 2018;61:293–307.

44. Vandenplas O, Ghezzo H, Munoz X, et al. What are the questionnaire items most useful in identifying subjects with occupational asthma? Eur Respir J. 2005;26:1056–63.

45. Grammer LC, Ditto AM, Tripathi A, Harris KE. Prevalence and onset of rhinitis and conjunctivitis in subjects with occupational asthma caused by trimellitic anhydride (TMA). J Occup Environ Med. 2002;44:1179–81.

46. Singh T, Bello B, Jeebhay MF. Risk factors associated with asthma phenotypes in dental healthcare workers. Am J Ind Med. 2013;56:90–9.

47. Gautrin D, Ghezzo H, Infante-Rivard C, Malo JL. Natural history of sensitization, symptoms and occupational diseases in apprentices exposed to laboratory animals. Eur Respir J. 2001;17:904–8.

48. Karjalainen A, Martikainen R, Klaukka T, et al. Risk of asthma among Finnish patients with occupational rhinitis. Chest. 2003;123:283–8.

49. Elliott L, Heederik D, Marshall S, et al. Progression of self-reported symptoms in laboratory animal allergy. J Allergy Clin Immunol. 2005;116:127–32.

50. Leynaert B, Neukirch F, Demoly P, Bousquet J. Epidemiologic evidence for asthma and rhinitis comorbidity. J Allergy Clin Immunol. 2000;106:S201–5.

51. Shaaban R, Zureik M, Soussan D, et al. Rhinitis and onset of asthma: a longitudinal population-based study. Lancet. 2008;372:1049–57.

52. Hytonen M, Kanerva L, Malmberg H, et al. The risk of occupational rhinitis. Int Arch Occup Environ Health. 1997;69:487–90.

53. Vandenplas O, Suarthana E, Rifflart C, et al. The impact of work-related rhinitis on quality of life and work productivity: a general workforce-based survey. J Allergy Clin Immunol Pract. 2020;8:1583–91.e5.

54. Folletti I, Forcina A, Marabini A, et al. Have the prevalence and incidence of occupational asthma and rhinitis because of laboratory animals declined in the last 25 years? Allergy. 2008;63:834–41.

55. Davies GE, Thompson AV, Niewola Z, et al. Allergy to laboratory animals: a retrospective and a prospective study. Br J Ind Med. 1983;40:442–9.

56. Cullinan P, Cook A, Gordon S, et al. Allergen exposure, atopy and smoking as determinants of allergy to rats in a cohort of laboratory employees. Eur Respir J. 1999;13:1139–43.

57. Gautrin D, Infante-Rivard C, Ghezzo H, Malo JL. Incidence and host determinants of probable occupational asthma in apprentices exposed to laboratory animals. Am J Respir Crit Care Med. 2001;163:899–904.

58. Elliott L, Heederik D, Marshall S, et al. Incidence of allergy and allergy symptoms among workers exposed to laboratory animals. Occup Environ Med. 2005;62:766–71.

59. Cullinan P, Cook A, Nieuwenhuijsen MJ, et al. Allergen and dust exposure as determinants of work-related symptoms and sensitization in a cohort of flour-exposed workers; a case-control analysis. Ann Occup Hyg. 2001;45:97–103.

60. Gautrin D, Ghezzo H, Infante-Rivard C, Malo JL. Incidence and host determinants of work-related rhinoconjunctivitis in apprentice pastry-makers. Allergy. 2002;57:913–8.

61. Walusiak J, Hanke W, Gorski P, Palczynski C. Respiratory allergy in apprentice bakers: do occupational allergies follow the allergic march? Allergy. 2004;59:442–50.

62. Skjold T, Dahl R, Juhl B, Sigsgaard T. The incidence of respiratory symptoms and sensitisation in baker apprentices. Eur Respir J. 2008;32:452–9.

63. Patiwael JA, Jong NW, Burdorf A, et al. Occupational allergy to bell pepper pollen in greenhouses in the Netherlands, an 8-year follow-up study. Allergy. 2010;65:1423–9.

64. Archambault S, Malo JL, Infante-Rivard C, et al. Incidence of sensitization, symptoms, and probable occupational rhinoconjunctivitis and asthma in apprentices starting exposure to latex. J Allergy Clin Immunol. 2001;107:921–3.

65. Ruoppi P, Koistinen T, Susitaival P, et al. Frequency of allergic rhinitis to laboratory animals in university employees as confirmed by chamber challenges. Allergy. 2004;59:295–301.

66. Scadding G, Hellings P, Alobid I, et al. Diagnostic tools in rhinology EAACI position paper. Clin Transl Allergy. 2011;1:2.

67. van Kampen V, de Blay F, Folletti I, et al. EAACI position paper: skin prick testing in the diagnosis of occupational type I allergies. Allergy. 2013;68:580–4.

68. Lux H, Lenz K, Budnik LT, Baur X. Performance of specific immunoglobulin E tests for diagnosing occupational asthma: a systematic review and meta-analysis. Occup Environ Med. 2019;76:269–78.

69. Gomez F, Rondon C, Salas M, Campo P. Local allergic rhinitis: mechanisms, diagnosis and relevance for occupational rhinitis. Curr Opin Allergy Clin Immunol. 2015;15:111–6.

70. Hytonen M, Sala E. Nasal provocation test in the diagnostics of occupational allergic rhinitis. Rhinology. 1996;34:86–90.

71. Gosepath J, Amedee RG, Mann WJ. Nasal provocation testing as an international standard for evaluation of allergic and nonallergic rhinitis. Laryngoscope. 2005;115:512–6.

72. Airaksinen L, Tuomi T, Vanhanen M, et al. Use of nasal provocation test in the diagnostics of occupational rhinitis. Rhinology. 2007;45:40–6.

73. Auge J, Vent J, Agache I, et al. EAACI Position paper on the standardization of nasal allergen challenges. Allergy. 2018;73:1597–608.

74. Airaksinen LK, Tuomi TO, Tuppurainen MO, et al. M. Inhalation challenge test in the diagnosis of occupational rhinitis. Am J Rhinol. 2008;22:38–46.

75. Vandenplas O, Suojalehto H, Aasen TB, et al. Specific inhalation challenge in the diagnosis of occupational asthma: consensus statement. Eur Respir J. 2014;43:1573–87.

76. Suojalehto H, Suuronen K, Cullinan P. Specific challenge testing for occupational asthma: revised handbook. Eur Respir J. 2019;54.

77. Pirila T, Nuutinen J. Acoustic rhinometry, rhinomanometry and the amount of nasal secretion in the clinical monitoring of the nasal provocation test. Clin Exp Allergy. 1998;28:468–77.

78. Nathan RA, Eccles R, Howarth PH, et al. Objective monitoring of nasal patency and nasal physiology in rhinitis. J Allergy Clin Immunol. 2005;115:S442–59.

79. Andre RF, Vuyk HD, Ahmed A, et al. Correlation between subjective and objective evaluation of the nasal airway. A systematic review of the highest level of evidence. Clin Otolaryngol. 2009;34:518–25.

80. Castano R, Theriault G, Maghni K, et al. Reproducibility of nasal lavage in the context of the inhalation challenge investigation of occupational rhinitis. Am J Rhinol. 2008;22:271–5.

81. Pignatti P, Pala G, Pisati M, et al. Nasal blown secretion evaluation in specific occupational nasal challenges. Int Arch Occup Environ Health. 2009;83:217–23.

82. Rimmer J, Hellings P, Lund VJ, et al. European position paper on diagnostic tools in rhinology. Rhinology. 2019;57:1–41.

83. Storaas T, Steinsvag SK, Florvaag E, et al. Occupational rhinitis: diagnostic criteria, relation to lower airway symptoms and IgE sensitization in bakery workers. Acta Otolaryngol. 2005;125:1211–7.

84. van der Walt A, Singh T, Baatjies R, et al. Work-related allergic respiratory disease and asthma in spice mill workers is associated with inhalant chili pepper and garlic exposures. Occup Environ Med. 2013;70:446–52.

85. Ahman M, Soderman E. Serial nasal peak expiratory flow measurements in woodwork teachers. Int Arch Occup Environ Health. 1996;68:177–82.
86. Meltzer EO. Allergic rhinitis: burden of illness, quality of life, comorbidities, and control. Immunol Allergy Clin North Am. 2016;36:235–48.
87. Segboer CL, Terreehorst I, Gevorgyan A, et al. Quality of life is significantly impaired in nonallergic rhinitis patients. Allergy. 2018;73:1094–100.
88. Vandenplas O, Vinnikov D, Blanc PD, et al. Impact of rhinitis on work productivity: a systematic review. J Allergy Clin Immunol Pract. 2018;6:1274–86.e9.
89. Groenewoud GC, de Groot H, Gerth van Wijk R. Impact of occupational and inhalant allergy on rhinitis-specific quality of life in employees of bell pepper greenhouses in the Netherlands. Ann Allergy Asthma Immunol. 2006;96:92–7.
90. Airaksinen LK, Luukkonen RA, Lindstrom I, et al. Long-term exposure and health-related quality of life among patients with occupational rhinitis. J Occup Environ Med. 2009;51:1288–97.
91. Brisman J, Jarvholm B. Bakery work, atopy and the incidence of self-reported hay fever and rhinitis. Eur Respir J. 1999;13:502–7.
92. Gerth van Wijk R, Patiwael JA, de Jong NW, et al. Occupational rhinitis in bell pepper greenhouse workers: determinants of leaving work and the effects of subsequent allergen avoidance on health-related quality of life. Allergy. 2011;66:903–8.
93. Maoua M, Maalel OE, Kacem I, et al. Quality of life and work productivity impairment of patients with allergic occupational rhinitis. Tanaffos. 2019;18:58–65.
94. Guerra S, Sherrill DL, Martinez FD, Barbee RA. Rhinitis as an independent risk factor for adult-onset asthma. J Allergy Clin Immunol. 2002;109:419–25.
95. Boutet K, Malo JL, Ghezzo H, Gautrin D. Airway hyperresponsiveness and risk of chest symptoms in an occupational model. Thorax. 2007;62:260–4.
96. Burte E, Bousquet J, Siroux V, et al. The sensitization pattern differs according to rhinitis and asthma multimorbidity in adults: the EGEA study. Clin Exp Allergy. 2017;47:520–9.
97. Castano R, Trudeau C, Castellanos L, Malo JL. Prospective outcome assessment of occupational rhinitis after removal from exposure. J Occup Environ Med. 2013;55:579–85.
98. Castano R. Persistent specific nasal reactivity to occupational allergens after removal from exposure. Ann Allergy Asthma Immunol. 2013;111:66–7.
99. Vandenplas O, Dressel H, Wilken D, et al. Management of occupational asthma: cessation or reduction of exposure? A systematic review of available evidence. Eur Respir J. 2011;38:804–11.
100. Slovak AJ, Orr RG, Teasdale EL. Efficacy of the helmet respirator in occupational asthma due to laboratory animal allergy (LAA). Am Ind Hyg Assoc J. 1985;46:411–5.
101. Merget R, Schulte A, Gebler A, et al. Outcome of occupational asthma due to platinum salts after transferral to low-exposure areas. Int Arch Occup Environ Health. 1999;72:33–9.
102. Vandenplas O, Jamart J, Delwiche JP, et al. Occupational asthma caused by natural rubber latex: outcome according to cessation or reduction of exposure. J Allergy Clin Immunol. 2002;109:125–30.
103. Bernstein DI, Karnani R, Biagini RE, et al. Clinical and occupational outcomes in health care workers with natural rubber latex allergy. Ann Allergy Asthma Immunol. 2003;90:209–13.
104. Eggleston PA, Ansari AA, Ziemann B, et al. Occupational challenge studies with laboratory workers allergic to rats. J Allergy Clin Immunol. 1990;86:63–72.
105. Quirce S, Swanson MC, Fernandez-Nieto M, de las Heras M, et al. Quantified environmental challenge with absorbable dusting powder aerosol from natural rubber latex gloves. J Allergy Clin Immunol. 2003;111:788–94.
106. Baur X, Akdis CA, Budnik LT, et al. Immunological methods for diagnosis and monitoring of IgE-mediated allergy caused by industrial sensitizing agents (IMExAllergy). Allergy. 2019;74:1885–97.
107. Moscato G. Specific immunotherapy and biological treatments for occupational allergy. Curr Opin Allergy Clin Immunol. 2014;14:576–81.
108. Bousquet J, Flahault A, Vandenplas O, et al. Natural rubber latex allergy among health care workers: a systematic review of the evidence. J Allergy Clin Immunol. 2006;118:447–54.
109. Vandenplas O, Larbanois A, Vanassche F, et al. Latex-induced occupational asthma: time trend in incidence and relationship with hospital glove policies. Allergy. 2009;64:415–20.
110. Cathcart M, Nicholson P, Roberts D, et al. Enzyme exposure, smoking and lung function in employees in the detergent industry over 20 years. Medical Subcommittee of the UK Soap and Detergent Industry Association. Occup Med (Lond). 1997;47:473–8.
111. Larsen AI, Cederkvist L, Lykke AM, et al. Allergy development in adulthood: an occupational cohort study of the manufacturing of industrial enzymes. J Allergy Clin Immunol Pract. 2020;8:210–8.e5.
112. Meijster T, Tielemans E, Heederik D. Effect of an intervention aimed at reducing the risk of allergic respiratory disease in bakers: change in flour dust and fungal alpha-amylase levels. Occup Environ Med. 2009;66:543–9.
113. Gordon S, Preece R. Prevention of laboratory animal allergy. Occup Med (Lond). 2003;53:371–7.

23

AIRWAY DISEASES DUE TO ORGANIC DUST EXPOSURE

Jill A. Poole,[1] Santiago Quirce,[2] Andrea Siracusa,[3] Maria Jesús Cruz Carmona,[4]
Amber N. Johnson,[5] Jean-Luc Malo,[6] and David I. Bernstein[7]
[1]Division of Allergy and Immunology, University of Nebraska Medical Center, Omaha, Nebraska, USA
[2]Department of Allergy, La Paz University Hospital, Universidad Autonoma de Madrid, Madrid, Spain
[3](Formerly) University of Perugia, Perugia, Italy
[4]Pulmonology Research Laboratory, Vall d'Hebron Research Institute (VHIR) and University of Barcelona, Barcelona, Spain
[5]Pulmonary and Critical Care Medicine, University of Nebraska Medical Center, Omaha, Nebraska, USA
[6]Hôpital du Sacré-Cœur de Montréal and Université de Montréal, Montréal, Québec, Canada
[7]Division of Immunology, Allergy and Rheumatology, University of Cincinnati College of Medicine, Cincinnati, Ohio, USA

Contents

CASE HISTORY

SWINE CONFINEMENT WORKER

1. A 35-year-old man has been employed for 15 years on a farm as a swine confinement unit manager. His duties included the daily care and feeding of the animals as well as cleaning the barns using a pressure washer.
2. He gradually developed a cough, chest tightness, wheezing, and dyspnea on exertion after being employed in this capacity for 15 years.
3. Pulmonary function tests revealed the presence of mild airway obstruction without reversibility with a short-acting beta-agonist bronchodilator.
4. His chest X-ray was normal.
5. The patient left his position because of his respiratory symptoms and took a job as a maintenance worker at a medical center. Pulmonary function tests performed 10 years later showed improvement in airway obstruction, but not complete normalization. At that point in time, he no longer had pulmonary symptoms at rest but occasionally with exercise.

Introduction

The agricultural environment may cause various acute and chronic airway inflammatory diseases including occupational asthma (OA), asthma-like disease, chronic obstructive pulmonary disease (COPD), and hypersensitivity pneumonitis (HP). Of the organic dusts, inflammatory insults from crop farming, animal farming industry, and cotton and other textile dusts have been studied more extensively. Acute respiratory symptoms and cross-shift declines in forced expiratory volume in 1 second (FEV_1) have been described among poultry, swine, and dairy workers,

TABLE 23.1 Comparisons of Manifestations of Hypersensitivity Pneumonitis (HP) and HP-Like Conditions

	Hypersensitivity Pneumonitis[a]	Airway Diseases Due to Organic Dust Exposure	Metal Fume Fever[b] (MFF)	ODTS[c]
Causal agents	Fungi, bacteria, bird proteins, chemicals	Grain and farming dust Cotton dust Swine confinement	Welding on zinc oxide and galvanized metal, but not exclusively	Various
Mechanism	IgG mediated response to various proteins	Unconfirmed: endotoxins, epithelial Toll-like receptors (TLR), water soluble agents with biologic activity, peptidoglycan (PGN), nucleotide oligomerization domain (NOD) proteins	Unknown	Unconfirmed: endotoxins
Clinical manifestations	Respiratory and systemic	Respiratory and systemic	Systemic Metallic taste	Systemic
Radiologic abnormalities	Frequent (acute and chronic forms)	Absent (except in long-term development of COPD)	Absent	Absent
Functional abnormalities	Frequent Mainly restrictive pattern and gas exchange	Obstructive pattern, mainly with long-term exposure	Absent (obstructive pattern in welders but not specific for MFF)	Absent
Diagnostic procedures	Various Assessment of specific IgG (recombinant antigens)	Clinical history Lung function tests WBC	Clinical history Lung function tests WBC	Clinical history Blood and sputum leukocytosis
Outcome	Possible respiratory long-term disability	Possible development of COPD	Possible OA (MFF may be a predictor) and COPD	Self-limited
Treatment	Avoidance of exposure Pharmacologic treatment if needed	Reduction in exposure to prevent long-term COPD	None (reduction in exposure improves symptoms)	None (reduction in exposure improves symptoms)

[a] See Chapter 24.

[b] See Chapter 16.

[c] ODTS: organic dust toxic syndrome; see Chapter 24.

Abbreviations: COPD, chronic obstructive pulmonary disease; WBC, white blood count.

slaughterhouse workers, and garbage handlers. Exposures in these environments are complex marked by a number of airborne bioaerosol contaminants including complex mixtures of organic dust, particulates, skin debris, feather, insect parts, aerosolized feed, animal respiratory secretions, excreta, bacteria, and fungi. The abundance and wide variety of gram-negative and gram-positive microbial components and fungal components in the organic dusts are likely responsible for the pathogenesis of the organic dust associated airway inflammatory diseases. Innate immune responses with engagement of Toll-like receptor signaling pathways and damage associated molecular signaling pathways are key to the initiation of the airway inflammatory and neutrophil predominant response. Adaptive immune responses with T cells and B cells with a Th1/Th17 polarized response in addition to key roles for macrophages are implicated in the chronic inflammatory response. Treatment strategies are limited and personal protective devices are strongly recommended to limit inhalation exposures. This chapter will review the organic dust exposures by environmental setting, immunopathogenesis, and the acute and chronic airway diseases associated with exposure.

A variety of occupational diseases affect the distal bronchioles and the lung parenchyma. This includes hypersensitivity pneumonitis (HP) (Chapter 24) with features that differ according to the offending agent (microorganisms, birds' proteins, metals, and chemicals). Exposure to organic dusts, which is covered in this chapter, and metal fumes (Chapter 16) as well as organic dust toxic syndrome (ODTS) (Chapter 24) can induce clinical, functional, and radiological manifestations with similarities and differences with HP, especially in the extent of involvement of lung parenchyma (Table 23.1).

Organic dust exposures by environmental setting

Crop farming and grain dust

Crop farming is the cultivation of plants for food, animal foodstuffs, or other commercial uses. Some plants are grown for food, like wheat, rice, and vegetables, whereas other plants are used to feed animals. A comprehensive review on the effect of food harvesting or processing in different settings reported that up 25% of occupational rhinitis and/or OA are due to food products or contaminants (1). Raw and processed vegetable products, microbes, additives and preservatives, and insect and mite contaminants are the main allergen sources (1).

Most of the studies of these farmers came from cross-sectional studies. In 1987, Dosman et al. (2) reported significantly lower lung function in farmers in Saskatchewan (Canada) compared with controls. European farmers were found to have lower prevalence of rhinitis and asthma than California farmers (12.7% vs 23.9% and 2.8% vs 4.7%), but they had a higher prevalence of chronic bronchitis and toxic pneumonitis than their California counterparts (10% vs 4.4% and 12.2% vs 2.7%) (3). The European farmers' project of 8000 farmers from several countries found an overall prevalence of work-related wheeze, breathlessness, and/or cough without phlegm of 22.1%, highest in Essex, United Kingdom (32.8%), and lowest in Germany, Saxony (18.3%) (4). In the Burden of Obstructive Lung Disease Study in the United States, among a random population sample of 1258 individuals, 288 were farmers; among these farmers, the prevalence of non-reversible airways obstruction was 30.2% (5). In addition, farming was significantly associated with airway obstruction Global Initiative for Chronic Obstructive Lung Disease (GOLD) stage 1 or higher with an odds ratio (OR) 1.5 (95% CI:1.1–2.0) (5).

Exposure to grain and flour dust is a frequent reported cause of OA (Chapters 3 and 12). The estimated annual incidence of cereal-induced asthma in the United Kingdom was 811 cases per million people employed over the period 1989–1997 (6), whereas in Norway, the incidence of OA among male and female bakers was 2.4 and 1 case per 1000 person-years, respectively (7). A Korean study in the bakery industry showed that the overall prevalence of wheat sensitization was 5.9% (8). Furthermore, this study confirmed that an IgE-mediated response is the major pathogenic mechanism for the induction of work-related symptoms in wheat-exposed workers, whereas wheat-specific IgG antibodies may represent current or previous exposure to wheat dust (8).

The relationship between lower and upper airway problems ("united airway disease") among 180 farmers from North Carolina has been investigated using a questionnaire. Lower airway symptom prevalence was 35%, and 66% had upper airway symptoms, whereas only 1% of farmers had physician-diagnosed rhinitis (9). Self-reported rhinitis and asthma symptoms were significantly correlated among farmers. This study points out that upper airway diseases are prevalent and should not be overlooked among farm workers, suggesting that early management of upper airway symptoms may prevent severe lower airway diseases (9).

Etiology and pathogenesis

Grain dust asthma has been widely reported, and can be mediated by allergic mechanisms to grain or contaminant-derived proteins or by nonallergic pathways due to inflammation from one or more of the toxins contaminating the dust. There is considerable evidence that exposures other than grain dust are associated with disease development. These exposures included dusts from animal feed, soil, and components of microorganisms such as endotoxin and fungi, which initiate inflammatory process in the airways and may ultimately lead to chronic airway disease. Moreover, workers handling cereal or vegetable seeds are at risk of exposure to high levels of endotoxin-containing seed dust. Occupational exposure to inhalable agricultural seed dust can induce inflammatory responses, and is a potential cause of organic dust toxic syndrome (ODTS) (Table 23.1) (Chapter 24). Exposure to flour allergens and endotoxins interact to induce allergic responses and respiratory symptoms. In addition, pesticides applied to crops are associated with respiratory symptoms. A study of the respiratory health of grain farmers in Alberta (Canada) conducted by telephone interview revealed that lifetime exposure to phenoxy herbicides is associated with an increased risk of asthma (10). The Agriculture Health Study in the United States demonstrated relationships between a number of pesticides with both allergic and nonallergic asthma, particularly among male farmers (11).

Animal farming

Farmers and farm owners constitute a large professional group, recognizing that their numbers have declined considerably in most developed countries. The last decades showed a strong tendency toward specialization and concentration, leading to fewer but larger farms, whereby the number of animals per farm has increased (Table 23.2). Farming practices are changing with large-scale enterprises gradually replacing smaller-scale traditional family farms. This rearing of farm animals that include beef cattle, dairy cows, swine, broilers (chickens raised for meat), and turkeys in intensive confinement facilities is associated with worker exposure to airborne dust, a wide variety and quantity of microbial agents, and gases. The respiratory health hazards in this agriculture industry have been associated with an increased risk of respiratory diseases as reviewed (12). Although recommendations to lower exposure levels have been published, there is little evidence that these have been achieved (13).

Etiology and pathogenesis

Animal farming exposures are complex and can vary based upon geographical location, type, size, and time of year of assessment. Most of the available data on these workplace exposure levels include evaluation of dust particulates, gram-positive

TABLE 23.2 Changing Structure of Cattle, Dairy, and Pig Farms from 2005–2010 in the European Union[a]

Animal Farming Type	2005	2010	% Change (2010/2005)
Cattle holdings × 1000	3757	2574	−31.5
Cattle × 1000			
Cattle: Animals/holding	90,018	88,146	−2.1%
Dairy holdings × 1000	25,151	23,162	−7.9%
Dairy: Animals/holding	8.9	13.6	+52.8
Pig holdings × 1000	3822	2755	−27.9
Pigs × 1000	154,625	151,808	−1.8
Pigs: Animals/holding	40.5	55.1	+36.0

[a] Directorate-General for Agriculture and Rural Development. Agriculture in the European Union, Statistical and Economic Information. European Union, Report 2013, December 2013.

(e.g. muramyl dipeptide/muramic acid and peptidoglycan) and gram-negative microbial components (e.g. endotoxins), and $(1\rightarrow3)$-β-d-glucans. The gases and fumes predominately originate from animal manure to include ammonia (NH_3); methane (CH_4), hydrogen sulfide (H_2S), and carbon dioxide (CO_2). Endotoxins are biologically active lipopolysaccharide produced by the cellular wall of gram-negative bacteria, and $(1\rightarrow3)$-β-d-glucans are polysaccharides that constitute a component of the cellular wall of molds, yeast, and some bacteria. Whereas dust, endotoxin, and $(1\rightarrow3)$-β-d-glucans are commonly measured in exposure settings, these exposures do not reflect the total bacterial burden. Culture-independent techniques utilizing gas chromatography mass spectrometry, polymerase chain reaction, denaturing gradient gel electrophoresis, and shotgun metagenomics sequencing techniques have provided information detailing the variety and abundance of gram-positive and gram-negative bacteria components that included several dominate bacterial families in swine environments: Bacteroides, Lactobacillus, Clostridium, Ruminococcus, Eubacterium, and Archeabacterium (14, 15). Proteases within swine dusts that can activate inflammatory responses have also been described (16). An overview image of the gases and components associated with the etiology and pathogenesis of organic dust-induced airway disease is shown in Figure 23.1.

Studies have shown great variations in personal exposures in different farm types. Pig and poultry farmers tend to have the highest exposure levels, whereas mixed production and mink farmers are less exposed (17). Despite efforts toward improving the exposure environment, no clear downward trends in dust and endotoxin exposure for the period 1985–2013 were observed, suggesting that the animal industry working environment is yet uncontrolled (18).

Animal models utilizing dust extracts primarily from swine facilities have demonstrated roles for Toll-like receptor (TLR) signaling pathways that recognize components of bacteria including endotoxin (TLR4), muramyl dipeptides (TLR2), and bacterial DNA (TLR9) with a central role for the adaptor protein myeloid differentiation factor 88 (MyD88), which is utilized by all TLR2s (except TLR3) (19). Scavenger receptor (20) and protease receptor (16) signaling pathways also mediate airway inflammatory responses to these dust extracts in mice. In humans, it has been demonstrated that swine confinement workers with polymorphisms of the *TLR2* and *TLR4* genes were associated with airway responses and lung function (21). Activation of lung macrophages with a prominent Th1/Th17 immune response has also been implicated (22).

Factors affecting exposure during farm work

There are many organic dust sources on indoor and outdoor animal farm working environments. Level of exposure is high during swine and dairy stable working tasks such as feeding, bedding, handling animals, and high pressure washing, and during work in milking parlors (23). Dust exposure was higher with automatic and lower with manual milking (24). Lower levels of organic dusts were found during field work of cattle and repair of stables. In confinement barns, the concentrations of organic dust, endotoxin, and ammonia increase during the winter. In pig farms,

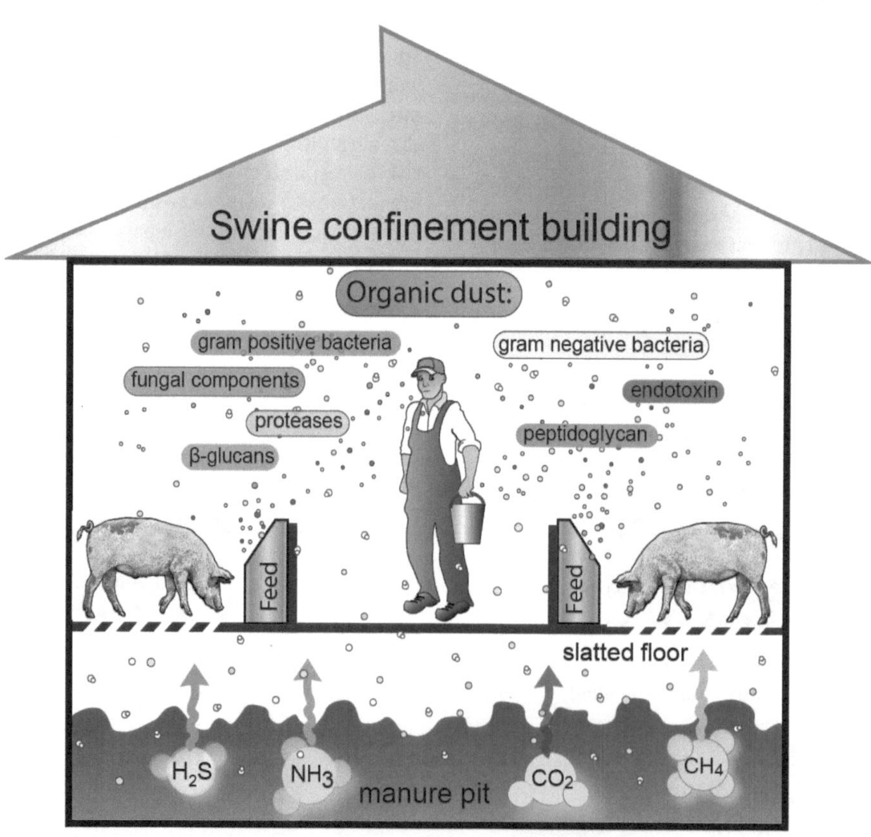

FIGURE 23.1 Overview image of the gases and components associated with etiology and pathogenesis of organic dust-induced airway disease attributed to work in a swine confinement. (Image is courtesy of Art Heires, University of Nebraska Medical Center, Omaha, Nebraska.)

feeding systems (e.g. dry feed and manual feeding), flooring (e.g. slatted floor coverage), and type of ventilation were predictors of indoor personal exposure levels to bioaerosol (25).

In poultry farmers factors such as the age of the chick involved and the housing system (e.g. aviary vs cage) seem to be relevant. In broiler poultry operations, total dust, endotoxin, and ammonia levels increased with flock age (26). Moreover, exposure to inhalable dust and endotoxins is higher in aviary barns than in conventional and enriched barns (27).

Cotton and other textile dusts

Byssinosis is a term that refers to acute and chronic airway disease among individuals with occupational exposure to textile/cotton dusts. The syndrome was first described in cotton workers and later described in those working with other fiber plants including hemp, flax, and jute (28). Cigarette smoking is an important factor contributing to accelerated progression of disease among textile workers (29, 30). Early recognition of the additive effect of cigarette smoke led to initial interest in campaigns to decrease smoking among textile workers; however, elimination of smoking does not eliminate occupational hazards of exposure to textile dusts.

Symptoms of acute byssinosis include fever, malaise, chest tightness, and dyspnea, with symptoms classically worse on Monday or the day after a vacation (29, 31). Chronically, byssinosis is associated with development of obstructive lung disease. Cotton mill workers demonstrate significant decrease in FEV_1, ratio of FEV_1 to forced vital capacity (FEV1/FVC), and peak expiratory flow rate as compared to controls (30, 31). There is a dose-response relationship in regards to lung function impairment with increased levels of cotton exposure correlating with decrease in FEV_1 and

FEV_1/FVC (30–32). Respiratory symptoms have also been shown to correlate with density of dust in the workplace and duration of exposure (29, 31, 33). In particular, work involving weaving, blowing, ginning, and spinning is associated with higher odds of developing respiratory symptoms (33). Cotton ginning has been found to have the highest burden of respiratory illnesses as compared to spinning and weaving, with more visible cotton dust observed in comparison to the other sectors (30). Inadequate ventilation in the workplace environment also increases odds of developing respiratory symptoms (33). Both acute change in FEV_1 over a single working shift and chronic decrease in FEV_1 after long-term exposure have been described. The magnitude of cross-shift drop in FEV_1 has been associated with annual decline in FEV_1, suggesting that cross-shift FEV_1 decline may predict long-term effect of occupational textile dust exposure (34).

A Byssinosis Grading System was first published by Schilling in 1955 demonstrating the correlation between respiratory symptoms and airway obstruction (35). Schilling's grading system was later replaced by a more extensive one developed by the World Health Organization in 1983 (Table 23.3).

Etiology and pathogenesis

Endotoxins derived from gram-negative bacteria present in textile dusts are thought to represent the major contributing factor to the pathogenesis of byssinosis, with chronic loss of lung function correlating more to endotoxin exposure than to dust exposure (2–7, 28, 29, 36–39). In a prospective cohort study aimed at delineating the effect of endotoxin exposure, symptoms of dyspnea and bronchitis correlated with recent exposure, but the effect of endotoxin exposure on FEV_1 correlated with cumulative

TABLE 23.3 World Health Organization Grading System of Byssinosis

Classification	Symptoms
Grade 0	No symptoms
Byssinosis	
Grade B1	Chest tightness and/or SOB on most of first days back at work
Grade B2	Chest tightness and/or SOB on the first and other days of the working week
Respiratory tract irritation	
Grade RT1 1	Cough associated with dust exposure
Grade RT1 2	Persistent phlegm (i.e. on most days during 3 mo of the year) initiated or exacerbated by dust exposure
Grade RT1 3	Persistent phlegm initiated or made worse by dust exposure either with exacerbations of chest illness or persisting for 2 years or more
Lung function	
1. Acute changes	
No effect	A consistent[a] decline in FEV_1 of less than 5% or an increase in FEV_1 during the work shift
Mild effect	A consistent[a] decline between 5% and 10% in FEV_1 during the work shift
Moderate effect	A consistent[a] decline between 10% and 20% in FEV_1 during the work shift
Severe effect	A decline of 20% or more in FEV_1 during the work shift
2. Chronic changes	
No effect	FEV_1[b] 80% of predicted value[c]
Mild to moderate	FEV_1 60%–79% of predicted value[c]
Severe effect	FEV_1[b] less than 60% of predicted value[c]

[a] A decline occurring in at least three consecutive tests made after an absence from dust exposure of 2 days or more.

[b] Predicted values should be based on the data obtained from local populations or similar ethnic and social class groups.

[c] By a pre-shift test after an absence from dust exposure of 2 days or more.

Abbreviation: Forced expiratory volume in 1 second (FEV_1); SOB: shortness of breath.

past exposure and effect on FEV$_1$ reduction waned over time since exposure in retired workers (40).

In a murine model, repeated low-dose endotoxin exposure leads to airway hyperresponsiveness and neutrophil infiltration, with increased levels of proinflammatory (CD11b+) dendritic cells and compensatory decreased percentage of lung macrophages (41). Consistent with the phenotypic upregulation of proinflammatory dendritic cells, gene expression of myeloid and antigen presenting cell markers were also shown to be upregulated in lung homogenates. As macrophages have been shown to inhibit dendritic cell antigen presentation and airway hyperresponsiveness in vivo, the inverted macrophage to dendritic cell phenotype may provide insight into the mechanism of endotoxin-induced airway inflammation and obstructive lung disease (41).

Genetic polymorphisms in microsomal epoxide hydrolase gene, tumor necrosis factor (TNF) gene, and lymphotoxin alpha LTA gene may modify the association between endotoxin and annual FEV$_1$ decline in cotton textile workers (36). Genetic variations in single nucleotide polymorphisms are associated with significant differences in rate of FEV$_1$ decline in newly hired female Chinese textile workers (37). Greater number or risk loci correlated with increased rate of FEV$_1$ decline, and subgroup analysis indicated that the effect of genetic risk on FEV$_1$ decline is impacted by both age and endotoxin level (37).

Immunopathogenesis

Innate immunity

Innate immunity plays a key role in the response to exposure to organic dust. Depending on its scale, this response and subsequent inflammation can lead to progressive lung function loss over time and to the development of respiratory diseases such as asthma. Bacterial components of organic dust such as liposaccharide (LPS), lipoproteins, peptidoglycans and bacterial DNA can activate macrophages and other cell types that play an important role in driving innate immune responses. These components act through the Toll-like receptors (TLRs); for instance, the effects of LPS are mediated by the activation of the CD14 receptor and TLR4 (42). Specifically, LPS stimulate a physical association between CD14 and TLR4; several in vitro studies have supported a role for TLR4 in LPS signaling (43), a process that activates the production of chemoattractants that are able to recruit inflammatory cells. The elevated expression of cytokines like TNF-a, IL-6, and particularly IL-8 increases the number of neutrophils inside the lung (44). The persistence of these neutrophils can lead to chronic inflammation and lung tissue damage. TLR2 has also been shown to recognize lipoproteins and peptidoglycans of gram-positive bacteria contained in organic dust, activating the production of neutrophils and cytokines and producing lung parenchyma inflammation (45). Moreover, some studies have demonstrated the role of TLR9 in recognizing bacterial DNA (46) and the involvement of TLR10, TLR1, and TLR6 in IL-6 production in the response to organic dust exposure (47). Exposure to organic dust also alters the production of surfactants A and B which play a key role in balancing immune responses in the lung (48).

Adaptive immunity

The existence of an adaptive immune response after repetitive exposure to organic dust is also well established. In a murine model, Poole et al. (49) showed that repetitive exposure to organic dust induces a mixed Th1 and Th17 immune response. It has been demonstrated that agricultural workers have strong Th17 and Th1 responses (49). The Th17 response has been associated with the development of nonallergic or neutrophilic asthma (50). More controversial is the role of the Th2 response and the possibility of developing allergic asthma. Agricultural workers present high exposure to allergens and it has been shown that specific IgE and IgG levels to these allergens are increased after repetitive exposure to organic dust (51). However, it appears that exposure to organic dust is related more to protection against the development of allergic asthma, although the results of the different studies are inconclusive (13). In fact, adaptation and the development of tolerance may occur following repeated exposure to organic dust (52). For instance, it has been demonstrated that farmers have less allergic disease compared with other communities, especially children who grow up on a farm (53). This is consistent with the hygiene hypothesis that states that early childhood exposure to particular microorganisms protects against allergic diseases by contributing to the development of the immune system. Moreover, L-selectin shedding may play a role in the downregulation of the inflammatory response.

Acute airway disease induced by organic dust exposures

Acute airway inflammatory reactions following exposure to organic dust environments have been demonstrated in healthy subjects and also in those with lung disease. In healthy subjects, a one-time exposure to organic dust environments can induce an increase in airway hyperresponsiveness to methacholine, airway inflammation predominately comprised of neutrophil influx, and a systemic reaction marked by increased body temperature, increased levels of circulating IL-6, and acute phase proteins (54, 55). These symptoms are usually self-limiting without requirement of evaluation or treatment by healthcare providers. However, more severe symptoms can occur from an acute or one-time exposure that can be fatal; this syndrome has been termed the organic dust toxic syndrome and is reviewed in Chapter 24. Acute febrile syndrome or grain fever is an acute illness occurring during or shortly thereafter high concentration of grain dust exposure, with high prevalence in the 1960s and 1970s (56, 57). Symptoms included facial warmth, headache, malaise, myalgia, fever, chilliness, throat and tracheal burning sensation, chest tightness, dyspnea, cough, and sputum production with laboratory changes reflecting increased neutrophils. Improvements in grain elevators and handling grain have reduced this disease burden.

The term *asthma-like syndrome* has also been used to describe the acute, nonallergic airway response arising from inhalation of various agents in the agricultural environment characterized by symptoms of chest tightness, wheeze, mucus production, and/ or dyspnea. This syndrome may or may not be associated with cross-shift decline in FEV$_1$ (usually less than 10%), which is dose related and associated with neutrophilic airway inflammation. As symptoms may occur on first exposure and specific antigens and antibodies have not been identified, the syndrome is likely to be an innate immune inflammatory response to the exposure environment and not an allergic reaction.

Special considerations are necessary for subjects with lung diseases such as asthma and COPD. Subjects with COPD experience more serious symptoms following acute exposure to pig barns than healthy, nonsmoking adults with symptoms similar to what COPD patients experience during acute exacerbations with substantial lung function impairment (58). Furthermore, just a 2-hour pig barn exposure increased matrix metallopeptidase 9 (MM9), tissue inhibitor of metalloproteinases (TIMP1), interleukin (IL)-6, CXCL8, and leukotriene B4 in sputum and MMP9 and IL-6 in blood in both healthy and COPD subjects (58). Serum C-reactive protein (CRP) increased more in COPD subjects than healthy controls following pig barn exposure. Cholinergic mechanisms to explain this heightened lung function impairment and symptoms in COPD subjects have been proposed (58). In addition, the risk for workplace-exacerbated asthma following organic dust exposures has also been observed. Among farm operators with asthma, 33% reported asthmatic exacerbations while doing farm work (59). In experimental studies, mice with established ovalbumin-induced asthma and then subsequently challenged with organic dust extracts from swine confinement facilities demonstrated increased airway hyperresponsiveness as well as increased numbers of dendritic cells, T cells, B cells, NK cells, and group 3 innate lymphoid cells as compared to ovalbumin alone or dust extract alone treated mice (60). Identifying subjects with asthma and/or COPD is important prior to the initiation of working in organic dust environments.

Chronic lung disease and organic dust exposures

Allergic and nonallergic asthma

Exposure to organic dust has been described as a potential risk factor for asthma. Several studies have shown that adult exposure to farming dust, soft paper dust, or cotton dust increases the likelihood of developing asthma symptoms (13). A recent meta-analysis demonstrated that paper/wood, flour/grain, and textile dust exposure could increase the asthma susceptibility rate by 48% (61). Furthermore, some studies have shown that reducing exposure to organic dust decreases asthma exacerbations (62).

Different phenotypes of asthma, as based on the immune response, have been identified, such as eosinophilic asthma in which an allergic response occurs, or noneosinophilic asthma, also known as nonallergic asthma, in which inflammation is usually neutrophilic. In general, exposure to organic dust elicits inflammatory and biological responses in a variety of cell types; in asthma, it appears to activate both Th1 and Th17 lymphocytes (49). However, it is not clear whether this exposure affects all exposed individuals equally depending on the immune mechanism involved in asthma, although it appears that a mixed inflammatory response occurs. Animal models of allergic asthma show that co-exposure to organic dust increases the Th2 allergic response but also produces neutrophilic inflammation (60). In nonallergic asthma, exposure to organic dust may aggravate the neutrophilic inflammation observed mainly in this type of response, by increasing IL17 in serum (49, 63). In this asthma phenotype, exposure to organic dust is able to induce neutrophilic pulmonary inflammation accompanied by a mixed lung infiltration of both Th1 and Th17 cells (49, 64).

Chronic bronchitis/COPD

The most frequent single causal factor for COPD is cigarette smoke, and the prevalence of COPD among nonsmokers varies between 2% and 4.2% (65). Occupational exposures including organic dust exposure among farm and cotton workers have been recognized as risk factors for development of COPD and chronic bronchitis (Chapter 25). A 2019 systematic review and meta-analysis found that ten studies showed a positive association between farming exposure and airflow limitation or chronic bronchitis, and 12 showed no association with an overall odds ratio of 1.77 (95% CI: 1.50 to 2.08, p<0.001) (66). Cattle, swine, poultry, and crop farming were associated with either airflow limitation or chronic bronchitis (66). In addition, in some circumstances, cigarette smoke and occupational exposure have been shown to have an additive or even a synergistic effect on the development of COPD.

Of the agriculture exposures, Eduard and colleagues demonstrated that livestock farmers were more likely to have chronic bronchitis (odds ratio of 1.9; 95% CI:1.4–2.6) and COPD (odds ratio 1.4, CI:1.1–1.7) as compared to crop farmers (67). Ammonia, hydrogen sulfide, and inorganic dust were the most strongly associated in their multiple regression models adjusted for co-exposures, but the effects of specific biological agents could not be appropriately assessed because they were too highly correlated. Farmers in this study that also had allergy had significantly lower FEV_1, and the effects of farming and specific agents on COPD were substantially greater in farmers with atopy (68). The dairy industry has experienced modernization with having a separation between the house and the cowshed or having a loose housing system for the animals, and these changes appear to have reduced COPD prevalence (69, 70). However, working in a traditional dairy farm remains a risk factor for COPD, and working in a traditional dairy farm plus current smoking was shown to have an additive effect in COPD prevalence (69).

In poultry work, prevalence rates of obstructive pulmonary disorders were found to be higher in individuals with longer exposure regardless of smoking status (71). The duration and intensity of farm work, farm tasks, livestock exposure, crop exposure and "other exposures" have been demonstrated to be independent entities and their clustering within a model was modified by the intensity units of exposure in determining COPD and chronic bronchitis risk (72). In cotton work, particularly those exposed to both jute and hemp dust, the frequency of chronic bronchitis in retired workers who previously smoked was higher (20%) as compared to currently smoking workers (17%) (29). Working in dense dust areas, active smoking, being older than 40 years of age, being an ex-smoker, and working in the factory for a period exceeding 15 years were significantly associated with bronchitis and emphysema development (29).

Asthma-COPD overlap

Subjects with COPD who show features of asthma and asthma patients with smoking history who develop non-fully reversible airflow obstruction are categorized as asthma-COPD overlap (ACO) (Chapter 25). These subjects have been usually described among subjects with COPD in whom a diagnosis of asthma is made based on highly reversible airflow obstruction, type 2 inflammation, airway and/or peripheral blood eosinophilia, or a previous physician diagnosis of asthma (73). However, the prevalence and clinical features of ACO among subjects with work-related asthma (WRA) such as with organic dust exposures remain largely unknown.

A telephone survey conducted in the United States (as part of the Behavioral Risk Factor Surveillance Survey) found that 51.9% of adults with WRA and 25.6% of adults with non-WRA had ever been diagnosed with COPD (74). Subjects with concurrent WRA and COPD had more severe asthma exacerbations and worse outcomes than those with non-WRA and no COPD (74). In a large retrospective study in Montreal (Canada), it was found 86.2% of those with ACO were diagnosed with OA and 13.8% with occupational ACO (75), which is similar to the lower prevalence estimates of ACO among asthma patients (73). Subjects with occupational ACO were older, received higher doses of ICS, and were less atopic than subjects with OA (75). Occupational ACO subjects had been exposed to the offending agent for a longer duration time and were more frequently exposed to low-molecular-weight agents (70% vs 52%) than OA subjects. A study from Finland showed that the risk of ACO was significantly related to presence of mold odor in the workplace, but not to other dampness indicators (76). Another Finnish study suggested that asthma patients with occupational exposure to vapors, gases, dust, or fumes develop ACO more often than subjects without such exposure (77).

Hypersensitivity pneumonitis

HP is an immune-mediated interstitial lung disease that develops following repeated exposures to inhaled environmental antigens including organic dusts, vapors, fungi, bacteria, molds, and chemicals. Well-known examples include farmer's lung disease, which involves repetitive exposure to various molds found in moldy hay and pigeon breeder's disease triggered by inhalation of antigens in bird droppings and feathers (Chapter 24). Signs and symptoms range from acute flu-like illness to irreversible pulmonary fibrosis (Chapter 24).

Diagnosis is made based on combination of antigen exposure and compatible clinical, laboratory, radiographic, and pathologic findings (Chapter 24) (78). Radiographic findings include groundglass opacities, centrilobular nodules, air trapping, fibrosis, and emphysema (79). Severity of bronchiectasis and honeycombing are associated with poorer prognosis (78). Bronchoalveolar lavage fluid is characterized by elevated lymphocytes (Chapter 24). In acute disease, typical pathological specimen involves lymphocytic alveolitis, non-necrotizing epithelial granulomas, intraalveolar fibrosis, and bronchiolitis, whereas chronic disease may lack these findings and instead demonstrate UIP-like or even NSIP-like patterns (80).

HP induces a proinflammatory response characterized by TNFα, IL-1β, IL-6, IL-8, IFN-γ, IL-17, and neutrophilic airway influx (80). With increased time from antigen exposure, alveolitis becomes increasingly characterized by lymphocytes and CD4+ and CD8+ T cells (81). IL-17 is associated with increased disease severity and collagen deposition in farmer's lung disease (81). Genetic polymorphisms in HLA and TNFα alleles have been associated with disease (Chapter 24). Currently, the mainstay of treatment is avoidance of inciting triggers. Corticosteroids and immunosuppressive drugs may shorten acute symptoms but have not been shown to affect long-term outcome (79).

Prevention and treatment

Early methods aimed at preventing development of byssinosis relied more heavily on employee-driven interventions such as cessation of smoking, since smoking is known to have an additive effect on development of disease, and use of a face mask. However, lung function decline has been noted in cotton textile mill workers despite use of a face mask (31), indicating more aggressive measures must be taken to avoid progression of disease. Inadequate ventilation in the workplace environment increases odds of developing respiratory symptoms (33), and therefore efforts to improve ventilation have occurred. Factories with improved, cleaner technology have been associated with improved respiratory indices as compared to older factories (28). Efforts have also been aimed at

bactericidal treatment, particularly of raw cotton to reduce endotoxin levels. There is no evidence that use of inhaled bronchodilators alleviates symptoms or slows progression of disease, and therefore efforts moved early on toward prevention rather than treatment of disease.

Research needs

Further research should focus on the following items:

* Elucidate the agents and signaling pathways causing airway and lung inflammation as well as disease manifestations.
* Further describe the complex acute and chronic pathologic, physiologic, and clinical consequences of exposure to various organic agents, and examine in what ways they differ.
* Develop new procedures and techniques to lower exposure; propose means by which the inflammatory process and its consequence can be reduced.

Summary

Organic dust exposures have been shown to induce not only acute airway disease such as asthma or asthma-like syndromes, but chronic exposure also gives rise to chronic airflow obstruction. They are recognized as complex with contribution from a diversity of gram-positive and gram-negative microbial components, particularly endotoxins and peptidoglycans. These components activate innate immune responses through highly conserved pattern recognition receptors to elicit airway inflammatory responses. However, these components alone do not appear to completely explain the airway inflammatory consequences observed, and thus, further research is necessary. Reduction of exposure so far is the only way to prevent this spectrum of disease.

References

1. Jeebhay MF, Moscato G, Bang BE, et al. Food processing and occupational respiratory allergy. A EAACI position paper. Allergy. 2019, Apr 6; doi:10.1111/all.13807.
2. Dosman JA, Graham BL, Hall D, et al. Respiratory symptoms and pulmonary function in farmers. J Occup Med. 1987;29:38–43.
3. Monso E, Schenker M, Radon K, et al. Region-related risk factors for respiratory symptoms in European and Californian farmers. Eur Respir J. 2003;21:323–31.
4. Radon K, Monso E, Weber C, et al. Prevalence and risk factors for airway diseases in farmers–summary of results of the European Farmers' Project. Ann Agric Environ Med. 2002;9:207–13.
5. Lamprecht B, Schirnhofer L, Kaiser B, et al. Farming and the prevalence of non-reversible airways obstruction: results from a population-based study. Am J Ind Med. 2007;50:421–6.
6. McDonald JC, Keynes HL, Meredith SK. Reported incidence of occupational asthma in the United Kingdom, 1989–97. Occup Environ Med. 2000;57:823–9.
7. Leira HL, Bratt U, Slastad S. Notified cases of occupational asthma in Norway: exposure and consequences for health and income. Am J Ind Med. 2005;48:359–64.
8. Hur GY, Koh DH, Kim HA, et al. Prevalence of work-related symptoms and serum-specific antibodies to wheat flour in exposed workers in the bakery industry. Respir Med. 2008;102:548–55.
9. Akpinar-Elci M, Pasquale DK, Abrokwah M, et al. United airway disease among crop farmers. J Agromedicine. 2016;21:217–23.
10. Cherry N, Beach J, Senthilselvan A, et al. Pesticide use and asthma in Alberta grain farmers. Int J Environ Res Public Health. 2018;15(3):526.
11. Hoppin JA, Umbach DM, London SJ, et al. Pesticide use and adult-onset asthma among male farmers in the Agricultural Health Study. Eur Respir J. 2009;34:1296–303.

12. Sigsgaard T, Basinas I, Doekes G et al. Respiratory diseases and allergy in farmers working with livestock: a EAACI position paper. Clin Transl Allergy. 2020; doi:org/10.1186/s13601-020-00334-x

13. Wunschel J, Poole JA. Occupational agriculture organic dust exposure and its relationship to asthma and airway inflammation in adults. J Asthma. 2016;53:471–7.

14. Poole JA, Dooley GP, Saito R, et al. Muramic acid, endotoxin, 3-hydroxy fatty acids, and ergosterol content explain monocyte and epithelial cell inflammatory responses to agricultural dusts. J Toxicol Environ Health A. 2010;73:684–700.

15. Stein MM, Hrusch CL, Gozdz J, et al. Innate immunity and asthma risk in Amish and Hutterite farm children. N Engl J Med. 2016;375:411–21.

16. Romberger DJ, Heires AJ, Nordgren TM, et al. Proteases in agricultural dust induce lung inflammation through PAR-1 and PAR-2 activation. Am J Physiol Lung Cell Mol Physiol. 2015;309:L388–99.

17. Basinas I, Sigsgaard T, Heederik D, et al. Exposure to inhalable dust and endotoxin among Danish livestock farmers: results from the SUS cohort study. J Environ Monit. 2012;(2):604–14.

18. Basinas I, Sigsgaard T, Kromhout H, et al. A comprehensive review of levels and determinants of personal exposure to dust and endotoxin in livestock farming. J Expo Sci Environ Epidemiol. 2015;25:123–37.

19. Poole JA, Wyatt TA, Romberger DJ, et al. MyD88 in lung resident cells governs airway inflammatory and pulmonary function responses to organic dust treatment. Respir Res. 2015;16(1):111.

20. Poole JA, Anderson L, Gleason AM, et al. Pattern recognition scavenger receptor A/CD204 regulates airway inflammatory homeostasis following organic dust extract exposures. J Immunotoxicol. 2015;12(1):64–73.

21. Gao Z, Dosman JA, Rennie DC, et al. Association of toll-like receptor 2 gene polymorphisms with lung function in workers in swine operations. Ann Allergy Asthma Immunol. 2013;110(1):44–50.e1.

22. Poole JA, Gleason AM, Bauer C, et al. CD11c(+)/CD11b(+) cells are critical for organic dust-elicited murine lung inflammation. Am J Respir Cell Mol Biol. 2012;47(5):652–9.

23. Davidson ME, Schaeffer J, Clark ML, et al. Personal exposure of dairy workers to dust, endotoxin, muramic acid, ergosterol, and ammonia on large-scale dairies in the high plains Western United States. J Occup Environ Hyg. 2018;15(3):182–93.

24. Basinas I, Sigsgaard T, Erlandsen M, et al. Exposure-affecting factors of dairy farmers' exposure to inhalable dust and endotoxin. Ann Occup Hyg. 2014;58(6):707–23.

25. Basinas I, Cronin G, Hogan V, et al. Exposure to inhalable dust, endotoxin, and total volatile organic carbons on dairy farms using manual and automated feeding systems. Ann Work Expo Health. 2017;61(3):344–55.

26. Senthilselvan A, Beach J, Feddes J, et al. A prospective evaluation of air quality and workers' health in broiler and layer operations. Occup Environ Med. 2011;68(2):102–7.

27. Arteaga V, Mitchell D, Armitage T, et al. Cage versus noncage laying-hen housings: respiratory exposures. J Agromedicine. 2015;20(3):245–55.

28. Saha A, Das A, Chattopadhyay BP, et al. A comparative study of byssinosis in jute industries. Indian J Occup Environ Med. 2018;22(3):170–6.

29. Er M, Emri SA, Demir AU, et al. Byssinosis and COPD rates among factory workers manufacturing hemp and jute. Int J Occup Med Environ Health. 2016;29(1):55–68.

30. Anyfantis ID, Rachiotis G, Hadjichristodoulou C, et al. Respiratory symptoms and lung function among Greek cotton industry workers: a cross-sectional study. Int J Occup Environ Med. 2017;8(1):32–8.

31. Dangi BM, Bhise AR. Cotton dust exposure: analysis of pulmonary function and respiratory symptoms. Lung India. 2017;34(2):144–9.

32. Ali NA, Nafees AA, Fatmi Z, et al. Dose-response of cotton dust exposure with lung function among textile workers: MultiTex study in Karachi, Pakistan. Int J Occup Environ Med. 2018;9(3):120–8.

33. Daba Wami S, Chercos DH, Dessie A, et al. Cotton dust exposure and self-reported respiratory symptoms among textile factory workers in Northwest Ethiopia: a comparative cross-sectional study. J Occup Med Toxicol. 2018;13:13.

34. Wang X, Zhang HX, Sun BX, et al. Cross-shift airway responses and long-term decline in FEV1 in cotton textile workers. Am J Respir Crit Care Med. 2008;177(3):316–20.

35. Schilling RS, Hughes JP, Dingwall-Fordyce I, et al. An epidemiological study of byssinosis among Lancashire cotton workers. Br J Ind Med. 1955;12(3):217–27.

36. Hang J, Zhou W, Wang X, et al. Microsomal epoxide hydrolase, endotoxin, and lung function decline in cotton textile workers. Am J Respir Crit Care Med. 2005;171(2):165–70.

37. Zhang R, Zhao Y, Chu M, et al. A large scale gene-centric association study of lung function in newly-hired female cotton textile workers with endotoxin exposure. PLOS ONE. 2013;8(3):e59035.

38. Zhang H, Hang J, Wang X, et al. TNF polymorphisms modify endotoxin exposure-associated longitudinal lung function decline. Occup Environ Med. 2007;64(6):409–13.

39. Wang XR, Zhang HX Sun BX, et al. A 20-year follow-up study on chronic respiratory effects of exposure to cotton dust. Eur Respir J. 2005;26(5):881–6.

40. Shi J, Mehta AJ, Hang JQ, et al. Chronic lung function decline in cotton textile workers: roles of historical and recent exposures to endotoxin. Environ Health Perspect. 2010;118(11):1620–4.

41. Lai PS, Fresco JM, Pinilla MA, et al. Chronic endotoxin exposure produces airflow obstruction and lung dendritic cell expansion. Am J Respir Cell Mol Biol. 2012;47(2):209–17.

42. Poole JA, Romberger DJ. Immunological and inflammatory responses to organic dust in agriculture. Curr Opin Allergy Clin Immunol. 201212(2):126–32.

43. Carrington JM, Poole JA. The effect of inhalant organic dust on bone health. Curr Allergy Asthma Rep. 2018;18(3):16.

44. Romberger DJ, Bodlak V, Von Essen SG, et al. Hog barn dust extract stimulates IL-8 and IL-6 release in human bronchial epithelial cells via PKC activation. J Appl Physiol (1985). 2002;93(1):289–96.

45. Poole JA, Wyatt TA, Kielian T, et al. Toll-like receptor 2 regulates organic dust-induced airway inflammation. Am J Respir Cell Mol Biol. 2011;45(4):711–9.

46. Dalpke A, Frank J, Peter M, et al. Activation of toll-like receptor 9 by DNA from different bacterial species. Infect Immun. 2006;74(2):940–6.

47. Smith LM, Weissenburger-Moser LA, Heires AJ, et al. Epistatic effect of TLR-1, -6 and -10 polymorphisms on organic dust-mediated cytokine response. Genes Immun. 2017;18(2):67–74.

48. Natarajan K, Meganathan V, Mitchell C, et al. Organic dust induces inflammatory gene expression in lung epithelial cells via ROS-dependent STAT-3 activation. Am J Physiol Lung Cell Mol Physiol. 2019;317(1):L127–140.

49. Poole JA, Gleason AM, Bauer C, et al. $\alpha\beta$ T cells and a mixed Th1/Th17 response are important in organic dust-induced airway disease. Ann Allergy Asthma Immunol. 2012;109(4):266–73.e2.

50. Sheats MK, Davis KU, Poole JA. Comparative review of asthma in farmers and horses. Curr Allergy Asthma Rep. 2019;19(11):50.

51. Warren KJ, Wyatt TA, Romberger DJ, et al. Post-injury and resolution response to repetitive inhalation exposure to agricultural organic dust in mice. Safety (Basel). 2017;3(1). doi:10.3390/safety3010010

52. Von Essen S, Romberger D. The respiratory inflammatory response to the swine confinement building environment: the adaptation to respiratory exposures in the chronically exposed worker. J Agric Saf Health. 2003;9(3):185–96.

53. May S, Romberger DJ, Poole JA. Respiratory health effects of large animal farming environments. J Toxicol Environ Health B Crit Rev. 2012;15(8):524–41.

54. Wang Z, Malmberg P, Larsson P, et al. Time course of interleukin-6 and tumor necrosis factor-alpha increase in serum following inhalation of swine dust. Am J Respir Crit Care Med. 1996;153(1):147–52.

55. Jagielo PJ, Thorne PS, Watt JL, et al. Grain dust and endotoxin inhalation challenges produce similar inflammatory responses in normal subjects. Chest. 1996;110(1):263–70.

56. Skoulas A, Williams N, Merriman JE. Exposure to grain dust. II. A clinical study of the effects. JOM. 1964;6:359–72.

57. Kleinfeld M, Messite J, Swencicki RE, et al. A clinical and physiologic study of grain handlers. Arch Environ Health. 1968;16(3):380–4.

58. Palmberg L, Sundblad BM, Ji J, et al. Cholinergic mechanisms in an organic dust model simulating an acute exacerbation in patients with COPD. Int J Chron Obstruct Pulmon Dis. 2018;13:3611–24.

59. Mazurek JM, White GE, Rodman C, et al. Farm work-related asthma among US primary farm operators. J Agromedicine. 2015;20(1):31–42.

60. Warren KJ, Dickinson JD, Nelson AJ, et al. Ovalbumin-sensitized mice have altered airway inflammation to agriculture organic dust. Respir Res. 2019;20(1):51.

61. Zhang Y, Ye B, Zheng H, et al. Association between organic dust exposure and adult-asthma: a systematic review and meta-analysis of case-control studies. Allergy Asthma Immunol Res. 2019;11(6):818–29.

62. Kim JL, Henneberger PK, Lohman S, et al. Impact of occupational exposures on exacerbation of asthma: a population-based asthma cohort study. BMC Pulm Med. 2016;16(1):148.

63. Kim YS, Choi EJ, Lee WH, et al. Extracellular vesicles, especially derived from gram-negative bacteria, in indoor dust induce neutrophilic pulmonary inflammation associated with both Th1 and Th17 cell responses. Clin Exp Allergy. 2013;43(4):443–54.

64. Wang D. Th1/Th17 cells in organic dust-induced airway disease. Ann Allergy Asthma Immunol. 2012;109(4):231–2.

65. Bang KM. Chronic obstructive pulmonary disease in nonsmokers by occupation and exposure: a brief review. Curr Opin Pulm Med. 2015;21(2):149–54.

66. Guillien A, Soumagne T, Dalphin JC, et al. COPD, airflow limitation and chronic bronchitis in farmers: a systematic review and meta-analysis. Occup Environ Med. 2019;76(1):58–68.

67. Eduard W, Pearce N, Douwes J. Chronic bronchitis, COPD, and lung function in farmers: the role of biological agents. Chest. 2009;136(3):716–25.

68. Eduard W, Pearce N, Douwes J. Chronic bronchitis, COPD, and lung function in farmers: the role of biological agents. Chest. 2009;136(3):716–25.

69. Marescaux A, Degano B, Soumagne T, et al. Impact of farm modernity on the prevalence of chronic obstructive pulmonary disease in dairy farmers. Occup Environ Med. 2016;73(2):127–33.

70. Jouneau S, Marette S, Robert AM, et al. Prevalence and risk factors of chronic obstructive pulmonary disease in dairy farmers: AIRBAg study. Environ Res. 2019;169:1–6.

71. Viegas S, Faisca VM, Dias H, et al. Occupational exposure to poultry dust and effects on the respiratory system in workers. J Toxicol Environmental Health A. 2013;76(4–5):230–9.

72. Weissenburger-Moser L, Meza J, Yu F, et al. A principal factor analysis to characterize agricultural exposures among Nebraska veterans. J Expo Sci Environ Epidemiol. 2017;27(2):214–20.

73. Christenson SA, Steiling K, van den Berge M, et al. Asthma-COPD overlap. Clinical relevance of genomic signatures of type 2 inflammation in chronic obstructive pulmonary disease. Am J Respir Crit Care Med. 2015;191(7):758–66.

74. Dodd KE, Mazurek JM. Prevalence of COPD among workers with work-related asthma. J Asthma. 2019:1–9.

75. Ojanguren I, Moulec G, Hobeika J, et al. Clinical and inflammatory characteristics of asthma-COPD overlap in workers with occupational asthma. PLOS ONE. 2018. 13(3):e0193144.

76. Jaakkola MS, Lajunen TK, Jaakkola JJK. Indoor mold odor in the workplace increases the risk of asthma-COPD overlap syndrome: a population-based incident case-control study. Clin Transl Allergy. 2020;10:3.

77. Tommola M, Ilmarinen P, Tuomisto LE, et al. Occupational exposures and asthma-COPD overlap in a clinical cohort of adult-onset asthma. ERJ Open Res. 2019;5(4); 00191–2019.

78. Wuyts W, Sterclova M, Vasakova M. Pitfalls in diagnosis and management of hypersensitivity pneumonitis. Curr Opin Pulm Med. 2015;21(5):490–8.

79. Soumagne T, Dalphin JC. Current and emerging techniques for the diagnosis of hypersensitivity pneumonitis. Expert Rev Respir Med. 2018;12(6):493–507.

80. Vasakova M, Morell F, Walsh S, et al. Hypersensitivity pneumonitis: perspectives in diagnosis and management. Am J Respir Crit Care Med. 2017;196(6):680–9.

81. Wang J, Yoon TW, Read R, et al. Genetic variability of T cell responses in hypersensitivity pneumonitis identified using the BXD genetic reference panel. Am J Physiol Lung Cell Mol Physiol. 2020;318(4):L631–143.

24

OCCUPATIONAL HYPERSENSITIVITY PNEUMONITIS AND ORGANIC DUST TOXIC SYNDROME

Anne-Pauline Bellanger,[1] Jean-Charles Dalphin,[*] Laurence Millon,[2] Gabriel Reboux,[3] Torben Sigsgaard,[4] Jean-Luc Malo,[5] and David I. Bernstein[6]

[1]*Parasitology-Mycology Department, University Hospital of Besancon, Besançon, France*
[2]*Parasitology-Mycology Department, University Hospital of Besançon, Besançon, France*
[3]*University Bourgogne Franche Comté, Parasitologie-Mycologie Department, University Hospital of Besançon, Besançon, France*
[4]*Department of Public Health, Section for Environment, Work & Health, Aarhus University, Aarhus C, Denmark*
[5]*Hôpital du Sacré-Cœur de Montréal and Université de Montréal, Montréal, Québec, Canada*
[6]*Division of Immunology, Allergy and Rheumatology, University of Cincinnati College of Medicine, Cincinnati, Ohio, USA*

[*]*Sadly, during the process of preparation of this new edition, the editors were informed of the unexpected passing of Professor Jean-Charles Dalphin from Besançon, France, who had enthusiastically and generously accepted to co-author this chapter. The editors want to pay tribute to him for his outstanding career, becoming a world authority in Hypersensitivity Pneumonitis.*

Contents

CASE HISTORY

A 62-year-old woman reports that she has previously worked in a metal industry. She is currently an employee on a pigeon breeding farm where her work has consisted of taking care of many birds of different species (parrots, canaries, budgerigars, parakeets) in the recent 5 years. She has been affected with dry coughing in the past 3–4 years. She also reports recurrent episodes of fever, dyspnea, arthralgia, and myalgia, mainly during the week at work. Her lung scan shows micronodules and ground glass shadows. She has slight hypoxemia at rest, which deteriorates on exercise. Lung function tests are as follows: slow vital capacity: 2.8 L (94% pred), forced vital capacity: 2.5 L (83% pred), FEV_1: 2.1 L (85% pred). She undergoes a bronchoalveolar lavage that shows a lymphocytic alveolitis (44%) with 136,000 cells/mL. Precipitin testing is positive with a clear response to various birds: 3 arcs with parakeet,

2 with pigeon, and 2 with poultry antigens. She also has increased serum specific IgG to these birds, using recombinant allergens.

A diagnosis of occupational bird fancier's lung is confirmed. The worker finds a new job with no exposure to birds but she decides to keep a parrot at home. Without specific drug treatment, her symptoms improve progressively and disappear in the 6 months that follow diagnosis even if she takes care of her parrot without protection (no gloves and no mask). A serology test then shows increased specific IgGs to pigeon, parakeet, canary, and budgerigar antigens but normal levels for parrot antigens.

She has become asymptomatic, keeping only her parrot at home.

Overview

A variety of occupational diseases affects the distal bronchioles and the lung parenchyma. This includes hypersensitivity pneumonitis (HP) with features that differ according to the offending agent (microorganisms, bird' proteins, metals, and chemicals) and organic dust toxic syndrome (ODTS). Exposure to organic dusts (Chapter 23) and metal fumes (Chapter 16) can induce clinical, functional, and radiological manifestations with similarities

and differences with HP, especially in the extent of involvement of lung parenchyma (Table 24.1).

The position paper of the European Academy of Allergy and Clinical Immunology proposed the following definition for occupational hypersensitivity pneumonitis (OHP) or occupational allergic alveolitis: "OHP is an immunologic lung disease with variable clinical presentation and outcome resulting from lymphocytic and frequently granulomatous inflammation of the peripheral airways, alveoli, and surrounding interstitial tissue which develops as the result of a non-IgE-mediated allergic reaction to a variety of organic or low molecular weight agents that are present in the work environment" (1). Causal agents include numerous fungi and microorganisms, animal and plant products, as well as chemicals. Farmer's lung due to moldy hay is the most widely known OHP. Symptoms, mainly shortness of breath and cough accompanied by chills and fever, occur according to various time frames, from acute to chronic. The syndrome is characterized by lymphocytic alveolitis that manifests by an interstitial lung disease associated with a restrictive and gas exchange functional defect as well as the production of specific IgG antibodies.

Epidemiology

The pitfalls of assessing the frequency of OHP have been discussed (2): vast variety of causal agents, tools to confirm the diagnosis that are often based on questionnaires only, reliability of assessment of

TABLE 24.1 Comparisons of Manifestations of Hypersensitivity Pneumonitis (HP) and HP-Like Conditions

	Hypersensitivity Pneumonitis	Airway Diseases Due to Organic Dust Exposure[b]	Metal Fume Fever[a] (MFF)	ODTS
Causal agents	Fungi, bacteria, bird proteins, chemicals	Grain and farming dust Cotton dust Swine confinement	Welding on zinc oxide and galvanized metal, but not exclusively	Various
Mechanism	IgG-mediated response to various proteins CD4+ T-cell mediated hypersensitivity	Unconfirmed: endotoxins, epithelial Toll-like receptors (TLR), water-soluble agents with biologic activity, peptidoglycan (PGN), nucleotide oligomerization domain (NOD) proteins	Unknown	Unconfirmed: endotoxins
Clinical manifestations	Respiratory and systemic	Respiratory and systemic	Systemic	Systemic Metallic taste
Radiologic abnormalities	Frequent (acute and chronic forms)	Absent (except in long-term development of COPD)	Absent	Absent
Functional abnormalities	Frequent Mainly restrictive pattern and gas exchange	Obstructive pattern, mainly with long-term exposure	Absent (obstructive pattern in welders but not specific for MFF)	Absent
Diagnostic procedures	Various Assessment of specific IgG (recombinant antigens)	Clinical history Lung function tests WBC	Clinical history Lung function tests WBC	Clinical history Blood and sputum leukocytosis
Outcome	Possible respiratory long-term disability	Possible development of COPD	Possible OA (MFF may be a predictor) and COPD	Self-limited
Treatment	Avoidance of exposure Pharmacologic treatment if needed	Reduction in exposure to prevent long-term COPD	None (reduction in exposure improves symptoms)	None (reduction in exposure improves symptoms)

[a] See Chapter 16.

[b] See Chapter 23.

Abbreviations: COPD, chronic obstructive pulmonary disease; OA, occupational asthma; ODTS, organic dust toxic syndrome; WBC, white blood count.

specific antibodies, lack of sensitivity of chest radiographs, cross-sectional studies only. In the general population, using a US administrative database in 150 million persons and a complex algorithm, it was found that the cumulative incidence rate of HP was 1.3 to 1.9 per 100,000 persons, 58% being women and more subjects being >65 years of age (3). This figure is slightly higher than the 0.9% per 100,000 incidence found in an earlier study of the British general population (4).

There are two types of causal agents for which frequency figures are more relevant for reasons of the number of exposed populations. First, the prevalence of farmer's lung, an occupational disease, is variable but is more frequent in humid areas. It has been examined in a large French population of more than 5000 dairy farmers with a participation of 83%. Prevalence of "clinical farmer's lung" defined as at least two symptomatic (cough and dyspnea) episodes during the past two winters was found to be 1.4% (1.1%–1.7%), being more frequent in nonsmokers (5). This figure may overestimate frequency as the suspected diagnosis was not confirmed. A 23-year surveillance program in the United States has shown that proportionate mortality ratio due to OHP was significantly elevated (8.1, 95% CI:6.4–10.2) for farmers, excluding horticulture (6).

Second, bird fancier's disease exists everywhere in the world but is rarely an occupational disease. Birds are more present in the general home environment. This condition may be commoner than farmer's lung although epidemiological studies have not been carried out in large populations.

Trimellitic anhydride exposure can induce a late respiratory systemic syndrome with features of OHP, although pulmonary infiltrates were not identified (7); it may therefore represent a toxic irritant reaction with an IgG response reflecting high exposure. Zeiss and coworkers found a 2.5% prevalence of this syndrome in 474 employees of a plant manufacturing trimellitic anhydride (7). Vandenplas et al. documented HP-like reactions by specific inhalation challenges (SICs) in nine workers exposed to MDI (8), representing 4.7% of 167 potentially exposed workers. All these subjects had increased specific IgG and all but one specific IgE to MDI-HSA conjugate. In a cross-sectional study performed in central Great Britain that collected data from 2002 to 2017, 206 cases of HP were identified and half of these were due to metalworking fluid (9), waste and recycling work representing an emerging cause (10). The frequency of OHP for most other causal agents has not been studied in sufficiently large population samples to make figures interpretable. In a case series of 317 workers with OA due to various agents as confirmed by SICs, 15 (5%) developed fever at the end of the day, of whom 11 showed a significant fall in forced vital capacity, nine also having a significant increase in peripheral neutrophil counts (11).

Epidemiological studies have documented a dose-response between exposure and the level of specific IgG antibodies and prevalence of OHP as reviewed (1). Promoter polymorphism gene MUC5B has been associated with chronic HP and the extent of fibrosis (12). The frequency of OHP is lower in smokers (1).

Clinical presentation

Besides systemic symptoms (chills, fever, fatigue, etc.), dyspnea at rest and on exercise and coughing are the most frequent symptoms in subjects with HP (13, 14) (see Case History). Inspiratory crackles are often heard on auscultation. Chest radiographs and more so CT scans mostly show ground glass abnormalities. A restrictive defect with gas exchange abnormalities, initially on exercise and progressively at rest, is the typical functional abnormality although an obstructive defect related to the occurrence of chronic bronchitis and emphysema can also be present (15). The type of exposure in terms of intensity and duration may influence the course of the disease (16) and a predominant radiological type of emphysema rather than that of fibrosis (15).

Diagnostic criteria

Clinical, radiological, functional, and laboratory tests are proposed in the investigation of subjects with potential HP (16, 17). In a multicenter study of 400 subjects referred for possible HP (116 confirmed HP and 284 controls), Lacasse and coworkers derived a predictive model with a high likelihood operative curve. This model contained: history of exposure to a known antigen, positive precipitating antibodies, recurrent episodes of symptoms, inspiratory crackles, symptoms occurring 4–8 hours after exposure, and weight loss (13).

Classification

HP has typically been classified as acute, subacute, and chronic (16) but a cluster analysis has shown that only two categories, acute and chronic, should be kept (18). The acute form is characterized by chills, myalgia, etc. occurring 4–8 hours after cessation of exposure and persisting for hours or days, a process that is considered as reversible after cessation of exposure. The chest radiograph mainly shows ground glass, centrilobular nodular and mosaic attenuation but may be normal in 30% of cases (18). Histopathology mainly shows lympho-plasmocytic inflammation with giant cells. In the chronic form of the disease, symptomatology has been present for more than 6 months and shows features of advanced interstitial lung disease with clubbing in 30% of cases and a restrictive functional defect and hypoxemia. Fibrosis is predominant on chest radiograph and on histopathology specimens.

The clinical, functional, pathological, and radiological features as well as the outcome of OHP due to fungi, bacteria, mycobacteria, bird proteins, and metalworking fluid are generally more pronounced than those described after exposure to chemicals (diisocyanates, trimellitic anhydride, etc.) for which the clinical outcome is often self-limited with no permanent sequelae. Moreover, in the latter instance, chest auscultation and chest radiographs are generally normal.

Differential diagnosis

The differential diagnosis of HP includes all conditions that have been seen in the control group of a multicenter study quoted above that included 284 controls with other interstitial lung diseases (13): sarcoidosis, interstitial pneumonia associated with collagen vascular disease, silicosis, bronchiolitis obliterans with organizing pneumonia, HIV-associated pneumonitis, cystic fibrosis associated with HP, drug-induced pneumonitis, and most acute lung infections. A local survey of 107 patient files containing a request for HP serology indicates that the diagnosis of respiratory disease was different from HP in 76.6% of patients. HP represents 4%–13% of interstitial lung diseases in Europe and is the third cause of such diseases after sarcoidosis and idiopathic pulmonary fibrosis (19). In addition, in the absence of radiological and functional abnormalities, other conditions with OHP-like manifestations should be considered (Table 24.1).

Pathology

The histopathological triad of HP in its acute form includes bronchiocentric lymphohistiocytic interstitial pneumonia with bronchiolitis and typical small poorly shaped nonnecrotizing granulomas (16, 20, 21). In chronic stages, there are fibrotic reactions predominating in the lower lung fields. Features of chronic stages include a pattern of overlapping usual interstitial pneumonia with subpleural patchy fibrosis and centrilobular fibrosis. At this stage there are fewer granulomas although giant interstitial cells are present. Emphysema can be present, the hypothesis being that it is related to exposure to microbial antigens. A fibrotic pattern may be a more prevalent outcome in case of exposure to avian proteins (15, 16). HP must be considered in all cases of diffuse lung disease and a detailed environmental exposure history is mandatory. Identification of a possible antigen can be difficult. Pathological material is therefore often required and obtained from open lung biopsies or transbronchial biopsies (reserved to a few centers with specific expertise) at which time a bronchoalveolar lavage (BAL) revealing lymphocytosis is also often carried out.

Diagnostic procedures

History and physical examination

OHP should be considered if a worker presents with recurrent episodes of fever and dyspnea, with a time schedule related to exposure at work, and in the investigation of interstitial lung disease of unknown etiology. A suspected source of possible antigen should be questioned by considering a job-exposure matrix scheme (see Chapters 6 and 10) and requesting safety data sheets (SDSs). A site visit to the workplace may be useful in identifying a source of exposure to microbial or chemical antigens. Inspiratory crackles are the most sensitive sign on physical examination as mentioned above.

Chest radiograph

Simple chest radiograph has lost some of its role with the more general use of CT scan. Although chest radiographs can show ground glass, nodular, ill-defined shadows, and nonspecific infiltrates, they can be normal in up to 20% of subjects (13), especially when the causal agents are metals and chemicals. Therefore, when chest radiograph shows diffuse ill-defined shadows or even if it is normal, it is relevant to ask for a CT scan. In the international multicenter study quoted above, 22 of the 199 patients with active HP (11%; 95% CI:7%–16%) had their initial chest radiograph interpreted as normal. Emphysema can also be present in farmer's lung, alone or associated with fibrosis (15).

Chest scan

Several articles with multiple photographs illustrate the spectrum of high-resolution CT scan in OHP with comparison with pathological examination (16, 22). The CT scan is a very sensitive means as only 4% of OHP subjects had normal CT scan in the aforementioned international multicenter study quoted above (13).

In acute OHP, the typical pictures show ground-glass shadows and small centrilobular nodules with mosaic attenuation (see Case History). In chronic OHP, CT scans mainly feature reticulation and distortion of the parenchyma. There are also cysts and emphysema in up to 20% of cases.

Pulmonary function tests

The typical lung function tests, in either the acute or the chronic form, show a restrictive pattern with, in most instances, an impairment in gas exchange (reduced DLCO) (see Case History). An extra obstructive defect has been described in the case of farmer's lung due to emphysema (15). With the progression of the disease, hypoxemia on exercise first and then at rest is a common occurrence. Results of lung function tests are used as guidance to adjust therapy, specifically the dose of oral steroid.

Specific antibodies

For the assessment of specific IgG antibodies, it is very important to compare results with satisfactory healthy control subjects. Some limitations are due to the type of precipitation technique used. For example, the double diffusion technique is no longer appropriate because the number of arcs is always low (23).

The presence of specific IgG antibodies should be considered as a supportive evidence of OHP (1) (see Case History) Asymptomatic exposed workers may show increased specific IgG antibodies and confirmed cases of OHP may have negative results. Moreover, the interpretation should take into account individual characteristics that influence the humoral response such as smoking, immunosuppression, and high doses of steroids (23). Also, the level of specific IgG antibodies can vary with exposure, farmers, for instance, being more exposed in winter. However, the seasonal variability is low and does not influence the diagnostic decision.

False negative results can occur because of the insufficient quantity and quality of the antigens used in testing. A "battery" of antigens should be assessed. In contrast, it was observed that for metalworking fluid-induced OHP some exposed healthy workers produce a significant number of precipitation arcs toward *Mycobacterium immunogenum* while remaining asymptomatic over years (24). Results of the multicenter international HP study demonstrate that positive serum antibodies are a significant predictor of HP (13).

For some types of OHP, antigens available for testing in most centers include some of those relevant for farmer's lung and humidifier lung. Many extracts are prepared locally. Information on the antigenicity of these extracts is often missing.

Rouzet and coworkers (25) as well as Bellanger and coworkers (26) make a proposal for an "à la carte" microbial analysis and production of customized antigens from the material provided by the patient. This "à la carte" strategy includes: (1) thorough questioning of workers about their private and occupational activity and possible visit at the workplace; (2) select a panel of six specific antigens for each type of exposure; (3) use enzyme-linked immunosorbent assay (ELISA) to test two highly specific recombinant antigens (these are available for farmer's lung, metalworking fluid, and bird fancier's lung; (4) if the test is negative and the diagnosis of OHP likely, examination of the worker's environment by culture or quantitative real-time polymerase chain reaction measurement and a microbial analysis of the suspect material at the workplace is obtained; and 5) "à la carte" antigens are produced for further testing. If the nature of the antigen cannot be found and detection of antibodies remains negative, at work exposure with biological and functional assessments to confirm the work-relatedness of the condition is suggested (see section "Specific Inhalation Challenge"). This "à la carte" strategic procedure is more and more developed (United States, France, Finland) and even if it is quite time-consuming, this is sometimes the only way to identify the offending antigens (26). Table 24.2 shows the type of panel that may be tested according to the type of exposure in a strategy proposed by Bellanger and coworkers (26).

TABLE 24.2 Strategy for Investigating Etiological Causes of Hypersensitivity Pneumonitis

Total extract, somatic and recombinant "à la carte" antigens for precipitins/antibodies research for each environmental circumstance/setting

Circumstance/Setting	Exposure	Total Extract Antigens		
Somatic Antigens				
Work environment				
Farmer, agricultural worker	Moldy material	Panel 1		
		Lichtheimia corymbifera	*Wallemia sebi*	*Eurotium amstelodami*
		Saccharopolyspora rectivirgula	*Thermoactinomyces Vulgaris*	*Saccharomonospora viridis*
		Panel 2		
		Fusarium solani	*Aspergillus versicolor*	*Aspergillus ochraceus*
		Penicillium chrysogenum	*Rhodotorula rubra*	mesophilic *Streptomyces*
Cheese maker	Molds growing on cheese	*Acarus siro*	*Penicillium camemberti*	*Penicillium roquefort*
		Mucor spinolosum	*Geotrichum candidum*	
Pork butcher	Molds on meat	*Penicillium nalgiovense*	*G. candidum*	
Metalworking	Molds in cooling water	*Mycobacterium immunogenum*	*Bacillus simplex* *Fusarium solani*	*Pseudomonas oleovorans*
Plaster maker	Molds in water	*S. rectivirgula*	*T. vulgaris*	*Aspergillus fumigatus*
		Penicillium frequentans	*P. chrysogenum*	*A. versicolor*
Sugarcane	Molds on vegetal substrate	*Lacevella sacchari* *T. vulgaris*	*Saccharomonospora viridis* *A. fumigatus*	*Thermocrispum municipale*
Woodworker	Molds on vegetal substrate	*P. chrysogenum*	*P. frequentans*	
Wine producer	Spores	*Botrytis cinerea*	*P. chrysogenum*	*Saccharomyces cerevisiae*
		Mucor racemosus	*A. versicolor*	
Wind instrument player	Contaminated instrument	*R. rubra*	*P. chrysogenum*	*Phoma glomerata*
		E. amstelodami	*F. oxysporum*	
Compost		*S. rectivirgula*	*S. rectivirgula*	*S. viridis*
		A. fumigatus	*Thermobifida fusca*	mesophilic *Streptomyces*
Home environment				
Housing	Moldy material	Panel 1		
		A. versicolor	*P. chrysogenum*	*Cladosporium sphaerospermum*
		Stachybotrys chartarum	*Mucor racemosus*	*Alternaria alternata*
		Panel 2		
		Schizophilum commune	*Trichoderma pseudokoningii*	*Fusarium oxysporum*
		Acremonium strictum	*R. rubra*	*L. sacchari*
Humidifier	Moldy reservoir	*C. sphaerospermum*	*A. strictum*	*Exophiala dermatitidis*
Jacuzzi user	Molds in hot water	*Mycobacterium avium*	*Mycobacterium phocaicum*	
Recombinant antigens				
Bird breeders	—	Immunoglobulin Lamda-likepolypeptide-1 (IGLL1)	Proproteinase E (ProE)	
Farmers	—	SR17 Hydroperoxidase	Dihydrolipoamide dehydrogenase (DLDH)	
Metalworking	—	Acyl-CoA-Dehydrogenase (Acyl-CoA)	Dihydrolipoyl dehydrogenase (DHDH)	

Modified from: Bellanger AP, Reboux G, Rouzet, A et al. Hypersensitivity pneumonitis: a new strategy for serodiagnosis and environmental surveys. *Respir Med.* 2019;150: 101–106, by permission.

Several methods for determination of precipitins or total IgG antibodies have been developed: radial immunodiffusion, immunoelectrophoresis, ELISA, and different antigen preparations have been described (23, 26). ELISA is usually the preferred method because automation is possible but unfortunately, the ELISA technique lacks standardization (27). Electrosyneresis is more challenging than the ELISA on several aspects: reading, interpretation, delay in reporting results; however, it is recognized as a performing technique (23).

As early as in 1959, Pepys suspected cross reactions between some microorganisms such as *Cladosporium* and *Penicillium* (28), this being confirmed using recombinant antigens (29). This antigen cross reactivity could at times throw doubts on the efficiency of serodiagnosis. Moreover, in case of multiple exposure, some antigens can induce a higher humoral response. Globally, the kinetic of the humoral response is estimated at 50% decrease over 5 years in case of eviction (29).

Recombinant antigens (RAg) issued from species involved in HP are useful tools to discriminate patients from exposed healthy subjects (26, 29). Few RAg are currently used for the diagnosis of metalworking fluid OHP (30), farmer's lung (31), and bird fancier's lung (32). The RAg can be carried out only by ELISA technique and is associated with sensitivity and specificity reaching 80% and 90%, respectively, for metalworking fluid HP (30), 83% and 77% for farmer's lung (31), and 76% and 100% for bird fancier's lung (32). However, RAg are not commercialized yet and specific RAg allowing the diagnosis of other OHP forms, such as hot tub lung remain to be identified.

Bronchoalveolar lavage

Lymphocytosis in BAL is a characteristic feature of HP, although it is not specific for the disease, being present in other conditions and in asymptomatic farmers and in other conditions (33) (see Case History). BAL is often done in the context of also performing a transbronchial lung biopsy in a subject with possible HP. BAL lymphocytosis in a patient with interstitial lung disease of unknown origin is at the best indicative of the possibility of OHP (34). Lymphocyte subsets expressed by the CD4/CD8 ratio are no longer indicative of a clear distinction between sarcoidosis and HP.

Specific inhalation challenge

SICs in the laboratory have initially been proposed in the case of bird fancier's lung, using pigeon and budgerigar sera (35). They can also be carried out in the laboratory in the case of various chemicals (viz. diisocyanates) that can cause either OA or OHP (see Chapter 8). For many other types of OHP in which microorganisms are the causal agents, there is a lack of standardized antigens. However, using commercial preparations of fungi (*Penicillium, Mucor, Aspergillus*), Munoz and coworkers found that SICs performed in the laboratory were 85% sensitive in confirming OHP (36). If the tests are negative or cannot be done in the laboratory, they can be carried out at the workplace by comparing biological and functional parameters during day(s) spent at work and away from work (see Chapter 8).

Transbronchial and open lung biopsy procedures

Most often, the diagnosis can be based on exposure to an agent known to cause OHP, the presence of specific IgG antibodies, results of BAL showing predominant lymphocytosis, and typical CT scans. However, in a relatively limited number of workers for whom a decision regarding diagnosis, management, and treatment needs to be made and that are proposed elsewhere (37), a procedure to obtain lung tissue specimens should be considered: either a transbronchial lung biopsy/cryobiopsy approach or an open-lung procedure. The use of video-assisted thoracoscopy to obtain good quality subpleural lung specimens has improved its safety. The diagnostic accuracy of open-lung biopsy is slightly better than for the transbronchial biopsy procedure, the latter intervention being associated with significant bleeding in 5% of cases and pneumothorax in 10% (38).

Offending environments, antigens, and relevance for laboratory testing

Antigens responsible of OHP originate from fungi, bacteria, mycobacteria, bird proteins, and chemicals. Quirce and coworkers propose a list of OHPs and responsible agents (1) and Soumagne and Dalphin focus on incriminated microorganisms and molds (39). The interested reader is referred to relevant tables included in these reviews. As regards microorganisms, OHP can occur in all environmental settings favorable for their growth and not necessarily in an agricultural setting. One interesting example of this is metalworking fluid first identified in 1995 as a cause of OHP in six workers by Bernstein and coauthors (40) and a current common cause of HP (9). Avian proteins present in droppings, blooms, and sera, best identified by recombinant antigen technique (32) play a major role, microorganisms present on various parts of birds being rarely responsible (25). Vegetal substrates (straw, hay, cotton) are not recognized as offending antigens per se, the microorganisms growing on them being implicated. Chemicals with higher predicted OA hazard, more lipophilic and protein cross-linkers are more likely to cause OHP (41). A seemingly "exhaustive" list, as presented above (39) may wrongly lead to the exclusion of favorable circumstances that are more rarely or not yet described.

To better identify offending antigens, microbial analysis of possible occupational agent present at the workplace and production of customized antigen from specific material brought by the workers are now more and more performed; this "à la carte" strategy is applied in several countries (Finland, United States, France) at an acceptable cost (26). This strategy is proposed in Table 24.2.

Treatment

In the case of OHP as for OA, once the diagnosis is confirmed, that is the disease is caused by work even if the responsible agent has not been identified, removal from exposure is the most relevant advice. Most medicolegal national systems offer compensation for OA and OHP (see Chapters 11A and 11B). In the case of farmer's lung, farmers do not adhere invariably to a national or private medicolegal insurance. As for OA (42), corticosteroids may hasten recovery from OHP after removal from exposure and may be justified in affected workers with severe symptoms and/or functional impairment. For a long time, patients with chronic HP and OHP were managed with corticosteroids, although there is no clear evidence to support recommendations for effective doses and duration of therapy. Fortunately, new alternative approaches for therapy, that are steroid-sparing, are now proposed using immunosuppressive agents such as rituximab, mycophenolate mofetil, and azathioprine (43, 44). The mechanism of action of Rituximab in chronic HP is explained by its high affinity for CD20 surface antigen of lymphocytes and its ability to act directly on B cells and on antibody production and cellular cytotoxicity (45). A Canadian multicenter retrospective study demonstrated that mycophenolate mofetil (MMF) and azathioprine (AZA) were well tolerated by patients with chronic HP and were associated with improved gas exchange and a reduction in prednisone dose (43). MMF exerts an immunosuppressive effect by inhibiting an enzyme (inosine monophosphate dehydrogenase) acting directly on the proliferation of lymphocytes while AZA limits the proliferation of lymphocytes by blocking the purine pathway (43). These immunosuppressive agents are very promising treatment options for long-term therapy for chronic HP.

Patients with progressive disease may also be evaluated early for lung transplantation. Lung transplantation in case of progressive HP is associated with good post-transplant medium-term survival (46).

Prevention

Primary prevention

Avoidance or reduction of exposure is the key recommendation as for OA (see Chapter 10). In the case of farmer's lung, preventive measures (mask, barn ventilation, avoidance of exposure, changing clothes) represent information readily made available to farmers. Practices vary according to the education level and the geographic area, being applied either generally or only in farmers with OHP.

Secondary prevention

As for OA, the avoidance or reduction of exposure to the causal agent is mandatory. In most instances, if several measures (hay handling and storage, use of products to diminish mold growth, adequate ventilation, mask wearing) (47) are taken along this line, most farmers affected with OHP can continue working on the farm they often own.

Outcome

The clinical and functional outcome of OHP is favorable in most cases (see Case History). The long-term outcome is conditioned by the presence of parenchymal fibrosis (48), outlining the importance of making an early diagnosis to prevent progression to chronic HP. A substantial number of subjects with idiopathic pulmonary fibrosis may rather be affected with HP (49). In addition, farmers may develop emphysema that also influences outcome (15). Mortality rates are also increased in HP, more so in subjects with fibrosis (3).

Organic dust toxic syndrome

Different terms have been proposed to describe the health effect of exposure on the farm: mycotoxicosis or organic dust toxic syndrome (ODTS), atypical farmer's lung, silo filler's disease, and inhalation fever. ODTS is a self-limited flu-like illness that follows exposure to organic dust (50). The characteristics of other conditions (OHP, diseases related to exposure to organic dust, metal fume fever) with similar manifestations are proposed in Table 24.1. It can occur whenever there is exposure to high concentrations of organic material and endotoxins such as in print shops, wood chip compost, recycling process, etc. This has been reported in agricultural workers handling seed dust, the elevated concentrations of endotoxins present being able to induce the release of high doses of cytokines (IL8, TNFα, IL6, and IL1β) by in vitro exposure to whole blood (51). This is currently a concern in the recycling process, especially with compost (9, 10).

Symptoms are similar to those described in HP (see section "Clinical Presentation"). However, chest radiographs and CT as well as lung function tests are usually normal as ODTS often occurs in an episodic context as a result of unusual contamination of a workplace. It is therefore detected early, causal agent being eliminated, and does not generally lead to permanent sequelae. The most relevant laboratory test that is a characteristic of the condition is neutrophilia as present in peripheral blood (52) and, even more so, in BAL or in induced sputum (values of one million cells/mL, JLM, personal finding).

It is hypothesized that exposure to toxins may induce the production of various cytokines (51). The hypothesis is that it represents a healthy response to a toxic environment. As a support to this hypothesis, the timing of the process is incompatible with an infectious or an allergic process, a sensitization period being absent. Besides presenting farmer's lung, many more farmers can temporarily be affected with ODTS presumably when the quantity of airborne organic dust is excessive (53).

ODTS is not difficult to distinguish from HP as in the former the physical examination is normal as well as chest radiographs and lung function tests. Moreover, it is self-limited. Most often, the source of contamination will be found rapidly, therefore preventing further exposure and the need for using pharmacological treatment.

Research needs

By comparison with OA, OHP is a rarer condition. If it is not diagnosed early and causal exposure stopped, it is as likely as OA for causing permanent sequelae.

Some research needs warrant being proposed:

- Identification of genetic markers
- Better quantification of environmental risk factors
- Development of recombinant antigen methodology with improved antigens to improve diagnosis

Complementary information

The authors refer the interested readers to other publications issued since the 4th edition of *Asthma in the Workplace* for documentary information on relevant radiographs, CT scans, and histopathological specimens: (1, 16, 20, 39, 54, 55).

References

1. Quirce S, Vandenplas O, Campo P, et al. Occupational hypersensitivity pneumonitis: an EAACI position paper. *Allergy*. 2016;71:765–79.
2. Bourke SJ, Dalphin JC, Boyd G, et al. Hypersensitivity pneumonitis: current concepts. *Eur Respir J Suppl*. 2001 Sep;32:81s–92s.
3. Fernandez Perez ER, Kong AM, Raimundo K, et al. Epidemiology of hypersensitivity pneumonitis among an insured population in the United States: a claims-based cohort analysis. *Ann Am Thorac Soc*. 2018;15:460–9.
4. Solaymani-Dodaran M, West J, Smith C, et al. Extrinsic allergic alveolitis: incidence and mortality in the general population. *QJM*. 2007;100:233–7.
5. Dalphin JC, Debieuvre D, Pernet D, et al. Prevalence and risk factors for chronic bronchitis and farmer's lung in French dairy farmers. *Br J Ind Med*. 1993;50:941–4.
6. Bang KM, Weissman DN, Pinheiro GA, et al. Twenty-three years of hypersensitivity pneumonitis mortality surveillance in the United States. *Am J Ind Med*. 2006;49:997–1004.
7. Zeiss CR, Wolkonsky P, Chacon R, et al. Syndromes in workers exposed to trimellitic anhydride. *Ann Intern Med*. 1983;98:8–12.
8. Vandenplas O, Malo JL, Dugas M, et al. Hypersensitivity pneumonitis-like reaction among workers exposed to diphenylmethane diisocyanate (MDI). *Am Rev Respir Dis*. 1993;147:338–46.
9. Walters GI, Mokhlis JM, Moore VC, et al. Characteristics of hypersensitivity pneumonitis diagnosed by interstitial and occupational lung disease multi-disciplinary team consensus. *Respir Med*. 2019;155:19–25.
10. Poole CJM, Basu S. Systematic review: occupational illness in the waste and recycling sector. *Occup Med (Lond)*. 2017;67:626–36.
11. Lemière C, Gautrin D, Trudeau C, et al. Fever and leucocytosis accompanying asthmatic reactions due to occupational agents: frequency and associated factors. *Eur Respir J*. 1996;9:517–23.
12. Ley B, Newton CA, Arnould I, et al. The MUC5B promoter polymorphism and telomere length in patients with chronic hypersensitivity pneumonitis: an observational cohort-control study. *Lancet Respir Med*. 2017;5:639–47.
13. Lacasse Y, Selman M, Costabel U, et al. Clinical diagnosis of hypersensitivity pneumonitis. *Am J Respir Crit Care Med*. 2003;168:952–8.
14. Hanak V, Golbin JM, Ryu JH. Causes and presenting features in 85 consecutive patients with hypersensitivity pneumonitis. *Mayo Clin Proc*. 2007;82:812–6.
15. Soumagne T, Chardon ML, Dournes G, et al. Emphysema in active farmer's lung disease. *PLOS ONE*. 2017;12:e0178263.
16. Vasakova M, Morell F, Walsh S, et al. Hypersensitivity pneumonitis: perspectives in diagnosis and management. *Am J Respir Crit Care Med*. 2017;196:680–9.
17. Richerson HB, Bernstein IL, Fink JN, et al. Guidelines for the clinical evaluation of hypersensitivity pneumonitis. *J Allergy Clin Immunol*. 1989;84:839–44.
18. Lacasse Y, Selman M, Costabel U, et al. Classification of hypersensitivity pneumonitis: a hypothesis. *Int Arch Allergy Immunol*. 2009;149:161–6.

19. Demedts M, Wells AU, Anto JM, et al. Interstitial lung diseases: an epidemiological overview. *Eur Respir J Suppl*. 2001;32:2s–16s.

20. Grunes D, Beasley MB. Hypersensitivity pneumonitis: a review and update of histologic findings. *J Clin Pathol*. 2013;66:888–95.

21. Takemura T, Akashi T, Ohtani Y, et al. Pathology of hypersensitivity pneumonitis. *Curr Opin Pulm Med*. 2008;14:440–54.

22. Silva CI, Churg A, Muller NL. Hypersensitivity pneumonitis: spectrum of high-resolution CT and pathologic findings. *AJR Am J Roentgenol*. 2007;188:334–44.

23. Reboux G, Piarroux R, Roussel S, et al. Assessment of four serological techniques in the immunological diagnosis of farmers' lung disease. *J Med Microbiol*. 2007;56(Pt 10):1317–21.

24. Tillie-Leblond I, Grenouillet F, Reboux G, et al. Hypersensitivity pneumonitis and metalworking fluids contaminated by mycobacteria. *Eur Respir J*. 2011;37:640–7.

25. Rouzet A, Reboux G, Dalphin JC, et al. Usefulness of a la carte antigens for bird fancier's lung serodiagnosis: total dropping extract and/or dropping's microflora antigens. *J Med Microbiol*. 2017;66:1467–70.

26. Bellanger AP, Reboux G, Rouzet A, et al. Hypersensitivity pneumonitis: a new strategy for serodiagnosis and environmental surveys. *Respir Med*. 2019;150:101–6.

27. Aberer W, Woltsche M, Woltsche-Kahr I, et al. IgG antibodies typical for extrinsic allergic alveolitis–an inter-laboratory quality assessment. *Eur J Med Res*. 2001;6:498–504.

28. Pepys J, Riddell RW, Citron KM, et al. Clinical and immunologic significance of aspergillus fumigatus in the sputum. *Am Rev Respir Dis*. 1959;80:167–80.

29. Millon L, Rognon B, Valot B, et al. Common peptide epitopes induce cross-reactivity in hypersensitivity pneumonitis serodiagnosis. *J Allergy Clin Immunol*. 2016;138:1738–41.e6.

30. Roussel S, Rognon B, Barrera C, et al. Immuno-reactive proteins from mycobacterium immunogenum useful for serodiagnosis of metalworking fluid hypersensitivity pneumonitis. *Int J Med Microbiol*. 2011;301:150–6.

31. Barrera C, Millon L, Rognon B, et al. Immunoreactive proteins of Saccharopolyspora rectivirgula for farmer's lung serodiagnosis. *Proteomics Clin Appl*. 2014;8:971–81.

32. Rouzet A, Reboux G, Dalphin JC, et al. An immunoproteomic approach revealed antigenic proteins enhancing serodiagnosis performance of bird fancier's lung. *J Immunol Methods*. 2017;450:58–65.

33. Cormier Y, Belanger J, Laviolette M. Persistent bronchoalveolar lymphocytosis in asymptomatic farmers. *Am Rev Respir Dis*. 1986;133:843–7.

34. Semenzato G, Bjermer L, Costabel U, et al. Clinical guidelines and indications for bronchoalveolar lavage (BAL): extrinsic allergic alveolitis. *Eur Respir J*. 1990;3:945-6, 961–9.

35. Hargreave FE, Pepys J, Longbottom JL, et al. Bird breeder's (fancier's) lung. *Lancet*. 1966;1:445–9.

36. Munoz X, Sanchez-Ortiz M, Torres F, et al. Diagnostic yield of specific inhalation challenge in hypersensitivity pneumonitis. *Eur Respir J*. 2014;44:1658–65.

37. King TE. Hypersensitivity pneumonitis (extrinsic allergic alveolitis): clinical manifestations and diagnosis. UptoDate. 2020.

38. Iftikhar IH, Alghothani L, Sardi A, et al. Transbronchial lung cryobiopsy and video-assisted thoracoscopic lung biopsy in the diagnosis of diffuse parenchymal lung disease. A meta-analysis of diagnostic test accuracy. *Ann Am Thorac Soc*. 2017;14:1197–211.

39. Soumagne T, Dalphin JC. Current and emerging techniques for the diagnosis of hypersensitivity pneumonitis. *Expert Rev Respir Med*. 2018;12:493–507.

40. Bernstein DI, Lummus ZL, Santilli G, et al. Machine operator's lung. A hypersensitivity pneumonitis disorder associated with exposure to metal-working fluid aerosols. *Chest*. 1995;108:636–41.

41. Seed MJ, Enoch SJ, Agius RM. Chemical determinants of occupational hypersensitivity pneumonitis. *Occup Med (Lond)*. 2015;65:673–81.

42. Malo JL, Cartier A, Côté J, et al. Influence of inhaled steroids on the recovery of occupational asthma after cessation of exposure: an 18-month double-blind cross-over study. *Am J Crit Care Respir Med*. 1996;153:953–60.

43. Morisset J, Johannson KA, Vittinghoff E, et al. Use of mycophenolate mofetil or azathioprine for the management of chronic hypersensitivity pneumonitis. *Chest*. 2017;151:619–25.

44. Fiddler CA, Simler N, Thillai M, et al. Use of mycophenolate mofetil and azathioprine for the treatment of chronic hypersensitivity pneumonitis-A single-centre experience. *Clin Respir J*. 2019;13:791–4.

45. Keir GJ, Maher TM, Ming D, et al. Rituximab in severe, treatment-refractory interstitial lung disease. *Respirology*. 2014;19:353–9.

46. Kern RM, Singer JP, Koth L, et al. Lung transplantation for hypersensitivity pneumonitis. *Chest*. 2015;147:1558–65.

47. Dalphin JC, Pernet D, Reboux G, et al. Influence of mode of storage and drying of fodder on thermophilic actinomycete aerocontamination in dairy farms of the Doubs region of France. *Thorax*. 1991;46:619–23.

48. Vourlekis JS, Schwarz MI, Cherniack RM, et al. The effect of pulmonary fibrosis on survival in patients with hypersensitivity pneumonitis. *Am J Med*. 2004;116:662–8.

49. Morell F, Villar A, Montero MA, et al. Chronic hypersensitivity pneumonitis in patients diagnosed with idiopathic pulmonary fibrosis: a prospective case-cohort study. *Lancet Respir Med*. 2013;1:685–94.

50. Seifert SA, Von Essen S, Jacobitz K, et al. Organic dust toxic syndrome: a review. *J Toxicol Clin Toxicol*. 2003;41:185–93.

51. Smit LA, Wouters IM, Hobo MM, et al. Agricultural seed dust as a potential cause of organic dust toxic syndrome. *Occup Environ Med*. 2006;63:59–67.

52. May JJ, Stallones L, Darrow D, et al. Organic dust toxicity (pulmonary mycotoxicosis) associated with silo unloading. *Thorax*. 1986;41:919–23.

53. Malmberg P, Rask-Andersen A, Hoglund S, et al. Incidence of organic dust toxic syndrome and allergic alveolitis in Swedish farmers. *Int Arch Allergy Appl Immunol*. 1988;87:47–54.

54. Spagnolo P, Rossi G, Cavazza A, et al. Hypersensitivity pneumonitis: a comprehensive review. *J Investig Allergol Clin Immunol*. 2015;25:237–50.

55. Jacob J, Bartholmai BJ, Brun AL, et al. Evaluation of visual and computer-based CT analysis for the identification of functional patterns of obstruction and restriction in hypersensitivity pneumonitis. *Respirology*. 2017;22:1585–91.

25

CHRONIC OBSTRUCTIVE AIRWAY DISEASE DUE TO OCCUPATIONAL EXPOSURE

Nicola Murgia,[1] Kjell Torén,[2] and Paul D. Blanc[3]
Editor Susan M. Tarlo[4]
[1]Section of Occupational Medicine, Respiratory Diseases and Toxicology, University of Perugia, Perugia, Italy
[2]School of Public Health and Community Medicine, Sahlgrenska Academy, University of Gothenburg, Gothenburg, Sweden
[3]School of Medicine, University of California, San Francisco, California, USA
[4]University Health Network and St Michael's Hospital, Toronto, Department of
Medicine, University of Toronto, Toronto, Ontario, Canada

Contents

CASE HISTORY

The patient is a 68-year-old man presenting with progressive dyspnea of 5-year duration and shortness of breath with one flight of stairs or with carrying groceries uphill. He denies dyspnea at rest, is without paroxysmal symptoms, and has only occasional complaints of wheezing.

He was an active cigarette smoker from age 14–30 years with a maximum of 1½ packs per day (24 pack-years total), quitting 40 years previously. He had done extremely dusty work with exposure to copious amounts of inorganic dust. This involved grinding large concrete display tanks as an exhibit preparer in an aquarium, work which he performed for 7 years. He reported less exposure over the following 5 years at which point he retired due to age. The work was sufficiently dusty that there was a spirometry-based workplace respirator-fit testing program as part of his employment, even though he did not use any personal protective equipment (PPE) on a routine basis. Because of abnormal findings on serial lung function testing, he was told at the time to consult his private physician regarding his results, but he did not do so.

On initial examination he is thin but not cachectic, with a prolonged expiratory phase but no wheezes or rhonchi. There is no increased pulmonic component to the second heart sound and no clubbing of the extremities. Initial pulmonary function testing (PFT) demonstrates obstruction without reversibility and a reduced diffusing capacity for carbon monoxide (DLco) that does not improve substantially adjusted for the observed lung volume (VA) (DLco, 59% height and age predicted; DLco/VA, 69% predicted). Follow-up PFTs after a course of systemic corticosteroids do not demonstrate any improvement. A computed tomography scan of the chest demonstrates bilateral lower lobe-predominant emphysema. A serum alpha-1-antitrypsin (A1AT) assay documents a "ZZ" phenotype and a quantified value of 24 units (normal ≥90).

Employment-based serial spirometry over 12 years of employment is available through his workplace respirator-fit surveillance program, along with nearly 5 years of subsequent follow-up data after his initial presentation for medical evaluation (following a 6-year data gap). Based on 18 serial measurements taken over 241 months, the patient's forced expiratory volume in 1 second (FEV_1) fell by 77 mL/yr. Using the US National Institute for Occupational Safety and Health (NIOSH) Spirometry Longitudinal Data Analysis (SPIROLA) software for analysis of lung function time trends, the change in FEV_1 during the employment exposure period (–128 mL/yr) demonstrates an accelerated decline relative to projected normal (–42 mL/yr), crossing the 95th percentile lower limit of normal (LLN) approximately midway in this dusty exposure period. After retirement and in the context of discontinued exposure, the FEV_1 remained below the LLN, but with a decline (–46 mL/yr) near the expected (1).

Introduction

Long before personal cigarette smoking was widespread, medical writers recognized that "dusty trades" were associated with various lung diseases. "Miner's phthisis" was prototypical of such diseases. This and related conditions (e.g. "grinder's rot") were associated with exposure to inorganic dusts and can best be understood by today's nosology as one or another of the pneumoconioses (with or without superimposed tubercular disease). Clinical syndromes consistent with chronic bronchitis or airway obstruction, in particular among persons experiencing heavy organic dust inhalation, were already well described throughout the nineteenth century (2).

By the mid-twentieth century, occupational exposures in the various dusty trades were generally presumed to be contributors to chronic bronchitis specifically and, by extension, to airway disease more broadly defined. For example, a key 1953 analysis of mortality data from the 1930s found that work in dusty trades, even within the same social class, was linked to bronchitis mortality (3). In 1958, Fletcher noted that "men who work in dusty trades, especially coal miners, have a higher prevalence of symptoms of bronchitis and emphysema...." (4). In the early 1960s, the "Dutch hypothesis" was articulated, holding that bronchitis and chronic airflow obstruction fell along a spectrum, with the ultimate pathophysiological manifestations of disease dependent on a combination of host and environmental factors (5). Fletcher's landmark studies, which came to downplay the role of chronic bronchitis in the progression of airway obstruction, coincided with the ascendancy of cigarette smoking as a major independent risk factor for airflow limitation-defined chronic obstructive pulmonary disease (COPD). This fits in with the "British hypothesis," which viewed COPD and asthma as separate processes with distinct causal pathways (6). The paramount importance of smoking in COPD tended to eclipse all other potential associations. This was especially true of consideration of possible links between occupational exposures and COPD, with or without concomitant chronic bronchitis.

Since the late 1960s and particularly throughout the 1970s, a number of industry-specific cohort studies, particularly of investigations of mining populations, accumulated data on progressive airflow decline associated with coal and inorganic dusts (predominantly silica, in particular the gold mining industry in South Africa, where COPD in this industry was recognized as work-related in the 1970s). Industry-specific occupational exposure to cadmium proved to be an important source of data relevant to emphysema pathogenesis (7).

Earlier, large population-based cross-industry studies of symptoms and lung function provided an important set of additional insights into the question of occupation in relation to COPD. These investigations treated occupational factors as little more than a controlling cofactor to be considered in multivariate modeling that focused on cigarette smoking and ambient air pollution. Despite this limitation, these studies yielded surprisingly consistent findings of a link between higher exposure jobs as a group and bronchitis or airflow obstruction. Thus, beginning in the mid-1980s, wider biomedical interest grew in the potential role of occupational exposures in the causation of chronic bronchitis, COPD, and emphysema. The seminal work of Dr. Margaret Becklake was critical in this regard. Early on, she had observed the association of airway obstruction of irritant gas inhalation among miners exposed to explosive blast fumes (8). Beginning in 1985, she authored a series of reviews

and informal meta-analyses systematically compiling the epidemiological evidence that had been accumulating in the medical literature (9–10). Initially, this work relied on findings reported from industry-specific cohort studies, in particular coal miners, showing airflow decline or pathologically confirmed emphysema. It later widened to multiple large population-based studies, all showing that a longitudinal decline in airflow or a greater prevalence of airflow obstruction was associated with work-related inhalation of gases and vapors or fumes and dust or both categories of exposure.

Other reviews followed on this work and a major systematic review by the American Thoracic Society (ATS) published in 2003, for which Dr. Becklake was a coauthor, marked a turning point in the general recognition of the occupational contribution to COPD (11). In 2019, an ATS/European Respiratory Society (ERS) task force updated this analysis, including multiple publications from the intervening two decades. The findings of that systematic review further support the conclusion that the occupational burden of COPD remains substantial (12).

Over time, the Dutch and British hypotheses have come to be seen less as polar opposites and more as constructs that both can be applied to questions of COPD and asthma, each construct yielding its own potential insights (13). The inclusion of a chapter devoted to chronic airway disease in this book on occupational asthma (OA), first introduced with the third edition of this text, underscores this more inclusive view. In this chapter, we will first present the epidemiological evidence linking occupation to COPD from a population-based perspective, including review of the population attributable fraction (PAF) of worked-related COPD and chronic bronchitis. Next, we will review the literature for industry-specific cohorts exposed to dusts and fumes. Organic dusts, such as cotton and grain, are addressed in a separate chapter in this volume (see Chapter 23) that considers both asthma-like responses and less reversible airflow obstruction in relation to such exposures.

COPD from an epidemiological perspective

Defining disease and measuring risk

COPD is defined by chronic airflow limitation that, in practical terms, requires spirometric assessment and the presence of persistent respiratory symptoms (14). The criteria for carrying out spirometry and the application of cut points for abnormality are discussed elsewhere in this volume and have been the focus of position papers by relevant international professional societies. Chronic airflow limitation can be assessed either by using a fixed ratio of forced expiratory volume in 1 second (FEV_1)/forced vital capacity (FVC) <0.70, or FEV_1/FVC less than the 5th percentile, the "lower limit of normal (LLN_5)." Beyond lung function-based definitions of airflow limitation, emphysema can be defined by computerized tomographic (CT) or pathological criteria (although inferences can also be drawn from lung volumes and diffusing capacity measurements) and chronic bronchitis can be defined by standardized questionnaire responses (although pathological criteria can be applied, for example, using airway biopsies). Despite these distinctions, the label "COPD" is often applied imprecisely in clinical practice and can be driven by diagnostic biases that are particularly relevant to occupationally related COPD. The clinical diagnosis of COPD is more likely to be given if linked to a history of cigarette smoke exposure. When another respiratory condition is present that might account for fixed airflow obstruction, for example, long-standing asthma in a nonsmoker, the concomitant diagnostic label of COPD may not be applied. When emphysema is present along with airflow obstruction, a patient may simply be told of the former diagnosis but not receive a label of "COPD." Of note, occupational factors in emphysema are generally not considered in clinical practice, even in the context of A1AT deficiency (exposure that was clearly relevant to the case scenario presented). When chronic bronchitis is combined with COPD, the latter diagnosis alone is frequently applied, and chronic bronchitis may not be captured even in medical records.

For epidemiological research studies that include the direct collection of spirometric data, airflow limitation can be quantified directly. In epidemiological research and clinical outcomes studies using other methods (e.g. questionnaire-based survey or interrogation of electronic medical record data), the case definition of COPD may have to take into account the clinical biases noted above, as well as the availability of ancillary data. Thus, COPD, emphysema, and chronic bronchitis, even though separate diagnostic entities, are sometimes studied together as a mixed diagnostic group, with condition-specific subcategories stratified insofar as the data allow. This is particularly relevant to the question of emphysema, given that even epidemiological studies that have included spirometric assessment may not have carried out systematic CT scanning. A related, more overarching category of chronic obstructive lung disease (COLD) includes asthma along with the previous three conditions. The COLD categorization will not be considered further in this discussion. Further complicating this topic, in recent years an "asthma-COPD overlap syndrome (ACOS)" has been categorized as a subtype of COPD. This syndrome has been defined by a persistent airflow limitation despite the administration of a short-acting beta2 agonist, an exposure to an offending agent (e.g. tobacco smoke, ambient air pollution, or, presumably, an occupational agent), a history of asthma before 40 years of age, and other features consistent with asthma, such as increased blood eosinophils. Only a few publications have appeared specially addressing the association between ACOS and occupational exposures (15–17). The role of ACOS as a distinct entity remains to be established, and will not be considered further here (14).

The epidemiological perspective on COPD in relation to occupational factors focuses on associations of risk, most through estimation of relative risk (RR) and a related measure, the odds ratio (OR). The study of occupationally related COPD has also been informed by estimations of population attributable risk percent, which is also known as the population attributable fraction (PAF). This measure integrates the magnitude of the RR or OR together with the prevalence of exposure to the risk factor in question among populations. For example, a putative risk factor (Exposure I) may be associated with a markedly elevated RR/OR for COPD, but this exposure may be limited to a small proportion of the population at large. Under that scenario, the actual number of COPD cases induced by (attributed to) Exposure I may be quite small. Were another risk factor for COPD (Exposure II) to have a much lower RR in absolute terms but be far more common, the number of cases induced by it could be far greater. The epidemiological calculation of the PAF can be performed using various algebraic equations and this can be done post hoc using published risk and exposure prevalence data. Whatever the method of calculation, the PAF provides an important estimate of disease caused, at least in part, by the factor in question. Another way of considering this question is to ask what burden of disease would

be removed were this factor eliminated. Further, because two factors may act upon each other to magnify risk, removing either one could reduce the burden of disease. Indeed, the PAF values estimated for multiple risk factors for the same outcome may yield a combined value of more than 100%. This is particularly relevant to considerations of combined occupational exposure and cigarette smoking in COPD causation.

The occupational burden of COPD, chronic bronchitis, and emphysema

As noted above, the ATS/ERS statement, the occupational burden of nonmalignant respiratory diseases, provided an updated (2002–2017) benchmark systematic review of the occupationally associated PAF for COPD and chronic bronchitis (CB) (12), emphasizing population-based studies across populations rather than industry-specific cohorts, as the previous ATS document (11).

Table 25.1 summarizes the ATS/ERS findings on the occupational PAF in relation to COPD (based mainly on spirometry) and chronic bronchitis (defined by self-reported symptoms). As the table shows, the epidemiological cohorts analyzed included a large subject pool and all the analyses were smoking adjusted or stratified. The ATS/ERS document concluded that 14% (95% CI:10%–18%) was an estimate of the work-related burden of COPD, similar to what was found before (15%) by the previous ATS statement (11). The occupational burden of COPD among never smokers, estimated from six studies including stratified data for smoking, produced a pooled PAF of 31% (95% CI:18%–43%) (12). Table 25.1 also presents the occupational burden of chronic bronchitis. The re-estimated PAF (13%) was also consistent with the findings in the previous ATS document.

Even since the publication of the latest ATS/ERS document, a number of additional studies and reviews have appeared on the question of occupational factors in COPD and chronic bronchitis. Among them, larger population-based studies are particularly relevant, such as one analyzing European Community Respiratory Health Survey follow-up, where the PAF for COPD for occupational exposures to vapor, gases, dusts, and fumes (VGDF) was 14.1% (18). Using the same survey, a separate estimate of the PAF for chronic bronchitis associated with VGDF was 6.8% (19). The Global Burden of Disease Study, studying COPD mortality, estimated the PAF associated with occupational exposure to particulate matter, gases, and fumes and secondhand smoke to be 15.6% (20). Other population studies have appeared, however, with lower PAF estimates, including an analysis of US national data (7.4% to 10.7% depending on the exposure definition) (21) and another of the UK Biobank cohort (4.8%) (22). Of note, additional ecological analyses of these latter two study populations have observed a higher prevalence

TABLE 25.1 ATS/ERS Findings on the Occupationally Associated PAF for COPD

Outcome Studied	PAF		Subjects	Studies
	Pooled estimate (%)	95% CI	N	N
COPD[a]	14	10–18	108,939	26
• In nonsmokers	31	18–43	13,526	6
Chronic bronchitis	13	6–21	26,741	7

[a] In 24 of 26 studies COPD was defined by spirometry.

Abbreviation: PAF, population attributable fraction.

of COPD in selected occupational groups (23,24). Moreover, another earlier ecological, population-level analysis from 45 sites of three international studies (the Burden of Obstructive Lung Disease study, the Latin American Project for the Investigation of Obstructive Lung Disease, and the European Community Respiratory Health Survey) included data from developing as well as developed economies, suggesting that a 20% reduction in the burden of COPD could be achieved by an 8.8% reduction in the prevalence of occupational exposures (25).

A number of studies have addressed the potential interaction between cigarette smoking and work exposures (frequently defined as regular contact with VGDF in one's longest held job). In one of the first such analyses (using a definition of disease based on physician-diagnosed COPD, emphysema, or CB and using nonsmoking, non-occupationally exposed subjects as the referent group), the OR for COPD was 1.4 for occupational exposure alone, 2.8 for smoking alone, and 6.2 for both risk factors combined; for COPD or emphysema, excluding chronic bronchitis alone, the effect was stronger, with estimated ORs of 2.4, 7.0, and 18.4, respectively (26). In another study that yielded an occupationally associated PAF for COPD between 13% and 33% (depending on the measure of exposure used), there was also a step-up in risk for combined occupational and smoking exposures: relative to no occupational exposure and no smoking, occupational factors doubled the risk of COPD, smoking alone carried a seven-fold excess risk, and combined exposure carried a 14-fold increased risk, a cross-product increase that is consistent with an additive effect (27).

In addition to occupation and smoking interactions, another topic of increasing interest has been the potential impact of occupational etiology and COPD severity. Limited data initially suggested a potential relationship (28). Further study has shown that prior occupational exposures are associated with worse COPD symptoms, quality of life, and exacerbation rate (29). Lung function decline has been extensively studied in occupational cohorts with interesting findings, but in population-based studies, results have been mixed: in some no association with VGDF exposure was observed (30), while in others there was an observed association, albeit limited to those carrying a specific predisposing genotype (31) or related to selected exposures only, such as solvents or pesticides (32,33).

As aforementioned, emphysema diagnosis is typically defined by pathology and/or radiographic findings, although it can be inferred from pulmonary function findings of an increased residual volume coupled with a reduction of diffusing capacity for carbon monoxide. Although previously very limited, the expanding availability of high-resolution CT-scan data in population-based studies has allowed the role of occupational exposure in emphysema to be more extensively evaluated. In the COPD gene study, emphysema and gas trapping were greater in those exposed to dust and fumes together, both in men and women (34). In a study considering Swedish adult population aged 50–64, the PAF related to occupational exposure to VGDF for CT-scan defined emphysema was 23% in the whole population, reaching 34% in males (35). In the SPIROMICS cohort, the percentage of lung volume occupied by emphysema was studied, finding that current or former smokers reporting exposure to VGDF in the longest held job had a larger percentage of emphysema than nonsmokers not exposed and smokers without an occupational exposure (36). Thus, the association between occupational exposures and emphysema at the population level appears to parallel that of COPD and chronic bronchitis.

Exposure to inorganic dusts, coal dust, metal fumes, and other agents

Occupational exposure to inorganic dust occurs in many work settings worldwide. Occupational inorganic and coal dust exposures can be broadly categorized as strongly fibrogenic dusts (silica, asbestos, and coal) and other inorganic dusts and metal fumes that may also be associated with adverse respiratory effects. Dust-induced pneumoconioses and associated tuberculosis have been the main noncancer causes of morbidity and mortality attributable to highly fibrogenic dust exposure. Industry-specific epidemiological studies have demonstrated, however, that exposure to inorganic dusts, primarily the more highly fibrogenic types of dusts, is also associated with obstructive lung function impairment and chronic bronchitis (10). These associations were also shown in those with lower exposures that may not lead to radiological signs of pneumoconiosis (37).

There may be multiple pathophysiological mechanisms by which highly fibrogenic dusts may potentially initiate lung injury leading to airflow obstruction, chronic bronchitis, or emphysema. Upon deposition, dust particles can reach two critical target cells in the lung: macrophages and epithelial cells (38). Macrophage ingestion of various dust particles (phagocytosis) has been shown to lead to macrophage activation and release of mediators causing tissue damage. The potential mechanisms of cell injury include cytotoxicity leading to generation of reactive oxygen/nitrogen species (39) and secretion of proinflammatory factors, cytokines, chemokines, elastase (40), and fibrogenic factors (41). Dusts analyzed in terms of these mechanisms and found to be toxic include not only crystalline silica and coal dust, but also kaolin, talc, bentonite, and feldspar.

In addition to macrophage-mediated effects, particles could react directly with epithelium. This may lead to increased mucus production in the bronchus leading to bronchitis (38) and emphysema (39,40,42). Particulates can also cause epithelial cell injury and localized fibrosis (43). The interaction between genetic background and environmental factors in the pathogenesis of COPD has been extensively studied for cigarette smoke and air pollution, but not for work-related toxicants. Heme oxygenase-1 polymorphism could play a role in the susceptibility to COPD in workers exposed to VGDF (44). As for cigarette smoke and environmental pollution, alpha 1 antitrypsin deficiency (AATD) plays a role in making more susceptible to lung function decline subjects exposed to VGDF (31). Little is known on other mechanisms involving the effect of occupational pollutants on the genome in the pathogenesis of COPD, even if DNA-methylation could play a role in workers exposed to VGDF (45).

Mineral dust airway disease (MDAD), defined by focal fibrosis in respiratory bronchioles associated with mineral dust exposure, has been reported as a pathological process causing airflow limitation in mineral dust-exposed workers (46). The following sections provide mainly epidemiological evidence relevant to the particular type of exposure and various COPD outcomes.

Silica

Despite the dramatic reduction of silica dust exposure levels in most developed countries during the last century, airflow limitation and associated COPD remain a worldwide health issues in workers exposed to silica (47). Epidemiological studies show that silica dust exposure can lead to airflow limitation in the absence of radiological signs of silicosis (10).

Large studies of hard rock miners demonstrated that the FEV_1, forced vital capacity (FVC), and FEV_1/FVC ratio, adjusted for age, height, and tobacco smoking, decreased with increasing cumulative respirable dust exposure in both smokers and nonsmokers. The average loss in lung function attributable to silica dust exposure, estimated for South African gold miners exposed for about 24 years to standard exposure levels, was equivalent to an average excess loss of 8–9 mL/yr of FEV_1 and 9.0 mL/yr of FVC (48).

Further epidemiological studies of morbidity have affirmed that silica dust exposure also constitutes a hazard for airflow limitation in many nonmining industries (general population study of silica exposure, granite crushers, tunnel workers, construction workers, brick-manufacturing workers, slate workers, stone carvers and grinders, ceramic workers, refractory ceramic fiber molders, and coremakers handling furan resin sand, silicon carbide industry, and iron foundry and smelter workers). A dose-dependent relationship between exposure (quantified duration of employment, dust level, or cumulative dust exposure) and lung function level or lung function decline was found in some of these studies. The effect of employment in silica dust-exposed occupations was even detected in a large general population-based cross-sectional study of Norwegian men of 30–46 years of age (49). Workers with 15 or more years of silica dust exposure had a statistically significant excess loss of FEV_1 of 4.3 mL [95% confidence interval (CI):1.1–7.5] with each year of exposure; the exposure-response relationship was similar among nonsmokers, exsmokers, and smokers.

Several mortality studies of cohorts of silica dust-exposed workers reported increased mortality from nonmalignant respiratory disease (NMRD) and COPD (50,51). Generally, NMRD combines deaths from pneumoconiosis and COPD. An exposure-response relationship between silica dust exposure and emphysema assessed on paper-mounted whole-lung sections at autopsy has also been observed (52). Silica dust exposure appears to be associated more with emphysema than asbestos dust (53). Nonetheless, the degree of emphysema found in silica dust-exposed miners with about 20 years of service who were never-smokers was relatively small and not correlated with lung function measured 5 years prior to death (54). Several new sources of exposure to crystalline silica have been described in the last 20 years in denim sandblasting, in goldsmiths, and among workers involved in cutting and processing artificial stone. Unfortunately, the data are limited relevant to COPD in these exposure categories. Workers involved in artificial stone processing, however, showed a reduction in FEV_1/FVC ratio compared to those not exposed, although the exposed were older and data were not adjusted for smoking (55).

In summary, the epidemiological evidence from large studies of hard rock miners demonstrate a positive exposure-response relation for airflow limitation and silica dust exposure that is not associated with the presence of silicosis.

Coal dust

Large epidemiological studies of British, US, and Italian coal miners have established an exposure-response relationship between cumulative coal dust exposure and decreased lung function, respiratory symptoms, and mortality (56–58). The association has been seen among smokers, exsmokers, and never-smokers, and across all age groups. Studies demonstrate that the severity of the impairment associated with coal mining dust exposure puts coal miners at an increased risk of clinical COPD comparable to smoking. Because of this evidence, COPD (i.e. chronic bronchitis and emphysema) became a compensable occupational disease among coal miners in some countries. Moreover, there is epidemiological evidence showing that current permissible concentrations of coal mining dust (2 mg/m^3 in the United States) can increase the risk of COPD, especially in the absence of coal worker's pneumoconiosis (CWP).

Several industry-wide surveys of more than 30,000 British coal miners, initiated during 1953–1958 with follow-up studies up to 1991, have shown excessive dose-dependent losses of FEV_1 with cumulative dust exposure independent of the presence of CWP; the loss was found to be greatest in younger men and in men with respiratory symptoms (56–59). Investigating the severity of the impairment associated with coal dust exposure, a study reported that the risks of having symptoms of chronic bronchitis and FEV_1 <80% predicted and <65% predicted were almost doubled in men with the highest exposure category of 348 gram-hours per cubic meter (ghm–^{3}) (57). The excess loss of FEV_1 persisted even after dust levels were substantially reduced in coal miners employed after 1970 (58). A British study of miners who did not have radiological signs of pneumoconiosis also found that adjusted FEV_1 was on average 155 mL (95% CI:74–236 mL) lower in miners than in population controls (59).

The findings of the National Study of Coal Workers' Pneumoconiosis (NSCWP) in US coal miners were similar (60); in addition, coal mining dust was also associated with higher rate of decline in lung function. In miners participating in the NIOSH coal worker health surveillance program, the prevalence of airway obstruction in never-smokers was 7.7% for the exposed, 16.4% among those with CWP, and 32.3% in those with progressive massive fibrosis (61). Furthermore, excessive decline in FEV_1 of 60 mL/yr or more was associated with early retirement from coal mining, increased risk of respiratory morbidity, and increased mortality from nonmalignant respiratory disease (62). A recent study shows a reduction of FEV_1 and FEV_1/FVC ratio associated with small opacities profusion in workers with CWP (63). Autopsy studies of coal miners find typical focal emphysema caused by coal dust deposition forming the coal macula and severity of emphysema in coal miners can be comparable to that of tobacco smoking (64). In summary, multiple studies show a positive exposure-response relationship between various outcomes of COPD (morbidity and mortality) and coal mining dust exposure. It has been estimated that 8.0% (95% CI:3.4%–13.7%) of nonsmoking coal miners with a cumulative respirable dust exposure of 123 ghm–^{3} (considered equivalent to 35 years of work with a mean respirable dust level at current allowed limits of 2 mg/m^3) could be expected to develop a clinically important (>20%) loss of FEV_1 attributable to dust (65). Among smoking miners, the estimate attributable to dust was 6.6% (95% CI:4.9%–8.4%) (65). The combined effect of dust and smoking can potentially account for a large number of cases of COPD (66). Coal mining dust contains predominantly coal dust, but it can also contain a high degree of silica complicating the interpretation of exposure-response relationships for coal dust and obstructive lung deficits.

Asbestos

Historically, occupational exposure to asbestos dust occurred most heavily in mining and quarrying, asbestos products manufacturing, and workplaces where asbestos was used for its heat insulation properties (e.g. shipyards). In the presence of asbestosis, lung function impairment associated with asbestos dust exposure is primarily a restrictive ventilator deficit. Nonetheless, epidemiological studies have shown that exposure to asbestos can be associated with obstructive as well as restrictive lung function impairment (67–68). This suggests that asbestosis-related functional changes can be coexistent with dust-related airway disease. In a longitudinal study, workers with heavy asbestos exposure had a steeper decline in both FEV_1 and FVC in comparison to workers exposed to cement and polyvinyl chloride; this steeper decline was found in nonsmokers and smokers (68).

Portland cement and other inorganic dusts

A variety of dusts that are less fibrogenic than coal, silica, and asbestos nonetheless have been found to be associated with airflow limitation. Some studies reported significantly lower $FEV_1\%$ values in workers exposed to cement in comparison to unexposed workers, suggesting that exposure to occupational factors in cement plants may lead to obstructive impairment (69). In other studies, however, no relationship between exposure to Portland cement dust and airflow limitation was found (70). These results suggest that exposure levels may play an important role in obstructive disease causation with Portland cement exposure. It should also be noted that Portland cement manufacture is also associated with irritant gas (sulfur dioxide) exposure; thus, cement exposure may be as relevant to the epidemiology of irritant gas as inorganic dust exposure. A recent study using CT-scan analysis, showed airway thickening and narrowing in workers exposed to cement dust with normal spirometry (71), suggesting that early changes in the airways could not be excluded with a normal spirometry. Finally, it is also important not to confuse cement with concrete dust exposure, the latter being a source of silica as well; the clinical relevance of concrete dust is highlighted by the clinical case scenario presented at the outset, specific to A1AT deficiency, but also generalizable.

Other agents

Airborne exposures associated with welding fumes include inorganic materials such as volatilized metal and submicron particles from both the welding rod and the base metal being welded; fumes from burning metal coatings, shielding gases, fluxes; and, often, dust or other airborne inorganic contaminants present in the surrounding workplace (historically, for example, asbestos from "welding blankets"). The nature and extent of exposures experienced by welders have been reviewed by many authors and have been shown to vary widely and are often in excess of regulated occupational exposure limits or guidelines. Most welding materials are alloy mixtures of metals characterized by different steels that may contain iron, manganese, chromium, and nickel. Animal studies have indicated that the presence and combination of different metal constituents is an important determinant in the potential pneumotoxic responses associated with welding fumes (72).

Gas inhalation can also be important in welding, especially exposure to oxides of nitrogen. Some welders experience acute airflow obstruction demonstrated by changes in airflow rates over a work shift (73).

Laboratory studies have provided evidence that welding exposure is linked to oxidative stress, thus providing mechanistic support for the hypothesis of inflammatory-mediated airway obstruction (74). Epidemiological studies have shown that welders experience increased cough and phlegm in association with measures of increased cumulative exposure to welding (75); however, one study found that bronchitis symptoms were reversible and not associated with lung function decline over a subsequent 3-year period (76). The possibility that the inflammatory response

to welding fume components may be lessened by the development of "tolerance" has been suggested (77).

Evidence of chronic airflow obstruction in relation to measures of welding exposure has been seen in most, but not all, studies designed to investigate this outcome and in one study functional changes in small airways among nonsmoking welders were reported (78). A longitudinal investigation of the same population of shipyard welders and burners in which welding-related functional abnormalities had been limited to smokers in cross-sectional analysis, Chinn and colleagues, found airflow obstruction in both smokers and nonsmokers that was linked to the nonuse of local exhaust ventilation while welding (79). Also relevant, a large cohort study observed a small but statistically significant welding-associated decline among nonsmokers but not current or exsmokers (80). On the contrary, a systematic review published in 2013, indicated that the difference with the nonexposed in FEV_1 decline was larger in smoker welders than in nonsmoker welders, suggesting smoking cessation as an effective preventive measure beside welding fumes exposure reduction (81).

In addition to welding fume, which includes a complex mix of metals as noted, certain individual metals have specific links to COPD. Vanadium is a metal that is a natural contaminant of fossil fuels and is also mined and milled for use in steelmaking and other industrial applications. Vanadium is associated epidemiologically with bronchitis (82). Moreover, the vanadium content in oil field fires has been suspected as a contributory factor in the adverse airway effects of the acrid smoke produced in such scenarios. Cadmium exposure is causally associated with airway inflammation and emphysema in experimental models (83) and is epidemiologically associated with lung function decrements (84) and emphysema in occupational exposure (85). A link between the cadmium content in cigarettes and smoking-related emphysema has been suggested (86). Moreover, cadmium blood levels were associated to a lung function decline also after a detailed adjusting for smoking (87) and in male never-smokers (86). Another metal under investigation for a possible association with emphysema is indium, where along with interstitial changes, emphysema progression at CT scan (88) and obstructive functional impairment were described (89). Furthermore, repeated exposure to irritants may have a role in causing chronic airway inflammation and airway impairment. Since the seminal study of Becklake on chronic airway effect of nitrous gases (8), other irritants seem to be involved in chronic and nonreversible airway damage, as in pulp mill workers experiencing repeated acute inhalation events due to sulfur dioxide and chlorine, that have been related to chronic bronchitis (90) and lung function impairment (91). More recently, an increased incidence of doctor-diagnosed COPD was found in nurses and it was associated with the use of disinfectants, including bleach, to clean surfaces and medical instruments (92). Workplace exposure to secondhand smoking (SHS) is considered another important risk factor for chronic bronchitis (93). A recent review evaluates the role of workplace SHS in lung function impairment finding limited evidence (94); however, the authors did not take into account the results of the COPD gene study, where the PAF of COPD attributable to SHS exposure for more than 20 years was 9% and work-related SHS exposure for 10 years increased the risk of COPD by 12% (95).

Future research needs

Many aspects of the relationship between COPD and occupational exposures await further investigation. For example, the relationship between occupational factors and COPD disease severity remains to be explored more fully. Research addressing systematic approaches to disease attribution on an individual basis for persons with COPD and multiple risk factors including occupational exposure could assist clinicians (96). Further, the role of occupational factors in emphysema (as opposed to airflow obstruction), defined by pathology or radiology is far from being fully delineated in occupational cohort and population-based studies. The detrimental impact of dusty work in A1AT deficiency, as highlighted in the Case Scenario presented at the outset, underscores the biological plausibility of this association, which has been further supported by miner autopsy studies and recent genetic studies. Beyond coal dust, silica, and asbestos, exposure-specific epidemiological studies in other cohorts, linked to experimental models, are needed to further clarify the pathophysiology of occupationally-related COPD and chronic bronchitis. This is also certainly true for organic dusts, as addressed elsewhere in this text. Clearly, much remains to be investigated regarding prevention. However, some attempts to review the available evidence on work-related COPD and chronic bronchitis prevention and to propose specific intervention have been made by national scientific societies (96, 97). For the entire range of occupationally related obstructive lung disease, further elucidation of the mechanisms of injury arising from diverse agents that can lead to such a heterogeneous group of responses remains a research priority.

Summary

Occupational exposures are relevant to obstructive airway diseases across a wide spectrum of diagnostic entities. For COPD and chronic bronchitis, the consistency of findings from multiple studies worldwide, using a variety of analytic approaches in heterogeneous populations and over a wide range of working conditions, strongly supports a causal association between occupational exposures and disease. Thus, it is reasonable to assume that 14% of COPD (3 in 20 cases) is attributable to work factors. Furthermore, as cigarette smoking declines, nonsmoking causes of COPD, including salaried and unsalaried working conditions (which can include biomass fuel cooking), will become even more prominent.

For selected mineral dusts and fumes, multiple epidemiological studies have shown an association between occupational exposure lung function impairment in both never-smokers and smokers, the latter after adjustment for smoking. There are likely to be various mechanisms by which such exposures can cause lung function impairment or chronic bronchitis. Whatever the underlying pathways, multiple epidemiological studies of large coal and hard rock mining cohorts have clearly established that both coal and silica dust are associated with obstructive impairment due to the effect of dust itself, independent of the presence of pneumoconiosis radiographically or a restrictive deficit physiologically. Data for other occupational factors are more limited due to smaller cohorts and more heterogeneous exposures.

Although beyond the scope of this chapter on COPD, chronic bronchitis, and emphysema, emerging awareness of occupational lung disease processes that target the terminal airways, in particular obliterative bronchiolitis obliterans (BO), may lead to better understanding of the role of work-related exposures across a range of pathologies. This pertains to the well-established association between diacetyl and BO (98), as well as the much less clear links between military service and BO (99).

Clinicians should be alert to the possibility that COPD, chronic bronchitis, and/or emphysema may be related to past or current occupational exposures. A history of smoking, in and of itself, does not preclude a link between work and obstructive lung disease. For fibrogenic dusts, the presence of interstitial disease radiographically or a restrictive ventilatory deficit by lung function testing does not exclude the presence of concomitant dust-related obstruction. Similarly, mixed obstructive and restrictive deficits may be seen with other scenarios as well, in particular in association with exposures suspected of causing bronchiolitis, potentially within a spectrum of pathological responses. When a clinical suspicion arises that a patient may have disease that is related to a novel exposure or may be part of a larger disease outbreak of occupationally related obstructive disease from an established risk factor, reporting to public health authorities may facilitate the recognition of a case cluster in a workplace and the prevention of further disease in coworkers.

References

1. Zutler M, Quinlan PJ, Blanc PD. Alpha-1-antitrypsin deficient man presenting with lung function decline associated with dust exposure: a case report. J Med Case Rep. 2011;5:154.
2. Thackrah CT. The Effects of Arts, Trades, and Professions, and of Civic States and Habits of Living, on Health and Longevity. 2nd ed. London: Longman; 1832. Edinburgh: Livingstone; 1957 (Reprint).
3. Goodman N, Lane RE, Rampling SB. Chronic bronchitis: an introductory examination of existing data. BMJ. 1953;2:237–43.
4. Fletcher CM. Disability and mortality from chronic bronchitis in relation to dust exposure. AMA Arch Ind Health. 1958;18:368–73.
5. Vestbo J, Prescott E. Update on the "Dutch hypothesis" for chronic respiratory disease. Thorax. 1998;53:S15–19.
6. Elias J. The relationship between asthma and COPD. Lessons from transgenic mice. Chest. 2004;126:111S–6S.
7. Davison AG, Newman Taylor AJ, Darbyshire J, et al. Cadmium fume inhalation and emphysema. Lancet. 1988;1:663–7.
8. Becklake MR, Goldman HI, Bosman AR, Freed CC. The long-term effects of exposure of nitrous fumes. Am Rev Tuberc. 1957;76:398–409.
9. Becklake M. Chronic airflow limitation: its relationship to work in dusty occupations. Chest. 1985;88:608–17.
10. Becklake MR. Occupational exposures: evidence for a causal association with chronic obstructive pulmonary disease. Am Rev Respir Dis. 1989;140:S85–91.
11. Balmes J, Becklake M, Blanc P, et al. American Thoracic Society statement: occupational contribution to the burden of airway disease. Am J Respir Crit Care Med. 2003;167:787–97.
12. Blanc PD, Annesi-Maesano I, Balmes JR, et al. The occupational burden of nonmalignant respiratory diseases. An official American Thoracic Society and European Respiratory Society statement. Am J Respir Crit Care Med. 2019;199(11):1312–34.
13. Eden E. Asthma and COPD in alpha-1 antitrypsin deficiency. Evidence for the Dutch hypothesis. COPD. 2010;7:366–74.
14. Global Strategy for the Diagnosis, Management and Prevention of COPD, Global Initiative for Chronic Obstructive Lung Disease (GOLD). 2020. https://goldcoped.org/
15. Jaakkola MS, Lajunen TK, Jaakkola JJK. Indoor mold odor in the workplace increases the risk of asthma-COPD overlap syndrome: a population-based incident case-control study. Clin Transl Allergy. 2020;10:3.
16. Tommola M, Ilmarinen P, Tuomisto LE, et al. Occupational exposures and asthma-COPD overlap in a clinical cohort of adult- onset asthma. ERJ Open Res. 2019;5(4):00191–2019.
17. Ojanguren I, Moullec G, Hobeika J, et al. Clinical and inflammatory characteristics of Asthma-COPD overlap in workers with occupational asthma. PLOS ONE. 2018;13(3):e0193144.
18. Lytras T, Kogevinas M, Kromhout H, et al. Occupational exposures and 20-year incidence of COPD: the European Community Respiratory Health Survey. Thorax. 2018;73(11):1008–15.
19. Lytras T, Kogevinas M, Kromhout H, et al. Occupational exposures and incidence of chronic bronchitis and related symptoms over two decades: the European Community Respiratory Health Survey. Occup Environ Med. 2019;76(4):222–229.

20. GBD 2016 Occupational Chronic Respiratory Risk Factors Collaborators; GBD 2016 occupational chronic respiratory risk factors collaborators. Global and regional burden of chronic respiratory disease in 2016 arising from non-infectious airborne occupational exposures: a systematic analysis for the Global Burden of Disease Study 2016. Occup Environ Med. 2020;77(3):142–50.

21. Doney B, Kurth L, Halldin C, et al. Occupational exposure and airflow obstruction and self-reported COPD among ever-employed US adults using a COPD-job exposure matrix. Am J Ind Med. 2019;62(5):393–403.

22. Sadhra SS, Mohammed N, Kurmi OP, et al. Occupational exposure to inhaled pollutants and risk of airflow obstruction: a large UK population-based UK Biobank cohort. Thorax. 2020;75(6):468–75.

23. Kurth L, Doney B, Halldin C, Hale J, Frenk SM. Airflow obstruction among ever-employed U.S. adults aged 18-79 years by industry and occupation: NHANES 2007-2008 to 2011-2012. Am J Ind Med. 2019;62(1):30–42.36.

24. De Matteis S, Jarvis D, Darnton A, et al. The occupations at increased risk of COPD: analysis of lifetime job-histories in the population-based UK Biobank Cohort. Eur Respir J. 2019;54(1).

25. Blanc PD, Menezes A-M B, Plana E, et al. Occupational exposures and COPD: an ecological analysis of international data. Eur Respir J. 2009;33:298–304.

26. Trupin L, Earnest G, San Pedro M, et al. The occupational burden of chronic obstructive pulmonary disease. Eur Respir J. 2003;22:1–9.

27. Blanc PD, Iribarren C, Trupin L, et al. Occupational exposures and the risk of COPD: dusty trades revisited. Thorax. 2009;64:6–12.

28. Blanc PD, Eisner MD, Trupin L, et al. The association between occupational factors and adverse health outcomes in chronic obstructive pulmonary disease. Occup Environ Med. 2004;61:661–7.

29. Paulin LM, Diette GB, Blanc PD, et al. Occupational exposures are associated with worse morbidity in patients with chronic obstructive pulmonary disease. Am J Respir Crit Care Med. 2015;191(5):557–65.

30. Sunyer J, Zock JP, Kromhout H, et al. Lung function decline, chronic bronchitis, and occupational exposures in young adults. Am J Respir Crit Care Med. 2005;172(9):1139–45.

31. Mehta AJ, Thun GA, Imboden M, et al. Interactions between SERPINA1 PiMZ genotype, occupational exposure and lung function decline. Occup Environ Med. 2014;71(4):234–40.

32. Alif SM, Dharmage S, Benke G, et al. Occupational exposure to solvents and lung function decline: a population based study. Thorax. 2019;74(7):650–8.

33. de Jong K, Boezen HM, Kromhout H, et al. Association of occupational pesticide exposure with accelerated longitudinal decline in lung function. Am J Epidemiol. 2014;179(11):1323–30.

34. Marchetti N, Garshick E, Kinney GL, et al. Association between occupational exposure and lung function, respiratory symptoms, and high-resolution computed tomography imaging in COPDGene. Am J Respir Crit Care Med. 2014;190(7):756–62.

35. Torén K, Vikgren J, Olin AC, et al. Occupational exposure to vapor, gas, dust, or fumes and chronic airflow limitation, COPD, and emphysema: the Swedish CArdioPulmonary BioImage Study (SCAPIS pilot). Int J Chron Obstruct Pulmon Dis. 2017;12:3407–13.

36. Paulin LM, Smith BM, Koch A, et al. Occupational exposures and computed tomographic imaging characteristics in the SPIROMICS cohort. Ann Am Thorac Soc. 2018;15(12):1411–9.

37. Hnizdo E, Vallyathan V. Chronic obstructive pulmonary disease due to occupational exposure to silica dust: a review of epidemiological and pathological evidence. Occup Environ Med. 2003;60:237–43.

38. Castranova V. From coal mine dust to quartz: mechanisms of pulmonary pathogenicity. Inhal Toxicol. 2000;12:7–14.

39. Vallyathan V. Generation of oxygen radicals by minerals and its correlation to cytotoxicity. Environ Health Perspect. 1994;102:111–5.

40. Zay K, Loo S, Xie C, et al. Role of neutrophils and alpha1-antitrypsin in coal- and silica-induced connective tissue breakdown. Am J Physiol. 1999;276:L269–79.

41. Dai J, Gilks B, Price K, Churg A. Mineral dust directly indices epithelial and interstitial fibrogenic mediators and matrix components in the airway wall. Am J Respir Crit Care Med. 1998;158:1907–13.

42. Churg A, Zay K, Li K. Mechanisms of mineral dust induced emphysema. Environ Health Perspect. 1997:1215–8.

43. Churg A. The uptake of mineral particles by pulmonary epithelial cells. State of the Art. Am J Respir Crit Care Med. 1996;154:1124–40.

44. Würtz ET, Brasch-Andersen C, Steffensen R, et al. Heme oxygenase 1 polymorphism, occupational vapor, gas, dust, and fume exposure and chronic obstructive pulmonary disease in a Danish population-based study. Scand J Work Environ Health. 2020;46(1):96–104.

45. van der Plaat DA, Vonk JM, Terzikhan N, et al. Occupational exposure to gases/fumes and mineral dust affect DNA methylation levels of genes regulating expression. Hum Mol Genet. 2019;28(15):2477–85.

46. Wright JL, Cagle P, Churg A, et al. Diseases of the small airways. Am Rev Respir Dis. 1992;146:240–62.

47. American Thoracic Society. Adverse effects of crystalline silica exposure. Am J Respir Crit Care Med. 1997;155:761–5.

48. Hnizdo E. Loss of lung function associated with exposure to silica dust and with smoking and its relation to disability and mortality in South African gold miners. Br J Ind Med. 1992;49:472–9.

49. Humerfelt S, Eide GE, Gulsvik A. Association of years of occupational quartz exposure with spirometric airflow limitation in Norwegian men aged 30–46 years. Thorax. 1998;53:649–55.

50. Vacek PM, Verma DK, Graham WG, et al. Mortality in Vermont granite workers and its association with silica exposure. Occup Environ Med. 2011;68:312–8.

51. Graber JM, Stayner LT, Cohen RA, et al. Respiratory disease mortality among US coal miners; results after 37 years of follow-up. Occup Environ Med. 2014;71(1):30–9.

52. Hnizdo E, Sluis-Cremer GK, Abramowitz JA. Emphysema type in relation to silica dust exposure in South African gold miners. Am Rev Respir Dis. 1991;143:1241–7.

53. Kinsella M, Muller N, Vedal S, et al. Emphysema in silicosis. A comparison of smokers with nonsmokers using pulmonary function testing and computed tomography. Am Rev Respir Dis. 1990;141:1497–500.

54. Hnizdo E, Sluis-Cremer GK, et al. Emphysema and airway obstruction in non-smoking South African gold miners with long exposure to silica dust. Occup Environ Med. 1994;51:557–63.

55. Ophir N, Shai AB, Alkalay Y, et al. Artificial stone dust-induced functional and inflammatory abnormalities in exposed workers monitored quantitatively by biometrics. ERJ Open Res. 2016;2(1):00086–2015.

56. Rogan JM, Attfield MD, Jacobsen M, et al. Role of dust in the working environments in development of chronic bronchitis in British coal miners. Brit J Ind Med. 1973;30:217–26.

57. Marine WM, Gurr D, Jacobsen M. Clinically important respiratory effects of dust exposure and smoking in British coal miners. Am Rev Respir Dis. 1988;137:106–12.

58. Soutar CA, Hurley JF, Miller BG, et al. Dust concentration and respiratory risks in coalminers: key risk estimates from British Pneumoconiosis Field Research. Occup Environ Med. 2004;61:477–81.

59. Lange AM. Characterization and measurements of the industrial environment. In: Merchant JA, ed. Mineralogy. Occupational Respiratory Disease. U.S. Dept of Health and Human Services (NIOSH) Publication No. 86–102, 1986.

60. Seixas NS, Robins TG, Attfield MD, Moulton LH. Longitudinal and cross sectional analyses of exposure to coal mine dust and pulmonary function in new miners. Brit J Ind Med. 1993;50:929–37.

61. Kurth L, Laney AS, Blackley DJ, et al. Prevalence of spirometry-defined airflow obstruction in never-smoking working US coal miners by pneumoconiosis status. Occup Environ Med. 2020;77(4):265–7.

62. Beeckman LA, Wang ML, Petsonk EL, Wagner GR. Rapid declines in FEV_1 and subsequent respiratory symptoms, illnesses, and mortality in coal miners in the United States. Am J Respir Crit Care Med. 2001;163:633–9.

63. Blackley DJ, Laney AS, Halldin CN, et al. Profusion of opacities in simple coal worker's pneumoconiosis is associated with reduced lung function. Chest. 2015;148(5):1293–9.

64. Kuempel ED, Wheeler MW, Smith RJ, et al. Contributions of dust exposure and cigarette smoking to emphysema severity in U.S. coal miners. Am J Respir Crit Care Med. 2009;180:257–64.

65. Oxman AD, Muir DCF, Shannon HS, et al. Occupational dust exposure and chronic obstructive pulmonary disease. Am Rev Respir Dis. 1993;148:38–48.

66. Hnizdo E, Baskind E, Sluis-Cremer GK. Combined effect of silica dust exposure and tobacco smoking on the prevalence of respiratory impairments among gold miners. Scand J Work Environ Health. 1990;16:411–22.

67. Kennedy SM, Vedal S, Muller N, et al. Lung function and chest radiograph abnormalities among construction insulators. Am J Ind Med. 1991;20:673–84.

68. Siracusa A, Cicioni C, Volpi R, et al. Lung function among asbestos cement factory workers: cross-sectional and longitudinal study. Am J Ind Med. 1984;5:315–25.

69. Saric M, Kalacic I, Holetic A. Follow-up of ventilatory lung function in a group of cement workers. Br J Ind Med. 1976;33:18–24.

70. Fell AKM, Thomassen TR, Kristensen P, et al. Respiratory symptoms and ventilatory function in workers exposed to Portland cement dust. J Occup Environ Med. 2003;45:1008–14.
71. Kim T, Cho HB, Kim WJ, et al. Quantitative CT-based structural alterations of segmental airways in cement dust-exposed subjects. Respir Res. 2020;21(1):133.
72. Antonini JM, Lewis AB, Roberts JR, Whaley DA. Pulmonary effects of welding fumes: review of worker and experimental animal studies. Am J Ind Med. 2003;43:350–60.
73. Fishwick D, Bradshaw LM, Slater T, Pearce N. Respiratory symptoms, across-shift lung function changes and lifetime exposures of welders in New Zealand. Scand J Work Environ Health. 1997;23:351–8.
74. Li GJ, Zhang LL, Lu L, et al. Occupational exposure to welding fume among welders: alterations of manganese, iron, zinc, copper, and lead in body fluids and the oxidative stress status. J Occup Environ Med. 2004;46:241–8.
75. Bradshaw LM, Fishwick D, Slater T, Pearce N. Chronic bronchitis, work related respiratory symptoms, and pulmonary function in welders in New Zealand. Occup Environ Med. 1998;55:150–4.
76. Beckett WS, Pace PE, Sferlazza SJ, et al. Airway reactivity in welders: a controlled prospective cohort study. J Occup Environ Med. 1996;38:1229–38.
77. Fine JM, Gordon T, Chen LC, et al. Characterization of clinical tolerance to inhaled zinc oxide in naive subjects and sheet metal workers. J Occup Environ Med. 2000;42:1085–91.
78. Hjortsberg U, Orbaek P, Arborelius M Jr. Small airways dysfunction among non-smoking shipyard arc welders. Br J Ind Med. 1992;49:441–4.
79. Chinn DJ, Cotes JE, el Gamal FM, Wollaston JF. Respiratory health of young shipyard welders and other tradesmen studied cross-sectionally and longitudinally. Occup Environ Med. 1995;52:33–42.
80. Thaon I, Demange V, Herin F, et al. Increased lung function decline in blue-collar welders exposed to welding fumes. Chest. 2012;142:192–9.
81. Szram J, Schofield SJ, Cosgrove MP, et al. Welding, longitudinal lung function decline and chronic respiratory symptoms: a systematic review of cohort studies. Eur Respir J. 2013;42(5):1186–93.
82. Irsigler GB, Visser PJ, Spangenberg PA. Asthma and chemical bronchitis in vanadium plant workers. Am J Ind Med. 1999;35:366–74.
83. Kirschvink N, Vincke G, Fiévez L, et al. Repeated cadmium nebulizations induce pulmonary MMP-2 and MMP-9 production and emphysema in rats. Toxicology. 2005;211:36–48.
84. Moitra S, Blanc PD, Sahu S. Adverse respiratory effects associated with cadmium exposure in small-scale jewelry workshops in India. Thorax. 2013;68(6):565–70.
85. Torén K, Olin AC, Johnsson Å, et al. The association between cadmium exposure and chronic airflow limitation and emphysema: the Swedish CArdioPulmonary BioImage Study (SCAPIS pilot). Eur Respir J. 2019;54(5):190096.
86. Oh CM, Oh IH, Lee JK, et al. Blood cadmium levels are associated with a decline in lung function in males. Environ Res. 2014;132:119–25.
87. Mannino DM, Holguin F, Greves HM, et al. Urinary cadmium levels predict lower lung function in current and former smokers: data from the Third National Health and Nutrition Examination Survey. Thorax. 2004;59:194–8.
88. Nakano M, Omae K, Uchida K, et al. Five-year cohort study: emphysematous progression of indium-exposed workers. Chest. 2014;146(5):1166–75.
89. Amata A, Chonan T, Omae K, et al. High levels of indium exposure relate to progressive emphysematous changes: a 9-year longitudinal surveillance of indium workers. Thorax. 2015;70(11):1040–6.
90. Andersson E, Murgia N, Nilsson T, et al. Incidence of chronic bronchitis in a cohort of pulp mill workers with repeated gassings to sulphur dioxide and other irritant gases. Environ Health. 2013;12:113.
91. Henneberger PK, Lax MB, Ferris BG Jr. Decrements in spirometry values associated with chlorine gassing events and pulp mill work. Am J Respir Crit Care Med. 1996;153(1):225–31.
92. Dumas O, Varraso R, Boggs KM, et al. Association of occupational exposure to disinfectants with incidence of chronic obstructive pulmonary disease among US female nurses. JAMA Netw Open. 2019;2(10):e1913563.218.
93. Pelkonen MK, Laatikainen TK, Jousilahti P. The relation of environmental tobacco smoke (ETS) to chronic bronchitis and mortality over two decades. Respir Med. 2019;154:34–9.
94. Lee PN, Forey BA, Coombs KJ, et al. Epidemiological evidence relating environmental smoke to COPD in lifelong non-smokers: a systematic review. F1000Res. 2018;7:146.
95. van Koeverden I, Blanc PD, Bowler RP, et al. Secondhand tobacco smoke and COPD risk in smokers: a COPD gene study cohort subgroup analysis. COPD. 2015;12(2):182–9.
96. Maestrelli P, Boschetto P, Carta P, et al. Linee Guida della Società Italiana di Medicina del Lavoro ed Igiene Industriale per la sorveglianza sanitaria di lavoratori esposti ad irritanti e tossici per l'apparato respiratorio. Tipografia PIME Editrice. 2009.
97. Fishwick D, Sen D, Barber C, et al. Occupational chronic obstructive pulmonary disease: a standard of care. Occup Med (Lond). 2015;65(4):270–82.
98. Hubbs AF, Kreiss K, Cummings KJ. Flavorings-related lung disease: a brief review and new mechanistic data. Toxicol Pathol. 2019;47(8):1012–1026.
99. Garshick E, Abraham JH, Baird CP, et al. Respiratory health after military service in southwest Asia and Afghanistan. An Official American Thoracic Society Workshop Report. Ann Am Thorac Soc. 2019;16(8):e1–e16.

26

BUILDING-RELATED ILLNESSES AND MOLD-RELATED CONDITIONS

Christopher Carlsten,[1] Brett J. Green,[2] Jean-Luc Malo,[3] and David I. Bernstein[4]
[1]Respiratory Medicine, Department of Medicine, Faculty of Medicine, University
of British Columbia, Vancouver, British Columbia, Canada
[2]National Institute for Occupational Safety and Health, CDC, Morgantown, West Virginia, USA
[3]Hôpital du Sacré-Cœur de Montréal and Université de Montréal, Montréal, Québec, Canada
[4]Division of Immunology, Allergy and Rheumatology, University of Cincinnati College of Medicine, Cincinnati, Ohio, USA

Contents

WORKPLACE/CASE SCENARIO

As a member of a workers' compensation committee, you are requested to offer expertise on chronic work-associated illnesses reported in eight teachers at the same elementary school. Maintenance of the 75-year-old elementary school building has been neglected in recent years. Water leaks originating from the roof, windows, and leaking pipes have damaged ceilings and walls. A report prepared by an industrial hygienist noted poor ventilation and growths of several mold species, including *Aspergillus versicolor* and *Chaetomium globosum* in air samples. Mushrooms have additionally been reported in washrooms and the basement. The teachers reported a variety of work-related symptoms including shortness of breath, cough, wheezing, watery and itchy eyes, and nasal congestion. Some teachers have lost weight and others have experienced fatigue and depression. Two teachers have a remote history of childhood asthma. Skin-prick testing showed that four of eight teachers were positive to various indoor mold species, house dust mite, or rodent and pet allergens. Baseline spirometry was normal in all teachers but four demonstrated increased nonspecific bronchial hyperresponsiveness (NSBH) to methacholine. A technician assessed serial spirometry during 2 days at work in all teachers and two exhibited progressive falls of ≥20% in forced expiratory volume in 1 second (FEV_1) at the end of a day at work.

What is the most likely diagnosis in these eight teachers?

Introduction

Background

Building-related illness refers to a complex of diseases that are "causally linked to indoor environmental exposures within a building and is applied to the nonindustrial environments such as office buildings, schools, or day care centers and where the causative agent or physiologic mechanism can be identified" (1). This includes various specific (Table 26.1) and nonspecific conditions that are related to infectious, allergic, inflammatory, irritant and/or nonspecific processes. The latter nonspecific type that is associated with mucous membrane complaints, headache, and cognitive difficulties is what is generally referred to as the sick building syndrome (SBS) or sick house syndrome, the latter referring to private dwellings. In a report published in 2018 (2), the World Health Organization estimated that around 4 million people die prematurely from illness attributable to household air pollution, particularly due to inadequate cooking practices with poorly vented stoves using solid fuels and kerosene; indoor air pollution may be associated with stroke, ischemic heart disease, chronic obstructive pulmonary disease (COPD), and lung cancer in adults as well as childhood pneumonia. Human beings currently spend approximately 90% of their time in indoor environments (3) and can be exposed to a broad diversity of chemicals, microorganisms, and particulate matter that may impact the health of the worker. The increased frequency of asthma has also been attributed, among other causes, to the augmentation of mites and pets in the indoor environment. Immediate skin-prick test (SPT) reactivity to one or more ubiquitous common allergens is now documented in nearly 50% of young adults living in developed countries with reactivity to house dust mites in one-third and pets in one-fourth of subjects (4).

Indoor air quality can have an impact on human health and is due to multiple factors including: moisture infiltration (leaking roof, pipes, and windows); house dust mite and microbial proliferation such as fungi due to high relative humidity (i.e. >50%); increasing allergen exposure load; inadequate air intake and filtration; mold; exposure to particulate matter from indoor and outdoor sources; various gases (organic and carbonyl compounds); and insufficient thermal control (1). Older and even newer buildings can be problematic (5). Whereas compliance with the presence of regulated compounds can be satisfactory, unregulated compounds can contribute substantially to levels of volatile organic compounds (VOCs) even in newly built nonindustrial environments (5). Indoor pollution may be related to socioeconomic status in developed countries, causing exposure disparities due to differences in housing construction and living behaviors (e.g. cooking with natural gas or propane) as previously mentioned (6).

Environmental intolerance is a syndrome that describes the "attribution of several, multisystem symptoms to specific environmental exposures, such as exposure to odorous/pungent chemicals, certain buildings, electromagnetic fields and everyday sounds" with overlap of symptoms caused by such exposures (7). Conditions such as building-related illnesses and SBS as well as multiple chemical sensitivity syndrome or idiopathic environmental intolerance (Chapter 19) are therefore related to this more general entity.

Health professionals in various fields may encounter patients with symptomatic features of SBS. The first important issue is to rule out other diseases that may mimic SBS symptomatology. In the investigation of SBS, environmental hygienists are often requested to offer their expertise in assessing for potential causal aspects either in individual dwellings or workplaces. In a retrospective survey of 239 participants with nonspecific building-related symptoms seen in a specialized clinic in Sweden, 50% of subjects had symptoms persist for at least 7 years while approximately one-third still reported eye, facial, and nasal mucosal symptoms. These symptoms were also more frequent than in the general population (8).

Definition

SBS is a "concept" (9) that appeared in the scientific literature in the 1970s, a syndrome that involves several symptomatic manifestations referable to the mucous membranes, causes upper and lower airway irritation, and is accompanied by nonspecific symptoms such as headache, fatigue, stress, somatization, as well as impaired adaptation to psychosocial situations. The pathophysiology of SBS has not been elucidated. It shares some features with irritant-induced asthma (Chapter 19) as exposure to low-molecular-weight (LMW) irritants is concerned, hypersensitivity pneumonitis (Chapter 24) and airway diseases due to organic dust exposure (Chapter 23) as exposure to molds and mold-derived products is relevant, and some others to sensitizer-induced occupational asthma (OA) (Chapter 4) as various allergenic products are also present. These various pathophysiological aspects are covered and presented in these respective chapters. In a broad sense, SBS is the general term describing health disturbances associated with exposure to the indoor environment (10). A cross-sectional study of more than 4000 US office workers found that headaches and migraines are frequent, affecting 38% and 21% subjects, respectively, on more than 1–3 days in the past 4 weeks (11).

Objective testing

Results of objective respiratory, nasal, ocular, and blood tests have been described in some studies (Table 26.1), although none have been validated as a diagnostic for SBS. These include spirometry, assessment of normal nonspecific bronchial hyperresponsiveness (NSBH) (Chapter 8), tear film stability (12) for ocular symptoms, nasal lavage, acoustic rhinomanometry (Chapter 22), allergen skin testing, and serum-specific IgE (Chapter 7), as well as other blood tests for eosinophils and eosinophil cationic protein (ECP). Analysis of nasal proteins obtained by lavage in 37 workers exposed in moldy and damp buildings showed alterations in some innate immunity proteins and alpha-1 antitrypsin, with a different profile depending on the presence of molds (13).

Frequency

Many cross-sectional and some longitudinal studies carried in recent years have attempted to assess the frequency of SBS. Table 26.1 lists some results of representative publications from 2010 onward. Professor Dan Norbäak, former contributor of *Asthma in the Workplace* (1), was involved in several of these surveys. Studies have been mainly carried out in several European countries and Asia. The prevalence/incidence of general, mucosal, dermal, and upper and lower respiratory symptoms is given from studies carried out in samples of the general population and on the occasion of an outbreak. Two longitudinal studies have shown an increased prevalence after 2 years of follow-up in Chinese pupils (Table 26.2, Zhang et al., 2011 and 2014). Sahlberg and coworkers (14) did not find an increased prevalence of symptoms in a 10-year prospective study from 1992–2002 carried out in Sweden. Objectively assessed dampness and visible indoor molds found in homes at baseline were predictors of generalized, mucosal, and dermal symptoms. The presence of NSBH, blood eosinophils, and total IgE was associated with increased incidence of SBS. Studies carried out on the occasion of an outbreak or in a specific workplace generally report a higher prevalence of symptoms.

Risk factors

Social and personal factors, psychosocial work environment

In a study of Swedish residents, social factors such as country of birth, education (number of years), and being unemployed were

TABLE 26.1 Selected Prevalence/Incidence Studies in SBS from 2010 Onward

Authors	Population	Prevalence/Incidence	Other Findings	References
Sahlberg et al., 2010	Random sample of 1000 people living in Sweden	General symptoms: 1991 prev: 48 2001 prev: 42 Mucosal symptoms: 1991 prev: 41 2001 prev: 43 (no significant increase)	Increased risk of onset of symptoms associated with dampness or molds in dwelling during f-up	*1. Sahhlberg, 2010*
Zhang et al., 2011	>1000 Chinese pupils followed for 2 yrs	General symptoms: 2004 prev: 28.1% 2006 prev: 44.3% Improvement while away from school: 27% inc 26%	Crowdedness, SO_2, NO_2, humidity, temperature positively or negatively associated with prevalent and incident symptoms	*2. Zhang, 2011*
Sahlberg et al., 2012	452 adults f-up for 10 yrs in the ECRHS survey (Uppsala part)	General symptoms: inc 8.5% Mucosal symptoms: inc 12.7% Dermal symptoms: inc 6.8%	Dampness or indoor molds at baseline were predictors of incident general, mucosal and dermal symptoms; women at risk; NSBH, eosinophils, ECP and physician diagnosis of asthma at baseline significant predictors	*3. Sahlberg, 2012*
Gomez-Acebo et al., 2013	357 hospital workers on the occasion of an outbreak; "cases" defined by the presence of at least 5 positive answers (mucosal and general symptoms)	192 (54%) identified as "ill" in the cluster analysis	Personal history of allergy, hypercholesterolemia, growing pains, intolerance to foods, symptoms worse with heat at the workplace all significantly predictive of being in the "ill" cluster	*4. Gomez-Acebo, 2013*
Zhang et al., 2014	2134 pupils (baseline) 1325 pupils (2-yr f-up)	General symptoms: prev (baseline) 20.4% Mucosal symptoms: prev (baseline) 22.7% Symptoms improvement away from school: prev (baseline) 39.2%. Increased prev at f-up	Environmental pollution (PM10, SO_2, O3, NO_2) "could increase" the prev and inc of SBS	*5. Zhang, 2014*
Azuma et al., 2015	Nationwide cross-sectional study of >3000 employees in 320 offices in Japan	General symptoms: prev: 14.4% Eye irritation: prev 12.1% Upper respiratory symptoms: prev 8.9%	Symptoms associated with several factors in a multiple logistic regression: unpleasant odors, amount of work, interpersonal conflicts, carpeting, etc. (mix of psychosocial and workspace conditions)	*6. Azuma, 2015*
Lim et al., 2015	695/2192 participants (32%) office workers in a Malaysian academic institution	Dermal symptoms: prev 11.9% Mucosal symptoms: prev 16% General symptoms: prev 23%	Positive skin tests (mite, cat) and high FeNO associated with symptoms; office temperature and humidity associated with office-related symptoms	*7. Lim, 2015*
Magnavita et al., 2015	>4000 workers in Latrium (Italy)	Any of 12 SBS symptoms: prev 27% 5 or more SBS symptoms: prev 3.8% Any of 18 work-related symptoms: prev 32%	In a multiple logistic regression, personal factors, environmental discomfort, job strains associated with SBS symptoms	*8. Magnavita, 2015*
Takaoka et al., 2015	>1000 students in Japan high schools	Mucosal symptoms: Prev 45% General symptoms: prev 39% Skin symptoms: prev 23%	Window condensation, floor dampness, odors, and atopy associated with mucosal, general, and skin symptoms	*9. Takaoka, 2015*

(Continued)

TABLE 26.1 Selected Prevalence/Incidence Studies in SBS from 2010 Onward (*Continued*)

Authors	Population	Prevalence/Incidence	Other Findings	References
Lu et al., 2015	417 randomly selected office workers in 87 office rooms of Taiwan	Eye symptoms: prev 23% Upper respiratory symptoms: prev 15% Nonspecific symptoms: prev 25%	CO_2 and VOC levels associated with some symptoms	*10. Lu, 2016*
Lu et al., 2016	>3000 randomly selected adults in China	Weekly fatigue: prev 15% Weekly headache: prev 4% Weekly eye/nose symptoms: prev 3%	Mold/dampness of floors/ceilings, moldy odors associated with general SBS symptoms; some outdoor factors associated with SBS symptoms but final model significant for indoor factors only	*11. Lu, 2016*
Lind et al., 2017	Population-based questionnaire in >8500 inhabitants in Sweden with >3000 participants	16% with allergy and asthma; 5% with "building intolerance" diagnosed by physician	Among subjects with allergy/asthma, 6% with physician-diagnosed building intolerance (OR: 11–13)	*12. Lind, 2017*
Lu et al., 2017	389 official employees of Taiwan	Nonspecific symptoms: prev 26% Upper respiratory symptoms: prev 16% Eye symptoms: prev 23%	High work pressure, low indoor airflow, CO_2, VOC, temperature more often significantly associated with nonspecific and lower respiratory symptoms	*13. Lu, 2017*
Belachew et al., 2018	Community-based in >3000 random residents of a town northwest Ethiopia	Prev: 21.7% (mainly general and mucosal)	SBS associated with fungal growth, unclean, no-window, charcoal cooking housing conditions	*14. Belachew, 2018*
Claeson et al., 2018	Two community-based populations of ˜5000 in Finland and Sweden	45 (0.09%) who satisfied criteria of building-related intolerance	BRI symptoms significantly associated with wheezing/asthma (OR: 18), eye irritation (OR: 8) + others	*15. Cleason, 2018*
Karvala et al., 2018	>4900 participants of Sweden and Finland	5.6 % fulfilled criteria for self-reported BRI of 12-yr mean duration; 2.5% with "wide-ranging symptoms"	Perceived health poorer and increased somatic and psychiatric comorbidities	*16. Karvala, 2018*
Nakayama et al., 2019	1500 subjects identified as "pre-sick" SBS	Eye symptoms: prev 7% Nasal symptoms: prev 13% Airway symptoms: prev 13%	Higher in 20–29 yrs old group, "condensation," "moisture odors"	*17. Nakayama, 2019*
Kim et al., 2019	314 store workers in 9 underground shopping centers of Seoul, Korea	Skin symptoms: prev 44% Eye symptoms: prev 66% General symptoms: prev 66%	SBS symptoms associated with indoor air quality perceptions and in clothing stores	*18. Kim, 2019*
Smajlovic et al., 2019	258 healthcare workers in Slovenia (response rate: 68%)	6 or more SBS symptoms: prev 12% 2–3 or more SBS symptoms: prev 19%	Lighting and noise problems at work	*19. Kalender Smajlovic, 2019*

Abbreviations: BRI, building-related intolerance; ECP, eosinophil cationic protein; f-up, follow-up; inc, incidence; NSBH, nonspecific bronchial hyperresponsiveness; prev, prevalence; SBS, sick building syndrome; VOC: volatile organic compound.

References: **1.** Sahlberg B, et al. *Scand J Public Health.* 2010;38(3):232–8; **2.** Zhang X et al. *Indoor Air.* 2011;21(6):462–71; **3.** Sahlberg B, et al. *Indoor Air.* 2012;22(4):331–8; **4.** Gómez-Acebo I, et al. *Int J Occup Med Environ Health.* 2013;26(4):563–71; **5.** Zhang X, et al. *PLOS ONE.* 2014;9(11):e112933; **6.** Azuma K, et al. Indoor air quality, and occupational stress. *Indoor Air.* 2015;25(5):499–511; **7.** Lim FL, et al.*Sci Total Environ.* 2015;536:353–61; **8.** Magnavita N, et al. *Int Arch Occup Environ Health.* 2015;88(2):185–96; **9.**Takaoka M, et al. *Glob J Health Sci.* 2015;8(2):165–77; **10.** Lu CY, et al. *Int J Environ Res Public Health.* 2015;12(6):5833–45; **11.** Lu C, et al. *Sci Total Environ.* 2016;560–561:186–96; **12.** Lind N, et al. *J Occup Environ Med.* 2017;59(1):80–4; **13.** Lu CY, et al. *Int J Environ Res Public Health.* 2017 Dec 22;15(1); **14.** Belachew H, et al. *Environ Health Prev Med.* 2018; 27;23(1):54; **15.** Claeson AS, et al. *J Occup Environ Med.* 2018 Apr;60(4):295–300; **16.** Karvala K, et al. *Int J Environ Res Public Health.* 2018;15(9); **17.** Nakayama Y, et al. *Environ Health Prev Med.* 2019;24(1):77; **18.** Kim J, Jang M, Choi K, et al. *BMC Public Health.* 2019;19(1):632; **19.** Kalender Smajlović S, et al. *Int J Environ Res Public Health.* 2019;16(17).

significantly associated with the SBS (15). Although this finding is not constant as previously presented (1), asthma and allergic conditions (i.e. rhinoconjunctivitis, atopic dermatitis) were identified as significant comorbidities of intolerance to chemicals and buildings in some studies (Table 26.1, Lind 2017 and Claeson 2018). Indicators of allergy and atopy were associated with increased presenteeism (reduced productivity at work) in nearly 7500 office workers in a US federal government building complex (16). Objective factors such as NSBR, blood eosinophils, and ECP have been identified as significant predictors of SBS in a prospective cohort (14) (Table 26.1).

Some psychological traits (tendencies to somatization, and neuroticism as well as anxiety and depression) (17) are more frequently found in subjects with SBS (1). Feeling depressed was reported by approximately 23% (work-related in about half) of more than 7500 office workers in a US federal government building complex (49% participation). Low social and supervisor support at work inducing stress seemed to play a role (18). In another

TABLE 26.2 Sources of Dampness and Moisture Infiltration in Buildings

Unsatisfactory management of water outside the building
Drainage, lawn watering, proximity of trees resulting in leaks
Following root or branch penetration of the basement and building envelope
Poor design of walls, roof, and ice dams
Thermal bridges or other design failures inside the floor or the wall construction (particularly if the wall is thick) resulting in condensation and chemical degradation of vinyl floor coverings
Inadequate management of water vapor from outdoors
Poorly installed air barriers in the exterior envelope
Condensation of humid air on cold surfaces
Wrong pressure relationships in conditions that make the building negative to outside air
Inadequate balance of airflows in and out
Sources of indoor moisture
Unsatisfactory air management
Inadequate dehumidification, with mold growth
Leaking roofs, plumbing, and window fixtures
Incorrectly sized air-conditioning systems
Failure of heating, ventilating, and air-conditioning (HVAC) systems

Legend: Table derived from the chapter by Norback D, Miller JD. Building-related illnesses and mold-Related conditions. In: Malo JL, Chan-Yeung M, Bernstein DI, eds. *Asthma in the Workplace*, 4th ed. Boca Raton FL: CRC Press; 2013.

study, psychosocial factors at the individual level but not at the workplace level were associated with the individual perception of indoor environment; these results suggested to the authors that there might be tendencies for overreporting (19).

Indoor climate and exposure in workplace buildings
Climate
Temperature and relative indoor humidity can influence the onset of symptoms. In a study that included objective assessments, tear film stability (used to assess dry eyes) was assessed in 173 university staff office workers and was found to be abnormal on days with higher air temperatures ($\geq$22.1 °C) (12). Neurobehavioral tests performed on 12 subjects conducting typical office work tasks at 22 °C and 30 °C showed that many physiological parameters were affected in the higher temperature test group and included increased heart rate, ventilation, end-tidal CO_2, and reduced tear film quality; all effects encountered in a thermally warm ambient environment (20). In addition, low humidity of less than 40% is the main determinant of altered precorneal tear film and suggests that dry eyes may be responsible for irritant eye symptoms noted by workers in low-humidity office building environments (21).

Ventilation
One of the most important factors to consider is the ventilation rates of buildings. A review of the scientific literature up to 2005 that included 27 peer-reviewed manuscripts concluded that higher rates of ventilation (25 L/s per person) in offices were associated with reduced prevalence of SBS (22). In the same article, the authors also review the historical background behind the concept of satisfactory home and building ventilation (22). Improving personal ventilation at individual workstations decreased the intensity of SBS symptoms induced by exposure to higher humidity and temperature conditions and improved the tear film stability test in 30 healthy subjects (23). In contrast, a study of 16 healthy adults showed that a reduction in ventilation rates over a 4-hour period did not elicit symptoms associated with SBS but reduced cognitive performance (24).

Workers exposed to indoor CO_2 levels >800 ppm were found to be more likely to report more eye irritation or upper respiratory symptoms as investigated in 111 office workers (25). Reducing the level of ambient CO_2 with a CO_2 demand-controlled ventilation system (variable flow) in computer classrooms slightly improved headaches and impressions of tiredness in 200 students (26).

Building dampness and respiratory disease
Moisture infiltration in the indoor environment can result in the growth and proliferation of microbial communities that can include bacteria and fungi. Water-damaged buildings have been previously determined in the peer-reviewed literature to be a common cause of a variety of health-related conditions. A list of outdoor and indoor causes of dampness and moisture in buildings is proposed in Table 26.2.

Bioaerosols that originate from fungi, pollen, and other eukaryotic or prokaryotic organisms (viz. bacteria) may cause immunological bronchial and lung diseases as well as infectious and nonspecific inflammatory effects (mycotoxins, endotoxins) (27). Various fungal species can infiltrate the indoor environment and proliferate on moisture damaged building materials. These fungi are typically hydrophilic, filamentous, and produce networks of hyphae as well as arrangements of asexual spores that vary in size and shape depending on the species. Biotic or abiotic disturbances result in the aerosolization of fungal spores, fragments, and potentially other components from the fungal culture. Airborne fungal spores and fragments can be collected with impaction devices (impactors and impingers) as well as dust sampling cassettes, deposited on slides and examined by a trained microbiologist to identify and quantify the collected fungal spores (28). Airborne fungal spores can be quantified using traditional methods such as cultivation and non-culture-based methods. Using these approaches, *Aspergillus* and *Penicillium* are common genera that are identified in contaminated buildings and houses whereas the outdoor fungal genus *Cladosporium* is predominant in buildings with satisfactory indoor air quality (29). Significant growth of *Aspergillus versicolor*, *Chaetomium globosum*, *Stachybotrys chartarum*, and *Ulocladium chartarum* have been associated with indoor dampness problems (27). Contemporary molecular methods such as quantitative polymerase chain reaction (qPCR) have been developed that allow the quantification of panels of fungi that occur in indoor environments. Internal transcribed spacer region (ITS) sequencing methods have also been developed and have provided a methodological approach to characterize the complete spectrum of fungi in indoor and outdoor environments. ITS sequencing analysis of a water-damaged building reported a much broader assemblage of fungi placed in the phyla Ascomycota and Basidiomycota (30). These studies have also shown that in addition to filamentous fungi, unicellular yeasts particularly placed in the Basidiomycota order, Tremellales, are abundant in air and dust samples and some studies have identified associations with adverse health effects (30). There is poor correlation between results provided by cultures and polymerase chain reaction (PCR) quantitation of species-specific DNA sequences which enable identification of a large variety of fungi and metabolites, suggesting each method offers complementary information (31). These methodological approaches have revealed a much broader assemblage of fungi and fungal products to contribute to nonindustrial working environments and these species should be considered in future investigations.

Type I (IgE dependent) immunological reactivity to molds was evaluated in a cohort study of 769 young apprentices; 15% had immediate SPT reactions to at least one of three common molds, including *Aspergillus* (4). Furthermore, hydrophilic fungi (mainly yeasts) quantification has been proposed as a measure of fungal biomass and a satisfactory marker of SBS in damp indoor environments (31).

Mycotoxins are toxic metabolites derived from molds. Hundreds of mycotoxins have been identified and examples include aflatoxins (metabolites of *Aspergillus*), ochratoxins (from *Aspergillus* and *Penicillium* genera), fumonisins (produced by *Fusarium* species), trichothecenes, and ergot alkaloids (28). Mycotoxins, particularly if absorbed through the ingestion of food or through the skin, can be teratogenic as well as carcinogenic, and are responsible for millions of deaths per year (32). In addition, fungi may also generate VOCs that are also implicated in SBS (33) and can induce inflammation in the lung (34). Gas chromatography-tandem mass spectrometry is a methodological approach that provides reliable assessment of the most frequently occurring airborne mycotoxins (35, 36). Aflatoxins and ochratoxins have also been detected in 11% of airborne samples in waste recycling and recovery facilities (37).

Association with asthma and rhinitis

Dampness and the resulting presence of molds and mites that grow well in humid environments have been implicated to increase the risk of onset and worsening of asthma (38). Jaakkola and coworkers estimated that the fraction of asthma attributable to workplace dampness and molds was 35% in a study of more than 500 adults with newly diagnosed asthma as compared to nearly twice the number of controls in (39). In a review of the scientific literature on the association of dampness and health effects (40 articles published from 1998 to 2000), Bornehag and coworkers concluded that dampness was associated with health effects, mainly atopic and nonatopic asthma and rhinitis; however, the precise causal agents (mites, molds, degraded building materials) could not be precisely ascertained (40). In a meta-analysis that included 33 studies, Fisk and coworkers estimated that the percent increase in unfavorable health outcomes (asthma as well as rhinitis and asthma-like symptoms) for all subjects in damp houses ranged from 30% to 52% (41). By reviewing scientific literature up to 2009, Mendell and coworkers concluded that there was strong evidence of an association between dampness and mold on the one hand and various respiratory conditions on the other hand (not including SBS), but only suggested that possible agents in dust (endotoxin, ergosterol) were also associated with symptoms (42). In the European Community Respiratory Health Survey (ECRHS) study, there was an excess of new asthma (documented by questionnaire and methacholine testing) in homes with reports of water damage (RR:1.5; 95% CI:1.1–1.9) and indoor molds at baseline (RR:1.3; 95%CI:1.0–1.7) as documented in more than 7000 young adults followed for 9 years (43).

The association of asthmatic symptoms with exposure to dampness and biological markers of moisture was also studied in schoolchildren who are considered more susceptible to indoor air pollutants. In a sample of approximately 200 schools in Finland, Spain, and the Netherlands, answers to a questionnaire showed that 24%–47% of all school buildings had different types of moisture problems (44). A large European study (HITEA) carried out in nearly 10,000 children in Spain, the Netherlands and Finland showed that cough at night was more frequent in schools with moisture damage in each of the three countries but the association with other respiratory symptoms was only significant in Finland (45). Examining data from the same HITEA study, Jacobs and coworkers found increased asthma symptoms in nearly 4000 children who attended "damaged schools" based on the number, extent, severity, and location of dampness and moisture damage observations (46). Levels of microbial markers (endotoxin, ergosterol, and *Penicillium chrysogenum* DNA levels) differed greatly between schools and countries, but were often higher in damaged schools (46). In a cross-sectional study of 330 Danish pupils aged 6–10 years old, Holst and coworkers reported that high classroom, but not bedroom dampness (assessed by a building engineer), was negatively associated with airway caliber (FEV$_1$, forced vital capacity) and positively associated with wheezing but not atopy. In the same study, dust microbial content did not influence any health outcome examined (47).

Exposure of animals to organic material containing molds and mold-derived agents has been particularly examined in relation to various airway diseases related to such exposure (Chapter 23). In a murine model, Poole and coworkers showed that inhalation of organic dust caused an influx of activated macrophages in the lung (48), as well as increased CD4+T cells and IL-17-producing CD4+T cells with a leading role of alpha/beta expressing T cells (49). Moreover, there is suggestion that exposure to organic dust can worsen asthmatic status. Warren and coworkers showed that exposure to organic dust increases NSBH as well as eosinophilic and neutrophilc counts in BAL in ovalbumin-sensitized mice (50). Also, bacterial components in indoor dust, represented by extracellular vesicles, can contribute to airway inflammation. These vesicles are internalized by airway epithelial cells and alveolar macrophages; intranasal installation of these vesicles in mice for 4 weeks elicited neutrophilic pulmonary inflammation (51). Beta-(1, 3)-glucan, a constituent of mold wall and mites, enhances eosinophilic, T helper 2, and house dust mite-specific T cells airway response in mice sensitized to house dust mites (52).

Working in damp and moldy buildings is also associated with a significant increase in proteins and alpha-1-antitrypsin in nasal lavage as shown in a sample of workers who reported two- to five-fold more mucosal irritation (including nasal symptoms) and general symptoms (13).

In a retrospective analysis of files of 2200 workers with respiratory symptoms related to damp and moldy working environment that were assessed at the Finnish Institute of Occupational Health from 1995 to 2004, Karvala reported on 201 with a probable and possible diagnosis of OA and 57 with unlikely OA (53). Among the 156 workers with probable OA, 20% had SPT reactivity and 16% had elevated specific IgE to molds (mainly *Aspergillus* and *Cladosporium*). Specific inhalation challenges (SICs), the reference standard to diagnose OA, were positive in 133 workers, with significant reactions to *Aspergillus* (n=85) and *Cladosporium* (n=26). A study of more than 2000 healthcare workers in New York City also showed that the frequency of asthma-related outcomes was higher for those participants who reported moisture or renovation in their work environment (54).

Causes of hypersensitivity pneumonitis

Hypersensitivity pneumonitis (HP) was first reported in farmers by Ramazzini in the eighteenth century (see Chapter 2) and later described as farmer's lung. A similar condition has also been documented in workers with occupational exposure to metal-working fluids (Chapter 24). HP can also be caused by molds in contaminated buildings or with chronic water infiltration (55).

Association with sick building syndrome

Signs of water damage, building moisture, moldy odor, or visible signs of indoor molds are almost invariably associated with symptoms of SBS. Such symptoms were reported by 22% of a random sample of the general Swedish population aged 20–65 years (466 subjects) (56). In a more recent cross-sectional study of nearly 1000 occupants living in 821 family houses across Sweden, a similar proportion (23%) of symptomatic participants was identified (57), and dampness problems were present in 40% of houses. In the follow-up aforementioned study of the Swedish population initially assessed by Norback and Edling (56) carried out 10 years later in 427 subjects, the authors found that there had been a general improvement in the home environment with regard to building dampness and indoor molds. However, the cumulative incidence of subjects with new onset of at least one symptom was 28% for mucosal symptoms and 25% for general symptoms, 10% for headache, and 15% for tiredness. In this cohort, the same group of investigators found that female gender and any type of building dampness at baseline were significant predictors of general and mucosal symptoms at the follow-up (14). Also, bronchial responsiveness to methacholine (a lower slope of the dose-response curve), ECP, and levels of eosinophils at baseline were also significant predictors of mucosal symptoms at follow-up (14). Dampness and molds in workplace buildings were examined in the same Swedish cohort over a 10-year period (1992–2002) and this study showed that the incidence of work-related symptoms (any symptom improving when away from the workplace) was 9.4% (58). Indices of the presence of dampness and molds in workplace buildings (signs of dampness in the floor construction, cumulative exposure to moldy odor, working in a remediated building) were associated with incident work-related symptoms and decreased remission of such symptoms (58) as well as increased bronchial responsiveness and higher levels of ECP. The authors concluded that dampness and molds in the workplace building exert an influence on the incidence and decreased remission of SBS as well as increasing bronchial responsiveness and eosinophilic inflammation (58).

In a sample of 100 office buildings in the United States and using the US Environmental Protection Agency's Building Assessment Survey and Evaluation Study (BASE) data, significant associations were identified between moisture indicators, building-related respiratory and mucous membrane symptoms, as well as fatigue/cognitive dysfunction and headaches (59).

Visual documentation of dampness is generally related to perceptions of odors and sensations of humid and dry air, the latter being also associated with SBS symptoms, as reported in a questionnaire survey of 4530 parents of Chinese children ages 1 to 8 years (60). Smedje and coworkers also showed that the absolute humidity had more influence on SBS symptoms than the relative humidity and moisture load (57).

Exposure to water damage in buildings is associated with an airway inflammatory reaction characterized by an increase in BAL lymphocytes, although there seems to be no change in the CD4/CD8 ratio, contrary to what has been reported in HP (61).

In a Cochrane review of 12 clinical and before-after trials, it was found that repairing houses damaged by dampness and molds significantly decreased asthma- and rhinitis-related symptoms in

adults and pupils' visits to physicians due to a common cold in children (62).

International (55) as well as national general (63) and occupational health (64) agencies have published building and remediation guidelines for improving the sanitary control of dampness and molds at home and at work.

Allergens in workplace buildings

The common indoor allergen sources are mite, molds, furry animals, and cockroaches, and can be present in excessive concentrations in workplace buildings and home environments. In a review, Pieckova outlined the importance of indoor fungal growth, promoted by indoor dampness, as associated with SBS through the indoor release of beta-D-glucan, mycotoxins causing inflammatory and hemorrhagic reactions in the respiratory tract, and VOCs causing inflammatory and hemorrhagic reactions in the respiratory tract (65). Although fungal spores remain in the upper respiratory tract, it seems highly probable that hyphal fragments are able to reach the alveoli (65). Saijo and coworkers (66) sampled more than 5000 newly built dwellings in six prefectures of Japan, with approximately 1500 residents living in 425 households participating. The prevalence of general symptoms was 2%, of mucous symptoms was 3% to 8%, and of respiratory symptoms, 7%. Mites were identified in more than 80% of dwellings. *Cladosporium*, *Penicillium*, and *Aspergillus* molds were commonly identified. A stepwise analysis showed that exposure to *Dermatophagoides* group 1 allergen was associated with nasal symptoms, *Aspergillus* with eye symptoms, and *Rhodotorula* with any reported symptoms. Cockroaches have a high sensitizing potential (67). In the National Health and Nutrition Examination Survey (NHANES) 2005–2006 study, sensitization to cockroach was found in approximately 10% of nearly 3000 children (68). It has been estimated that at least half of urban, low-income homes have a clinically relevant level of cockroach allergen for which environmental interventions can be considered and judged as efficacious (69).

Settled and indoor house dust can be examined for chemical contents (see sections "Volatile Organic Compounds" and "Chemical Components in Settled Dust") and also for microbial content assessed by quantifying a cell wall component that is muramic acid and endotoxins (lipopolysaccharides) as well as fungal presence through the quantification of beta-D-glucan, ergosterol, and fungal DNA measurements done by PCR. New onset of various SBS symptoms was found to be either negatively or positively (depending on the factor) associated with muramic acid as well as total and specific lipopolysaccharides contents in a 2-year prospective study of more than 1000 Chinese pupils (70). In this study, the authors concluded that exposure to bacterial cell wall components can protect against adverse mucosal and general symptoms, whereas fungal DNA concentrations were shown to result in increased school-related symptoms (70). *Acanthamoeba* is an opportunistic protozoan pathogen that has been detected in the ventilation system of commercial buildings and factories in Malaysia. It was found to be significantly correlated with ambient total fungus count and respirable particulates as well as with SBS symptoms, with a five-fold probability of symptoms if present (71).

Air filters can be useful to lower inhalable dust and the concentration of common indoor allergens such as cat and mite allergens (72).

Airborne particles

Particulate matter represents a significant portion of indoor and outdoor air pollution (73). The mean aerodynamic diameter is the index of classification of particulate matter; coarse particles (2.5–10 micron) are deposited in the large airways, whereas fine (<2.5 micron) and ultrafine (<0.1 micron) particles can reach the alveoli and be absorbed in the systemic circulation (73). Standards specifically related to air particles, which can be assessed by filter sampling or direct reading instruments, have been proposed by WHO (74) with regards to hourly and daily exposure. Guidelines for ozone, NO_2, and SO_2 are also presented in this document (74). As a rule, larger particles are mainly present indoors whereas fine particles are a concern in outdoor environments. Particles derived from cooking and heating and generated by fuel and biomass combustion represent an important source of indoor pollution. Indoor cooking is of particular concern in developing countries (2), whereas outdoor origin of pollution and cigarette smoke (currently less so) play a more important role in developed countries. Such exposures have deleterious health effects, causing ischemic cardiovascular disease, COPD, pneumonia, bronchiolitis, and worsening of asthma in children. Prevention of childhood pneumonia by promoting the use of cleaner burning biomass-fueled cookstoves instead of open fires may represent a relevant target for interventions although a community-level open randomized controlled trial in rural Malawi did not show significantly positive results (75). In a study carried out in more than 5000 subjects (65% participation) living in Bejing, Li and coworkers found that living near a highway and environmental tobacco smoke were associated with general and mucosal symptoms of SBS, an effect attributed to particulate pollutants, NO_2, and SO_2 as well as by noise (76). The inflammatory respiratory effect of exposure to particulate matters has been thoroughly reviewed (73) and affects both innate and adaptive immunity. This involves oxidative stress (Chapters 4 and 19), production and release of inflammatory mediators (interleukins, TNF-alpha), as well as modification in the proportion of T cells.

Volatile organic compounds

VOCs are chemicals that, due to their physical properties, evaporate or sublimate easily, being therefore volatile. VOCs include various solvents (toluene, benzene, xylene, terpene, etc.) and formaldehyde, a strong irritant. In the US BASE study carried out in 34 office buildings, high ozone levels, considered alone or combined with polyester/synthetic material, were associated with general and mucosal symptoms of SBS (77). In a longitudinal study carried out in Chinese pupils, ozone levels were significantly associated with skin symptoms related to SBS at baseline (Table 26.1, Zhang 2014). Formaldehyde levels were significantly related to an increased risk of asthma (OR:1.8, 95%CI:1.2–2.8) in a meta-analysis that included 13 studies (78). However, Glas and coworkers compared the levels of formaldehyde, NO_2, ozone, and terpenes in office buildings where workers presented with and without SBS (in nearly equal numbers) and did not find significant exposure differences (79). Salonen and coworkers examined irritant potentials of various VOCs, identifying formaldehyde as substance most likely to enhance sensory irritation; however, no relationships were found between the presence of symptoms in more than 1000 workers and exposure levels of 50 VOCs including formaldehyde (80). Kwon and coworkers assessed 34 workers who had moved into a new building. The level of VOC and xylene metabolites in the urine was associated with incident ocular symptoms (81). Formaldehyde and other chemicals were also present in newly built homes (82). One VOC measured in family homes, 1-octen 3-ol, has been associated with reported mucosal symptoms in 620 Japanese residents (83). This VOC has

also been reported to be produced by fungi and in a Drosophila model, Inamdar and colleagues showed that 1-octen 3-ol was able to cause dopamine neuron degeneration and disrupt dopamine homeostasis (84). Semivolatile compounds including plasticizers have also been shown to be associated with SBS symptoms in occupants of residential dwellings (85). Exposure to phthalates enhances the immediate asthmatic reaction induced by allergens, similar to other pollutants (e.g. ozone), and favors the recruitment of macrophages (86). It is thus likely that such an exposure can enhance respiratory symptoms found in allergic patients presented with SBS symptoms.

Besides the effect of increased exposure to indoor allergens as well as to molds and mold-derived products, exposure to various VOCs may also play a role in inducing SBS. In a mouse model, it has been shown that chronic exposure to VOCs that originated from PVC flooring increases eosinophilic lung inflammation as detected in BAL, with a decrease in Th1cytokine IFN-gamma and an increase of Th2 cytokine production. In addition, in this study, the two VOCs that were emitted at the highest concentrations (N-methyl-2-pyrrolidone and trimethyl-pentanediol diisobutyrate) reduced IL-12 production and induced oxidative stress (87).

Chemical components in settled dust

Settled dust can be examined in terms of quantity and size of particles. It can also be evaluated with more sophisticated means such as high-resolution mass spectrometry capable of detecting noxious chemicals (88). A so-called exposome that represents an atlas of chemicals measured in indoor dust has been published (89) and includes 511 chemicals with defined toxicity. The European Commission has developed a relevant information platform, IPCHEM, that can be used as a resource for chemical monitoring of indoor air (90).

In a study of 462 students from 8 randomly selected secondary schools in Malaysia, Norback and coworkers found a significant association between the amount of fine dust and ocular symptoms, whereas endotoxin was inversely associated with symptoms (91). Due to concern regarding health effects of hormone-disrupting chemicals, some have been examined in the indoor environment (92). Epidemiological studies provide weak support for associations of allergic diseases and exposure to phthalate (93). Experimental studies in animals suggest that these are immune adjuvants (93). The levels of organophosphate and phthalate esters (including PVC) were examined in multistory buildings in Stockholm, with high and low prevalence of SBS and little or no differences in concentrations of the target substances were detected (94).

Cases of indoor and building-related asthma

Indoor allergens (e.g. house dust mites, furry animals including rodents) can either cause or exacerbate asthma and allergic rhinoconjunctivitis in domestic workers (Chapter 20). Landscape workers are exposed and sensitized to outdoor aeroallergens and are at risk of developing allergic rhinoconjunctivitis and asthma symptoms (95). This also applies to the domestic use of cleaning products that can cause acute or chronic irritant-induced asthma (Chapter 19) and in epidemiological studies, has been associated with enhanced risk of asthma and COPD (Chapter 17). In addition, worsening of asthma due to excessive dampness has been discussed above. Therefore, the clinician or expert sitting on a workers' compensation board (WCB) may face a situation such as the one proposed in the Section Workplace/Case Scenario, in which the differential diagnoses could include OA, occupational rhinitis, work-exacerbated asthma, or SBS.

COMMENTS ON WORKPLACE/CASE SCENARIO

Among eight teachers presenting with work-related symptoms, a diagnosis of OA or work-exacerbated asthma was confirmed in two teachers with NSBH and skin reactivity to mold and mite allergens who exhibited significant falls in FEV_1 during 2 days spent at work. Two other teachers with NSBH and skin reactivity to mold and/or mite allergens had no decrement in FEV_1 in the workplace but reported nasal symptoms; a diagnosis of occupational rhinitis was proposed. SBS was used to define symptoms reported by the four other teachers.

How to improve the indoor environment in workplace buildings

If employees report symptoms compatible with SBS, inexpensive means such as reducing ambient temperature or improving local ventilation in specific rooms would be appropriate. In many instances, such simple approaches are successful. Documents on guidance for cleaning and disinfecting public spaces, workplaces, businesses, schools, and homes for developing, implemental, and maintaining cleaning plans are available from the US Environmental Protection Agency (https://www.epa.gov/sites/production/files/2020-04/documents/316485-c_reopeningamerica_guidance_4.19_6pm.pdf). Concerning the key topic of prevention, the US Occupational Safety and Health Administration (OSHA) has issued a document on "Tips for Prevention" (96) (https://ohsonline.com/articles/2016/10/01/sick-building-syndrome.aspx) with the following suggestions:

1. Clean up wet or damp areas;
2. Install high-volume, low-speed fans for ventilation;
3. Perform regular heating, ventilation, and air-conditioning (HVAC) maintenance;
4. Install air cleaners or filters;
5. Open windows to improve natural air circulation;
6. Choose interior materials carefully.

Interventions at a work-area level seem preferable to those with a more generalized building-wide approach (16), a suggestion that can favor improvement of personal rather than general ventilation (see above in the same section). Invasive investigations to identify and remove hidden mold growth sites can be costly. The promotion of health behavior offered in three sessions by one specialist in occupational medicine and two by psychologists was unsuccessful in a randomized controlled trial in 55 patients with work-related respiratory symptoms and moisture-damaged workplaces (97).

Besides reducing environmental impacts, the design of green buildings aims at improving health. In a review of initial scientific evidence, Allen and coworkers state that green buildings improve general indoor environmental quality (lower levels of VOCs, formaldehyde, allergens, and other factors) and health of occupants (98). In a study by Colton and coworkers, participants living in green homes experienced 47% fewer SBS symptoms and fewer reports of mold, pests, inadequate ventilation, and air stuffiness (99). In a subsequently published study, the same group of authors confirmed these observations and found that asthmatic children were less symptomatic with fewer hospital visits and school absences (100). The fungal microbiomes able to grow and proliferate on green and nongreen buildings have also been shown to differ (101).

Research needs

Future research might:

- Explore the health consequences of social disparities of indoor exposure in various countries;
- Develop and improve objective means to characterize SBS, in particular the effects on mucous membranes;
- Provide a convincing link between epidemiological evidence and experimental findings; and
- Document the effect of outdoor pollution on indoor quality of air.

Acknowledgments

The findings and conclusions in this study are those of the authors and do not necessarily represent the official position of the National Institute for Occupational Safety and Health, Centers for Disease Control and Prevention.

References

1. Norback D, Miller JD. Building-related illnesses and mold-related conditions. In: Asthma in the Workplace. 4th ed. Boca Raton: CRC Press, Taylor & Francis; 2013.
2. WHO. Household air pollution and health. 2018. https://wwwwhoint/news-room/fact-sheets/detail/household-air-pollution-and-health
3. Diffey BL. An overview analysis of the time people spend outdoors. Br J Dermatol. 2011;164(4):848–54.
4. Gautrin D, Infante-Rivard C, Dao TV, et al. Specific IgE-dependent sensitization, atopy and bronchial hyperresponsiveness in apprentices starting exposure to protein-derived agents. Am J Respir Crit Care Med. 1997;155:1841–7.
5. Suzuki N, Nakaoka H, Hanazato M, et al. Indoor air quality analysis of newly built houses. Int J Environ Res Public Health. 2019;16(21):4142.
6. Ferguson L, Taylor J, Davies M, et al. Exposure to indoor air pollution across socio-economic groups in high-income countries: a scoping review of the literature and a modelling methodology. Environ Int. 2020;143:105748.
7. Palmquist E, Claeson AS, Neely G, et al. Overlap in prevalence between various types of environmental intolerance. Int J Hyg Environ Health. 2014;217(4–5):427–34.
8. Edvardsson B, Stenberg B, Bergdahl J, et al. Medical and social prognoses of non-specific building-related symptoms (Sick Building Syndrome): a follow-up study of patients previously referred to hospital. Int Arch Occup Environ Health. 2008;81(7):805–12.
9. Norback D. An update on sick building syndrome. Curr Opin Allergy Clin Immunol. 2009;9(1):55–9.
10. Miyajima E, Tsunoda M, Sugiura Y, et al. The diagnosis of sick house syndrome: the contribution of diagnostic criteria and determination of chemicals in an indoor environment. Tokai J Exp Clin Med. 2015;40(2):69–75.
11. Tietjen GE, Khubchandani J, Ghosh S, et al. Headache symptoms and indoor environmental parameters: Results from the EPA BASE study. Ann Indian Acad Neurol. 2012;15(Suppl 1):S95–9.
12. Bakke JV, Norbäck D, Wieslander G, et al. Symptoms, complaints, ocular and nasal physiological signs in university staff in relation to indoor environment—temperature and gender interactions. Indoor Air. 2008;18(2):131–43.
13. Wahlen K, Fornander L, Olausson P, et al. Protein profiles of nasal lavage fluid from individuals with work-related upper airway symptoms associated with moldy and damp buildings. Indoor Air. 2016;26(5):743–54.
14. Sahlberg B, Norbäck D, Wieslander G, et al. Onset of mucosal, dermal, and general symptoms in relation to biomarkers and exposures in the dwelling: a cohort study from 1992 to 2002. Indoor Air. 2012;22(4):331–8.

15. Barmark M. Social determinants of the sick building syndrome: exploring the interrelated effects of social position and psychosocial situation. Int J Environ Health Res. 2015;25(5):490–507.

16. Lukcso D, Guidotti TL, Franklin DE, et al. Indoor environmental and air quality characteristics, building-related health symptoms, and worker productivity in a federal government building complex. Arch Environ Occup Health. 2016;71(2):85–101.

17. Bjornsson E, Janson C, Norback D, et al. Symptoms related to the sick building syndrome in a general population sample: associations with atopy, bronchial hyper-responsiveness and anxiety. Int J Tuberc Lung Dis. 1998;2(12):1023–8.

18. Runeson-Broberg R, Norbäck D. Sick building syndrome (SBS) and sick house syndrome (SHS) in relation to psychosocial stress at work in the Swedish workforce. Int Arch Occup Environ Health. 2013;86(8):915–22.

19. Brauer C, Mikkelsen S. The influence of individual and contextual psychosocial work factors on the perception of the indoor environment at work: a multilevel analysis. Int Arch Occup Environ Health. 2010;83(6):639–51.

20. Lan L, Wargocki P, Wyon DP, et al. Effects of thermal discomfort in an office on perceived air quality, SBS symptoms, physiological responses, and human performance. Indoor Air. 2011;21(5):376–90.

21. Wolkoff P. "Healthy" eye in office-like environments. Environ Int. 2008;34(8):1204–14.

22. Sundell J, Levin H, Nazaroff WW, et al. Ventilation rates and health: multidisciplinary review of the scientific literature. Indoor Air. 2011;21(3):191–204.

23. Melikov AK, Skwarczynski MA, Kaczmarczyk J, et al. Use of personalized ventilation for improving health, comfort, and performance at high room temperature and humidity. Indoor Air. 2013;23(3):250–63.

24. Maddalena R, Mendell MJ, Eliseeva K, et al. Effects of ventilation rate per person and per floor area on perceived air quality, sick building syndrome symptoms, and decision-making. Indoor Air. 2015;25(4):362–70.

25. Tsai DH, Lin JS, Chan CC. Office workers' sick building syndrome and indoor carbon dioxide concentrations. J Occup Environ Hyg. 2012;9(5):345–51.

26. Norbäck D, Nordström K, Zhao Z. Carbon dioxide (CO2) demand-controlled ventilation in university computer classrooms and possible effects on headache, fatigue and perceived indoor environment: an intervention study. Int Arch Occup Environ Health. 2013;86(2):199–209.

27. Eduard W, Heederik D, Duchaine C, et al. Bioaerosol exposure assessment in the workplace: the past, present and recent advances. J Environ Monit. 2012;14(2):334–9.

28. Švajlenka J, Kozlovská M, Pošiváková T. Biomonitoring the indoor environment of agricultural buildings. Ann Agric Environ Med. 2018;25(2):292–5.

29. Cabral JP. Can we use indoor fungi as bioindicators of indoor air quality? Historical perspectives and open questions. Sci Total Environ. 2010;408(20):4285–95.

30. Green BJ, Lemons AR, Park Y, et al. Assessment of fungal diversity in a water-damaged office building. J Occup Environ Hyg. 2017;14(4):285–93.

31. Park JH, Cox-Ganser JM, Kreiss K, et al. Hydrophilic fungi and ergosterol associated with respiratory illness in a water-damaged building. Environ Health Perspect. 2008;116:45–50.

32. Omotayo OP, Omotayo AO, Mwanza M, et al. Prevalence of mycotoxins and their consequences on human health. Toxicol Res. 2019;35(1):1–7.

33. Polizzi V, Adams A, De Saeger S, et al. Influence of various growth parameters on fungal growth and volatile metabolite production by indoor molds. Sci Total Environ. 2012;414:277–86.

34. Wong J, Magun BE, Wood LJ. Lung inflammation caused by inhaled toxicants: a review. Int J Chron Obstruct Pulmon Dis. 2016;11:1391–401.

35. Jargot D, Melin S. Characterization and validation of sampling and analytical methods for mycotoxins in workplace air. Environ Sci Process Impacts. 2013;15(3):633–44.

36. Saito R, Park JH, LeBouf R, et al. Measurement of macrocyclic trichothecene in floor dust of water-damaged buildings using gas chromatography/tandem mass spectrometry-dust matrix effects. J Occup Environ Hyg. 2016;13(6):442–50.

37. Schlosser O, Robert S, Noyon N. Airborne mycotoxins in waste recycling and recovery facilities: occupational exposure and health risk assessment. Waste Manag. 2020;105:395–404.

38. Caillaud D, Leynaert B, Keirsbulck M, et al. Indoor mould exposure, asthma and rhinitis: findings from systematic reviews and recent longitudinal studies. Eur Respir Rev. 2018;27(148):170137.

39. Jaakkola MS, Nordman H, Piipari R, et al. Indoor dampness and molds and development of adult-onset asthma: a population-based incident case-control study. Environ Health Perspect. 2002;110:543–7.

40. Bornehag CG, Sundell J, Bonini S, et al. Dampness in buildings as a risk factor for health effects, EUROEXPO: a multidisciplinary review of the literature (1998-2000) on dampness and mite exposure in buildings and health effects. Indoor Air. 2004;14(4):243–57.

41. Fisk WJ, Lei-Gomez Q, Mendell MJ. Meta-analyses of the associations of respiratory health effects with dampness and mold in homes. Indoor Air. 2007;17:284–96.

42. Mendell MJ, Mirer AG, Cheung K, et al. Respiratory and allergic health effects of dampness, mold, and dampness-related agents: a review of the epidemiologic evidence. Environ Health Perspect. 2011;119(6):748–56.

43. Norback D, Zock JP, Plana E, et al. Mould and dampness in dwelling places, and onset of asthma: the population-based cohort ECRHS. Occup Environ Med. 2013;70(5):325–31.

44. Haverinen-Shaughnessy U, Borras-Santos A, Turunen M, et al. Occurrence of moisture problems in schools in three countries from different climatic regions of Europe based on questionnaires and building inspections—the HITEA study. Indoor Air. 2012;22(6):457–66.

45. Borràs-Santos A, Jacobs JH, Täubel M, et al. Dampness and mould in schools and respiratory symptoms in children: the HITEA study. Occup Env Med. 2013;70:681–7.

46. Jacobs J, Borràs-Santos A, Krop E, et al. Dampness, bacterial and fungal components in dust in primary schools and respiratory health in schoolchildren across Europe. Occup Environ Med. 2014;71:704–12.

47. Holst G, Høst A, Doekes G, et al. Allergy and respiratory health effects of dampness and dampness-related agents in schools and homes: a cross-sectional study in Danish pupils. Indoor Air. 2016;26(6):880–91.

48. Poole JA, Gleason AM, Bauer C, et al. CD11c(+)/CD11b(+) cells are critical for organic dust-elicited murine lung inflammation. Am J Respir Cell Mol Biol. 2012;47(5):652–9.

49. Poole JA, Gleason AM, Bauer C, et al. αβ T cells and a mixed Th1/Th17 response are important in organic dust-induced airway disease. Ann Allergy Asthma Immunol. 2012;109(4):266–73.e2.

50. Warren KJ, Dickinson JD, Nelson AJ, et al. Ovalbumin-sensitized mice have altered airway inflammation to agriculture organic dust. Respir Res. 2019;20(1):51.

51. Kim YS, Choi EJ, Lee WH, et al. Extracellular vesicles, especially derived from Gram-negative bacteria, in indoor dust induce neutrophilic pulmonary inflammation associated with both Th1 and Th17 cell responses. Clin Exp Allergy. 2013;43(4):443–54.

52. Hadebe S, Kirstein F, Fierens K, et al. β-Glucan exacerbates allergic airway responses to house dust mite allergen. Respir Res. 2016;17:35.

53. Karvala K, Toskala E, Luukkonen R, et al. New-onset adult asthma in relation to damp and moldy workplaces. Int Arch Occup Environ Health. 2010;83(8):855–65.

54. Rollins SM, Su FC, Liang X, et al. Workplace indoor environmental quality and asthma-related outcomes in healthcare workers. Am J Ind Med. 2020;63(5):417–28.

55. WHO. WHO Guidelines for Indoor Air Quality – Dampness and Mold. 2nd ed. Copenhagen: World Health Organization; 2009.

56. Norback D, Edling C. Environmental, occupational, and personal factors related to the prevalence of sick building syndrome in the general population. Br J Ind Med. 1991;48(7):451–62.

57. Smedje G, Wang J, Norback D, et al. SBS symptoms in relation to dampness and ventilation in inspected single-family houses in Sweden. Int Arch Occup Environ Health. 2017;90(7):703–11.

58. Zhang X, Sahlberg B, Wieslander G, et al. Dampness and moulds in workplace buildings: associations with incidence and remission of sick building syndrome (SBS) and biomarkers of inflammation in a 10 year follow-up study. Sci Total Environ. 2012;430:75–81.

59. Mendell MJ, Cozen M, Lei-Gomez Q, et al. Indicators of moisture and ventilation system contamination in U.S. office buildings as risk factors for respiratory and mucous membrane symptoms: analyses of the EPA BASE data. J Occup Environ Hyg. 2006;3(5):225–33.

60. Wang J, Li B, Yang Q, et al. Odors and sensations of humidity and dryness in relation to sick building syndrome and home environment in Chongqing, China. PLOS ONE. 2013;8(8):e72385.

61. Wolff CH. Innate immunity and the pathogenicity of inhaled microbial particles. Int J Biol Sci. 2011;7(3):261–8.

62. Sauni R, Verbeek JH, Uitti J, et al. Remediating buildings damaged by dampness and mould for preventing or reducing respiratory tract symptoms, infections and asthma. Cochrane Database Syst Rev. 2015;2:CD007897.

63. Health Canada. Addressing moisture and mould in your home. https://wwwcanadaca/en/health-canada/services/publications/healthy-living/addressing-moisture-mould-your-homehtml. 2014.

64. NIOSH (National Institute for Occupational Safety and Health). Dampness and mold assessment tool-General Buildings. 2018.

65. Pieckova E. Adverse health effects of indoor moulds. Arh Hig Rada Toksikol. 2012;63(4):545–9.

66. Saijo Y, Kanazawa A, Araki A, et al. Relationships between mite allergen levels, mold concentrations, and sick building syndrome symptoms in newly built dwellings in Japan. Indoor Air. 2011;21(3):253–63.

67. Oldenburg M, Latza U, Baur X. Occupational health risks due to shipboard cockroaches. Int Arch Occup Environ Health. 2008;81:727–34.

68. McGowan EC, Peng R, Salo PM, et al. Cockroach, dust mite, and shrimp sensitization correlations in the National Health and Nutrition Examination Survey. Ann Allergy Asthma Immunol. 2019;122(5):536–8.e1.

69. Ahluwalia SK, Matsui EC. Indoor environmental interventions for furry pet allergens, pest allergens, and mold: looking to the future. J Allergy Clin Immunol Pract. 2018;6(1):9–19.

70. Zhang X, Zhao Z, Nordquist T, et al. A longitudinal study of sick building syndrome among pupils in relation to microbial components in dust in schools in China. Sci Total Environ. 2011;409(24):5253–9.

71. Ooi SS, Mak JW, Chen DK, et al. The correlation of Acanthamoeba from the ventilation system with other environmental parameters in commercial buildings as possible indicator for indoor air quality. Ind Health. 2017;55(1):35–45.

72. Punsman S, van der Graaf T, Zahradnik E, et al. Effectiveness of a portable air filtration device in reducing allergen exposure during household chores. Allergo Journal International. 2019;28:299–307.

73. Wu W, Jin Y, Carlsten C. Inflammatory health effects of indoor and outdoor particulate matter. J Allergy Clin Immunol. 2018;141:833–44.

74. WHO. WHO Air Quality Guidelines for Particular Matter, Ozone, Nitrogen Dioxide and Sulphur Dioxide. Global update 2005. Copenhagen: Summary of Risk Assessment World Health Organization; 2005.

75. Mortimer K, Ndamala CB, Naunje AW, et al. A cleaner burning biomass-fuelled cookstove intervention to prevent pneumonia in children under 5 years old in rural Malawi (the cooking and pneumonia study): a cluster randomised controlled trial. Lancet. 2017;389(10065):167–75.

76. Li L, Adamkiewicz G, Zhang Y, et al. Effect of traffic exposure on sick building syndrome symptoms among parents/grandparents of preschool children in Beijing, China. PLOS ONE. 2015;10(6):e0128767.

77. Buchanan IS, Mendell MJ, Mirer AG, et al. Air filter materials, outdoor ozone and building-related symptoms in the BASE study. Indoor Air. 2008;18(2):144–55.

78. Yu L, Wang B, Cheng M, et al. Association between indoor formaldehyde exposure and asthma: A systematic review and meta-analysis of observational studies. Indoor Air. 2020;30:682–90.

79. Glas B, Stenberg B, Stenlund H, et al. Exposure to formaldehyde, nitrogen dioxide, ozone, and terpenes among office workers and associations with reported symptoms. Int Arch Occup Environ Health. 2015;88(5):613–22.

80. Salonen H, Pasanen AL, Lappalainen S, et al. Volatile organic compounds and formaldehyde as explaining factors for sensory irritation in office environments. J Occup Environ Hyg. 2009;6(4):239–47.

81. Kwon JW, Park HW, Kim WJ, et al. Exposure to volatile organic compounds and airway inflammation. Environ Health. 2018;17(1):65.

82. Takigawa T, Wang BL, Saijo Y, et al. Relationship between indoor chemical concentrations and subjective symptoms associated with sick building syndrome in newly built houses in Japan. Int Arch Occup Environ Health. 2010;83(2):225–35.

83. Araki A, Kawai T, Eitaki Y, et al. Relationship between selected indoor volatile organic compounds, so-called microbial VOC, and the prevalence of mucous membrane symptoms in single family homes. Sci Total Environ. 2010;408(10):2208–15.

84. Inamdar AA, Hossain MM, Bernstein AI, et al. Fungal-derived semiochemical 1-octen-3-ol disrupts dopamine packaging and causes neurodegeneration. Proc Natl Acad Sci USA. 2013;110(48):19561–6.

85. Kanazawa A, Saito I, Araki A, et al. Association between indoor exposure to semi-volatile organic compounds and building-related symptoms among the occupants of residential dwellings. Indoor Air. 2010;20(1):72–84.

86. Maestre-Batlle D, Huff RD, Schwartz C, et al. Dibutyl phthalate augments allergen-induced lung function decline and alters human airway immunology: a randomized crossover study. Am J Respir Crit Care Med. 2020;202:672–80.

87. Bönisch U, Böhme A, Kohajda T, et al. Volatile organic compounds enhance allergic airway inflammation in an experimental mouse model. PLOS ONE. 2012;7(7):e39817.

88. Moschet C, Anumol T, Lew BM, et al. Household dust as a repository of chemical accumulation: new insights from a comprehensive high-resolution mass spectrometric study. Environ Sci Technol. 2018;52(5):2878–87.

89. Dong T, Zhang Y, Jia S, et al. Human indoor exposome of chemicals in dust and risk prioritization using EPA's ToxCast database. Environ Sci Technol. 2019;53(12):7045–54.

90. Kephalopoulos S, Bopp SK, Costa SD, et al. Indoor air monitoring: sharing and accessing data via the information platform for chemical monitoring (IPCHEM). Int J Hyg Environ Health. 2020;227:113515.

91. Norbäck D, Hashim JH, Markowicz P, et al. Endotoxin, ergosterol, muramic acid and fungal DNA in dust from schools in Johor Bahru, Malaysia–Associations with rhinitis and sick building syndrome (SBS) in junior high school students. Sci Total Environ. 2016;545-546:95–103.

92. Rudel RA, Perovich LJ. Endocrine disrupting chemicals in indoor and outdoor air. Atmos Environ (1994). 2009;43(1):170–81.

93. Bølling AK, Sripada K, Becher R, et al. Phthalate exposure and allergic diseases: review of epidemiological and experimental evidence. Environ Int. 2020;139:105706.

94. Bergh C, Magnus Åberg K, Svartengren M, et al. Organophosphate and phthalate esters in indoor air: a comparison between multi-story buildings with high and low prevalence of sick building symptoms. J Environ Monit. 2011;13(7):2001–9.

95. Gautrin D, Vandenplas O, DeWitte JD, et al. Allergenic exposure, IgE-mediated sensitization and related symptoms in lawn cutters. J Allergy Clin Immunol. 1994;93:437–45.

96. Heinkel N. Sick Building Syndrome: What It Is and Tips for Prevention (https://ohsonline.com/articles/2016/10/01/sick-building-syndrome.aspx). Occup Health Saf. 2016;85(10):62,4.

97. Vuokko A, Selinheimo S, Sainio M, et al. Decreased work ability associated to indoor air problems–An intervention (RCT) to promote health behavior. Neurotoxicology. 2015;49:59–67.

98. Allen JG, MacNaughton P, Laurent JG, et al. Green buildings and health. Curr Environ Health Rep. 2015;2(3):250–8.

99. Colton MD, MacNaughton P, Vallarino J, et al. Indoor air quality in green vs conventional multifamily low-income housing. Environ Sci Technol. 2014;48(14):7833–41.

100. Colton MD, Laurent JG, MacNaughton P, et al. Health benefits of green public housing: associations with asthma morbidity and building-related symptoms. Am J Public Health. 2015;105(12):2482–9.

101. Coombs K, Vesper S, Green BJ, et al. Fungal microbiomes associated with green and non-green building materials. Int Biodeterior Biodegradation. 2017;125(0):251–7.

27

OCCUPATIONAL URTICARIA AND ALLERGIC CONTACT DERMATITIS

D. Linn Holness,[1] Victoria H. Arrandale,[2] Karin Pacheco,[3] Jean-Luc Malo,[4] and David I. Bernstein[5]

[1]*Dalla Lana School of Public Health and Department of Medicine, University of
Toronto, St. Michael's Hospital, Toronto, Ontario, Canada*
[2]*Dalla Lana School of Public Health, University of Toronto, Toronto, Ontario, Canada*
[3]*Division of Environmental & Occupational Health Sciences, Department of Medicine, National Jewish Health, and Division
of Environmental & Occupational Health, University of Colorado School of Public Health, Aurora, Colorado, USA*
[4]*Hôpital du Sacré-Cœur de Montréal and Université de Montréal, Montréal, Québec, Canada*
[5]*Division of Immunology, Allergy and Rheumatology, University of Cincinnati College of Medicine, Cincinnati, Ohio, USA*

Contents

Introduction

Occupational skin disease (OSD) is one of the most common occupational diseases worldwide. There are a variety of OSDs caused by chemical, physical, biological, and mechanical trauma. Common OSDs include contact dermatitis (CD), infections, cancer, pigmentary changes, and aggravation of preexisting skin disease.

Occupational contact dermatitis (OCD) is an eczematous eruption caused by irritation or a type IV allergic response to a workplace agent. Occupational contact urticaria (OCU) is an urticarial response caused by a type I allergic or nonimmunologic response to a workplace agent.

OCU and OCD can be caused by exposure to a variety of proteinic material and chemicals in the workplace. Of interest is the fact that exposures that may cause OCU and/or OCD may also cause occupational asthma (OA). Therefore, it is important to consider the possibility of both skin and respiratory effects with exposure to some workplace chemicals. We will describe some

of the challenges in estimating the burden of OSD, discuss OCD and OCU separately, explore the possible co-occurrence of occupational lung and skin exposures and response, and end with a discussion of prevention of dermal exposure.

Evidence-based practice—Challenges in occupational skin diseases

A challenge with many occupational diseases is to find reliable sources of data related to the burden of illness. Sources of such information include administrative data (insurance or government reporting systems, workers' compensation authorities, government-operated reporting schemes) and workplace- or population-based studies. It is well recognized that OSDs are underrecognized and underreported. A further challenge for all the sources of incidence and prevalence information is the accuracy of the diagnostic information that underpins the reporting.

It can be difficult to obtain accurate epidemiological data both for general CD and contact urticaria (CU) and for those cases associated with work. Key issues may include a lack of standard case definitions, a lack of a standard application of these definitions, and challenges in the diagnosis of the work-relatedness. Cases may be defined using a variety of criteria including: the self-reporting of current or past episodes of urticaria or dermatitis in the workplace, histories of urticaria or dermatitis associated with specific occupational exposure or work activity, objective signs of urticaria or dermatitis on clinical examination, and evidence of specific immunoglobulin E (IgE) to suspect occupational antigens (e.g. radioallergosorbent test (RAST) or skin-prick testing) for urticaria and patch testing for dermatitis. The accuracy of diagnosis of OCD and OCU is also challenging. The diagnosis is based on the medical and exposure history, physical findings, and in vitro or in vivo testing. In the allergic contact urticarial syndromes particularly, the lack of standardized occupational test allergens also contributes to the problem. All these difficulties may lead to potential misclassification of OCD and OCU, which can result in either over- or underestimation of disease frequency.

Much of the literature on urticaria and dermatitis in the workplace is anecdotal case reports and case series. Many of these cases in the literature are based upon clinical presentations where the urticaria or dermatitis is diagnosed based upon a "probable" occupational exposure and a "probable" allergic or nonallergic mechanism.

There are additional problems in assessing the epidemiology of occupational urticaria, dermatitis, and other OSDs:

- OCD and OCU are not a reportable disease in all jurisdictions.
- OCD and OCU are not diseases that commonly lead to mortality or hospitalizations; thus, death certificates or hospital records are not valuable data sources.
- OCD and OCU are diseases seen and treated (though not always specifically diagnosed) by medical professionals in multiple specialties.
- OCD and OCU are diseases that often go undiagnosed and untreated; thus, many cases may never be documented in any data source.
- Unique exposures may occur in different populations and industries, making the epidemiology of OCU and OCD in one population or workforce unique and not necessarily generalizable.
- The evaluation of past exposures causing OCU and OCD may be difficult, as this will rely on historical information and patient recollection, which are subject to biases.
- An OCU or OCD case, especially if treated by a company's own occupational health personnel, may not involve lost wages or any costs to the workers. Thus, there would be no workers' compensation claim, reducing the utility of this already limited data source.

While there are such clear limitations, there have been several systematic reviews including one focused on OCD and OCU (1).

Occupational urticaria

Although OCU is much less common than OCD (2, 3), urticaria carries a significant risk of anaphylactic reactions (hazard ratio: 2.5 in a study [4]). Moreover, urticaria has a significant impact on well-being, capacity to work, and quality of life (5).

Definition and description

According to an international guideline, urticaria is a condition characterized by the development of wheals (hives), angioedema, or both (6). Urticaria can be classified according to its acute (≤6 weeks) or chronic incidence and spontaneous or inducible occurrence (6). Other relevant features may include: clinical distribution (localized, generalized), etiology (occupational, idiopathic), route of exposure (direct contact, oral), and mechanisms, as proposed (immunologic or not) (7). Contact urticaria (CU) and protein-CD are "immediate contact skin reactions that manifest as itching wheals and/or eczema following skin contact with the causative agent" (8). The manifestations of elevated erythematous lesions are transient, peaking in minutes/hours and disappearing usually in the 24 hours following contact. The key feature that distinguishes these skin lesions from CD is their timing: rapid onset within minutes to hours after exposure, limited duration, and complete resolution within 24 hours, although new lesions may appear in close proximity to older ones. When the edema extends into the subcutaneous tissue, it is referred to as angioedema and the overlying erythema may not be visible, for example, swollen eyelids and lips. Angioedema may be followed by anaphylaxis.

Urticaria is an inflammatory disease in which mast cells play a key role by releasing histamine, platelet-activating factors, and cytokines (6). Skin barrier that regulates transepidermal water loss, the main protective component being located in the stratum corneum, plays a central role (9).

CU is defined as urticaria that occurs after direct skin contact with a substance. There are four types of CU (10):

1. Nonallergic (nonimmunologic; primary urticariogenic agents): occur at first contact, without prior sensitization, usually nonspecific histamine release; rarely prostaglandins, leukotrienes, or substance P.
2. Allergic (immunologic): typically, IgE mediated, rare cases of specific IgG or IgM activating complement.
3. Combined allergic and nonallergic.
4. Combined allergic eczematous and urticarial.

Since most allergic CU is caused by airborne exposures that trigger symptoms by specific IgE, many agents have also been associated with respiratory disease. Von Krogh and Maibach (11) have proposed a staging system for the CU syndrome that delineates increasing systemic symptoms as follows:

Stage 1. Localized urticaria with nonspecific symptoms of itching, tingling, and/or burning.
Stage 2. Generalized urticaria with or without angioedema.
Stage 3. Urticaria along with extra cutaneous involvement: rhinoconjunctivitis, bronchospasm, orolaryngeal or gastrointestinal symptoms.
Stage 4. Urticaria with anaphylactic shock.

Every presentation of CU should include a thorough clinical history documenting any extracutaneous involvement that could progress to systemic anaphylaxis.

OCU is a subset of CU, and is caused by exposure to one or more substances or physical agents in the workplace. Workplace conditions may also aggravate urticaria, or cause nonimmunologic physical urticarias such as pressure/vibration, solar, aquagenic, heat-induced or cold-induced types, depending on the environment. OCU may present in the context of an irritant or immunological CD affecting the skin barrier. Whereas some agents can affect normal skin, others may require damaged, eczematized or fissured skin to cause hives (12).

Epidemiology

Urticaria is a relatively rare condition in the general population. Its chronic spontaneous form, that is recurrent (6 weeks or longer), is considered to affect 230 persons/100,000 (prevalence of 0.3%) according to a US-based study (13), a figure close to a prevalence of 0.4% reported in a large population-based study carried out in Italy (14) but less than the corresponding prevalence in South Korea (4.5% for the period 2010–2014) (15). It has been estimated that in a lifetime 5%–23% of the US population may have had an episode of acute urticaria (16). A questionnaire survey of nearly 5000 respondents in Poland showed that 11.2% had reported at least one episode of urticaria in their lives, the frequency being higher in women (17).

Data from three German cohorts with more than 150,000 patients (18) showed that nearly 0.3% were cases of CU, women representing the majority of subjects. One-third had an occupational cause and lesions affected principally the hand and face (18). Asthma and rhinoconjunctivitis were significant associated factors.

In nearly 2500 patients with anaphylactic reactions, a workplace cause was reported in 3.5% (18). In the United Kingdom, from 2002 to 2005, the rate per million was 3.1 (by dermatologists) to 12.6 (by occupational physicians) according to two databases, suggesting that most workers with OCU are not seen by specialists (2). In ~40% of OCU cases, there was a codiagnosis of OCD (2). Urticarial symptoms were reported by 13% of 455 young Turkish hairdressers, jewelers, and workers in car mechanics (19). A report by the French National Network for Occupational Disease Vigilance and Prevention identified 251 cases from 2001 to 2010, half being cases due to latex that diminished by 19%/year with no decrease for other causes (20). In 2018, the Bureau of Labor Statistics (BLS) recorded 25,000 skin diseases at a rate of 2.2 per 10,000 employees. Allergic CD, of which CU is a component, constitutes from 20% to 25% of all OCD although the incidence and prevalence of CU is thought to be severely underreported (https://www.cdc.gov/niosh/docs/96-115/diseas.html, accessed 9/1/2020). Table 27.1 lists the causes of immunological and nonimmunological CU.

In the German cohort aforementioned above, the most frequent occupations of patients with CU were: nurses, dental assistants, hairdressers, bakers, and cleaners (18). Cosmetics, gloves, disinfectants, rubber, and foods, therefore more often high-molecular-weight (HMW) than low-molecular-weight (LMW) agents, represent common causes. Food industry workers are at particularly high risk for OCU, and foods are the most common cause of immunological CU, including seafood, meat, vegetables, and fruits (21). Statistics of the Finnish Institute of Occupational Health that reported 570 cases from 2005 to 2016 (11% of all reported cases of skin diseases) show that cow dander and proteins of plant origins (flour, foods, grains, animal feed, ornamental plants) as well as persulfates were the most common agents and occupations at risk were bakers, cooks, farmers, veterinarians, gardeners, and hairdressers (22).

Among the principal causes of occupational anaphylaxis reactions as reviewed in a database, Moscato lists drugs, foods, latex, insect and animal bites, and various chemicals (23).

A personal and familial history of atopic conditions is recognized as significantly associated with CU (18, 24).

TABLE 27.1 Causes of Occupational Contact Urticaria

Immunological

Proteins 1. Bourrain, 2006

Fruits, vegetables, spices, plants, and woods

Animal-derived proteins: hair, blood, brains

Dairy products

Eggs

Meat

Seafood

Worms/larvae/parasites (Anisakis simplex)

Grains

Enzymes

Nonproteins 2. Amaro, 2008

Abietic acid	Methylhexahydrophthalic anhydride
Acetylsalicylic acid	Methyl methacrylate
Bacitracin	Nickel
Benzoyl peroxide	Neomycin
Chlorhexidine	Oleic acid
Colophony	O-phenylphenate
Copper	Penicillins
Di 2-ethylhexyl phthalate	Persulfates
Diethyltoluamide	Phenylmercuric acetate
Diglycidyl ether of bisphenol A (DGEBA)	Platinum salts
Epoxy resin	
Formaldehyde	Polyethylene
Fragrances	Polyfunctional aziridine hardener
Lindane	Rifamycin
Menthol	Xylene
	Wool alcohol

Nonimmunological 3. Walter, 2019

Foods

Foods that cause direct mast-cell activation: alcohol, strawberries, tomatoes

Foods that contain histamine: matured cheeses, pickled herring, pineapple, red wine, sauerkraut, contaminated tuna, yeast

Other: flavoring agents, preservatives, food additives such as benzoic acid, sorbic acid, cinnamic acid, cinnamic aldehyde, Balsam of Peru

Chemicals 1. Bourrain, 2006

Acetic acid	Chloroform
Amyl alcohol	Cobalt chloride
Balsam of Friar	Diethyl fumarate
Benzaldehyde	Ethyl alcohol
Butyl alcohol	Isopropyl alcohol
Butyric acid	Nicotinic acid
Capsaicin	Sodium benzoate
Chlorocresol	Tar

References: **1.** Bourrain JL. *Clin Rev Allergy Immunol.* 2006; 30:39–46; **2.** Amaro C, et al. *Contact Dermatitis.* 2008;58:67–75; **3.** Walter A. *Clin Rev Allergy Immunol.* 2019;56:19–31.

Diagnosis

Although a diagnosis of urticaria is easy to establish if the patient presents with active lesions, that is not often the case. More likely is the patient presenting with a history of transient skin lesions, and it is up to the clinician to distinguish urticaria from CD on the basis of the patient's history describing the appearance, symptoms, onset, and duration of the rash. A checklist published by Cherrez-Ojeda and colleagues provides a useful set of questions and conditions that can be used to elicit an efficient clinical history (25). Occupation and exposure at work are among the important questions to be addressed for diagnosis (25, 26). It is however important to note that no cause can be found in the majority of cases of chronic urticaria.

Nicholson et al. (1) suggest that the two evidence-based components of the clinical evaluation include: (1) a temporal relationship between the onset or aggravation of symptoms and work, and (2) a focused and detailed history, clinical examination, and prick testing. For patients presenting with a history that suggests CU, it may also be important to consider the possibility of CD and include patch testing in the investigation. Although no general consensus yet exists, a review of the best documented cases of OCU suggests seven helpful criteria to establish the diagnosis (Table 27.2).

Allergy tests can be useful in the diagnostic process, as reviewed (27), and are relevant for the evaluation of food, aeroallergens, as well as some drugs and chemicals. Commercially available extracts for skin-prick testing (SPT) are obtainable for many foods, but not produced for many other preservatives or chemicals. Oral food challenges are generally not recommended for foods causing CU, as the food allergens may also be altered by cooking and digestion (28). A variation called the scratch chamber test has been developed and is particularly useful for solids such as food substances (29). With this procedure, the test substance is placed into a large patch test device and then taped to the skin over a 7- to 8-mm-long scratch and observed for a response over 15 to 30 minutes. If chemicals are tested in this way, results may not be interpretable as they can cause nonspecific irritation.

Open or closed patch testing is the preferred test for the evaluation of systemic urticaria thought to be caused by skin exposure, as it most closely approximates the conditions under which exposure occurs in the workplace. In the open patch test, the suspected agent is placed directly on the skin "as is," and the test site is observed for up to 60 minutes for erythema or a wheal and flare reaction. In the closed patch test, the suspected causal agent is placed on a standard commercial patch test device, and occluded against the skin for 15–30 minutes. The device is then removed, and the test site observed for a reaction for an additional 40 minutes (total 60 minutes). The preferred test sites include the ventral forearm, upper outer arm, or upper back. Because the test concentrations are not standardized, the interpretation of a test as "positive" should ideally be supported by at least 20 negative controls.

As presented in Chapter 7, serum-specific IgE assays are not commercially available for most workplace chemicals. Where available, the RAST can be helpful, especially in the presence of generalized urticaria. Total IgE levels and peripheral blood eosinophilia are suggestive of allergy, but not specific for any causal agent. Skin biopsies are seldom helpful in establishing a diagnosis of urticaria, which is usually made on clinical grounds alone, unless urticarial vasculitis is suspected. Diagnostic criteria have been proposed for anaphylaxis (30).

TABLE 27.2 Criteria to Establish the Diagnosis of Occupational Contact Urticaria

- 1. *The clinical diagnosis of urticaria has been documented by medical examination*

The pathognomonic lesion of urticaria is the wheal, a circumscribed, pruritic, raised, pink to erythematous effervescent swelling of the superficial dermis. The wheal usually lasts only a few hours—rarely more than 24 hours. A skin biopsy is not usually helpful or necessary to confirm the diagnosis of urticaria, but may sometimes be useful to exclude these other dermatologic conditions.

- 2. *Exposure has occurred in the workplace to an agent that has been documented as a potential cause of urticaria, based on published medical or toxicological studies*

Rigorous or convincing proof is often lacking; skin tests allegedly supporting a causal relationship may or may not have adequate standardization or controls.

- 3. *The temporal relationship between cutaneous allergen exposure and elicitation of urticarial responses should be consistent with an immediate hypersensitivity reaction*

Hives should develop within 30–60 minutes of exposure to the putative causal agent in the workplace. However, there is no general consensus concerning the typical period of time between the initial exposure (i.e. latency period of sensitization) and the first occurrence of urticaria.

- 4. *Associated medical symptoms and anatomical localization of urticaria must be consistent with the clinical route of exposure to the alleged causal agent*

If skin is the primary route of exposure, the skin should be the first to develop hives. Although hives may remain localized to the primary areas of direct contact (CU), generalized urticaria may develop if sufficient percutaneous absorption occurs. If the primary route of exposure is airborne, urticaria may be associated with additional allergic symptoms of rhinitis, conjunctivitis, or asthma.

- 5. *Urticaria should occur only in the workplace and should resolve away from work*

As urticaria is a common disorder in general, care should be taken to distinguish urticaria that may be aggravated by nonspecific workplace conditions (i.e. work-aggravated urticaria) such as hot environments, vibration, pressure, and heavy physical exercise, from hives caused by an exposure that occurs only at work.

- 6. *Nonoccupational causes of urticaria should be excluded*
- 7. *Medical testing should support a causal relationship between urticaria and a workplace exposure.* Tests may be employed to establish an occupational exposure as the cause of contact or systemic urticaria.

Management

Treatment follows the same therapeutic principles used in the management of nonoccupational chronic urticaria. Guidelines provide evidence-based recommendations for management (6).

Second-generation antihistamines are the preferred first-line medication for symptomatic treatment. Additional options include omalizumab (31), antileukotrienes, corticosteroids, as well as non-steroidal anti-inflammatory and immunomodulating therapies.

Prevention of OCU follows the same hierarchy of controls as other occupational diseases. Where a specific causal agent can be identified, the treatment of choice is avoidance of the offending agent. In some cases, a nonallergenic substance may be substituted and the affected worker kept in the same job as illustrated by the successful management of latex-induced occupational diseases (e.g. substitution of nitrile gloves for natural rubber latex [NRL] gloves). Redeployment to a low-exposure area, or the introduction of exposure controls, may lead to improvement or resolution in some workers. In other cases, the affected worker will have to be removed from exposure, even if it ultimately means changing jobs. Workers with OCU in conjunction with other allergic manifestations, such as rhinoconjunctivitis or asthma, are at the highest risk of progression of disease and risk of anaphylaxis, and should be removed from exposure. However, medical recommendations should be supported by adequate objective medical findings, including tests that specifically identify the causal agent.

Impact of disease/outcomes

The health and social burden of urticaria is significant as reviewed (6). A 6-month follow-up of 1048 patients diagnosed with an OSD identified 155 with CU. These workers had some of the best outcomes, in that 54 (35%) had healed their skin disease at follow-up. Of the remainder, 23% were on sick leave, 17% had changed work tasks but remained in the same job, 14% had changed jobs or occupation, and 14% had lost their job due to unemployment or retirement (32). In one study, nearly 50% of employees with hand eczema and/or OCU had to change their profession and leave the workplace, this principally being the case (71%) for cleaners (33). In a cohort of nearly 200 patients recognized as having contact allergy due to rubber, latex, and epoxy by the Danish National Board of Industrial Injuries and recontacted 2 years later, 31% were still exposed to the relevant allergen. Of 59 subjects no longer exposed, 76% reported an improvement of their skin condition, significantly more so than those who were still exposed. Subjects with OCU had a poorer prognosis (34).

Quality of life (QOL) has been examined in some studies. One QOL study assessed 21 untreated patients with general chronic urticaria (not specifically occupational), comparing them to patients with respiratory allergy using the SF-36 and the Satisfaction Profile (SAT-P) (35). CU patients had significantly lower scores in physical functioning, bodily pain, general health, and emotional functioning compared to those with respiratory allergy, and in all scores (including vitality, social functioning, and mental health) compared to a reference sample, with similar findings using the SAT-P. In the study by Clemenssen and coworkers, aforementioned above, the dermatologic life quality index was significantly impaired in one-third of subjects (34).

Occupational contact dermatitis

Definition and description

CD is defined as "an (eczematous) inflammatory skin reaction to direct contact with noxious agents in our environment" (36). In the case of OCD, it is a noxious agent in the workplace. There are two major types of CD: irritant contact dermatitis (ICD) and allergic contact dermatitis (ACD). ICD is the result of a direct toxic effect of the chemical agent on the skin. ACD is the result of a cell-mediated, type IV immunologic response.

Epidemiology

OCD is the most common OSD in developed countries and accounts for 70%–90% of reported cases (1) although its incidence diminished, as for OA, in 10 countries of Europe from 2000 to 2012 (37). Generally, occupational irritant CD occurs more commonly than occupational allergic CD (1).

Information about common causative agents and industries and jobs at risk comes from several sources including national registries, surveillance systems, and patch test databases. An example of a national registry is the Finnish Register of Occupational Diseases. Aalto-Korte et al. reported on occupational skin disease included in the Finnish Register of Occupational Diseases (2005–2016) including common occupations and causative allergens (3,38). Another source of information is national surveillance systems. In the United Kingdom there are several surveillance systems including EPIDERM and the Occupational Physicians Reporting Activity (OPRA) (39). These systems have provided opportunities to examine specific allergens and their trends over time. An example is the decrease in occupational allergic CD when latex exposure was reduced accompanied by an increase in occupational irritant CD related to more handwashing (40). One advantage when studying occupational allergic CD versus occupational allergic CU is the availability of large patch test databases. Clinicians, using standardized protocols and allergens, pool their individual results providing a large population and the ability to explore not only the most common allergic contactants in these populations but also common work-related allergens. Results have been reported from several large groups including the North American Contact Dermatitis Group (NACDG) (41) and the European Surveillance System on Contact Allergy (ESSCA) (42). The results from these and other studies have been synthesized in several systematic reviews that provide information on the key causative agents, industries, and jobs (1). Major groups of chemicals associated with occupational allergic CD include metals, rubber-related materials, epoxies, resins and acrylics, organic dyes, plants, foods, medications, and biocides and germicides and industries at risk are agriculture, beauticians, chemical workers, cleaners, construction workers, cooks and caterers, electronics workers, hairdressers, healthcare and social care workers, machine operators, mechanics, metalworkers, and vehicle assemblers. A number of occupational agents are both irritants and allergens.

Diagnosis

The diagnosis of OCD is based on exposure history, temporal relationships between the disease and exposures, as well as physical examination findings consistent with the diagnosis. In the case of occupational allergic CD, patch test results indicating an allergic response to the causative agent are also important.

Mathias (43) proposed the following criteria for the diagnosis of OCD:

1. Is the clinical appearance consistent with CD?
2. Are there workplace exposures to potential cutaneous irritants or allergens?
3. Is the anatomic distribution of the dermatitis consistent with the form of cutaneous exposure in relation to the job task?

4. Is the temporal relationship between exposure and onset consistent with CD?
5. Are nonoccupational exposures excluded as likely causes?
6. Does removal from exposure lead to improvement of the dermatitis?
7. Do patch tests or provocation tests implicate a specific workplace exposure?

There are two additional criteria that may be used to evaluate *aggravation* of CD:

1. Has new dermatitis occurred on skin surfaces not previously affected by preexisting dermatitis?
2. Has dermatitis become more severe on skin surfaces already affected by preexisting dermatitis even though no new skin surfaces are involved?

The Mathias criteria have been recently validated in a clinical population showing very high sensitivity and specificity (44). One concern is the time it takes for a worker to receive an accurate diagnosis. There is evidence that workers often spend several years before diagnosis and that the presence of symptoms for a longer time prior to diagnosis tends to result in poorer outcomes (45). It is important to increase awareness of the potential for OCD among physicians to improve the timeliness of referral to specialized centers for appropriate diagnosis including patch testing.

The approach to diagnosis is well described in the British Association of Dermatologists' guidelines (46). Patch testing is a specialized diagnostic test used to identify contact allergy. It is important to patch test individuals not only with a history suggestive of allergic CD but also with persistent dermatitis as the clinical features alone are unreliable to distinguish allergic CD from other causes of dermatitis (46). Patch testing should be undertaken by physicians formally trained in CD and patch testing and, if available, in a specialized clinic (47) and in accordance with international guidelines such as those of the International Contact Dermatitis Research Group (48). Most patch testing is done using commercially available allergens. Particularly in the case of occupational exposures, it may be important to test with the worker's own workplace materials. The methods for testing with workplace materials are described elsewhere (48). Several studies have demonstrated the added value of testing with workplace products (49,50). It is particularly important that testing with workplace materials be done by experienced specialists as there is the possibility of causing severe reactions or even sensitizing the worker. De Groot's book *Patch Testing* provides valuable information on the suggested concentrations for testing with workplace agents (51).

Management

The key to management is early and accurate diagnosis followed by medical and exposure management. Several recent reviews provide evidence-based guidelines for the medical management of hand dermatitis (4652). Key components of medical management include topical corticosteroids with second-line therapies including phototherapy, oral retinoids, and immunosuppression.

Avoidance of exposure can lead to recovery, but in some instances, despite avoidance of exposure, disease may persist (1). Redeployment may lead to improvement in some but not all workers (1). Glove or protective clothing use may improve or prevent symptoms in some workers who continue to have exposure to the causative agents (1). Education may also improve outcomes

(1,53). Several interventions have shown increased knowledge by employees about skin hazards, improved work habits, and health outcomes (54).

On a larger scale, modifications in legislation and regulation can have a positive impact and impressive favorable lessons can be deduced in the specific cases of latex in health personnel and chromate in construction workers, as shown in some exposure control studies (54).

Impact of disease/outcomes

OCD may have a large impact on the affected worker. Outcomes vary widely. Disease persists in many individuals, even with workplace interventions and exposure reduction. In some settings, reasonable exposure control and job retention are possible (1). Up to half of workers with OCD have time off because of their disease, and job loss or a complete change of employment is unfortunately common (1). The majority of workers with OCD manage to continue working in some capacity, though sometimes with altered employment (1,55). Between 29% and 72% of individuals with CD due to various agents are reported to have changed their job because of their skin disease, often with significant lost time from work and economic consequences (1).

Another concern relates to workers' compensation. A low percentage of OCD cases apply for workers' compensation (56). While it is recognized that particular requirements of the workers' compensation system may exclude certain groups, there appears to be underutilization of the compensation system in the case of OCD.

Connections between the skin and respiratory systems in the workplace

Introduction

The co-occurrence of skin and respiratory symptoms and disease, and more specifically the possibility that asthma may develop following sensitization via skin exposure, continues to be a topic of investigation. One of the challenges in finding information on the co-occurrence of skin and respiratory symptoms and diseases is the fact that they are often investigated, in either a research protocol or a clinical setting, in organ system silos. There is some observational evidence of coexisting skin and respiratory outcomes, but most arises from case reports.

Allergic inflammation can affect the mucosa of various organs: skin, eye, and nose, as well as the bronchial tree, in a synchronous or progressive way. The process that has been described as a primary defect of the epithelial barrier (57) can occur simultaneously or follow an "allergic march" in the same way as an "atopic march" has been proposed in describing the progression from atopic dermatitis that mainly occurs in childhood to allergic rhinitis and asthma (57). An example of such an "allergic march" was illustrated in the description of a worker with OCD who later developed occupational rhinitis and OA to ammonium persulfate (58).

Experimental studies in animal models

As reviewed in Chapter 4, skin exposure to LMW (chemicals) is currently the predominant route for inducing sensitization in animal models of asthma. For this, animals are first exposed to the sensitizer through the skin, followed by respiratory manifestations that are examined (airway inflammation, caliber, and NSBR). In a systematic research of PubMed and Embase on chemical-induced asthma up to 2017, Tsui and coworkers identified 22 LMW agents with evidence of skin exposure-induced NBBR (59). The authors concluded that the "ability of a chemical to cause sensitization via skin exposure should be regarded as constituting a risk of adverse respiratory reactions." The evidence for a sensitization potential was judged by the same authors as high for diisocyanates (60, 61) and trimelletic anhydride (62) and moderate for ammonium persulfate (59). It has also been shown that cutaneous and not (only) airway latex exposure can induce allergic lung inflammation and NBBR in mice (63). All of these exposures are known to cause both OA and CD (64). Interestingly and in an alternate way, inhalation exposure to isocyanate may lead to skin reactions (65) and cutaneous contact with some allergens, specifically the halogenated dinitrobenzenes, may lead to inflammatory responses in the airways (59), suggesting that the two organ systems are connected.

Epidemiological studies

Whereas the occurrence of concomitant nasal and bronchial manifestations at work has often been reported in epidemiological studies, this has less often been the case as regards skin symptoms except for agents such as latex and polyisocyanates (see sections, respectively, on natural rubber latex and isocyanates). Seven of ten common causes of OCD are agents that can also cause OA (64). The evidence for such an association was mainly documented in individual case studies or case series (Table 27.3 and Table 27.4) but less often in epidemiological studies. Table 27.5 shows results obtained in selected cross-sectional studies or in databases for workers exposed to various HMW and LMW agents, except for latex and isocyanates (see sections, respectively, on "Natural Rubber Latex" and "Isocyanates"). The prevalence of skin symptoms is generally higher than the prevalence of work-related asthma (WRA) symptoms or OA. In some studies, a significant association was found between skin manifestations and WRA, or between skin manifestations and skin reactivity by prick testing. In a review of OCU and OCD (protein CD) cases from 2005–2011 (n=291) in Finland, 21% of cases also had OA and 38% had occupational rhinitis (8).

We now highlight two occupational exposures for which there is evidence of a connection between the skin and respiratory symptoms in terms of sensitization and the development of OA: NRL and isocyanates.

Natural rubber latex

NRL (Chapter 18) is a HMW antigen that is known to cause a type I immediate hypersensitivity reaction, in both the skin (urticaria) and the lungs (asthma).

Whereas anaphylactic reactions to NRL were often reported before the 1990s, involving skin or visceral contact, reactions due to airborne exposure became an important health issue afterward with description of cases of OA and OR in healthcare

TABLE 27.3 Exposures Reported in Published Case Studies to Cause Both Occupational Asthma and Occupational Contact Urticaria

Exposure	Occupation	References
Latex	Nurse	*1. De Zotti, 1992*
	Condom production	*2. Rask-Andersen, 2000*
Nickel	Metal production	*3. Estlander, 1993*
Potato	Homemaker	*4. Jeannet-Peter, 1999*
Welding fumes	Welder	*5. Kaplan, 1963*
Sesame seed	Baker	*6. Keskinen, 1991*
Piperacillin	Pharmaceutical production	*7. Moscato, 1995*
Lilium longiflorum (lilies)	Florist	*8. KeskiPiirila, 1999*
Limonium tataricum	Florist	*9. Quirce, 1993*
Chamomile	Cosmetician	*10. Rudzki, 2003*
Platinum	Various	*11. Santucci, 2000*
Nematode (*Askaris simplex*)	Fish processing	*12. Scalla, 2001*
Diphenylmethane diisocyanate (MDI)	Chemical manufacturing	*13. Stingeni, 2008*
	Plastics manufacturing	*14. Valks, 2003*
Compositae	Florist	*15. Uter, 2001*
Cockroaches	Research technicians	*16. Zschunke, 1978*
3-(Bromomethyl)-2-chloro-4-(methylsulfonyl)-benzoic acid (BCMBA)	BCMBA manufacturing	*17. Suojalehto, 2017*
Oxidative hair dyes	Hairdresser	*18. Helaskoski, 2014*
Squid	Food manufacturing	*19. Wiszniewska, 2013*
Gum arabic	Candy manufacturing	*20. Viinanen, 2011*

References: **1.** De Zotti R, et al. *Br J Ind Med.* 1992;49(8):596–8; **2.** Rask-Andersen, et al. *Allergy.* 2000;55:836–41; **3.** Estlander T, et al. *Clin Exp Allergy.* 1993;23(4):306–10; **4.** Jeannet-Peter N, et al. *Am J Contact Dermatitis.* 1999;10:40–2; **5.** Kaplan I, et al. *Arch Dermatol.* 1963;88:188–9; **6.** Keskinen H, et al. *Clin Exp Allergy.* 1991;21(5):623–4; **7.** Moscato G, et al. *Eur Respir J.* 1995;8:467–9; **8.** Piirila P, et al. *Allergy.* 1999;54(3):273–7; **9.** Quirce S, et al. *Allergy.* 1993;48(4):285–90; **10.** Rudzki E, et al. *Contact Dermatitis.* 2003;49:162; **11.** Santucci B, et al. *Contact Dermatitis.* 2000;43(6):333–8; **12.** Scala E, et al. *Eur J Dermatol.* 2001;11:249–50; **13.** Stingeni L, et al. *Contact Dermatitis.* 2008;58:112–3; **14.** Valks R, et al. *Contact Dermatitits.* 2003;49:166–7; **15.** Uter W, et al. *Am J Contact Dermat.* 2001;12:182–4; **16.** Zschunke E. *Contact Dermatitis.* 1978;4(5):313–4; **17.** Suojalehto H, et al. *Occ Env Med.* 2017;75:277–82; **18.** Helaskoski E, et al. *Ann Allergy, Asthma, Immunol.* 2014;112:46–52; **19.** Wiszniewska M, et al. *Occup Med.* 2013;63:298–300; **20.** Viinanen A, et al. *J Allergy (Cairo).* 2011;841508.

TABLE 27.4 Exposures Reported in Published Case Studies to Cause Both Occupational Asthma and Occupational Contact Dermatitis

Exposure	Occupation	References
Diagnosed OA (SIC) and OCD (Patch Test)		
2-hydroxyethyl methacrylate (HEMA)	Beautician	*1. Moulin, 2009*
Diclycidyl ether of bisphenol A (DGEBA)	Resin applier	*1. Moulin, 2009*
Potassium dichromate	Cement floorer	*2. deRaeve, 1998*
Aziridine hardener	Painter and varnisher	*3. Kanerva, 1995*
Onion	Homemaker	*4. Valdivieso, 1994*
Nickel	Manual grinding of metal castings	*5. Estlander, 1993*
Spiramycin	Poultry breeder	*6. Paggiaro, 1979*
Diagnosed OA and OCD (No SIC and No Patch Test)		
Nematode (*Anisakis simplex*)	Fish processing	*7. Barbuzza, 2009*
Limodene	Laborer	*8. Guarneri, 2008*
Peptide coupling reagents	Laboratory workers	*9. Vandenplas, 2008*
Ortho-phthalaldehyde	Nurse	*10. Fujita, 2006*
Sapele wood	Carpenter	*11. Ivarez-Cuesta, 2004*
Ammonium persulfate	Hairdresser	*12. Krautheim, 2004*
Leek	Agricultural worker	*13. Cadot, 2001*
Aziridine crosslinker	Spray painter	*14. Leffler, 1999*
Sodium metabisulfite	Photographic technician	*15. Jacobs, 1995*
Green bean	Homemaker	*16. Igea, 1994*
DGEBA	Insulation manufacturing	*17. Kanerva, 1991*
Acrylates	Nail technician	*18. Vaccaro, 2014*

References: **1.** Moulin P, et al. *J Occup Health.* 2009;51:91–6; **2.** deRaeve H, et al. *Am J Ind Med.* 1998;34:169–76; **3.** Kanerva L et al. *Clin Exp Allergy.* 1995;25:432–9; **4.** Valdivieso R, et al. *J Allergy Clin Immunol.* 1994;94:928–30; **5.** Estlander T, et al. *Clin Exp Allergy.* 1993;23(4):306–10; **6.** Paggiaro PL, et al. *Clin Allergy.* 1979;9:571–4; **7.** Barbuzza O, et al. *Contact Dermatitis.* 2009;60:239–40; **8.** Guarneri F, et al. *Contact Dermatitis.* 2008;58:315–6; **9.** Vandenplas O, et al. *Occup Environ Med.* 2008;65:715–6; **10.** Fujita H, et al. *J Occup Health.* 2006;48:413–6; **11.** Ivarez-Cuesta C, et al. *Contact Dermatitis.* 2004;51:88–98; **12.** Krautheim AB, et al. *Contact Dermatitis.* 2004;50(3):113–6; **13.** Cadot P, et al. *Allergy.* 2001;56(2):192–3; **14.** Leffler CT, et al. *Environ Health Perspect.* 1999;107(7):599–601; **15.** Jacobs MC, et al. *Contact Dermatitis.* 1995;33:65–6; **16.** Igea JM, et al. *J Allergy Clin Immunol.* 1994;94(1):33–5; **17.** Kanerva L, et al. *Scand J Work Environ Health.* 1991;17(3):208–15; **18.** Vaccaro M, et al. *Int J Occup Med Env Health.* 2014; 27:137–140.

workers and description of significant frequency in cross-sectional studies (66–68). OA due to latex accounted for 3%–24% of the reported cases in the 1990s (69). Since the last edition of this chapter, the frequency of OA and OR due to latex has been substantially reduced in most countries with a highly successful environmental control (reduction of proteins in latex gloves, use of nonpowdered and latex-free gloves) as reviewed (69). Physician-based self-reporting programs conducted in the United Kingdom from 1993 to 1999 had shown that OCD represented 80% of all cases of occupational diseases, and occupational urticaria, 4% (70). Latex had become the leading cause (14%) of OCD (71). A reassessment of the same UK data (EPIDERM) from 1996 to 2012 showed an annual diminution of 1.2% of cases of OCD associated with rubber products (71). In more than 8500 patients assessed in a dermatology clinic of a University Hospital in Denmark from 2002 to 2013, there was also a decrease in sensitization to latex (from 6.1% at the beginning of this period to 1.9% at the end) and in clinical manifestations of this allergy (from 1.3% to 0.6%) (72). In the same study and in others, subjects sensitized to latex reported frequent allergic reactions to bananas, kiwis, and avocados (72).

The natural history of NRL allergy includes localized urticaria, progressing to generalized urticaria, wheezing and respiratory complaints, and possibly asthma, facial swelling, and anaphylaxis in rarer cases (73). This progression may result from occupational and/or nonoccupational exposure to latex-containing glove powders; skin (glove use) and airborne exposures (latex containing glove powder) can occur simultaneously during glove use.

De Zotti et al. (74) reported on an interesting case of a health-care worker with both OCU and OA, performing skin exposure challenge. The worker wore a latex glove on one hand while monitoring FEV_1. The results showed a marked decrease in FEV_1 as well as itching on the glove-wearing hand and weals on her head and neck. In this case, the latex skin contact appears to have been sufficient to elicit both a dermal and a respiratory response.

Isocyanates

Isocyanates are still a significant cause of OA (Chapter 14), although less frequently so. Animal and epidemiological studies have shown that skin and not only airborne exposure play a role in the sensitizing process as reviewed (75). Skin exposure to polyisocyanates can be a common exposure in some workplaces, being reported in 53% of 73 employed in two plants producing hexamethylene diisocyanate (HDI) (76). Isolated airway exposure to toluene diisocyanate (TDI) can result in skin sensitization

TABLE 27.5 Frequency of Occupational Skin Diseases and Work-Related Asthma in Selected Studies

First Author, Year	Agent/ Type of Study	Frequency of Skin Symptoms	Frequency of Work-Related Asthma	Comment	References
High-molecular-weight agents					
Cartier et al., 1984	Snow-crab. Cross-sectional assessment of 313 snow-crab processing workers	Skin rash at work: 24%	Confirmed by objective tests: 16%	Skin rash at work significantly associated with immediate skin tests to crab	*1. Cartier, 1984*
Malo et al., 1990	Psyllium. 193 nurses in chronic care hospitals	Skin redness or itching: 5%	OA confirmed by SIC: 4%	Skin reactivity to psyllium: 3%; increased specific IgE: 12%	*2. Malo, 1990*
Malo et al., 1990	Guar gum. Carpet manufacturing	Skin redness or itching: 11%	OA confirmed by SIC or highly probable: 2%	Skin reactivity to guar gum: 5%; increased specific IgE: 8%	*3. Malo, 1990*
Simoneti et al., 2017	Laboratory animals. Cross-sectional study of 453 exposed volunteers	51% with skin symptoms in sensitized group and 29% in nonsensitized group	27% confirmed asthma (NBHR) in sensitized group and 3% in nonsensitized group	16% of the total of 51% with skin symptoms also had confirmed asthma	*4. Simoneti, 2017*
Low-molecular-weight agents					
Bernstein et al., 1993	Urethane (MDI) mold plant. Cross-sectional study in a plant with minimal exposure	1% urticaria/ angioedema	4% with WRA symptoms, 1% with confirmed OA	Low prevalence of occupational respiratory disease attributed to low levels of exposure	*5. Bernstein, 1993*
Lynde et al., 2009	Professional cleaners. Cross-sectional study of 549 workers (participation: 39%) control group of 593 nonexposed building workers	21% rash in the past 12 months vs 11% in controls	32% with WRA symptoms; 60% in workers with rash and 30% in workers without rash	Cleaners with a rash in the past 12 months more likely to report WRA symptoms	*6. Lynde, 2009*
Espuga et al., 2011	Hairdressers. 174 workers with suggestive OA from ˜1300 hairdressers	23%–24% with skin rash or eczema	72/1334 (5%) with possible OA	Rhinitis and/or dermatitis associated with possible OA (OR: 7.8, 95% CI:3.3–18.3)	*7. Espuga, 2011*
Meza et al., 2013	Machining fluid. Cross-sectional study of 407 workers at an aircraft manufacturing plant	22% with contact dermatitis in the past 12 months	20% with WRA	Airborne concentrations of machining fluid below norms	*8. Meza, 1990*
Kwok et al., 2014	Beauticians. UK THOR Database 1996–2011	257 beauticians with contact dermatitis (33%)	4% with OA	Acrylates as the most common suspected	*9. Kwok, 2014*
Foss-Skiftesvik, 2017	Hairdressers. 3-yr prospective study in 248 apprentices and 816 controls	Incidence of hand eczema, urticaria: 42–68/1000 person-yrs	Incidence of wheezing: 51/1000 person-yrs	Skin diseases responsible for leaving in 47% of cases	*10. Foss-Skiftesvik, 2017*
Suojalehto et al., 2019	Epoxy compounds. Retrospective analysis of 113 subjects referred in clinic and with a history of WRA	Contact dermatitis: 22%	NA	2/15 (13%) subjects with confirmed OA had contact dermatitis	*11. Suojalehto, 2019*

(Continued)

TABLE 27.5 Frequency of Occupational Skin Diseases and Work-Related Asthma in Selected Studies (*Continued*)

First Author, Year	Agent/ Type of Study	Frequency of Skin Symptoms	Frequency of Work-Related Asthma	Comment	References
High- and low-molecular-weight agents					
Arrandale et al., 2013	Surveillance programs in Ontario, Canada			Exposure-response relationships for itchy and dry skin, significant in body shop workers	*12. Arrandale, 2013*
	723 in bakeries	17%, itchy skin	2% with WRA		
	473 in auto body shops	8.5%, itchy skin	4% with WRA		
Helaskoski et al., 2017	Retrospective analysis of 291 accepted cases at the Finnish Institute of Occupational Health (1995–2011)	Contact urticaria: 232 Protein contact dermatitis: 59. Most common agents: flour and grains (21%), cow dander (18%), latex (15%), various chemicals (14%)	Concomitant OA: 21% Concomitant OR: 38%		*13. Helaskoski, 2017*

Abbreviations: NA, not assessed; NSBR, nonspecific bronchial hyperresponsiveness; OA, occupational asthma; OR, occupational rhinitis; SIC, specific inhalation challenge; WRA, work-related asthma.

References: **1.** Cartier A, et al. *J Allergy Clin Immunol.* 1984;74:261–9; **2.** Malo JL, et al. *Am Rev Respir Dis.* 1990;142:1359–66; **3.** Malo JL, et al. *J Allergy Clin Immunol.* 1990;86:562–9; **4.** Simoneti CS, et al. *Clin Exp Allergy.* 2017;47:1436–44; **5.** Bernstein DI, et al. *J Allergy Clin Immunol.* 1993;92:387–96; **6.** Lynde CB, et al. *Occup Med (Lond).* 2009;59:249–54; **7.** Espuga M, et al. *Int Arch Allergy Appl Immunol.* 2011;155:379–88; **8.** Meza F, et al. *Am J Ind Med.* 2013;56(12):1394–401; **9.** Kwok C, et al. *Clin Exp Dermatol.* 2014;39:590–5; **10.** Foss-Skiftesvik MH, et al. 2017;76(3):160–6; **11.** Suojalehto H, et al. 2019;7(1):191–8; **12.** Arrandale V, et al. *Int Arch Occup Environ Health.* 2013;86:167–75; **13.** Helaskoski E, et al. 2017;77(6):390–6.

shown by patch testing in a guinea pig model (65). An outbreak of eczema in 16 workers (of whom, 13 reacted by patch testing) exposed to polymeric methylene diphenyl diisocyanate (MDI) was described (77), followed by a report of four workers with OCD due to HDI (78). Engfeldt estimated that 5 of 100 workers exposed to polymeric MDI had or previously had occupation-related skin problems (OCD) (79). OCD can occur after a single intense exposure (80). Skin-related work symptoms were examined in a group of 300 Polish workers exposed to MDI in a vehicle equipment factory (81). Of 21 subjects who reported skin symptoms, a diagnosis of occupational allergic CD was proposed in 7 workers, occupational irritant CD in 10, and joint allergic and irritant in 3 others (81). Positive patch tests were found in 10 workers, mostly to phenylenediamine and diaminodiphenylmethane (MDA) but not to MDI (82). In a cross-sectional study at a plant with low levels of exposure to MDI, only 1% of 243 workers reported urticaria/angioedema (Table 27.3) (82).

The animal evidence of skin sensitization contributing to the development of an asthma-like response upon subsequent respiratory exposure is accepted for various isocyanates including TDI, MDI, and HDI (Chapter 4) (59). Unlike latex, the mechanism through which isocyanates cause OA has not been conclusively determined (Chapter 14). Isocyanates can also cause skin sensitization through a type IV delayed hypersensitivity mechanism (83). There are reported cases of workers with both asthma and OCU related to isocyanates (Tables 27.2, 27.3, and 27.4). Epidemiological studies among isocyanate-exposed workers demonstrate that they have both skin and airborne exposures to isocyanates as reviewed (75) (Chapter 14).

In conclusion of this section, there is compelling evidence that workers are likely to have both skin and airborne exposures at the same time, and that these exposures can, at a minimum, lead to local sensitization and allergic disease independently. When assessing the risk of exposure in workplaces, all routes of potential exposure should be considered. In cases where there is possible or probable airborne or skin exposure, employers, physicians, and occupational health and safety professionals should seek to reduce both routes of exposure.

Prevention

The principles of primary prevention to reduce or eliminate skin exposure are similar for both OCU and OCD. An excellent source for prevention is *Controlling Skin Exposure to Chemicals and Wet Work—A Practical Book* by Sithamparanadarajah (84). Hazard identification is a vitally important step. Safety data sheets (SDSs) and labels may contain useful information on potential skin hazards and safety practices. There are a number of "hazard" phrases to help identify chemicals that have potential skin effects. Although these systems should theoretically identify potential skin effects, a review indicated that a number of known skin sensitizers were not identified as such in commonly used occupational hygiene reference documents (64).

The standard hierarchy of occupational hygiene controls can be applied to substances that may cause skin sensitization. These include elimination or substitution, engineering, administrative, and personal protective equipment (PPE). Examples of successful substitution include the replacement of NRL gloves with the use of synthetic rubber gloves, and the removal of chromium from cement (1, 85).

Engineering controls, including ventilation improvements or the enclosure of exposure sources to prevent splashes and spills, may be applicable in some circumstances and are especially important for agents that are airborne. Exposure monitoring is possible, but dermal exposure monitoring is less frequently employed than airborne exposure monitoring. Education is another valuable administrative control strategy, and while general health and safety education may be delivered, education specific to skin exposures and protection may be less commonly provided (86). Appropriately targeted and sustained educational programs can induce important behavioral changes (1, 85).

Administrative controls may also include job or task rotation. PPE, specifically the use of gloves and respirators, is a less desirable strategy, but is often the one most frequently used in dermal exposure. Limited wearing of gloves can reduce the incidence of ICD when coupled with other preventive measures (1). Wearing cotton liners can prevent impairment of skin barrier function (1, 87).

Another approach to skin protection is "APC." This stands for *Avoid* contact with the skin, *Protect* the skin, and *Check* for early signs of disease. Avoidance involves elimination and substitution, engineering controls, maintaining a safe working distance from exposure sources, changes to work handling and processes, administrative controls, and PPE. Protecting the skin is as important and also includes PPE and chemical protective clothing, but includes both personal hygiene and skin care. This may include pre- and postwork skin care as well as emollient creams. Some prework creams may help, but generally they are not an effective preventive measure (1, 87). Regular application of emollients can help prevent OCD (1, 87). Finally, checking for early signs of disease is recommended, although there is minimal reporting of such activity in the literature.

Research needs

Further research on OCU and OCD is needed to better elucidate the burden of illness, risk factors, prevention strategies, and successful return to work. In addition, the inclusion of both respiratory and cutaneous perspectives in research is needed. For the clinician, the key message is awareness: that workers presenting with either lung disease or skin disease may also have disease in the other system that may require investigation and management as well. For the workplace, the message is the importance of ensuring that prevention measures address both the skin and the respiratory system.

References

1. Nicholson PJ, Llewellyn D, English JS, Guidelines development group. Evidence-based guidelines for the prevention, identification and management of occupational contact dermatitis and urticaria. Contact Dermatitis. 2010;63(4):177–86.
2. Turner S, Carder M, van Tongeren M, et al. The incidence of occupational skin disease as reported to The Health and Occupation Reporting (THOR) network between 2002 and 2005. Br J Dermatol. 2007;157(4):713–22.
3. Aalto-Korte K, Koskela K, Pesonen M. 12-year data on dermatologic cases in the Finnish Register of Occupational Diseases I: distribution of different diagnoses and main causes of allergic contact dermatitis. Contact Dermatitis. 2020;82(6):337–42.
4. Yong SB, Chen HH, Huang JY, et al. Patients with urticaria are at a higher risk of anaphylaxis: a nationwide population-based retrospective cohort study in Taiwan. J Dermatol. 2018;45(9):1088–93.
5. Vietri J, Turner SJ, Tian H, et al. Effect of chronic urticaria on US patients: analysis of the National Health and Wellness Survey. Ann Allergy Asthma Immunol. 2015;115(4):306–11.
6. Zuberbier T, Aberer W, Asero R, et al. The EAACI/GA²LEN/EDF/WAO guideline for the definition, classification, diagnosis and management of urticaria. Allergy. 2018;73(7):1393–414.
7. Holness DL, Arrandale VH, Mathias CG. Occupational urticaria and allergic contact dermatitis. In: Asthma in the Workplace. 4th ed. Boca Raton: CRC Press, Taylor & Francis; 2013.
8. Helaskoski E, Suojalehto H, Kuuliala O, et al. Occupational contact urticaria and protein contact dermatitis: causes and concomitant airway diseases. Contact Dermatitis. 2017;77(6):390–6.
9. Kasemsarn P, Bosco J, Nixon RL. The role of the skin barrier in occupational skin diseases. In: Agner T, ed. Skin Barrier Function. Curr Probl Dermatol. 2016;49:135–43.
10. Taylor JS, Leow YH, Fisher AA. Contact urticaria. In: Adams RM, ed. Occupational Skin Disease. 3rd ed. Philadelphia: WB Saunders; 1999:111.
11. von Krogh G, Maibach HI. The contact urticaria syndrome–an updated review. J Am Acad Dermatol. 1981;5(3):328–42.
12. Reitschel RL, Fowler JF. Contact urticaria. In: Reitschel RL, Fowler JF, eds. Fisher's Contact Dermatitis. 6th ed. Hamilton: BC Decker; 2008:615.
13. Wertenteil S, Strunk A, Garg A. Prevalence estimates for chronic urticaria in the United States: a sex- and age-adjusted population analysis. J Am Acad Dermatol. 2019;81(1):152–6.
14. Lapi F, Cassano N, Pegoraro V, et al. Epidemiology of chronic spontaneous urticaria: results from a nationwide, population-based study in Italy. Br J Dermatol. 2016;174(5):996–1004.
15. Seo JH, Kwon JW. Epidemiology of urticaria including physical urticaria and angioedema in Korea. Korean J Intern Med. 2019;34(2):418–25.
16. Greaves MW. Chronic urticaria. N Engl J Med. 1995;332(26):1767–72.
17. Raciborski F, Kłak A, Czarnecka-Operacz M, et al. Epidemiology of urticaria in Poland—nationally representative survey results. Postepy Dermatol Alergol. 2018;35(1):67–73.
18. Süß H, Dölle-Bierke S, Geier J, et al. Contact urticaria: frequency, elicitors and cofactors in three cohorts (Information Network of Departments of Dermatology; Network of Anaphylaxis; and Department of Dermatology, University Hospital Erlangen, Germany). Contact Dermatitis. 2019;81(5):341–53.
19. Aktas E, Esin MN. Skin disease symptoms and related risk factors among young workers in high-risk jobs. Contact Dermatitis. 2016;75(2):96–105.
20. Bensefa-Colas L, Telle-Lamberton M, Faye S, et al. Occupational contact urticaria: lessons from the French National Network for Occupational Disease Vigilance and Prevention (RNV3P). Br J Dermatol. 2015;173(6):1453–61.
21. Lukács J, Schliemann S, Elsner P. Occupational contact urticaria caused by food—a systematic clinical review. Contact Dermatitis. 2016;75(4):195–204.
22. Pesonen M, Koskela K, Aalto-Korte K. Contact urticaria and protein contact dermatitis in the Finnish Register of Occupational Diseases in a period of 12 years. Contact Dermatitis. 2020;83(1):1–7.
23. Moscato G, Pala G, Crivellaro M, et al. Anaphylaxis as occupational risk. Curr Opin Allergy Clin Immunol. 2014;14(4):328–33.
24. Śpiewak R, Góra-Florek A, Horoch A, et al. Risk factors for work-related eczema and urticaria among vocational students of agriculture. Ann Agric Environ Med. 2017;23;24(4):716–21.
25. Cherrez-Ojeda I, Robles-Velasco K, Bedoya-Riofrío P, et al. Checklist for a complete chronic urticaria medical history: an easy tool. World Allergy Organ J. 2017;10(1):34.
26. Antia C, Baquerizo K, Korman A, et al. Urticaria: a comprehensive review: epidemiology, diagnosis, and work-up. J Am Acad Dermatol. 2018;79(4):599–614.
27. Magerl M, Altrichter S, Borzova E, et al. The definition, diagnostic testing, and management of chronic inducible urticarias—The EAACI/GA(2) LEN/EDF/UNEV consensus recommendations 2016 update and revision. Allergy. 2016;71(6):780–802.
28. Brancaccio RR, Alvarez MS. Contact allergy to food. Dermatol Ther. 2004;17:302–13.
29. Lachapelle JM, Maibach HI. Patch Testing and Prick Testing. 2nd ed. Berlin: Springer; 2009:33–70.
30. Sampson HA, Muñoz-Furlong A, Campbell RL, et al. Second symposium on the definition and management of anaphylaxis: summary report–Second National Institute of Allergy and Infectious Disease/Food Allergy and Anaphylaxis Network symposium. J Allergy Clin Immunol. 2006;117(2):391–7.
31. Eghrari-Sabet J, Sher E, Kavati A, et al. Real-world use of omalizumab in patients with chronic idiopathic/spontaneous urticaria in the United States. Allergy Asthma Proc. 2018;39(3):191–200.
32. Mälkönen T, Jolanki R, Alanko K, et al. A 6-month follow-up study of 1048 patients diagnosed with an occupational skin disease. Contact Dermatitis. 2009;61(5):261–8.
33. Caroe TK, Ebbehøj NE, Bonde JP, et al. Occupational hand eczema and/or contact urticaria: factors associated with change of profession or not remaining in the workforce. Contact Dermatitis. 2018;78(1):55–63.

34. Clemmensen KK, Carøe TK, Thomsen SF, et al. Two-year follow-up survey of patients with allergic contact dermatitis from an occupational cohort: is the prognosis dependent on the omnipresence of the allergen? Br J Dermatol. 2014;170(5):1100–5.

35. Baiardini I, Giardini A, Pasquali M, et al. Quality of life and patients' satisfaction in chronic urticaria and respiratory allergy. Allergy. 2003;58(7):621–3.

36. Lachapelle JM. Historical aspects. In: Rycroft RJG, Menne T, Frosch PJ, Benezra C, eds. Textbook of Contact Dermatitis. Berlin: Springer-Verlag; 1992:7.

37. Stocks SJ, McNamee R, van der Molen HF, et al. Trends in incidence of occupational asthma, contact dermatitis, noise-induced hearing loss, carpal tunnel syndrome and upper limb musculoskeletal disorders in European countries from 2000 to 2012. Occup Environ Med. 2015;72:294–303.

38. Aalto-Korte K, Koskela K, Pesonen M. 12-year data on skin diseases in the Finnish Register of Occupational Diseases II: risk occupations with special reference to allergic contact dermatitis. Contact Dermatitis. 2020;82(6):343–9.

39. McDonald JC, Beck MH, Chen Y, et al. Incidence by occupation and industry of work-related skin diseases in the United Kingdom, 1996–2001. Occup Med (Lond). 2006;56(6):398–405.

40. Turner S, McNamee R, Agius R, et al. Evaluating interventions aimed at reducing occupational exposure to latex and rubber glove allergens. Occup Environ Med. 2012;69(12):925–31.

41. Rietschel RL, Mathias CG, Fowler JF, et al. Relationship of occupation to contact dermatitis: evaluation in patients tested from 1998 to 2000. Am J Contact Dermat. 2002;13(4):170–6.

42. Pesonen M, Jolanki R, Larese Filon F, et al. Patch test results of the European baseline series among patients with occupational contact dermatitis across Europe—analyses of the European Surveillance System on Contact Allergy network, 2002–2010. Contact Dermatitis. 2015;72(3):154–63.

43. Mathias CG. Contact dermatitis and workers' compensation: criteria for establishing occupational causation and aggravation. J Am Acad Dermatol. 1989;20(5 Pt 1):842–8.

44. Gomez de Carvallo M, Calvo B, Benach J, et al. Assessment of the Mathias criteria for establishing occupational causation of contact dermatitis. Actas Dermosifiliogr. 2012;103(5):411–21.

45. Holness DL, Nethercott JR. Is a worker's understanding of their diagnosis an important determinant of outcome in occupational contact dermatitis? Contact Dermatitis. 1991;25(5):296–301.

46. Johnston GA, Exton LS, Mohd Mustapa MF, et al. British Association of Dermatologists' guidelines for the management of contact dermatitis 2017. Br J Dermatol. 2017;176(2):317–29.

47. Bourke J, Coulson I, English J. Guidelines for the management of contact dermatitis: an update. Br J Dermatol. 2009;160(5):946–54.

48. Lachapelle JM, Maibach HI. Patch Testing and Prick Testing. 3rd ed. Berlin: Springer; 2020.

49. Slodownik D, Williams J, Frowen K, et al. The additive value of patch testing with patients' own products at an occupational dermatology clinic. Contact Dermatitis. 2009;61(4):231–5.

50. Houle MC, Holness DL, Dekoven J, et al. Additive value of patch testing custom epoxy materials from the workplace at the occupational disease specialty clinic in Toronto. Dermatitis. 2012;23(5):214–9.

51. De Groot AC. Patch Testing. 4th ed. The Netherlands: Acdegroot Publishing; 2018.

52. Fonacier L, Bernstein DI, Pacheco K, et al. Contact dermatitis: a practice parameter-update 2015. J Allergy Clin Immunol Prac. 2015;3(3 Suppl):S1–39.

53. Zack B, Arrandale VH, Holness DL. Workers with hand dermatitis and workplace training experiences: a qualitative perspective. Am J Ind Med. 2017;60(1):69–76.

54. Keefe AR, Demers PA, Neis B, et al. A scoping review to identify strategies that work to prevent four important occupational diseases. Am J Ind Med. 2020;63(6):490–516.

55. Agner T, Andersen KE, Brandao FM, et al. Hand eczema severity and quality of life: a cross-sectional, multicentre study of hand eczema patients. Contact Dermatitis. 2008;59(1):43–7.

56. Holness DL. Health care services use by workers with work-related contact dermatitis. Dermatitis. 2004;15(1):18–24.

57. Zheng T, Yu J, Oh MH, et al. The atopic march: progression from atopic dermatitis to allergic rhinitis and asthma. Allergy Asthma Immunol Res. 2011;3:67–73.

58. Poltronieri A, Patrini L, Pigatto P, et al. Occupational allergic "march". Rapid evolution of contact dermatitis to ammonium persulfate into airborne contact dermatitis with rhinitis and asthma in a hairdresser. Med Lav. 2010;101:403–8.

59. Tsui HC, Ronsmans S, De Sadeleer LJ, et al. Skin exposure contributes to chemical-induced asthma: what is the evidence? A systematic review of animal models. Allergy Asthma Immunol Res. 2020;12(4):579–98.

60. Tarkowski M, Vanoirbeek JA, Vanhooren HM, et al. Immunological determinants of ventilatory changes induced in mice by dermal sensitization and respiratory challenge with toluene diisocyanate. Am J Physiol Lung Cell Mol Physiol. 2007;292(1):L207–14.

61. Vanoirbeek JA, Tarkowski M, Vanhooren HM, et al. Validation of a mouse model of chemical-induced asthma using trimellitic anhydride, a respiratory sensitizer, and dinitrochlorobenzene, a dermal sensitizer. J Allergy Clin Immunol. 2006;117(5):1090–7.

62. Arts J, de Koning M, Bloksma N, et al. Respiratory allergy to trimellitic anhydride in rats: concentration-response relationships during elicitation. Inhal Toxicol. 2004;16(5):259–69.

63. Lehto M, Haapakoski R, Wolff H, et al. Cutaneous, but not airway, latex exposure induces allergic lung inflammation and airway hyperreactivity in mice. J Invest Dermatol. 2005;125(5):962–8.

64. Arrandale VH, Liss GM, Tarlo SM, et al. Occupational contact allergens: are they also associated with occupational asthma? Am J Ind Med. 2012;55:353–60.

65. Ebino K, Ueda H, Kawakatsu H, et al. Isolated airway exposure to toluene diisocyanate results in skin sensitization. Tox Letters. 2001;121:79–85.

66. Tarlo SM, Wong L, Roos J, et al. Occupational asthma caused by latex in a surgical glove manufacturing plant. J Allergy Clin Immunol. 1990;85:626–31.

67. Lagier F, Vervloet D, Lhermet I, et al. Prevalence of latex allergy in operating room nurses. J Allergy Clin Immunol. 1992;90:319–22.

68. Vandenplas O, Delwich JP, Evrard G, et al. Prevalence of occupational asthma due to latex among hospital personnel. Am J Respir Crit Care Med. 1995;151:54–60.

69. Vandenplas O, Raulf M. Occupational latex allergy: the current state of affairs. Curr Allergy Asthma Rep. 2017;17:14.

70. Cherry N, Meyer JD, Adisesh A, et al. Surveillance of occupational skin disease: EPIDERM and OPRA. Br J Dermatol. 2000;142(6):1128–34.

71. Warburton KL, Urwin R, Carder M, et al. UK rates of occupational skin disease attributed to rubber accelerators, 1996–2012. Contact Dermatitis. 2015;72(5):305–11.

72. Blaabjerg MS, Andersen KE, Bindslev-Jensen C, et al. Decrease in the rate of sensitization and clinical allergy to natural rubber latex. Contact Dermatitis. 2015;73(1):21–8.

73. Shah D, Chowdhury MM. Rubber allergy. Clin Dermatol. 2011;29(3):278–86.

74. De Zotti R, Larese F, Fiorito A. Asthma and contact urticaria from latex gloves in a hospital nurse. Br J Ind Med. 1992;49(8):596–8.

75. Redlich CA. Skin exposure and asthma: is there a connection? Proc Am Thorac Soc. 2010;2:134–7.

76. Hathaway JA, Molenaar DM, Cassidy LD, et al. Cross-sectional survey of workers exposed to aliphatic diisocyanates using detailed respiratory medical history and questions regarding accidental skin and respiratory exposures. J Occup Environ Med. 2014;56(1):52–7.

77. Frick M, Bjorkner B, Hamnerius N, et al. Allergic contact dermatitis from dicyclohexylmethane-4,4'-diisocyanate. Contact Dermatitis. 2003;48(6):305–9.

78. Aalto-Korte K, Pesonen M, Kuuliala O, et al. Contact allergy to aliphatic polyisocyanates based on hexamethylene-1,6-diisocyanate (HDI). Contact Dermatitis. 2010;63(6):357–63.

79. Engfeldt M, Isaksson M, Zimerson E, et al. Several cases of work-related allergic contact dermatitis caused by isocyanates at a company manufacturing heat exchangers. Contact Dermatitis. 2013;68(3):175–80.

80. Engfeldt M, Pontén A. Contact allergy to isocyanates after accidental spillage. Contact Dermatitis. 2013;69(2):122–4.

81. Kieć-Świerczyńska M, Swierczyńska-Machura D, Chomiczewska-Skóra D, et al. Occupational allergic and irritant contact dermatitis in workers exposed to polyurethane foam. Int J Occup Med Environ Health. 2014;27(2):196–205.

82. Bernstein DI, Korbee L, Stauder T, et al. The low prevalence of occupational asthma and antibody-dependent sensitization to diphenylmethane diisocyanate in a plant engineered for minimal exposure to diisocyanates. J Allergy Clin Immunol. 1993;92:387–96.

83. Donovan JC, Kudla I, DeKoven JG. Rapid development of allergic contact dermatitis from dicyclohexylmethane-4,4'-diisocyanate. Dermatitis. 2009;20(4):214–7.

84. Sithamparanadarajah R. Controlling Skin Exposure to Chemicals and Wet-Work, a Practical Book. Stourbridge: RMS Publishing; 2008.

85. Plus NHS/Royal College of Physicians. Dermatitis: Occupational Health Aspects of Management: A National Guideline. London: Royal College of Physicians; 2009.

86. Gupta T, Arrandale VH, Kudla I, et al. Gaps in workplace education for prevention of occupational skin disease. Ann Work Expo Health. 2018;62(2):243–7.

87. Saary J, Qureshi R, Palda V, et al. A systematic review of contact dermatitis treatment and prevention. J Am Acad Dermatol. 2005;53(5):845.